Epidemiology and Control of Schistosomiasis (Bilharziasis)

Epidemiology and Control of Schistosomiasis (Bilharziasis)

Edited by N. ANSARI, World Health Organization, Geneva

Contributors
A. DAVIS, M. FAROOQ, N. G. HAIRSTON, G. MACDONALD, D. B. McMULLEN,
L. J. OLIVIER, L. S. RITCHIE, M. A. STIREWALT, K. UEMURA and W. H. WRIGHT

69 figures and 70 tables

Published on behalf of the World Health Organization by
University Park Press · Baltimore · London · Tokyo · 1973

Originally published by S. Karger AG, Basel, Switzerland
Distributed exclusively in the United States of America and Canada by University
Park Press, Baltimore, Maryland
Library of Congress Catalog Card Number LC 72-12707
International Standard Book Number (ISBN) 0-8391-0578-9

Contents

Chapter 1: Historical Development
(M. FAROOQ)

Chapter 2: Important Features of Schistosomes
(M. A. STIREWALT)

Chapter 3: Geographical Distribution of Schistosomes and their Intermediate Hosts
(W. H. WRIGHT)

Chapter 4: *The Dynamics of Transmission*
(N. G. Hairston)

Contents

Chapter 5: The Public Health and Economic Importance of Schistosomiasis – Its Assessment
(G. MACDONALD and M. FAROOQ)

Chapter 6: Measurement of the Clinical Manifestations of Schistosomiasis
(G. MACDONALD)

Contents XI

Chapter 7: Review of National Control Programmes
(M. Farooq)

Chapter 8: General Considerations in the Control of Schistosomiasis
(M. Farooq)

Chapter 9: Planning and Organization of Control Programmes
(M. Farooq)

Chapter 10: Chemical Control of Snails
(L. S. Ritchie)

Contents

Chapter 11: *Biological and Environmental Control of Snails* (D. B. McMullen)

Contents

Chapter 12: Chemotherapy in Control
(A. DAVIS)

Chapter 13: Evaluation of Control Programmes
(L. J. OLIVIER)

Chapter 14: Techniques, Statistical Methods and Recording Forms

A. Techniques (L. J. OLIVIER)

B. Statistical Methods (K. UEMURA)

Contents

C. Recording Forms (L. J. Olivier and K. Uemura)

Foreword

Schistosomiasis is estimated to affect two hundred million people in the world. In view of its prevalence, its wide distribution over three continents and the extent of the morbidity it causes, schistosomiasis ranks among the most important public health problems of the tropics and subtropics, coming next to malaria as a parasitic disease. If the necessary preventive measures are not taken, it is bound to become an even greater problem in many developing countries where the harnessing of water resources for irrigation and motive power production as well as large population movements have created ideal conditions for the propagation of schistosomiasis. There are known examples to testify to the reality of such ecological boomerang effects.

Interest of investigators which, for a long time, was concentrated mainly on clinical, pathological and parasitological aspects of schistosomiasis, has shifted in the last three decades more and more to ways of attacking the disease at its sources and to its epidemiology, the indispensable basis of any control work. While in former times field workers were satisfied to establish the existence and prevalence of schistosome infection in population groups, it was soon realized that other quantitative data, obtained by reliable techniques, were needed to assess the public health importance of the disease and investigate a given epidemiological situation.

When a young investigator first devotes himself to field work on schistosomiasis, he is confronted with a maze of practical, administrative and scientific hurdles. The required literature, scattered in numerous single articles published in various journals or reports, is not readily available to him. Neither do existing textbooks nor academic courses help him to overcome his difficulties. The manual on the *Epidemiology and Control of Schistosomiasis* is intended to fill this gap by providing the reader with both the basic scientific knowledge and understanding of its practical application in field work. It is an excellent guide for correct planning of projects and evaluation of results.

The manual was prepared under the sponsorship of the World Health Organization which, since its inception, has accorded a high priority to schistosomiasis in its programme of work. By calling upon experts from all over the world to assist governments in the planning and implementation of surveys and control projects, to recommend the most promising approaches for research and field activities and to participate in collaborative laboratory and operational programmes, the World Health Organization has gathered considerable information and experience which have been condensed in this publication.

Dr. N. ANSARI, Chief of the Parasitic Diseases unit in WHO and Editor of the present manual, has long felt the need for such a comprehensive guide. It is to his credit that he not only conceived this work but also brought it to completion, and special recognition is, therefore, due to him and to his collaborators.

HANS VOGEL
Professor of Tropical Medicine,
Bernhard Nocht Institute for
Maritime and Tropical Diseases,
Hamburg

Preface

The purpose of this manual on the epidemiology and control of schistosomiasis is to provide broad practical guidance in the planning and conduct of epidemiological surveys and operations designed to control schistosomiasis. To avoid any ambiguity, let it be said that several degrees of control may be achieved by a wide range of measures. The objective may be the simple containment of the spread of infection, a reduction in the morbidity, or a significant reduction in transmission resulting in decreased morbidity, severity and prevalence. In optimum circumstances, total interruption of transmission may be feasible and eradication attempted.

If epidemiology and control are given equal prominence in this publication, this is by a deliberate choice. Experience has shown the absolute necessity of correctly carrying out epidemiological investigations not only in order to assess the infection and the disease in a given community or area but also to identify the local and regional epidemiological patterns, select the most appropriate control methods and evaluate their results on the basis of well-defined parameters. In the past, the lack of uniform methods in schistosomiasis has often prevented the proper assessment of operational programmes, with the result of needlessly discouraging both public and official support. It is hoped that the present manual will in part at least meet this deficiency.

It is realized that, in schistosomiasis, the methodology for epidemiological assessment and control has not yet reached such a stage of sophistication as to allow a simple solution to be offered to meet the needs of every situation. In fact, were guidance of this type attempted, it would probably impede the exercise of independent judgement and the development of new methods. On the other hand, the valuable experience gained in schistosomiasis

control over the past decades suggests that certain guide-lines may con-
structively channel efforts in directions that give indications of being most
fruitful. This experience has been acquired through national programmes and
through WHO-assisted pilot projects in different parts of the world. Much
information and inspiration has also emanated from the deliberations and
recommendations of various conferences, scientific groups and expert committees sponsored by WHO since 1949.

For whom then is the present manual intended? In the lesser industrialized countries where resources for public health activities may be particularly
scarce, a reasonable choice must be made between alternatives among health
programmes. Such a choice must be based upon both knowledge of past
successes and failures and an accurate assessment of the existing situation.
Responsible officials in organizations or government agencies interested in
initiating schistosomiasis control will, therefore, find useful the comparative
information contained in this book for establishing national and local
priorities in control of schistosomiasis.

By providing broad guide-lines in epidemiology and control of schistosomiasis, the intention has also been to assist the 'worker in the field' who has
little access to the specialized literature and no time to waste on learning by
trial and error. Within this frame of reference are included the investigating
epidemiologist, the aquatic biologist, the parasitologist and the irrigation
engineer, as well as other field personnel and the associated laboratory
technicians who should be in a position to share in and profit from the
experiences of past efforts.

Further progress in the epidemiology and control of schistosomiasis will
depend on advances made in the many fields of tropical medicine and of
related research – epidemiology, biology, chemotherapy, immunology,
clinical medicine, preventive medicine, molluscicides, sanitary engineering,
etc. To people already engaged or interested in such fields, the manual gives an
opportunity to acquire a greater familiarity with concrete problems raised in
the current practice of the epidemiology and control of schistosomiasis.

By incorporating accepted and recommended methods for the epidemiological assessment of schistosomiasis the present manual considerably
enlarges upon a previous WHO monograph which was limited to snail
control[1]. Most of the information contained in the latter has been revised in
the light of knowledge gained in the intervening period and integrated into
the present manual.

1   *Snail control in the prevention of bilharziasis.* World Health Organization Monograph
Series No. 50 (Geneva 1965).

This manual would not have been possible were it not for the voluntary co-operation of prominent specialists who, depending on the subject covered, undertook singly or with the assistance of other experts, to summarize and assess the data and experience acquired over the last two decades by numerous individual scientists and laboratories as well as information collected in national and WHO-supported research and control programmes, or by survey teams and consultants. Special acknowledgement is, therefore, due to the principal authors of the fourteen chapters of the manual for this arduous task.

In a brief historical introduction, Dr. M. FAROOQ chose to review past events that led to the present knowledge of epidemiology and control of schistosomiasis, thereby paying tribute to the insight and effort of many predecessors.

Of the schistosome species causing disease in man, Dr. M. A. STIREWALT describes those features in their life-cycle that are of importance for their identification and for evaluation of their role in epidemiological assessments.

Dr. W. H. WRIGHT'S review of the geographical distribution of schistosomes and their intermediate hosts attempts to condense current knowledge of the subject into one and the same report. To facilitate its use according to needs, the information is presented on three scales: first on a world basis, then area by area, and finally for each area country by country. For further details, numerous reference lists have been appended.

The same chapter also includes a discussion of the schistosome-intermediate host complex in Africa, Southwest Asia, the Orient and the Americas, which deals with the relative susceptibilities to the human schistosome species of proved or potential molluscan intermediate hosts, and of their significance in the transmission of the disease. Factors having an influence in gradually limiting or increasing its spread are considered in the concluding section on future trends of the disease.

In the preparation of certain parts of this chapter, Dr. WRIGHT was able to enlist the co-operation of a number of specialists possessing authoritative knowledge of a particular area or problem, namely: Dr. N. AYAD, Prof. J. FRAGA DE AZEVEDO, Dr. F. S. BARBOSA, Dr. V. DE V. CLARKE, Dr. M. FAROOQ, Dr. J. H. S. GEAR, Dr. J. GILLET, Dr. H. F. HSÜ, Dr. P. JORDAN, Prof. Y. KOMIYA, Dr. F. S. MCCULLOUGH, Prof. G. S. NELSON, Dr. W. L. PARAENSE, Dr. R. J. PITCHFORD and Dr. G. WEBBE. Their individual contributions, which have been integrated into the text and will be easily recognized by the expert, are herewith gratefully acknowledged, and so is Mrs. J. BERNARD-KIRUKHINE'S help in the tracing and checking of source material.

The mere knowledge of the factors and the chain of events leading to transmission of schistosomiasis in a given area is not sufficient to permit the development of a sound plan for the control of the disease. A quantitative approach is needed to effect such measurements as will assist in the selection of appropriate control methods and in monitoring their results during and after control proper. In the chapter on the dynamics of transmission Prof. N. G. HAIRSTON describes how such quantitative studies are carried out, the problems that are encountered and the ways in which results may be interpreted. This chapter also demonstrates the usefulness of descriptive models of schistosomiasis transmission such as the one developed by Prof. HAIRSTON, which provides a logical frame of reference to epidemiological research.

Apart from the question of availability of funds and staff, any decision to initiate schistosomiasis control must be based on a reliable assessment of the public health importance of this disease. The relevant problems are taken up in the chapter by Prof. G. MACDONALD and Dr. M. FAROOQ. They also describe the organization and types of investigation required for such an assessment. Although estimation of the economic effects of parasitic diseases in conditions obtaining in developing countries is still hampered by the lack of an accepted methodology, suggestions and examples are given which may prove useful in broadly evaluating the cost of schistosomiasis as compared to the cost of its control.

Few investigations have been carried out to ascertain the severity of schistosomiasis but where this has been done the results revealed that schistosomiasis is a far greater cause of morbidity than was suspected. Such studies need to be encouraged. The interested investigator will find in Prof. MACDONALD's résumé of the report of two WHO scientific groups (one convened under his chairmanship) a description of the essential pathological and clinical manifestations of the three main forms of human schistosomiasis wherein those features lending themselves to quantitative analysis are singled out. Procedures and working criteria for comparative studies are also presented.

The three following chapters by Dr. M. FAROOQ provide information on the various approaches followed and the results achieved in past and current national control programmes, on the considerations upon which to base a decision to initiate control, and on the planning and organization of a control programme which can attain the chosen objective.

It is now generally accepted that control of schistosomiasis is best achieved by the use of a combination of control measures. However, specialists have generally agreed that snail destruction is still the most effective single control measure. Dr. L.S. RITCHIE, with the collaboration of Prof. E. PAULINI, Mr. W.R. JOBIN, Dr. V. DE V. CLARKE and Mr. A. E. H. HIGGINS, presents an up-to-date review on the chemical control of snails which includes: descriptions of laboratory and field methods used for screening and evaluating promising molluscicides; a summary of the properties of available and candidate molluscicides; and practical guidance on the choice of a molluscicide as well as on the strategy, planning and equipment for molluscicide application.

The two other ways to control the snail intermediate hosts are 'biological control' using the harmful effects to snails of predators, parasites and competitors, and 'environmental control' aimed at rendering habitats unsuitable to the snails. These are dealt with in a chapter prepared by Dr. D.B. McMULLEN with the collaboration of Mr. Z. BUZO, Prof. E. CHERNIN and Dr. F.F. FERGUSON. While biological control has distinct limitations, a wide range of engineering measures are known to be very effective when applied to such widely varying habitats as streams, ponds, marshes, drains and irrigation schemes. The difficulties encountered in the use of these control measures and the methods to be used in overcoming them, are discussed in this chapter.

Mass administration of drugs for the purpose of reducing transmission of schistosomiasis should not be attempted without a clear appreciation of its precise indications, careful scientific planning and strict working criteria. The reasons, both technical and pharmacological, are explained by Dr. A. DAVIS in the chapter on chemotherapy in control which also contains general information related to drugs presently used or showing promise in the control of schistosomiasis.

Whatever the methods chosen to control schistosomiasis, it is essential that their efficacy be evaluated during the attack phase of the control programme to allow operational mistakes to be corrected and to allow judgement of the results achieved on the basis of reliable data. In discussing this subject, Dr. L.J. OLIVIER examines the various parameters and procedures that can be used to obtain direct or indirect evidence of the efficacy of control work.

The last chapter, prepared by Dr. L.J. OLIVIER and Mr. K. UEMURA, is entirely devoted to descriptions of techniques, statistical methods and recording forms used for schistosomiasis surveys and for control operations. They are illustrated by examples and figures from field epidemiological and control programmes or laboratory work.

Many other specialists, by participating in the work of WHO expert and scientific meetings, by offering advice and comments, have contributed, although indirectly, to the preparation of the present manual. Their names have been mentioned in the special acknowledgements that close this book, as an expression of our gratitude.

Dr. W.H. WRIGHT, Prof. P.C. BEAVER, Dr. B.A. SOUTHGATE and Mrs J. SOTIROFF have read and edited the manuscript in part or *in toto*. Appreciation for their invaluable guidance and assistance is due to each of them.

Finally, we wish to thank Karger S.A. for agreeing to publish this work which, it is hoped, will stimulate interest in the epidemiology and control of schistosomiasis, a disease that impairs the health of millions of people and is a heavy burden in the economic struggle of many developing countries.

N. ANSARI

Contributors

Authors

Dr. A. DAVIS, Director, World Health Organization/(British) Medical Research Council/ Tanzania Bilharziasis Chemotherapy Centre, Tanga, Tanzania.

Dr. M. FAROOQ†, Former Senior WHO Adviser (Epidemiologist), Egypt-49 Project, World Health Organization Regional Office for the Eastern Mediterranean, Alexandria, Egypt, United Arab Republic.

Prof. N.G. HAIRSTON, Director, Museum of Zoology, University of Michigan, Ann Arbor, Mich., USA.

Prof. G. MACDONALD†, Former Director, Ross Institute of Tropical Hygiene, London School of Hygiene and Tropical Medicine, London, United Kingdom.

Dr. D.B. McMULLEN†, Former Scientific Adviser, Walter Reed Army Institute of Medical Research, Washington, D.C., USA.

Dr. L.J. OLIVIER, Parasitic Diseases Adviser, Pan American Health Organization and World Health Organization Regional Office for the Americas, Washington, D.C., USA. Formerly: Laboratory of Parasitic Diseases, National Institutes of Health, Bethesda, Md., USA.

Dr. L.S. RITCHIE, Senior Scientist, Puerto Rico Nuclear Center operated by the University of Puerto Rico for the US Atomic Energy Commission, San Juan, Puerto Rico; Walter Reed Army Institute of Research, Washington, D.C., USA.

Dr. M.A. STIREWALT, Acting Director, Department of Parasitology, Naval Medical Research Institute, National Naval Medical Center, Bethesda, Md., USA.

Mr. K. UEMURA, Chief, Health Statistical Methodology, Division of Health Statistics, World Health Organization, Geneva, Switzerland.

Dr. W.H. WRIGHT, Former Chief, Laboratory of Tropical Diseases, National Institutes of Health, Bethesda, Md., USA.

Other Contributors

Dr. N. AYAD, Former Director-General, Bilharziasis and Endemic Diseases Department, Ministry of Public Health, Cairo, Egypt, United Arab Republic.

Prof. J. FRAGA DE AZEVEDO, Chair of Entomology and Helminthology, Escola Nacional de Saude Publica e de Medicina Tropical, Lisbon, Portugal.

Dr. F. S. BARBOSA, Medical Officer, Parasitic Diseases, Division of Communicable Diseases, World Health Organization, Geneva, Switzerland. Formerly: Head, Department of Preventive Medicine, University of Pernambuco, Recife, Brazil.

Mr. Z. BUZO, Regional Adviser in Environmental Health, World Health Organization Regional Office for South East Asia, New Delhi, India.

Prof. E. CHERNIN, Department of Tropical Public Health, Harvard School of Public Health, Boston, Mass., USA.

Dr. V. DE V. CLARKE, Director, Blair Research Laboratory, Salisbury, Rhodesia.

Dr. F. F. FERGUSON, Chief, San Juan Laboratories, Ecological Investigations Program, National Communicable Disease Center, US Public Health Service, Old San Juan, Puerto Rico.

Dr. J. H. S. GEAR, Director, South African Institute for Medical Research, Johannesburg, South Africa.

Prof. J. GILLET, Director, Public Health School, Université Catholique de Louvain, Brussels, Belgium.

Mr. A. E. H. HIGGINS, Senior Lecturer, Department of Zoology and Applied Entomology, Imperial College Field Station, Ascot, Berkshire, United Kingdom.

Prof. H. F. HSÜ, Chair of Parasitology, Department of Preventive Medicine and Environmental Health, College of Medicine, University of Iowa, Iowa City, Iowa, USA.

Mr. W. R. JOBIN, Public Health engineer, Foxboro, Mass., USA.

Dr. P. JORDAN, Director, Research and Control Department, Castries, St. Lucia, West Indies.

Prof. Y. KOMIYA, Director, National Institute of Health, Tokyo, Japan.

Dr. F. S. McCULLOUGH, WHO Adviser, World Health Organization Regional Office for Africa, Brazzaville, People's Republic of the Congo; Bilharziasis Pilot Control Project, Mwanza, Tanzania.

Prof. G. S. NELSON, Head, Department of Medical Helminthology, London School of Hygiene and Tropical Medicine, London, United Kingdom.

Dr. W. L. PARAENSE, Director, Instituto Central de Biologia, Universidade de Brasilia, Brasilia, D. F., Brazil.

Prof. E. PAULINI, Chief, Department of Chemical Engineering, Universidade Federal de Minas Gerais; Centro de Pesquisas René Rachou, Belo Horizonte, Minas Gerais, Brazil.

Dr. R. J. PITCHFORD, Director, Bilharzia Field Unit, Medical Research Council, Nelspruit, South Africa.

Dr. G. WEBBE, Reader in Medical Parasitology, London School of Hygiene and Tropical Medicine; Scientific Director, Winches Farm Field Station, St. Albans, United Kingdom.

Editors

Dr. N. ANSARI, Chief, Parasitic Diseases, Division of Communicable Diseases, World Health Organization, Geneva, Switzerland.

Prof. P. C. BEAVER, Department of Tropical Medicine and Public Health, Tulane University School of Medicine, New Orleans, La., USA.

Mrs. J. SOTIROFF, Parasitic Diseases, Division of Communicable Diseases, World Health Organization, Geneva, Switzerland.

Dr. B. A. SOUTHGATE, Senior Lecturer, Ross Institute for Tropical Hygiene, London School of Hygiene and Tropical Medicine, London, United Kingdom.

Dr. W. H. WRIGHT, Former Chief, Laboratory of Tropical Diseases, National Institutes of Health, Bethesda, Md., USA.

Chapter 1

Epidemiology and Control of Schistosomiasis, pp. 1–16
(Karger, Basel and University Park Press, Baltimore 1973)

Historical Development

M. FAROOQ

Introduction

From the course of events which has revealed the essential features of the life cycle, morphology and biology of the human schistosomes, much can be learned about the distribution and control of schistosomiasis in different parts of the world. Speculation on the possible original centres of infection and important routes and modes of spread also help us to understand the present distribution of schistosomiasis.

In the following brief review, the most important landmarks in the study and control of *Schistosoma haematobium, S. mansoni* and *S. japonicum,* the three major species of the parasite which infect man, will be indicated, and many of the individuals to whom we owe much of our knowledge of the epidemiology of these infections will be mentioned. This review will also serve to remind us that discoveries in medical history are rooted in the thoughts and efforts of many men. As has frequently been the case in important contributions to science, the same problem has been attacked simultaneously by several workers without their knowledge of one another's investigations, and often honours should be equally shared.

Epidemiology

Schistosoma haematobium

A chronic endemic disease, characterized by blood in the urine and by various bladder troubles, has been known to occur in Egypt and Mesopotamia since earliest times, associated with the agricultural civilizations of the great river valleys. Haematuria is described in the Gynaecological Papyrus of Kahun, one of the oldest papyrus fragments found in the ruins of the town of Kahun (near the entrance to the Fayoum), written during the middle of the XIIth dynasty period, about 1900 BC. Since many remedies for haematuria have been recorded (20 in Ebers Papyrus, 11 in Berlin Papyrus and 9 in Hearst) it can be assumed that the condition was widespread and constituted a serious problem among the Egyptians in ancient times. Remedies 'to kill worms in the body that have been caused by *âaâ* disease' are given in 'Papyrus Ebers' of about 1500 BC.[1] For a long time it was believed that *âaâ* disease was hookworm disease, the 'Egyptian chlorosis', until PFISTER [1913] refuted it and EBBELL [1927] showed convincingly that *âaâ*

did not designate a disease but an important symptom, *haematuria*. This also explains why a phallus is used as determinative of the word.

The symbol may, in fact, represent the concept of haematuria. The treatment recommended to cure haematuria lends further support to this belief. It consists of pronouncing a magic formula of

on a phallus made of cake dough on which some names have been written. The phallus must then be wrapped with fat meat and given to a cat. Since the symbolic treatment is accompanied by a representation of a phallus, it may be presumed that the disease is related to the penis. Usually where such symbolic treatment was given, the affected part of the body was represented.

Direct evidence of the presence of the parasite by one of the foremost pioneers in the field of palaeopathology [RUFFER, 1910] was furnished by the demonstration of a large number of calcified ova of the parasite, situated for the most part among the straight tubules in the kidneys of two Egyptian mummies of the XXth dynasty (1250–1000 BC).

To the ancient Egyptian physicians the symptom, as a rule, was the disease and when several symptoms were observed the disease was named

1   This leads one to wonder if the Egyptians knew that haematuria was caused by a trematode worm. Though EBBELL [1927] considers that such a hypothesis would appear bold, he points out that the one definite passage in Ebers' Papyrus states that haematuria produces the worms '*hrt*'. If '*hrt*' means platyhelminth related to haematuria, the Egyptians could have made an error and confused the effect with the cause. However, it is significant that worms are mentioned in relation to haematuria.

after the chief symptom. Since haematuria is one of the chief symptoms of urinary schistosomiasis and since palaeopathological findings confirm the occurrence of the disease in antiquity, we may assume that the passages in the medical papyrus refer to this disease.

Historians of mediaeval Egypt, mostly Arabs, told the story of a disease among Egyptian males which made them 'menstruate'. In his memoirs, LARREY [1812–1817] also notes that symptoms of the disease were frequent among the French troops during the Napoleonic invasion of Egypt, 1799–1801.

Pathognomonic symptoms of urinary infection have also been described in Babylonian inscriptions and in mediaeval medical literature, and by AVICENNA (IBN SINA) in the 10th century.

It was not, however, until 1851 that THEODOR BILHARZ found at the Kasr el Aini Hospital in Cairo, the causative agent *(Distoma haematobium, a blood-fluke)* in the mesenteric vein during a *post mortem* examination. The parasite bears the generic name *Schistosoma* and the disease it causes in man is called schistosomiasis.[2]

LEIPER identified the intermediate hosts of *S. haematobium* at El Margh village near Cairo during the spring and summer of 1915. By exposing mice to cercariae it was possible to demonstrate that those developing in *Bulinus* always produced worms which gave rise solely to terminal-spined eggs.

The original centre of *S. haematobium* infection has usually been assumed to lie in the upper Nile basin but sometimes the northern Nile valley, where it has long been prominent and which certainly has served as one focus from where it has spread, has been favoured. The dispersal of schistosomiasis haematobia from the Great Lake plateau region has been repeatedly commented upon, and in recent years WRIGHT [1961] has postulated the evolutionary origin of the host-parasite relationships of the human schistosomes in the area. He suggests that not only was East Africa one of the centres of man's evolutionary origin but it was also the place of origin of the bulinid hosts for *S. haematobium*. Thus, throughout the early

2   By a decision of the International Commission on Zoological Nomenclature [Opinions and declarations of zoological nomenclature, 1954, Opinion 226, supplement to Opinion 77, vol. 4, pp. 176–200], the generic name of the group to which the human blood flukes belong is *Schistosoma* Weinland, 1858, and not *Bilharzia* Meckel von Hemsbach, 1856, nor yet *Bilharzia* Cobbold, 1859; but the same body recommends that the term 'bilharziasis' should continue to be used for the diseases which they cause in man. However, a WHO expert committee recommended in December 1966 that the term 'schistosomiasis' be adopted by the World Health Organization for the disease in man and animals [*Wld Hlth Org. techn. Rep. Ser. 372:* 33 (1967)].

stages of human evolution both of the hosts necessary to the schistosome life cycle were continually in close contact under conditions ideally suited to transmission of the parasite. In these circumstances it was possible for the very specific host-parasite relationships of the human schistosomes to have evolved there.

It is apparent that areas of long-established and pronounced endemicity coincide largely with the Islamic cultural orbit. No doubt Arab colonization, trade routes, slave-raiding practices and religious traditions of pilgrims have contributed materially to the firm entrenchment of this infection within their sphere of influence. It has been suggested that the wide wanderings of the Bantus in the early part of the last century were instrumental in the southward spread of the disease, and the present distribution limits in the Cape Province seem to coincide well with their movements. As regards the westward spread, the infection has infiltrated, within living memory, from Zambia into south-eastern Katanga. In many regions now recognized as affected, the disease was not noted before the first quarter of the 20th century. In certain instances, the present situation has resulted from reintroduction, or an increase in prevalence of pre-existing but diffuse centres. This may, for instance, have been the case in Rhodesia and Zambia, where the disease was not noticed a century ago. It may also apply to northern Sudan, a region previously conquered by ancient Egypt and overrun by a wave of Arab conquest in the 14th century, where schistosomiasis flared up in the 19th century in the wake of the conquering Ottoman and Egyptian armies.

Cultivation in the valley of the twin rivers (Tigris-Euphrates) has been largely dependent upon perennial irrigation and *S. haematobium* has, in all probability, been endemic in the area for many thousands of years. Since the destruction of the original irrigation system in the 13th century it has been a health problem of relatively minor importance until the present century, when first the military operations during the First World War and then the progressive restoration of the irrigation system, brought it into prominence once more.

Schistosoma mansoni

In 1898 MANSON suggested, on the grounds of dissimilar geographical distribution, that vesical and intestinal forms of the disease were of separate origin. In 1902, he found lateral-spined eggs in the faeces of a West Indian patient in London and postulated the existence of a second species of blood fluke. LOOSS, however, disagreed with this hypothesis and maintained that the lateral-spined eggs were *S. haematobium* eggs produced partheno-genetically in the absence of males. Four years of controversy followed and SAMBON, in the teeth of opposition from LOOSS, named the new species after MANSON in 1907, 'in appreciation of this one of his many genial intuitions'. The SAMBON-LOOSS controversy, which reached a stalemate by 1915, was finally settled by the work of LEIPER in 1915 in Egypt; he established beyond doubt the presence of two distinct species and that the snail intermediate hosts belonged not only to two different genera but to two different sub-families.

Comparatively little is known of the history of this infection. It is usually assumed that the parasite was spread westward from the African Lake plateau region by various Bantu tribes. *S. mansoni* infection, probably no less ancient than *S. haematobium,* is found in south-western Arabia, a region traversed by a principal overland pilgrim route to Mecca. The infection was doubtless carried to the New World with the slaves, from endemic foci in East, Central and West Africa in the 16th, 17th and 18th centuries, and became established in those areas in the West Indies and South America where appropriate snails existed in water contaminated by human excreta. Although large numbers of infected African slaves were imported into other regions of the Americas (viz. continental USA, Mexico. Central American countries, Cuba, etc.), the absence or lack of abundance of susceptible snails prevented development of *S. mansoni* in those countries, just as *S. haematobium* in imported Africans failed to become established in the Americas, due to lack of appropriate snails.

The credit for the discovery of *S. mansoni* in the New World is attributed to PIRAJA DA SILVA who, in 1904, found 'worm eggs bearing a lateral spine' in the stools of patients in Bahia (Brazil). By 1908, he had become aware of the discussions going on in the Old World over the identity of the parasites and succeeded in discovering new and important facts and, in the same year, published details of his findings, including the anatomical characteristics of adult *S. mansoni* recovered at necropsy.

The first reference to the occurrence of the disease in Venezuela was made by SOTO in 1906. Shortly afterwards it was proved in Egypt that *S. mansoni* was transmitted through a snail intermediate host, ITURBE and GONZÁLES [1917] incriminated *Biomphalaria glabrata* in Venezuela and ITURBE at the same time carried out epidemiological studies on *S. mansoni* infection in that country.

GONZALEZ MARTINEZ discovered rectal schistosomiasis in Puerto Rico in 1904, but definite proof of transmission of the infection was not confirmed until the demonstration of the *S. mansoni* cercariae in the planorbid snail host by HOFFMAN in 1927.

Schistosoma japonicum

The earliest recorded account of infection caused by *Schistosoma japonicum* is that of FUJII in 1847 who described the disease occurring in a village situated at the foot of a hill, Katayama, in Hiroshima Prefecture. Katayama, also called 'Urishi' which means 'lacquer', was the site where a typhoon wrecked a ship loaded with 'Urishi'. The skin eruptions on hands and feet, 'Kabure', later followed by other symptoms of the 'Katayama syndrome' among the inhabitants of the village, were locally believed to be due to the lacquer in the rice-field water.

BAELZ [1883] was the first to mention the disease in a language other than Chinese or Japanese. While working in Japan he described the clinical features of 'Okayama' disease (enlargement of the liver and spleen, bloody diarrhoea, anaemia, fever, cachexia, ascites and oedema) but attributed them to *Clonorchis sinensis,* a trematode he found in the liver of some of his patients. YAMAGIWA [1890] described a case of Jacksonian epilepsy in which ova were found in the brain. He attributed his findings to the lung fluke, *Paragonimus westermani.*

The first relationship of the true causative agent to the disease was reported by KATSURADA in 1904. He recovered worms from the portal system of a cat and named the species *Schistosoma japonicum.* He gave an accurate description of the eggs found in man and in the cat. FUJINAMI [1907], who investigated the infection in cows, described the pathological anatomy of the infected tissues, the morphology of the adult worms and their distribution in the definitive host, but it was not until FUJINAMI and NAKAMURA [1909] conducted careful field experiments with animals in the Katayama endemic area that the route of infection by way of the skin was established.[3]

---

3   Apparently ALLEN [1888] was the first investigator to theorize that the infection was acquired through the skin. Working in Natal, South Africa, he formulated the belief that 'nearly all the youths bathing in the Umsindusi and Dorspruit are infected, while the girls, who do not bathe, remain free of the disease'. The skin route of infection was likewise supported by LOOSS, although he came to the conclusion that the schistosome was a monogenetic

Clinical phases of the infection were described by others in Japan and by 1911 cattle, horses, dogs and cats were shown to be hosts of the parasite. Guinea pigs, monkeys and rats were found to be susceptible to experimental infection with *S. japonicum*.

FUJINAMI, NAKAMURA and MIYAGAWA between 1909 and 1913 worked out the path of migration of schistosome larvae through the body. MIYAIRI and SUZUKI established that *Oncomelania nosophora* was the intermediate host of the parasite in Kyushu Island in 1913–1914. They were able to infect mammals with cercariae obtained from this snail and observed the penetration of miracidia into the same species and followed the development of the parasite in the intermediate host. This work, which was studied by LEIPER and ATKINSON in Japan, provided a basis for LEIPER's later work and discoveries in Egypt.

The infection was recognized in China by LOGAN [1905], in the Philippines by WOOLLEY [1906], in Formosa by TAKEGAMI [1914], in Celebes by BRUG and TESCH [1937] and in Laos by VIC DUPONT *et al.* and GALLIARD [1957]; infection was reported by CHAIYAPORN and his associates in a patient in Thailand in 1959, in 1960 HARINASUTA and KRUATRACHUE found a small focus in the southern province of Nakornsrithamaraj. Reports of clinical cases treated in Paris [BARBIER, 1966], New York [MOST, 1966], Bangkok [LEE *et al.*, 1966] and Pnom-Penh [AUDEBAUD *et al.*, 1968] led to various investigations which established or confirmed the presence of endemic foci in the Mekong river basin, namely at Ubol, Thailand [DESOWITZ *et al.*, 1967], in Khong Island, Laos [BARBIER, 1966; IIJIMA and GARCIA, 1967] and Kratie, Cambodia [KRIOUTCHOV, 1968; BAZILLIO, 1969; IIJIMA, 1970; JOLLY *et al.*, 1970].

The *Oncomelania* intermediate hosts were discovered in China by FAUST and MELENEY [1924], first in Soochow in Kiangsu Province and later in Chekiang Province and in the Pearl River delta in South China. YOKOGAWA first discovered *O. formosana* to be the intermediate host in Formosa in 1915. In the Philippines *O. quadrasi* was found to be responsible for transmission by TUBANGUI in 1932. The intermediate hosts in Celebes, in Thailand and in Laos have not yet been identified.

---

trematode and the free-living miracidium directly invaded man without the intercalation of the sporocyst generation in an intermediate host. LOOSS dogmatically maintained this belief against heavy odds for nearly 20 years, until the demonstration of the complete life-history by MIYAIRI and SUZUKI [1913, 1914], MIYAGAWA [1913], and LEIPER and ATKINSON [1915]. These investigations proved that the schistosomes had a cercarial stage and that their larvae penetrated the skin.

Early Work in Prevention and Control

There is a widespread belief among South African tribes, probably handed down from time immemorial, that haematuria is caused by something that enters the body through the orifice of the penis during bathing. To prevent this, certain tribes such as Zulus wear a basket-like protection (Kaffir cock-box). A similar belief and like form of protection prevailed among the ancient Egyptians. Its mode of use is figured on the walls of some of the ancient temples of Egypt. The concept that water was the source of the cause of haematuria, therefore, goes back into antiquity. No such belief exists amongst Egyptians today but LEIPER was told that troops proceeding to Egypt were instructed to wear penile sheaths while bathing in canals to prevent schistosomiasis. LEIPER believed that small leeches, which sometimes gained entrance into the urethra and caused profuse urethral bleeding, had been mistaken for the cause of the haematuria.

The theory that infection takes place through the skin was put forward by various South African writers. Many, however, were reluctant to accept this; some believed that infection was limited to the tender skin of the prepuce and advocated universal circumcision. RUFFER and others believed the infection was due to entrance of cercariae through the anus.

In proving that the skin was the portal of entry of the parasite, FUJINAMI and NAKAMURA demonstrated for the first time in 1909 a means of preventing the infection. In their experiments, calves known to be susceptible to the infection were provided with waterproof leggings which prevented their becoming infected when immersed in 'infected water'. It remained for LEIPER [1915], after visiting the Orient and observing and confirming the work of Japanese investigators, to study the problem in Egypt.

FUJINAMI and NAKAMURA [1911] attempted to prevent infection by killing molluscan hosts. MIYAGAWA [1913] and others found that chemicals such as unslaked lime and calcium cyanamide could be utilized to kill the snails and also possessed fertilizing properties for crops. Chlorinated lime and copper sulphate, though efficacious, were found to be injurious to crops; calcium phosphate and ammonium sulphate were less efficacious against snails but, since they were good fertilizers, they were also considered. With the discovery of the intermediate host and the coincident recognition of the role of the cercariae it was demonstrated that these chemicals, acting both on the intermediate host and the parasite, served a dual purpose in preventing the infection.

In the Katyama area, FUJINAMI and SUEYASU [1919] used calcium oxide in 0.1-percent concentrations in rice fields and later experimented with the application of first hot water and then live steam pumped from a boiler through a hose under heavy canvas spread upon the dykes bordering rice fields. In the coastal endemic area of Shizuoka, tidal waters were utilized to inundate snail-infested lands and found to be effective.

The possibility of control of the disease by killing eggs in human faeces (extensively used as fertilizer in Japan) was studied by MIYAGAWA [1916]. Practical application was made of the fact that eggs failed to hatch in urine-faeces mixture after 16 days and that the chemicals which killed the intermediate host and the cercariae also killed the miracidia. This was supplemented by the prevention of promiscuous defaecation by children and, when the role of other mammalian hosts was discovered, attempts were made to control them. The possession of cats and dogs was discouraged, and oxen were replaced by horses as farm animals when FUJINAMI and NAKAMURA [1913] demonstrated that the latter rarely passed eggs in their faeces. Rearing ducks was encouraged in the hope that they would eat and eliminate snails.

In 1914, when knowledge which discredited the LOOSS hypothesis had just been acquired by Japanese workers, the First World War began. LEIPER, in charge of the first Wandsworth Expedition of the London School of Tropical Medicine, was investigating the mode of spread of trematode infections of man in the Far East at the time, and was commissioned to Egypt 'to investigate bilharzia disease in that country and advise as to the preventive measures to be adopted in connection with the troops'. During a period of six months he produced the monumental work referred to previously which proposed the first rational approach to the control of schistosomiasis on the African continent. LEIPER, in 1915, was the first to see the relationships between the introduction of perennial irrigation and schistosomiasis in Egypt and the need for proper water management to discourage snail breeding. He concluded that 'in order to break the life cycle of the bilharzia worm one must find some simple means of destroying it during the free-swimming infective stage, or of depriving it of its essential intermediate host'. The former he considered was the line of attack suited to the conditions in urban centres and the latter in the rural areas of Egypt. The suggested measures included the replacement of the small agricultural drains by piping or by 'mole' drains, together with the proper utilization of canal clearance and the periodic drying of the small canals during the summer 'rotations', although it was realized that the snails would not be entirely destroyed by these means. It was also recommended that the small collections of residual water should be treated chemically to destroy the surviving molluscs; ammonium sulphate was advised because it killed snails and was a good fertilizer. Suitable siting of new villages in relation to canals in reclaimed areas was suggested. The relationship of schistosomiasis control to agricultural practices was not lost sight of and improvements were proposed which, while discouraging snail breeding, would improve the yield of cotton. The benefits of abolishing open drains were emphasized and the cost estimates provided were reasonable. The administrative need for the public health services and the department of irrigation to establish a suitable liaison through a medical zoologist was emphasized. LEIPER'S exceptional insight and rational approach to the problem, advocated half a century ago, undoubtedly blazed the trail for schistosomiasis control.

Chronology of Important Events

1847 AD FUJII, Y., described 'Katayama disease' from Katayama endemic area in Hiroshima Province, Japan.

1851   BILHARZ, T., discovered a bisexual distome, named *Distoma haematobium*, and established relationship between this trematode worm and the symptoms of dysentery and haematuria.

1859   COBBOLD, T.S., showed that schistosomes in Africa were not confined to man when he discovered '*Bilharzia magna*' in a West-African monkey.

1864   HARLEY, J., ascribed the endemic haematuria in Cape of Good Hope and Natal, 'Cape haematuria', as due to *Bilharzia*. He named the parasite '*Bilharzia capensis*'.

1870   COBBOLD, T.S., first attempted to trace the life cycle through an invertebrate intermediate host.

1888   ALLEN, J.F., in South Africa, formulated the hypothesis that a larval stage of the parasite might enter the body through the skin.

1898   MANSON, P., suggested the existence of vesical and intestinal forms of the disease.

1901 (onward) SYMMERS, W.St.C. [1901]; GOEBEL, C. [1903]; FAIRLEY, N.H. [1919]; GIRGES, R. [1929]; GELFAND, M. [1948]; ERFAN, M. and associates [1949]; MAKAR, N. [1952] among others made valuable contributions to clinico-pathological studies in schistosomiasis.

1902   MANSON, P., found lateral-spined eggs in a patient from Antigua (West Indies).

1904   KATSURADA, F., discovered *S. japonicum* in Japan. He described the parasite and the pathology which it produces.

1904   PIRAJA DA SILVA first detected *S. mansoni* infection in the New World.

1904   CATTO, J., discovered *S. japonicum* infection in a Chinese in Singapore, who had come from the coastal province of Fukien in China.

1904   GONZALES-MARTINEZ, I., discovered *S. mansoni* infection in Puerto Rico.

1905   LOGAN, O.T., confirmed the presence of *S. japonicum* in China.

1906   WOOLLEY, P. G., described the occurrence of *S. japonicum* in the Philippines.

1907   SAMBON, L. W., named the laterally-spined ovum-producing agent of intestinal schistosomiasis as '*Schistosoma mansoni*'.

1907   FUJINAMI, A., worked out the pathological anatomy of the infected tissue in *S. japonicum*.

1909   FUJINAMI, A. and NAKAMURA, H., showed conclusively that the route of infection was by way of skin and that cattle, horses, dogs and cats, as well as man, were found to be natural hosts of *S. japonicum*.

1910   RUFFER, M. A., demonstrated the presence of calcified ova of *S. haematobium* in the kidneys of two Egyptian mummies of the XXth dynasty (1250–1000 BC).

1912–13 MIYAGAWA, Y., worked out the path of migration of *S. japonicum* larvae through the body.

1913–14 MIYAIRI, K. and SUZUKI, M., found the intermediate host of *S. japonicum* (classified as belonging to the family *Hydrobiidae*) in Kyushu, observed the penetration of hatched miracidia into the snail and infected mammals with cercariae obtained from the snail.

1914   TAKEGAMI, K., reported the presence of *S. japonicum* from Formosa.

1915   LEIPER, R. T., established that *S. haematobium* and *S. mansoni* were transmitted by two different snails, *Bulinus contortus* and *Planorbis boissyii* respectively.

1915   LEIPER, R. T. worked out the basis of prophylactic work in Egyptian rural and urban areas.

1915   YOKOGAWA, S., located an endemic area of *S. japonicum* in Formosa and reported on the presence of its intermediate host.

1915   LEIPER, R. T., and ATKINSON, E. L., repeated and confirmed the work of MIYAIRI and SUZUKI and of MIYAGAWA from Japanese material. Existence of an alteration of generations, as in other digenetic trematodes with a parthenogenetic generation intercalated between the miracidium and the cercaria, was confirmed.

1918   CHRISTOPHERSON, J. B., introduced tartar emetic as a cure for schistosomiasis in Khartoum, Sudan.

1918   Lime first used as molluscicide in Japan (Hiroshima).

1919   CORT, W. W., presented a full description of the cercaria of *S. japonicum*, forming the basis for the differentiation between non-schistosome fork-tailed, non-mammalian schistosome and human schistosome cercariae.

1920   CHANDLER, A. C., in the USA demonstrated the molluscicidal properties of copper sulphate.

1924   FAUST, E. C. and MELENEY, H. E., surveyed endemic areas in China and discovered the molluscan host in the Soochow, Kashing, and Shaohsing areas in China.

1924   FAUST, E. C. and MELENEY, H. E., provided detailed information on the egg-miracidium phase of the life cycle; the developmental cycle of *Schistosoma japonicum* within the molluscan host, the cercarial stage and its development within its definitive host and the route of migration, and provided a detailed description of the pathological anatomy divided into various stages of the development of the parasite and related clinical course of the disease. The status of treatment with emetine and other preparations of antimony were reviewed and regimens recommended.

1927   KHALIL, M., first applied copper sulphate in Rashda village in Dakhla Oasis for the eradication of *Bulinus*.

1927   EBBELL, B., showed that *âaâ* disease represented haematuria.

1928   SCHMIDT, H., of Bayer, developed stibophen intramuscular treatment for schistosomiasis in Cairo.

1930–37 SCOTT, J. A., of the Rockefeller Foundation, conducted extensive comprehensive surveys on the prevalence and distribution of *S. haematobium* and *S. mansoni* in Egypt.

1932   TUBANGUI, M. A., discovered the intermediate host of schistosomiasis in Palo, Leyte Island, Philippines.

1937   BARLOW, C. H., advocated repeated weed clearance from canals as a method of snail control in Egypt.

1937   BRUG, S. L. and TESCH, J. W., reported *S. japonicum* infection in Lake Lindoê area in Celebes.

1938   A Bilharzia Snail Destruction (Eradication) Section was created in Egypt.

1942   Schistosomiasis control programme started in Venezuela.

1944   Calcium cyanamide used as molluscicide in Japan (Hiroshima).

1944–45 Numerous cases of schistosomiasis in American and Australian troops following the invasion of Leyte, Philippines, in October 1944.

1945   WRIGHT, W. H., and associates, discovered new endemic areas in Mindanao, Philippines.

1945   MCMULLEN, D. B., screened several molluscicides in the Philippines and in Japan in 1951; field tested promising ones with American and Japanese collaborators and recommended NaPCP DN-1 and D-111 as most potent against *Oncomelania nosophora*.

1946   Antibilharziasis Section created in the Ministry of Health, Venezuela.

1946   Molluscicide screening programme inaugurated in National Institutes of Health, Bethesda, Md., USA; first field tests in 1949, with NaPCP and other halogenated hydrocarbon compounds.

1947   First schistosomiasis control programme initiated in Puerto Rico (OLIVER-GONZÁLEZ).

1949   Joint OIHP/WHO Study Group on Bilharziasis in Africa held in Cairo.

1949   Bilharzia Section established in Iraq.

1950   Large-scale experiment with NaPCP started in Fukuoka Prefecture, Japan.

1951   Division of Schistosomiasis created in the Philippines.

1951   First snail control programme started in Rhodesia using $CuSO_4$.

1952   First WHO-assisted Bilharziasis Control Project – Pilot Project (Egypt 10) started near Cairo.

1952   First WHO Expert Committee on Bilharziasis met in San Juan, Puerto Rico.

1952   WHO-assisted Bilharziasis Control Project (Syria-4) established in Kamichlie, Syrian Gezireh.

1953   Programme of cementing ditches in the endemic areas in Japan was begun.

1953   WHO-assisted Bilharziasis Control Project (Philippines-9) established in Palo, Leyte.

1953   Chemical barrier with continuous application of 0.125 ppm $CuSO_4$ was started in the Sudan.

1953   An experiment in eradication of schistosomiasis from an endemic area along the Chikugo River of Fukuoka Prefecture by Japanese workers.

1954   Study Group on the Identification and Classification of the Bilharzia Snail Vector (Equatorial and South Africa) met in Paris.

1954–58   BERRY, E.G. and WRIGHT, W.H., demonstrated the efficacy of NaPCP in the control of transmission of *S. haematobium* and *S. mansoni* in Warraq el Arab near Cairo.

1956   WHO-assisted Bilharziasis Control Pilot Project established in Tarmiah in Iraq.

1956   An eradication programme of 7 to 12 years was started in China (Mainland).

1957   WHO Study Group on the Ecology of the Intermediate Snail Hosts of Bilharziasis met in Paris.

1957   WHO African Conference on Bilharziasis held in Brazzaville, Congo.

1957   GALLIARD, H., diagnosed an autochthonous case of *S. japonicum* from Pakse, Laos along the Mekong River.

1958   WHO Inter-Regional Training Course (Inter-Regional 17) held in Cairo.

1958   A WHO Bilharziasis Advisory Team established with headquarters in Geneva.

1959   CHAIYAPORN, V., and associates reported *S. japonicum* infection from Thailand.

1959   WHO-assisted Bilharziasis Control Project (Iran-38) started in Dizful, Khuzistan.

1959   Meeting of the Scientific Group on Research in Bilharziasis (Molluscicides).

1960   Second African Conference on Bilharziasis (WHO/CCTA) held in Lourenço Marques, Mozambique.

1960   Second WHO Expert Committee on Bilharziasis (Molluscicides) met in Geneva.

1960   Meeting of the Scientific Group on Research in Bilharziasis (Assessment of Medical and Public Health Importance), Geneva.

1960   HARINASUTA, C. and KRUATRACHUE, M. found a focus of *S. japonicum* in Thailand.

1961   WHO/UNICEF-assisted Schistosomiasis Control Pilot Project and Training Centre (Egypt-49) started near Alexandria in Egypt.

1961   Meeting of the WHO Scientific Group on Research in Bilharziasis (Immuno-Biological Diagnosis of Bilharziasis), Geneva.

1962   Scientific Group on Research in Bilharziasis (Pathobiology and Immunity), Geneva.

1962   WHO-assisted Bilharziasis Control Pilot Project (Ghana-5) launched at Wa, Ghana.

1964   WHO Scientific Group on Research in Bilharziasis (Chemotherapy), Geneva.

1964   Third WHO Expert Committee on Bilharziasis met in Geneva.

1965   Meeting of the WHO Scientific Group on Research in Bilharziasis (Measurement of the Public Health Importance), Geneva.

1965   Evidence of interruption of transmission of *S. haematobium* and *S. mansoni* following the use of niclosamide obtained from the Egypt-49 Project (FAROOQ and HAIRSTON).

References

ALLEN, J. F.: Practitioner *40:* 310 (1888).
AUDEBAUD, G.; TOURNIER-LASSERVE, C.; BRUMPT, V.; JOLLY, M.; MAZAUD, R.; IMBERT, X., and BAZILLIO, R.: Bull. Soc. Path. exot. *61:* 778 (1968).
BAELZ, E.: Berl. klin. Wschr. *20:* 234 (1883).
BARBIER, M.: Bull. Soc. Path. exot. *59:* 974 (1966).
BARLOW, C. H.: Amer. J. Hyg. *25:* 327 (1937).
BAZILLIO, R.: La bilharziose à *S. japonicum* au Cambodge. Premières observations et premières études épidémiologiques. Thèse, Faculté royale de Médecine de Phnom Penh (1969).
BILHARZ, T.: Z. wiss. Zool. *4:* 53 (1852).
BRUG, S. L. and TESCH, J. W.: Geneesk. T. Ned.-Ind. *77:* 2151 (1937).
CATTO, J.: Brit. med. J. *ii:* 663 (1904).
CHAIYAPORN, V.; KOONVISAL, L., and DARMADHACH, A.: J. med. Ass. Thailand *42:* 438 (1959).
CHANDLER, A. C.: J. agric. Res. *20:* 193 (1920).
CHRISTOPHERSON, J. B.: Lancet *ii:* 325 (1918).
COBBOLD, T. S.: Trans. Linn. Soc. London *22:* 363 (1859).
COBBOLD, T. S.: Brit. med. J. *ii:* 89 (1872).
CORT, W. W.: Univ. Calif. Publ. (Zool.) *18:* 485 (1919).
DESOWITZ, R.; HARINASUTA, C.; KRUATRACHUE, M.; CHESDAPHAN, C., and JETANASEN, S.: Trans. roy Soc. trop. Med. Hyg. *61:* 153 (1967).
EBBELL, B.: Z. Aegypt. Sprache *62:* 16 (1927).
ERFAN, M., *et al.:* Gaz. Fac. Med. Cairo *23:* 1 (1957).
FAIRLEY, N. H.: Proc. roy. Soc. Med. *13:* 1 (1919).
FAROOQ, M.; HAIRSTON, N. G., and SAMAAN, S. A.: Bull. Wld Hlth Org. *35:* 369 (1966).
FAUST, E. C. and MELENEY, H. E.: Amer. J. Hyg., Monogr. Ser. 3, pp. 1–268 (1924).
FUJII, Y.: Chugai Iji Shimpo (Int. med. J.) *691:* 55 (1847) (in Japanese).
FUJINAMI, A.: Kyoto Igakkai Zasshi (J. Kyoto med. Ass.) *4:* 1 (1907) (in Japanese with German abstract).
FUJINAMI, A. and NAKAMURA, H.: Kyoto Igakkai Zasshi (J. Kyoto med. Ass.) *6:* 224 (1909) (in Japanese).
FUJINAMI, A. and NAKAMURA, H.: Chugai Iji Shimpo (Int. med. J.) *753:* 1009–1027 (1911) (in Japanese).
FUJINAMI, A. and NAKAMURA, H.: Kyoto Igakkai Zasshi (J. Kyoto med. Ass.) *10:* 262 (1913) (in Japanese with German abstract).
FUJINAMI, A. and SUEYASU, Y.: Nishin Igaku (Jap. J. med. Progr.) *9:* 433 (1919) (in Japanese).
GALLIARD, H.: Personal communication to Dr. N. ANSARI, WHO (1957).
GELFAND, M.: Schistosomiasis in South Central Africa. A clinico-pathological study (Juta, Cape Town, 1950).
GIRGES, R.: Schistosomiasis (Bale-Sons-Danielsson, London 1934).
GOEBEL, C.: J. trop. Med. Hyg. *6:* 106, 127, 143 (1903).
GONZALEZ-MARTINEZ, I.: Memoria leída en la Asamblea General de la Associación Médica de Puerto Rico, 3 de Abril 1904, Tip Boletin, p. 32 (1904).
HARINASUTA, C. and KRUATRACHUE, M.: Ann. trop. Med. Parasit. *56:* 314 (1962).

HARLEY, J.: Med-Chir. Trans. *47:* 55 (1864).

HOFFMAN, W. A.: Puerto Rico Rev. publ. Hlth trop. Med. *3:* 223 (1927).

IIJIMA, T.: Assignment report 1968–69 to Cambodia. WHO unpublished document WPR/ 059/70 (1970).

IIJIMA, T. and GARCIA, R. G.: Preliminary survey for schistosomiasis in South Laos. Unpublished document WHO/BILH/67.64 (1967).

ITURBE, J. and GONZALES, E.: Vargas *8:* 134 (1917).

Joint OIHP/WHO Study Group on Bilharziasis in Africa. Wld Hlth Org. techn. Rep. Ser. *17* (1950).

JOLLY, M.; BAZILLIO, R.; AUDEBAUD, G.; BRUMPT, V., and BOU SOPHINN: Méd. trop. *30:* 462 (1970).

KATSURADA, F.: Annot. Zool. Japan *5:* 146 (1904).

KHALIL, M.: Lancet *ii:* 1235 (1927).

KRIOUTCHOV, V. S.: Rapport de fin de mission, Cambridge 0505. WHO unpublished document (1968).

LARREY, D. J.: (Haematurie) Mémoires de chirurgie militaire et campagnes, (Smith, Paris 1812–1817).

LEE, H.-F.; WYKOFF, D. E., and BEAVER, P. C.: Amer. J. trop. Med. Hyg. *15:* 303 (1966).

LEIPER, R. T.: J. roy. Army med. Cps *25:* 1; *26:* 147, 253 (1915).

LEIPER, R. T. and ATKINSON, E. L.: Brit. med. J. *i:* 201 (1915a).

LEIPER, R. T. and ATKINSON, E. L.: Chin. med. J. *29:* 143 (1915b).

LOGAN, O. T.: J. trop. Med. Hyg. *9:* 294 (1906).

LOOSS, A.: Ann. trop. Med. Parasit. *2:* 153 (1908).

LOOSS, A.: in MENSE Handbuch der Tropenkrankheiten; 2. Aufl., vol. 2, pp. 331–374 (Leipzig 1914).

MAKAR, N.: Acta Un. int. Cancer *8:* 323 (1952).

MANSON, P.: Tropical diseases. A manual of the diseases of warm climates; rev. ed., pp. 605–606, 639 (Cassell, London 1898/1903).

MANSON, P.: N. Y. med. J. *77:* 121 (1903).

MCMULLEN, D. B.; ISHII, N., and MITOMA, Y.: J. Parasit. *34:* suppl., vol. 95 (1948).

MIYAGAWA, Y.: Tokyo Iji Shinshi (Tokyo med. J.) *1736:* 1–4 (1911) (in Japanese).

MIYAGAWA, Y.: Tokyo Iji Shinshi (Tokyo med. J.) *1833:* 1–3 (1913) (in Japanese).

MIYAGAWA, Y.: Mitt. med. Fak. Univ. Tokyo *15:* 453 (1916) (in Japanese).

MIYAIRI, K. and SUZUKI, M.: Tokyo Iji Shinshi (Tokyo med. J.) *1836:* 1 (1913) (in Japanese).

MIYAIRI, K. and SUZUKI, M.: Mitt. med. Fak. Kais. Univ. Kyushu (Fukuoka) *1:* 187 (1914).

MOST, H.: Personal communication to Dr. N. ANSARI, WHO (1966).

NAKAMURA, H.: Kyoto Igakkai Zasshi (J. Kyoto med. Ass.) *7:* 239 (1910) (in Japanese).

NAKAMURA, H.: Kyoto Igakkai Zasshi (J. Kyoto med. Ass.) *8:* 1 (1911a) (in Japanese)

NAKAMURA, H.: Nippon Byorigakkai Kaishi (Trans. Jap. Path. Soc.) *1:* 1, 61, 63, 66 (1911b) (in Japanese).

PFISTER, E.: Arch. Gesch. Med. *6:* 12 (1913).

RUFFER, M. A.: Brit. med. J. *i:* 16 (1910).

SAMBON, L. W.: J. trop. Med. Hyg. *10:* 303 (1907).

SAMBON, L. W.: J. trop. med. Hyg. *12:* 1 (1909).

SCHMIDT, H.: Indian med. Gaz. *63:* 643 (1928).

SCOTT, J. A.: J. Parasit. *18:* 129 (1931).

SCOTT, J. A.: J. Parasit. *20:* 145 (1933).

SCOTT, J. A.: Amer. J. Hyg. *25:* 566 (1937a).

SCOTT, J. A.: J. trop. Med. Hyg. *40:* 125 (1937b).

SILVA, M. PIRAJA DA: J. trop. Med. Hyg. *12:* 159 (1909).

SOTO, V. R.: Naturaleza de la disenteria en Caracas; Tesis de doctorado No. 63 (1906).

SYMMERS, W. ST. C.: J. Path. Bact. *9:* 237 (1903).

TAKEGAMI, K.: Taiwan Igakkai Zasshi (J. Formosa med. Ass.) *137:* 183–201 (1914) (in Japanese).

TUBANGUI, M. A.: Philipp. J. Sci. *49:* 295 (1932).

VIC DUPONT; BERNARD, E.; SOUBRANE, J.; HALLÉ, B., and RICHIR, C.: Bull. Soc. méd. Hôp., Paris *73:* 933 (1957).

WHO: Expert Committee on Bilharziasis, San Juan, Puerto Rico, 1952. First report. Wld Hlth Org. techn. Rep. Ser. *65* (1953).

WHO: Bilharzia Snail Vector Identification and Classification (Equatorial and South Africa). Report of a study group, Paris 1954. Wld Hlth Org. techn. Rep. Ser. *90* (1954).

WHO: Study Group on the Ecology of Intermediate Snail Hosts of Bilharziasis, Paris 1956. Report. Wld Hlth Org. techn. Rep. Ser. *120* (1957a).

WHO: African Conference on Bilharziasis, Brazzaville 1956. Report. Wld Hlth Org. techn. Rep. Ser. *139* (1957b).

WHO/CCTA: Second African Conference on Bilharziasis, Lourenço Marques, Mozambique, 1960. Report. Wld Hlth Org. techn. Rep. Ser. *204* (1960).

WHO: Molluscicides. Second Report of the Expert Committee on Bilharziasis, Geneva 1960. Wld Hlth Org. techn. Rep. Ser. *214* (1961).

WHO: WHO Expert Committee on Bilharziasis, Geneva 1964. Third report. Wld Hlth Org. techn. Rep. Ser. *299* (1965).

WHO: Chemotherapy of Bilharziasis. Report of a WHO Scientific Group, Geneva 1964. Wld Hlth Org. techn. Rep. Ser. *317* (1966).

WHO: Measurement of the Public Health Importance of Bilharziasis. Report of a WHO Scientific Group, Geneva 1965. Wld Hlth Org. techn. Rep. Ser. *349* (1967a).

WHO: Epidemiology and Control of Schistosomiasis. Report of a WHO Expert Committee, Geneva 1966. Wld Hlth Org. techn. Rep. Ser. *372* (1967b).

WOOLLEY, P. G.: Philipp. J. Sci. *1:* 83–90 (1906).

WRIGHT, C. A.: Trans. roy. Soc. trop. Med. Hyg. *55:* 225 (1961).

WRIGHT, W. H.; DOBROVOLNY, C. G., and BERRY, E. G.: Bull. Wld Hlth Org. *18:* 963 (1958).

WRIGHT, W. H.; McMULLEN, D. B.; FAUST, E. C., and BAUMAN, P. M.: J. Parasit. *32:* suppl., vol. 12 (1946).

YAMAGIWA, K.: Tokyo Igakkai Zasshi (Z. Tokio-med. Ges.) *4:* 21 (1890). (in Japanese).

YOKOGAWA, S.: Tokyo Iji Shinshi (Tokyo med. J.) *1918:* 9 (1915) (in Japanese).

Chapter 2

Epidemiology and Control of Schistosomiasis, pp. 17–31
(Karger, Basel and University Park Press, Baltimore 1973)

Important Features of the Schistosomes[1]

M. A. STIREWALT

Introduction

With the accumulation of information resulting from extensive bio-medical studies of the schistosomes in the past two decades, it is obvious that these parasites comprise a group of trematodes with diverse biological characteristics and features. Although basic morphology and taxonomic considerations are of great importance in certain aspects of biology of the schistosomes, the present manual is concerned primarily with the relationship of the parasites to public health. In the following account, emphasis will be given to different aspects of the life cycle with notes on the eggs, miracidia, cercariae, schistosomules and adults. Although the schistosomes belong to the trematoda, they are not typical flukes in all respects. They do, however, possess the following characteristics of digenetic trematodes:

(1) They develop in a complicated life cycle through a succession of stages; egg, miracidium, first generation sporocyst, second generation sporocyst, cercaria, schistosomule, adult. Neither redial nor metacercarial stages are known.

(2) An alternation of generations occurs in which there are a sexual generation parasitic in definitive vertebrate hosts including man, a short-lived free-swimming stage infective for molluscs, an asexual generation parasitic in molluscs, and a short-lived free-swimming stage infective for vertebrate hosts.

(3) Adult schistosomes have a basic bilateral symmetry; suckers; a

---

1   The opinions and assertions contained herein are those of the author and are not to be construed as official or reflecting the views of the Navy Department or the Naval service at large.

body covering which is a syncytial integument with sunken cytons; a blind alimentary system consisting of mouth, oesophagus and bifurcated caeca; the area between the integument and alimentary canal filled with a loose cellular network; musculature of circular, oblique, longitudinal and special fibres; and an excretory or water-balance system based on flame cells [DAWES, 1946; FAUST and RUSSELL, 1964; YAMAGUTI, 1958].

Schistosomes are atypical digenetic trematodes in that the sexes are separate; the adults are not leaf-shaped but worm-like; the female is not dorsoventrally flattened; a muscular pharynx is absent; eggs are not operculated but are characterized by the presence of a spine or knob and are passed from man with a fully developed miracidium.

For convenience in discussing the epidemiological and control aspects associated with schistosome infections, the parasites have been grouped into three large categories:

(a) The species causing human schistosomiasis include: *Schistosoma haematobium, S. japonicum, S. mansoni, S. intercalatum, S. mattheei, S. margrebowiei, S. rodhaini* and *S. bovis.* Of these, only three *(S. haematobium, S. japonicum* and *S. mansoni)* are of major public health significance but *S. intercalatum* is of concern in a few foci in Africa.

(b) Schistosomes causing cercarial dermatitis and non-patent infections in subhuman primates without the development of adult parasites include: *S. spindale, Schistosomatium douthitti* and *Heterobilharzia americana.*

It should be noted that some of the species listed in (a) and (c) are also responsible for cercarial dermatitis.

(c) Schistosomes of veterinary significance and possibly of concern in meat production include species such as *S. nasalis, S. indicum, S. spindale* and *Orientobilharzia turkestanicum.* Spurious infections may be reported as a result of consumption of animals infected with the above-named species, and can lead to serious confusion when found in faecal samples of man in some areas.

It is important to note that the eggs of the schistosomes of some of the lower vertebrates may be confused with the schistosomes of man. Examples are *S. margrebowiei* eggs resembling those of *S. japonicum* and *Orientobilharzia harinasutai* eggs which could be mistaken for those of *S. mansoni.*

Human exposure to animal schistosomes may possibly influence the severity of natural infections by the more pathogenic species, by a process of non-specific resistance. In some endemic areas of Africa there are far more cercariae of the schistosomes of cattle and wild antelope in natural waters than there are cercariae of *S. mansoni* and *S. haematobium.* Man is continually exposed to infection with these schistosomes. Laboratory studies have shown that previous infections with heterologous strains or species can confer some degree of immunity against species or strains of schistosomes which are more pathogenic. Recent laboratory studies in England and the USA indicate that *S. bovis* and *S. mattheei* can confer some degree of protection against challenging infections with *S. mansoni* and *S. haematobium* in rhesus monkeys.

Eggs

Schistosome eggs are important as pathogenic agents and as diagnostic stages of infection. They are laid in an immature condition as the paired worms push as far as possible into small venules of the intestinal or bladder

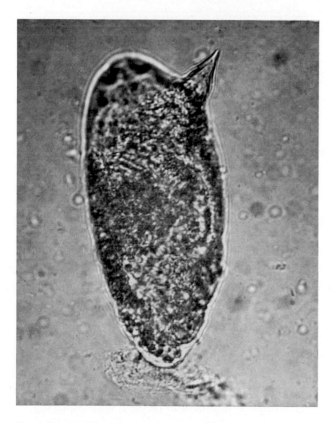

Fig. 1. Egg of *Schistosoma mansoni.* × 450.

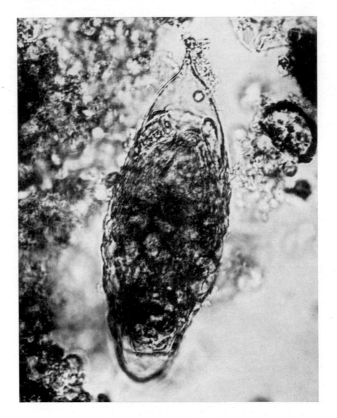

Fig. 2. Egg of *Schistosoma haematobium.* × 605.

wall and the females stretch out of the gynaecophoral canal of the male to extend the body sufficiently to free the genital pore.

Eggs are produced and laid singly by *S.mansoni* and in groups by *S.haematobium* and *S.japonicum*. They are oval or fusiform, golden-brown, non-operculated and possess terminal or lateral spines or rudiments of spines (Fig. 1, 2 and 3). Those of *S.mansoni* measure about 114 to 175 μm by 45 to 68 μm, are elongate-ovoid in shape and have a broad-based lateral spine. *S.haematobium* eggs are a little smaller and more spindle-shaped with a terminal spine; they measure about 112 to 170 μm by 40 to 70 μm. The smallest eggs are those of *S.japonicum*, 70 to 100 μm by 50 to 65 μm; they are ovoid and their spine, when visible, is a rudimentary knob often within a depression [FAUST and MELENEY, 1924; FAUST *et al.*, 1934; YAMAGUTI, 1958].

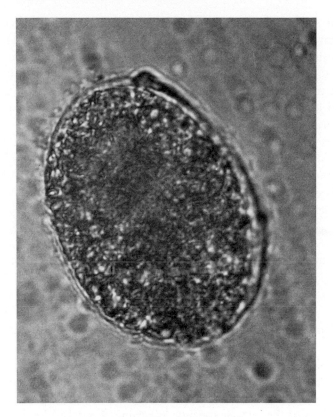

Fig. 3. Egg of *Schistosoma japonicum.* × 900.

The eggs retained in host tissues are surrounded by host cells either in the intestinal or bladder wall, liver or, more rarely, in the spleen or almost any other tissue to which they may be swept by the flow of venous blood; the miracidia within them generally die within three weeks or less and the eggs become dark and finally calcified. Eggs destined to play a part in the life cycle of the parasite usually contain completely developed miracidia within several days of their deposition, so that by the time they are passed from the host motile miracidia are visible within them. Under suitable environmental conditions and dilution of faeces or urine with fresh water, miracidia move rapidly in the egg and finally break through the egg shell, shed the embryonic membranes and begin to swim.

For epidemiological evaluation and for the diagnosis of infection, attention must be given to the characteristic outline of the eggs of parasites in the different schistosome complexes. Experiences by various investigators in certain parts of Africa have emphasized the unusual problems associated with the recognition of terminally-spined schistosome eggs. In this respect PITCHFORD [1965] has recently suggested a method of measurement to facilitate differentiation of eggs of *S. bovis*, *S. haematobium* and *S. mattheei* and he has recommended that the measurement of the width of eggs be taken at a point 40 μm from the tip of the spine.

Attention is drawn to the fact that staining techniques may be employed for the differentiation of eggs of the *S. mansoni* group from those of the *S. haematobium* complex [BRYGOO and RANDRIAMALALA, 1959]. This method is particularly useful in histopathology.

Epidemiologically there has been concern regarding the viability of schistosome eggs in excreta. Under certain circumstances longevity in viability of eggs could be an important factor in maintenance of the parasite cycle. Further information is needed to determine the survival time of schistosome eggs under natural conditions.

Miracidia and Snail Stages

Miracidia of the human schistosomes [FAUST and HOFFMAN, 1934; OTTOLINA, 1957; FAUST and RUSSELL, 1964; PAN, 1965] are similar in behaviour and morphology, but they differ slightly in size. Those of *S. mansoni* are the largest of the human species, averaging about 160 by 62 μm after fixation.

The shape of a miracidium varies greatly with the environment and activity of the organism. In swimming miracidia, it is conico-cylindrical, but at other times it may be almost ovoid. The body may be tapered at either end or at both ends simultaneously. Usually the oral end comes to a point in the constantly-moving spiny terebratorium (fig. 4).

Miracidial bodies are covered with cilia which are essentially equal in length except for those in the vicinity of the papillae. Cilia are borne in epidermal plates arranged in four tiers. With these, miracidia swim rapidly in straight lines. When deflected, they back away, turn, and set out on a new straight-line course. Longevity has been reported to be as brief as 6 h or as long as 72 h.

In transverse section, layers of the body consist of epidermal plates bearing cilia, a subepithelium interrupted by the alimentary and excretory openings and those of the ducts of the gland cells, circular and longitudinal

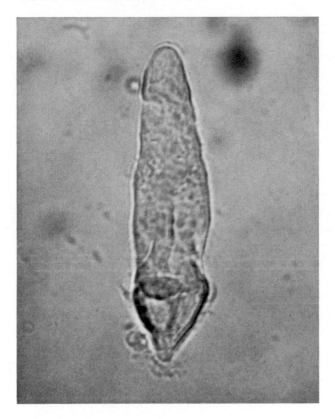

Fig. 4. Miracidium of *Schistosoma mansoni.* × 450.

muscle layers, and a network of undifferentiated somatic cells within which lie the internal organs.

Alimentary organs are the mouth within the terebratorium and a sac described sometimes as solid, non-functional and possessing four nuclei, sometimes as bilobed with granular contents. On each side of the alimentary sac is a large unicellular periodic acid-Schiff staining gland, often called a cephalic penetration gland. Each opens anterolaterally by a duct at the base of the terebratorium. Medially and aborally are the neural cell cluster and a group of cells which have been said to secrete mucus through laterally-opening ducts. Lateral in position are four flame cells, the collecting tubules and aboral ampullae and pores of the excretory system. Finally, germinal cells are present, arranged, according to some reports, in an aborally positioned cell cluster; according to others, in cords near the miracidial body wall.

Miracidia are equipped specifically to find and infect snail hosts. They are chemo-sensitive, presumably attracted to certain snails, and able to penetrate their soft tissues quickly [MACINNIS, 1965]. Whether penetration is by muscular effort alone or with the aid of lytic secretions is not known. After penetration, the ciliated coat disappears, the muscles degenerate and, within a few days, the larva reorganizes into a first generation sporocyst, usually in the immediate vicinity of its penetration site.

First generation sporocysts [FAUST and MELENEY, 1924; OTTOLINA, 1957; PAN, 1965] are essentially non-motile, opaque, elongated, convoluted sacs, several hundred μm in length [OLIVIER and MAO, 1949], with germinal cells arranged in layers along the sporocyst wall. The central cavity of the sporocyst, divided into chambers by the convolutions of the organism, contains the germ balls of second generation sporocysts. The latter are present from about two to six weeks post penetration, after which only degenerating organisms are found in first generation sporocysts.

Second generation sporocysts are opaque, elongated, worm-like, motile sacs with a snout-like spine-covered anterior end. They may become larger than the parent sporocyst and, unlike it, migrate to mature usually in the snail liver or ovotestis. Cercarial germ balls are recognizable in the central cavity of sporocysts over 15 days old, and continue to be produced for the duration of the infection. This is often for the life of the snail and may be more than a year.

Cercariae which emerge from the sporocysts migrate through the snail tissues and accumulate in sinuses and dilated veins. From as early as 20 days post infection, often for the life of the snail, cercariae migrate from the sinuses to the epithelial layer at the mantle collar. Time required for development of stages of the parasites in the snails varies with the environmental temperature, being shorter at temperatures of 26 to 28° C and longer as the temperature decreases. Cercariae emerge daily, generally in large but variable numbers. Main emergence of cercariae of *S. mansoni* and *S. haematobium* is between 9.30 a. m. and 2.00 p. m. and of *S. japonicum* between 10.30 p. m. and 2.00 a. m.

The reaction of snails to infection depends on the species and strain of schistosome and host. Some infected snails suffer pathological changes [OTTOLINA, 1957; PAN, 1965] which include oedema, congestion of blood vessels, tissue degeneration especially of the liver and ovotestis, loss of pigmentation, formation of granulomata, shell erosion and thinning, loss of sand grains in the gizzard, and gradual inhibition of reproduction. Tissue responses may be both focal and generalized.

Studies on the survival of infected snails are referred to in the paper by HAIRSTON (pp. 290 to 293 and 309 to 310).

Cercariae

Cercariae, like miracidia, are morphologically and physiologically adapted for the special purpose of host invasion, and must accomplish this within a matter of hours. To this end, locomotion may be by swimming, in which case the tail pulls the body along, or by a looping, inchworm movement along surfaces.

The behaviour patterns of cercariae of different species are distinctive. *S. mansoni* and *S. haematobium* tend to distribute themselves more freely in the water than *S. japonicum*, which tends to hang at the surface. Since the cercariae of *S. japonicum* tend to stick to glassware, special techniques must be employed for handling.

Cercariae of the three human species are similar in appearance (fig. 5). They are furcocercous, lack eyespots and a pharynx, and are somewhat less than 1 mm long. The ratio of length to diameter changes with activity. Cercarial shape is that of a spindle with an obvious constriction separating the body and the bifurcated tail. Oral and ventral suckers are present, the heavily-muscular oral sucker occupying about one third of the body and being eversible. The ventral sucker, protruding from the body wall about one half the distance from the aboral end, is smaller.

A mucous film over a tegument with scattered minute spines and hairs, considered to be sensory in function, covers the cercaria. Below are a layer of circular and a layer of longitudinal muscles. Special muscle fibres are numerous.

Internal organs are embedded in a loose mesenchymatous tissue most evident along the body wall and between the acetabular glands and oral sucker. A subterminal mouth, an oesophagus which leads through the oral sucker, and a small bisacculate dorsally-placed gut make up the alimentary system. Dorsal to the oesophagus is a neuropile, a mass of nerve fibres from which anterior and posterior nerve trunks extend. Flame cells, collecting tubules and a posterior excretory bladder and pore constitute the excretory or water-balance system in the body. Four pairs of flame cells are present in the body in cercariae of *S. mansoni* [VOGEL, 1932] and of *S. haemato-*

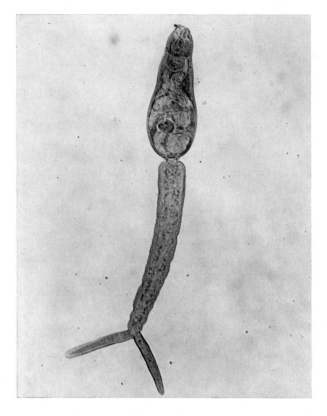

Fig. 5. Cercaria of *Schistosoma mansoni.* × 90.

bium [GORDON *et al.,* 1934], whereas there are three pairs in *S. japonicum* [CORT, 1919]. One pair of flame cells with collecting tubules is present in the tail. These caudal tubules empty at the tips of the furci.

Dominating the internal organs are the large unicellular glands whose processes serve as ducts [GORDON *et al.,* 1934; STIREWALT and KRUIDENIER, 1961]. Two pairs are pre-acetabular and three or four pairs, post-acetabular. These glands occupy the posterior two thirds of the body. Their contents are emptied through ducts which open at the anterior rim of the oral sucker. These ducts, in two lateral bundles, lead circuitously from the glands with a great dorsal arch to pierce the oral sucker laterally and end in protrusible duct tips. The arches provide for adaptation of the ducts to elongation and contraction of the body. A sixth pair of unicellular glands called escape glands and situated in the anterior portion of the body can be seen only in un-emerged cercariae. A 'head gland' lies within the oral sucker.

The post-acetabular glands are the smaller of the two types. They contain finely granular, periodic acid-Schiff staining contents, minute quantities of which are secreted at each attachment of the oral sucker. These deposits swell in water to provide a sticky mucus for attachment first of the oral and then of the ventral sucker, as the cercariae loop over surfaces and begin to penetrate. This material may also serve to protect the cercariae and direct and conserve secreted enzymes [STIREWALT, 1959; STIREWALT and KRUIDENIER, 1961].

The pre-acetabular glands contain alkaline, macrogranular, alizarin-staining material. Calcium has been demonstrated in them histochemically. Very small quantities of secretion from the pre-acetabular glands are demonstrable in some mucus deposits, but most of it is emitted only when the oral end of a penetrating cercaria has reached the keratogenous zone immediately below the horny layer of the skin. It permeates the skin and appears to aid in penetration and migration by softening the keratin of the host's horny layer by its alkalinity, and by altering the acellular cement and ground substances of epidermis and dermis [LEWERT and LEE, 1954; STIREWALT, 1966].

At present, apart from the number of flame cells, there are no reliable methods for distinguishing the cercariae of the different schistosomes infecting man, but morphological studies and staining techniques have shown some promise [FAINet al., 1953; VERCAMMEN-GRANJEAN, 1951].

Schistosomules

Post-penctration larvae or schistosomules differ in several ways from cercariae [STIREWALT, 1963]. As opposed to the latter, they are usually tailless, have lost a precise shape and assumed a worm-like appearance, and their acetabular glands are empty. They have become adapted to saline and serum, but are unable to live in water even for a brief time. They can no longer form pericercarial sero-envelopes in antiserum.

Those destined for successful host infection enter peripheral venous or lymphatic vessels within one to several days, reach the lungs by way of the right heart and, from them, the portal system. From skin to lungs there is little question that migration is by way of the blood vessels. From lungs to the portal circulation there is less certainty that the route must be circulatory. An increasing body of information suggests that some young schistosomes may follow a direct path through the tissues to the portal vein. In the latter, or its hepatic branches, development proceeds rapidly and by five or six weeks the schistosomes are mature and egg-laying begins.

Adult Schistosomes

Adult schistosomes [FAUST and MELENEY, 1924; FAUST *et al.*, 1934; YAMAGUTI, 1958] are dioecious though hermaphroditism has occasionally been reported (fig. 6). Female worms are held within the gynaecophoral canal of males. Both sexes of worms have oral and ventral suckers, the former terminal and usually larger, the latter subterminal. Body openings

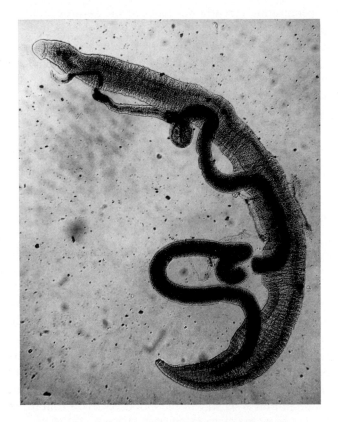

Fig. 6. Paired adult *Schistosoma japonicum.* × 22.5.

are a mouth surrounded by the oral sucker, a postero dorsal excretory pore and a gonopore slightly posterior to the ventral sucker. The integument bears spines, tubercles or hairs, or all three.

As seen in transverse section, the body consists of the integument, circular, longitudinal and special muscles, and a network of mesenchymal cells surrounding the internal organs.

The alimentary system is a simple one composed of mouth, short oesophagus with a circle of gland cells, and an intestine which lacks lateral diverticula but bifurcates at the level of the ventral sucker and unites again posterior to the testes or ovary to form a single blind tube. Flame cells, collecting tubules and an excretory bladder with a terminal pore make up the excretory or water-balance system.

Male human schistosomes have a short, cylindrical pre-acetabular portion of the body and a wide, flattened post-acetabular portion with the edges inrolled ventrally to form a gynaecophoral canal. They possess fewer than 10 testes in one or two rows beginning at the anterior end of the gynaecophoral canal. The seminal vesicle is pre-testicular; a gonopore lies immediately post-acetabular. There is no cirrus pouch.

The female body is filiform, essentially round in transverse section, and longer than that of the male. The single ovary is median, elongate, and usually about the level of the transverse midbody line. A seminal receptacle lies at its posterior end. There is one pair of lateral vitellaria. An oviduct and a pair of vitelline ducts open anteriorly into the oötype, from which the uterus leads to the gonopore just behind the acetabulum. There is no Laurer's canal.

It has been estimated that each female *S. mansoni* produces 100 to 300 eggs/female/day, whereas in *S. japonicum* there may be 1,400 to 3,500 eggs/female/day. As yet, there have been no reliable estimations of the egg output for *S. haematobium*.

Specific characteristics of the schistosomes, in addition to geographical distribution, include the habitat of choice in the human host, size, integumentary tuberculation, number of testes, shape and position of several organs, and the number of well-developed eggs in the uterus (table I) [YAMAGUTI, 1958; FAUST and RUSSELL, 1964]. Since *S. japonicum* is found most frequently in the portal, superior and inferior mesenteric veins, eggs are passed in faeces. *S. haematobium* may be encountered in these veins but occurs in the greatest numbers in the vesicle and pelvic plexuses, so eggs are more common in urine. However, rectal biopsies invariably show the presence of *S. haematobium* eggs in heavy infections. Since *S. mansoni*

Table I. Differential characteristics of the schistosomes of man

	S. haematobium	S. japonicum	S. mansoni
Male			
Length, mm	10–14	12–20	6–12
Number of testes	4	7	6–9
Posterior union of intestinal caeca	about midbody	caudad to midbody	cephalad to midbody
Cuticle	finely tuberculate	non-tuberculate	grossly tuberculate
Female			
Length, mm	16–20	16–28	7–17
Number of eggs in uterus	20–100	50 or more	usually 1
Position of ovary	caudad to midbody	about midbody	cephalad to midbody

frequents the veins draining the small and large intestines near the ileo-caecal junction, eggs occur in faeces. Unmated females, however, are often in the haemorrhoidal veins, and unmated males in hepatic veins.

Recent studies have indicated that the pathological patterns in *S. mansoni* infections are closely associated with the number of parasites present and their distribution in the host. The latter is especially applicable in *S. haematobium* infections.

Strain Differences in Schistosomes

One of the recent developments in schistosomiasis is the recognition of variations in the biological characteristics and potentials of schistosomes of the same species endemic in different geographical areas. These differences are manifest in the infection in the intermediate as well as in the definitive hosts. An example of geographical variations is found in the case of *S. japonicum* in Taiwan when compared with the parasite of the same species in Japan and the Philippines [KUNTZ, 1955]. The Taiwan *S. japonicum,* a zoophilic strain, is capable of infecting a wide range of lower mammals but is unable to infect man [HSÜ and HSÜ, 1956]. Comparative studies with *S. mansoni* [SAOUD, 1965] from different areas have shown that there are races differing in their morphology as well as in their infectivity and pathogenicity in the definitive hosts. Differences have also been detected in the *S. haematobium* complex and it has been suggested that these differences justify the separation of the two extreme forms under specific status, i.e. the South African form being known as *S. capense* to distinguish it from the type recognized in Egypt. This separation, however, is not yet justified in the light of new knowledge on the range of variability of the individual species. These intraspecific variations have obvious epidemiological significance.

References

BRYGOO, E. R. and RANDRIAMALALA, J. C.: Bull. Soc. Path. exot. *52:* 26 (1959).

CORT, W. W.: Univ. Calif. Publ. Zool. *18:* 485 (1919).

DAWES, B.: The Trematoda (Cambridge University Press, Cambridge 1946).

FAIN, A.; THIENPONT, D.; HERIN, U., and DERAMÉE, O.: Ann. Soc. belge Méd. trop. *33:* 423 (1953).

FAUST, E. C. and HOFFMAN, W. A.: Puerto Rico J. publ. Hlth *10:* 1 (1934).

FAUST, E. C. and MELENEY, H. E.: Studies on schistosomiasis japonica. Amer. J. Hyg., Monogr. Ser. *3:* 1–268 (1924).

FAUST, E. C. and RUSSELL, P. F.: in CRAIG and FAUST Clinical parasitology (Lea & Febiger, Philadelphia 1964).

FAUST, E. C.; JONES, C. A., and HOFFMAN, W. A.: Puerto Rico J. publ. Hlth *10:* 133 (1934).

GORDON, R. M.; DAVEY, T. H., and PEASTON, H.: Ann. trop. Med. Parasit. *28:* 323 (1934).

HSÜ, H. F. and HSÜ, S. Y. L.: Amer. J. trop. Med. Hyg. *5:* 521 (1956).

KUNTZ, R. E.: Amer. J. trop. Med. Hyg. *4:* 383 (1955).

LEWERT, R. M. and LEE, C. L.: J. infect. Dis. *95:* 13 (1954).

MacINNIS, A. J.: J. Parasit. *51:* 731 (1965).

OLIVIER, L. and MAO, C. P.: J. Parasit. *35:* 267 (1949).

OTTOLINA, C.: Rev. Sanid. Asist. soc. *22:* 1 (1957).

PAN, C. T.: Amer. J. trop. Med. Hyg. *14:* 931 (1965).

PITCHFORD, R. J.: Bull. Wld Hlth Org. *32:* 105 (1965).

SAOUD, M. F. A.: J. Helminth. *39:* 101 (1965).

STIREWALT, M. A.: Exp. Parasit. *8:* 199 (1959).

STIREWALT, M. A.: Exp. Parasit. *13:* 395 (1963).

STIREWALT, M. A.: Skin penetration mechanisms of helminths; in SOULSBY Biology of parasites, p. 41 (Academic Press, New York/London 1966).

STIREWALT, M. A. and KRUIDENIER, F. J.: Exp. Parasit. *11:* 191 (1961).

VERCAMMEN-GRANJEAN, P. H.: Ann. Parasit. hum. comp. *26:* 412 (1951).

VOGEL, H.: Arch. Schiff. Tropenhyg. *36:* 108 (1932).

YAMAGUTI, S.: Systema helminthum. I. The digenetic trematodes of vertebrates (Interscience, New York 1958).

Chapter 3

Epidemiology and Control of Schistosomiasis, pp. 32–249
(Karger, Basel and University Park Press, Baltimore 1973)

Geographical Distribution of Schistosomes and their Intermediate Hosts

W. H. WRIGHT

with the collaboration of N. AYAD, J. FRAGA DE AZEVEDO, F. S. BARBOSA, V. DE V. CLARKE, M. FAROOQ, J. H. S. GEAR, J. GILLET, H. F. HSÜ, P. JORDAN, Y. KOMIYA, F. S. MCCULLOUGH, G. S. NELSON, W. L. PARAENSE, R. J. PITCHFORD and G. WEBBE

Introduction

This chapter provides information on the geographical distribution of the human schistosomes and their intermediate hosts, area by area and country by country. There are many limitations in the current data and undoubtedly there are endemic foci of schistosomiasis which remain undiscovered; this is especially true for isolated areas which lack health facilities. Only in recent years has an intensive effort been made to secure more information on the distribution of the parasites and to arrive at a better understanding of the medical, economic and public health importance of the disease.

Knowledge concerning the molluscs involved in the transmission of schistosomiasis is rather more restricted than information concerning distribution of the disease. However, great progress has been made towards better definition of those snails serving as intermediate hosts and in bringing some order into their classification.

Data concerning the prevalence of infection in some areas are also given. Few intensive surveys of countries have been conducted to secure such data and for this reason, it is not possible to provide specific figures on a countrywide basis. Even in a limited area prevalence rates vary considerably from place to place in relation to the transmission pattern and the extent of exposure of the human population.

General Distribution of the Human Schistosomes

Schistosoma haematobium, S. mansoni and *S. japonicum,* the three major species of schistosomes which infect man, are widely distributed: *S. haematobium* occurs in Africa and South-West Asia, and a small focus is present in India; *S. mansoni* is distributed in parts of Africa, South-West Asia and the western hemisphere; and *S. japonicum* is an oriental species. In addition, *S. intercalatum* has been reported from localized foci in Central and West Africa; and *S. bovis* and *S. mattheei,* lower mammal schistosomes, have been reported in man in parts of Africa, with the latter species reaching a prevalence of 40% in some parts of the Transvaal.

S. haematobium and *S. mansoni* are widely distributed in Africa. In North Africa, the former is found in Morocco, Algeria, Tunisia, Libya and Egypt. *S. mansoni* is also endemic in Egypt and one focus occurs in Libya. *S. haematobium* occurs in Mauritius. Both species are found in almost all other African countries, although *S. haematobium* is more widely distributed.

In South-West Asia, *S. mansoni* occurs in Israel, Yemen, Southern Yemen and Saudi Arabia, while *S. haematobium* has been reported from Southern Yemen, Saudi Arabia, Yemen, Israel, Lebanon, Syria, Turkey, Iraq and Iran. The focus of schistosomiasis in Maharashtra State in India, apparently due to *S. haematobium,* represents the only occurrence of this species in South-Central and South-East Asia, although it is possible that other foci may yet be found.

In the western hemisphere, *S. mansoni* is endemic in the Dominican Republic, Puerto Rico, Vieques, French St Martin, Antigua, Guadeloupe, Martinique and St Lucia. In Venezuela, the species is distributed in the States of Aragua, Carabobo, Miranda, Maracay and the Federal District. It is found in Surinam and occurs in Brazil in the States of Pará, Maranhão, Piauí, Ceará, Rio Grande do Norte, Paraíba, Pernambuco, Alagoãs, Sergipe, Bahia, Minas Gerais, Espirito Santo, Rio de Janeiro, Guanabara, São Paulo and Paraná.

In South-East Asia, *S. japonicum* has recently been discovered in Thailand, Laos and Cambodia. There is a focus of long standing in the Celebes. In the Philippines, this species occurs in the islands of Luzon, Leyte, Samar, Mindoro, Mindanao and Bohol. *S. japonicum* is found in mammals in Taiwan (Formosa), but human cases have not been discovered. In Japan, the parasite occurs on the main island of Honshu and on the island of Kyushu.

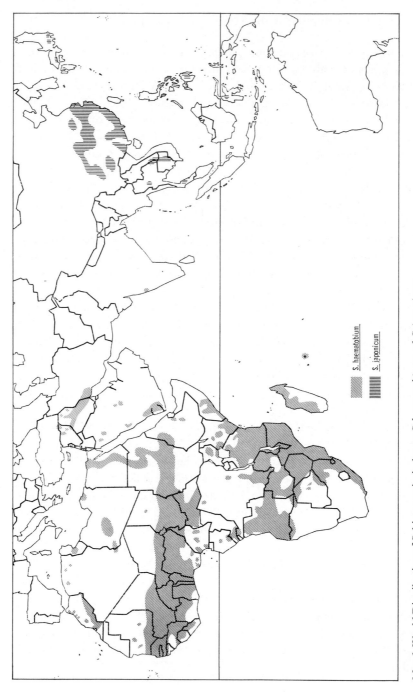

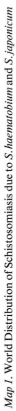

Map 1. World Distribution of Schistosomiasis due to *S. haematobium* and *S. japonicum*

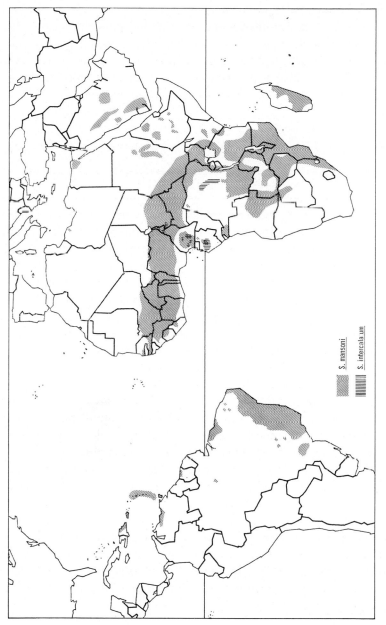
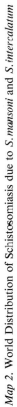

Map 2. World Distribution of Schistosomiasis due to *S. mansoni* and *S. intercalatum*

In China (Mainland), *S. japonicum* is endemic in the Provinces of Kiangsu, Chekiang, Hupeh, Hunan, Kiangsi, Anhwei, Kwangtung, Fukien, Szechwan and Yunnan. It is also present in the Municipality of Shanghai and the autonomous region of Kwangsi.

With this extensive distribution, it is highly probable that the disease may occur in additional localities, especially in isolated areas not yet supplied with health facilities. Extension of the disease to free areas is possible in certain instances, since some molluscan intermediate hosts are known to occur outside the presently recognized endemic areas.

Identity and Geographical Distribution of the Intermediate Hosts

Until very recently, there was considerable disagreement about the identification and nomenclature of certain molluscs involved in the transmission of schistosomiasis. This confusion had adversely affected efforts to arrive at a better understanding of the epidemiology of the disease and to promote more effective control measures. The establishment by WHO of a central laboratory of malacology in Copenhagen was a major step in helping to bring order out of the chaos surrounding snail identification. A similar facility for the western hemisphere has been located at Belo Horizonte, Brazil[1]. A working group, under the aegis of the Pan American Health Organization/WHO Regional Office for the Americas, has prepared an introductory guide for the intermediate hosts of schistosomiasis in that part of the world. The recommendations of these agencies are being followed in this publication.

In spite of these salutary developments, more knowledge is required concerning the identification and distribution of the molluscan intermediate hosts. Some African species show certain anatomical variations, and further study may indicate the advisability of separating them into subspecies or varieties. In the Americas, a species complex or group is recognized and continued study of more material is needed to evaluate properly the anatomical design of the forms involved.

Another factor of importance in the epidemiology of the disease is the varying susceptibility of known host species to schistosome strains. Certain strains of known molluscan hosts have been shown to be almost completely resistant to infection with some strains of schistosomes. A more detailed discussion of this phenomenon follows later in this chapter.

1   Now in Brasilia, Brazil.

Table I. Molluscan intermediate hosts

S. mansoni in the Americas	
Biomphalaria glabrata (syn. *Australorbis glabratus*)	Dominican Republic, Puerto Rico, Vieques, French St Martin, Antigua, Guadeloupe, Martinique, St Lucia, Venezuela, Surinam, Brazil
B. tenagophila (syn. *Australorbis tenagophilus, A. nigricans*)	Brazil
B. straminea (syn. *Tropicorbis stramineus, T. centimetralis*)	Brazil
S. mansoni in Africa	
Biomphalaria pfeifferi	Africa south of the Sahara, Madagascar
B. choanomphala	Lake Victoria
B. smithi	Lake Edward
B. stanleyi	Lake Albert
B. alexandrina	Egypt
B. angulosa	Tanzania, Zambia, Republic of South Africa
B. camerunensis	Cameroon, Nigeria
B. sudanica	Sudan, Uganda, Kenya, Tanzania, Central African Republic, Ghana, Zaire
S. haematobium in Africa	
Bulinus (Physopsis) africanus	Cameroon, Ethiopia?, Kenya, Tanzania, Mozambique, Zambia, Rhodesia, Republic of South Africa
B. (Ph.) globosus	Africa south of the Sahara
B. (Ph.) nasutus	Uganda, Kenya, Tanzania
B. (Ph.) abyssinicus	Ethiopia, Somalia
B. (Ph.) jousseaumei	Gambia, Senegal, Portuguese Guinea, Chad
Bulinus (Bulinus) truncatus	Morocco, Algeria, Tunisia, Egypt, Sudan, Ethiopia, Mauritania, Mali, Chad, Ghana, Nigeria, Cameroon, Zaire
B. (B.) guernei	Gambia, Senegal
B. (B.) coulboisi	Burundi?
B. (B.) cernicus	Mauritius
B. (B.) forskalii	Nigeria?
B. (B.) obtusispirus	Madagascar
B. (B.) camerunensis	Cameroon
B. (B.) senegalensis	Gambia, Senegal
Planorbarius metidjensis	Morocco
S. intercalatum in Africa[1]	
Bulinus (Ph.) globosus	Zaire
B. (Pyrgophysa) forskalii	Cameroon, Gabon

Table I (Continued)

S. haematobium in Europe	
Planorbarius metidjensis	Portugal
S. mansoni in South-West Asia	
Biomphalaria alexandrina	Israel (now no longer found)
B. pfeifferi	Yemen, Saudi Arabia, Southern Yemen
S. haematobium in South-West Asia	
Bulinus (B.) truncatus	Turkey, Lebanon, Syria, Israel, Iraq, Iran, Yemen, Saudi Arabia
B. (B.) reticulatus	Southern Yemen
B. (B.) beccarii	Southern Yemen
S. haematobium in South Central Asia	
Ferrissia tenuis	India
S. japonicum in the Orient	
Oncomelania nosophora	Japan
O. hupensis	China (Mainland)
O. formosana	China (Taiwan)
O. quadrasi	Philippines
?	Thailand, Laos, Cambodia

1 Under investigation for confirmation.

The molluscan intermediate hosts named herein (table I) include those species considered to be involved in the transmission of the disease on the basis of natural or experimental infection or epidemiological evidence. Some of the more important intermediate hosts are illustrated in figures 1, 2 and 3. Certain other snails outside known endemic areas have been shown experimentally to be susceptible to infection.

References to the most important published papers covering the subject matter of this chapter are given for most of the areas covered, and a considerable amount of unpublished material made available in the Parasitic Diseases Unit, World Health Organization, has been utilized in the preparation of the chapter.

References

ABBOTT, R. T.: Bull. Mus. comp. Zool., Harvard College *100:* 245 (1948).
MANDAHL-BARTH, G.: Bull. Wld Hlth Org. *16:* 1103; *17:* 1 (1957).
MANDAHL-BARTH, G.: Bull. Wld Hlth Org. *22:* 565 (1960).
Pan American Health Organization: A guide for the identification of the snail intermediate hosts of schistosomiasis in the Americas. Scientific Publication No. 168 (Washington 1968).

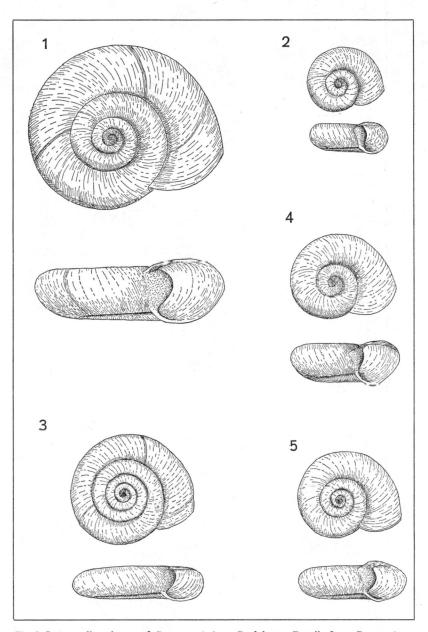

Fig. 1. Intermediate hosts of *S. mansoni.* 1 = *B. glabrata*, Brazil; 2 = *B. straminea*, Brazil; 3 = *B. sudanica*, Uganda; 4 = *B. pfeifferi*, Rhodesia; 5 = *B. alexandrina*, Egypt. × 2 natural size.

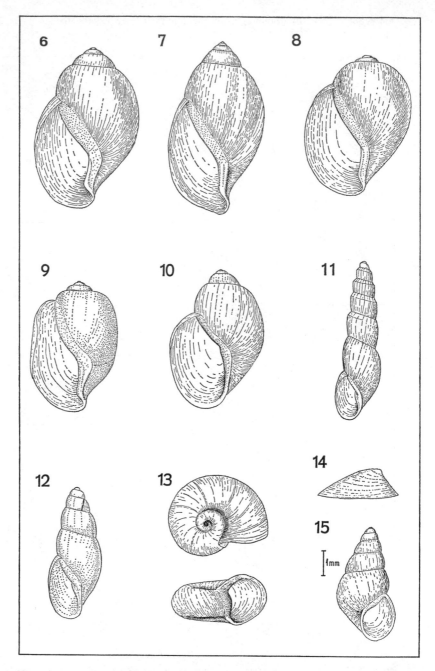

Fig. 2. Intermediate hosts of *S. haematobium* and *S. japonicum*. 6 = *B. (Ph.) africanus*, Kenya; 7 = *B. (Ph.) nasutus*, Tanzania; 8 = *B. (Ph.) globosus*, Angola; 9 = *B. (Ph.) abyssinicus*, Somalia; 10 = *B. (B.) truncatus*, Egypt; 11 = *B. (B.) forskalii*, Sudan; 12 = *B. (B.) senegalensis*, Gambia; 13 = *Planorbarius metidjensis*, Portugal; 14 = *Ferrissia tenuis*, India; 15 = *Oncomelania quadrasi*, Philippines. No. 6–10 and 13: × 2.5; No. 11 and 12: × 3; No. 14 and 15: × 6.5 natural size.

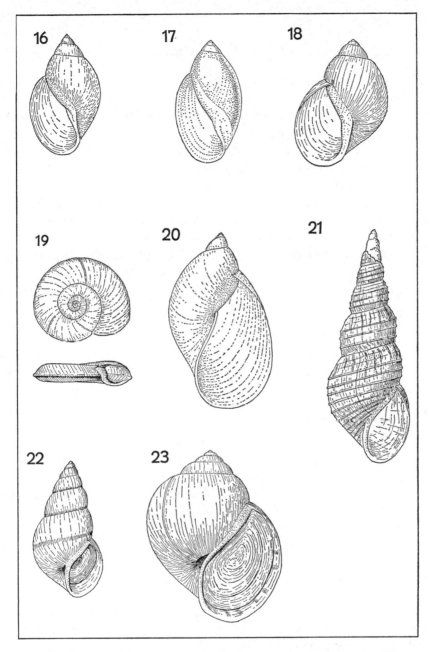

Fig. 3. Accompanying species. 16 = *Physa acuta*, Egypt; 17 = *Ph. waterloti*, Ghana; 18 = *Bulinus tropicus*, Rhodesia; 19 = *Planorbis planorbis*, Egypt; 20 = *Lymnaea natalensis*, Kenya; 21 = *Melanoides tuberculata*, Uganda; 22 = *Cleopatra bulimoides*, Egypt; 23 = *Pila ovata*, Uganda. No. 16–22: × 2.5 natural size; No. 23: natural size.

Schistosomes and Intermediate Hosts in Africa

Knowledge concerning the distribution of the human schistosomes in most African countries is far more limited than that available for the majority of other endemic areas of the world. This situation is due to a number of factors, among which are:

(1) the relative magnitude of the problem;
(2) the inaccessibility of many areas;
(3) the paucity of skilled workers; and
(4) the comparative limitation of health staffs and health facilities.

For these reasons, the information in the following summaries may be regarded as insufficient for many countries in providing a satisfactory analysis of the schistosomiasis problem. The sectional divisions employed here are purely arbitrary and for convenience only.

North Africa

S. haematobium is the predominant species in North Africa. *S. mansoni* is an important parasite in lower United Arab Republic (Egypt) but elsewhere in the region it has been reported only from Taurorga in Libya.

United Arab Republic
Distribution of Human Schistosomiasis

Relative to prevalence and gravity, schistosomiasis heads the list of endemic diseases in the UAR.

A survey in 1935 by SCOTT [1937] in which he examined about 40,000 persons from various villages in different localities showed an over-all prevalence rate of 48% *S. haematobium* infection in rural Egypt. *S. mansoni* infection was absent from upper Egypt south of Giza, with an over-all prevalence rate of 32% in the Nile Delta.

About 20 years later, another survey was carried out by the Egyptian Ministry of Public Health, using the same methods employed by SCOTT and in the same villages surveyed by him but, this time, involving 124,253 persons taken by random sampling. The over-all *S. haematobium* prevalence rate was found to be 38%, autochthonous *S. mansoni* cases were still absent from upper Egypt, and an over-all prevalence rate of only 9% existed in the Nile Delta. The results of this survey and their comparison with the findings of 1935 are given in table II. It is shown that:

Table II. Prevalence and distribution of human schistosomiasis in various parts of rural Egypt in 1935 and 1955, according to the 1935 and 1955 spot surveys

Province	S. haematobium 1935 (Scott)			S. haematobium 1955 (MPH)			S. mansoni 1935 (Scott)			S. mansoni 1955 (MPH)		
	number examined	number positive	%	number examined	number positive	%	number examined	number positive	%	number examined	number positive	%
Beheira	2,901	1,543	53	7,473	3,453	46		1,568	54		2,305	31
Gharbiya	3,095	1,608	52	12,058	6,131	51		1,196	39		2,032	17
Dakahliya	1,743	931	53	10,518	5,220	50		659	38		978	9
Sharkiya	2,102	1,384	66	6,571	3,437	52		575	27		322	5
Qualyubiya	3,057	1,879	61	14,554	4,478	31		791	26		435	3
Minufiya	1,162	737	63	11,709	5,297	45		44	4		85	1
Giza	1,148	617	54	8,095	2,726	34		7	1		273	3
Fayum	1,510	1,340	89	10,450	3,966	38		1	–		–	–
Beni-Suef	1,191	981	82	6,615	2,399	36		–	–		–	–
Minya	3,022	1,371	45	8,597	3,331	39		–	–		–	–
Assiut	2,546	548	22	9,670	1,537	16		–	–		–	–
Suhag	1,633	51	3	12,776	5,377	42		–	–		–	–
Qena	1,508	57	4	4,138	176	4		–	–		–	–
Aswan	676	91	13	1,029	239	23		–	–		–	–
Total	27,294	13,138	48	124,253	47,767	38	15,208	4,841	32	70,978	6,430	9

(1) the over-all prevalence rate of both types of human schistosomiasis fell in *S. haematobium* infection from 48 to 38%, and in *S. mansoni* infection from 32 to 9%;

(2) the improvement in the prevalence of *S. mansoni* was much greater than in *S. haematobium* and involved all provinces of lower Egypt, falling to about one quarter of its previous prevalence;

(3) the general prevalence of *S. haematobium* also fell, but to a lesser extent (21%). This was general in lower Egypt and in the areas of perennial irrigation in upper Egypt as far south as Assiut. In those areas it fell from 55 to 41%, i.e. a reduction of about 30%. South of Assiut, i.e. in the southern three provinces of Suhag, Qena and Aswan, the prevalence rose, particularly in Suhag province where it rose from 3% in 1935 to 42% in 1955. This is attributable to the change of basin or flood irrigation (only during the Nile flood) into perennial or all-year-round irrigation, leading to more availability of water for the snails and also more opportunity for the propagation of infection.

This important influence of systems of irrigation on the spread of human schistosomiasis can also be seen from a study of the prevalence of urinary schistosomiasis in different districts of the same governorate in these southern areas. This is shown in table III, the data being derived from the 1955 records of the endemic diseases hospitals of the Ministry of Public Health which are located in different districts of Assiut, Suhag and Qena governorates in relation to the methods of irrigation used. The table shows that the prevalence of urinary schistosomiasis in 1955 among persons visiting those hospitals in areas under perennial irrigation in these southern governorates was higher, varying from 56 to 69%, while in areas under basin irrigation in the same governorates in the same year it was much lower, varying from 9 to 17%, i.e. only one tenth to one fifth that of the former areas;

(4) the prevalence of schistosomiasis is generally higher in males than in females, and rises with age until it reaches a maximum at 10 to 15 years of age, remains high in the next age group and starts to fall gradually after the age of 20 years. This has been verified in a study of 60,197 cases taken by random sampling in surveys made in 23 villages distributed in different parts of the UAR in 1955. The data are summarized in table IV, which shows that the over-all prevalence of urinary schistosomiasis in these 60,197 cases was 40%. In males it was 45% and in females 35%. This sex relativity may be explained by the greater degree of exposure to infection in males due to occupational and social factors.

Table III. The prevalence of urinary schistosomiasis in areas under different methods of irrigation in three southern provinces in 1955

Province	District	Number examined	Number positive	%	Main irrigation method
Assiut	Dairut	12,228	8,252	67	perennial mainly
	El-Badari	6,815	4,721	69	perennial mainly
	Manfalut	7,278	1,271	17	basin
	Abnub	5,637	704	12	basin
	Assiut	9,024	2,176	24	basin
	Abu Teeg	7,656	1,329	17	basin
Suhag	Akhmeem	8,225	4,575	56	perennial
	Girga	10,157	6,934	68	perennial
	El-Balyana	12,995	7,917	61	perennial
	Tima	1,892	242	13	basin
	Tahta	3,281	298	9	basin
Qena	Nage Hammadi	11,586	7,218	62	pumps (perennial)
	Qus	5,874	637	11	basin
	Luxor	7,106	1,055	15	basin

Table IV. Prevalence of urinary schistosomiasis by age and sex among 60,197 persons surveyed in 23 villages in different locations in Egypt

Age groups year	Males number examined	number positive	%	Females number examined	number positive	%	Total number examined	number positive	%
0– 1	38	0	0	35	0	0	73	0	0
2– 4	866	120	14	768	165	21	1,634	285	17
5– 9	4,642	2,343	50	4,478	1,951	44	9,120	4,294	47
10–14	4,296	2,929	68	3,782	1,977	52	8,078	4,906	60
15–19	3,223	2,013	62	2,775	1,361	49	5,998	3,374	56
20–29	4,615	2,310	50	5,372	2,071	39	9,987	4,381	44
30–39	5,213	2,098	40	5,602	1,501	27	10,815	3,599	33
40–49	3,826	1,048	27	3,867	753	19	7,693	1,801	23
50	3,400	757	22	3,399	603	18	6,799	1,360	20
Total	30,119	13,618	45	30,078	10,382	35	60,197	24,000	40

As regards age, the prevalence rises from 17% in the 2- to 4-year age group to 47% in the age group of 5 to 9 years and reaches a peak of 60% at 10 to 14 years. From 15 years onwards it starts to decline until it reaches 20% at 50 years and over. This trend is observed in both males and females.

Since 1955, the only prevalence rates available are 'hospital returns' from the endemic diseases hospitals all over the country, covering more than one million people annually. It is important to note, however, that the over-all rates according to the spot surveys of 1935 and 1955 were analogous with the hospital returns of the corresponding years (for the 1955 hospital returns see table V and its footnote 2).

Table V shows the percentage of the prevalence and distribution of schistosomiasis according to hospital returns from the endemic diseases hospitals in 1955 and 1965. The number of people examined was 1,326,979 and 1,254,258 respectively. It is shown that:

(1) the over-all incidence of both types of human schistosomiasis has again decreased, in *S. haematobium* infection from 43.7% to 37.0% and in *S. mansoni* infection from 6.1 to 4.3%;

(2) the improvement in the prevalence of *S. mansoni* is still greater than in that of *S. haematobium;*

(3) the tendency for the prevalence of *S. haematobium* to rise in the southern three provinces of Suhag, Qena and Aswan has stopped. In fact, a drop has occurred, especially in Suhag and Aswan. However, a recent investigation of the health aspects of the Lake Nasser Development scheme showed that 20% of 376 primary school-children in Gharb Aswan and 19% of 103 persons examined on Atig island were infected with *S. haematobium*. So far, there do not seem to be any cases of *S. mansoni* in the Aswan, Qena and Suhag governorates, but vigorous measures must be taken to prevent the introduction of the infection into the Lake Nasser area [SATTI, 1970].

The Distribution of the Molluscan Intermediate Hosts

Bulinus (B.) truncatus, the snail intermediate host of *S. haematobium* in the UAR, occurs throughout the country, both in irrigation channels and in drains. It is also present, though to a lesser degree, in the main feeder canals and even in the Nile itself and its Rosetta and Damietta branches, especially in backwater baylets containing vegetation or in residual pools left when the water recedes. An unexplained phenomenon is the presence of *B.(B.) truncatus* in some of the Egyptian oases in the Western Desert,

Table V. Percentage of prevalence and distribution of human schistosomiasis in the UAR according to hospital returns from the endemic diseases hospitals in 1955 and 1965

Governorate[1]	S. haematobium		S. mansoni		Notes
	1955	1965	1955	1965	
Beheira	41.1	35.7	21.3	20.0	
Gharbiya	42.1	37.0	11.5	5.0	
Kafr el Sheikh	43.4	45.3	25.5	20.8	previously part of Gharbiya
Dakahliya	51.3	41.9	13.4	10.5	
Damietta	43.2	23.7	29.5	18.5	previously part of Dakahliya
Sharkiya	56.1	51.0	4.4	2.0	
Qalyubiya	41.1	38.8	1.7	0.9	
Minufiya	51.4	37.7	0.7	0.3	
Giza	45.8	40.0	0.3	0.08	
Fayum	56.6	48.4	–	–	
Beni-Suef	51.5	41.4	–	–	
Minya	51.1	40.0	–	–	
Assiut	37.9	37.0	–	–	
Suhag	60.3	40.4	–	–	
Qena	30.2	28.8	–	–	
Aswan	36.6	26.9	–	–	
Cairo	36.3	31.1	0.4	0.4	⎫
Alexandria	14.8	21.0	1.9	7.0	⎪ urban and, therefore, not
Port Said	22.6	14.5	4.1	2.1	⎬ cited in the 1935 and 1955
Ismailiya	31.0	20.3	2.3	2.7	⎪ spot surveys
Suez	20.3	29.0	1.9	1.1	⎭
Total	43.7	37.0	6.1[2]	4.3[3]	

1 Governorates were previously called provinces. Some provinces have been subdivided; hence the newly established Kafr el Sheikh and Damietta governorates.
2 This is the *S. mansoni* average prevalence rate for the country, the figure for rural lower Egypt being 9.2.
3 This is the *S. mansoni* average prevalence rate for the country, the figure for rural lower Egypt being 8.3.

about 450 km away from the Nile valley. Their water supply is drawn from artesian wells which have no connexion with the Nile. The snails might either have been carried to the oases by human agency, or they might represent a remnant stock from the humid Pleistocene period before the advent of desert conditions. In the New Valley governorate, comprising

Dakhla and Kharga Oases, repeated generalized snail control through the use of copper sulphate has succeeded in stamping out *B.(B.) truncatus* since 1952. However, the snail still exists in Baharya Oasis, now part of Matruh governorate.

Biomphalaria alexandrina, the snail intermediate host of *S.mansoni* in the UAR, is common in lower Egypt, especially in the lowlands in the northern part of the Nile Delta. Two forms of *B.alexandrina* occur in Egypt, one highly susceptible, the other almost insusceptible, to *S.mansoni.* In Pharaonic times the low portions of the Delta formed vast sweet-water marshes and swamps which may have been the nursery maintaining the present-day stock. They are usually more abundant in drains than in irrigation channels, but in an irrigation network they are more plentiful towards the distal ends of the network because they thrive more in the slower current. They were entirely absent in upper and middle Egypt as far north as Cairo, although ecological conditions do not appear to be particularly unfavourable to them, and dead *Biomphalaria* shells were actually discovered in the previously swampy area of El Gharaq in the south-western part of Fayum governorate, when reclaimed by a drainage project of pumps using hydro-electric power.

It is worthy of mention that *Biomphalaria,* and even to a lesser extent *Bulinus,* are present in the brackish water lakes in the northernmost parts of the Delta, especially near the outlets of the main fresh-water drains into these lakes.

References

SATTI, M. H.: Lake Nasser Development Centre (Health Aspects). WHO unpublished document, EM/EPID/19 (1970).
SCOTT, J. A.: Amer. J. Hyg. *25:* 566 (1937).

Libya

Schistosomiasis occurs in isolated foci in a few areas on the Mediterranean coast and in Fezzan, where local conditions are favourable for the molluscan intermediate hosts.

S.haematobium is the species mainly involved. It probably occurs at Dabusia and Lathrum west of Derna in the extreme north-east; cases have been reported from the latter city, but BERRY [1964] determined that infection in these cases was acquired in Fezzan and Egypt. However, according to HAMAMI [1965] during the period from 22 January 1964 to 10 March 1965, 20 cases of schistosomiasis in children were treated at the

Derna Hospital. All cases were indigenous with no history of having been outside the town. HALAWANI [1966] reported positive urine specimens in 16 of 240 schoolboys in Derna and in two of 120 inhabitants of adjoining El Maghak.

The infection occurs in all the valleys of Fezzan, with the exception of the Gufrah and Hikmah valleys [EL GINDY, 1969]. GIORDANO [1935] reviewed the findings of previous investigators and detected cases at Al Mahruqah and El Gedid in West-Central Libya and at El Barcat near Gat in the south-west, near the Algerian border. BERRY [1964] reported a high prevalence rate at Al Mahruqah and a focus at Brach, 75 km north of Sebha. The disease is also endemic at Tmessa south-east of Sebha.

HALAWANI [1966] reported prevalence rates of S. haematobium of 24% at Drak, 12% at Temzawa, 25% at Temenhint, 10% at Mourzouk, 62.5% at Tragen, 8,2% at Khelef, and 2% at El Gerefa. There was a low prevalence at El Abiad but a high rate at Ben Hareth. According to HALAWANI, examinations at the Sebha Central Hospital revealed prevalence rates among school-children of 86% at El Birkat, 55% at Mahrouga and 61% at Gregia. At El Gedid, HALAWANI obtained a rate of 11% in school-boys.

The only reported focus of infection with S. mansoni is in the area of Taurorga on the Mediterranean coast west of Misurata.

B. (B.) truncatus is the molluscan intermediate host of S. haematobium in most of the endemic foci. However, BERRY [1964] collected Bulinus at Sebha and Brach, which he believed to be a new species but which may fall within the variation range of B. (B.) truncatus. YASURAOKA [1966] found Bulinus at Samnon, 60 km south-east of Sebha.

At Taurorga, a species of Biomphalaria is the intermediate host. This was thought by BERRY [1964] to represent a new species. HALAWANI [1966] believed the species to be B. alexandrina.

References

BERRY, E. G.: Investigations of the snail intermediate hosts of bilharziasis in Libya. WHO unpublished document, PA/230.64 (1964).

GINDY, M. S. EL: Field report. Libya schistosomiasis control project. WHO Regional Office for the Eastern Mediterranean, unpublished document (1969).

GIORDANO, M.: Arch. ital. Sci. med. colon. 16: 510 (1935).

HALAWANI, A. A. EL: Summary report. A survey of bilharziasis in the Kingdom of Libya, 15 December 1965–27 February 1966. WHO unpublished document, EM/BIL/34, LIBYA, 24/TA (1966).

HAMAMI, A. A.: Report on a visit to Libya, 7–16 March 1965. WHO Regional Office for the Eastern Mediterranean, unpublished document (1965).

YASURAOKA, K.: Assignment report. A survey of the snail vectors of bilharziasis in Libya, 11 January–11 March 1966. WHO unpublished document, EM/BIL/35, LIBYA 24/TA (1966).

Tunisia

S. haematobium is the sole species involved in schistosomiasis in Tunisia. A number of endemic areas exist. VERMEIL [1957] described in detail the foci at Gafsa and its environs. In Gafsa city and Sidi Mansour, VERMEIL found 69% of 75 boys and 16% of 52 girls infected. At El Ksar 52% of 50 boys, and at Lalla 39% of the same number of boys were infected.

COUMBARAS [1960] conducted a survey in Nefzaoua in the region of Kebili-Douz in the south of Tunisia. From 12 villages a total of 919 school-children were examined, of whom 572, or 62%, were positive. The infection rate varied with age, the lowest rate being 22% in the 6-year-old group and the highest 64% in the age group 13 to 14 years.

COUMBARAS [1961] reviewed the schistosomiasis situation in Tunisia. In addition to the areas mentioned above, the disease is endemic in the region of Tozeur (Djerid), El Hamma, Matmata and Zarat. At El Hamma, 11% of 88 school-children were positive, as were 8% of 93 at Matmata. An examination of 100 children from 7 to 14 years of age at Zarat and nearby Cedria revealed 29 positives.

In a survey conducted by random sampling in the Gabès and Gafsa governorates AZAR [1968] found a prevalence rate of 21% in the area of Kabili. The whole of Gafsa town and its surroundings are considered to be infected, with particularly high rates in Lalla, Gafsa-Nord and El Ksar. The foci in Degueche, Kebili and Douz form a belt along Chott Djerid.

The molluscan intermediate host of *S. haematobium* in Tunisia is *B. (B.) truncatus*. It is found in drainage areas around artesian wells and in irrigation canals.

References

AZAR, J.E.: La bilharziose en Tunisie. Rapport de mission, 1967. WHO unpublished document, EM/BIL/41 (1968).
COUMBARAS, A.: Arch. Inst. Pasteur Tunis *37:* 313 (1960).
COUMBARAS, A.: Arch. Inst. Pasteur Tunis *38:* 255 (1961).
VERMEIL, C.: Arch. Inst. Pasteur Tunis *34:* 167 (1957).

Algeria

Limited foci of *S. haematobium* exist in Algeria but *S. mansoni* has not been reported to be endemic. DESCHIENS [1952] reviewed the literature and summarized available data. Foci are present at St Aimé de la Djidioua, Foundouk [MARILL *et al.,* 1949] and Biskra, all in northern Algeria, and in the oasis of Djanet in the far south near the Libyan border. At St Aimé de la Djidioua, a survey in 1939 disclosed 42 positive individuals in 96 examined. In the oasis of Djanet, 85 % of 148 inhabitants were positive.

The molluscan intermediate host of *S.haematobium* in Algeria is *B. (B.) truncatus.* According to DESCHIENS, it is found in all of the endemic foci and in addition it has been reported from Macta, Mazafran, Mirabeau, the Oued Souman near Bougie and Lake Oubeira. *Planorbarius metidjensis* has also been reported from a number of areas including the focus at Foundouk.

References

DESCHIENS, R.: Le problème sanitaire des bilharzioses dans les territoires de l'Union française. Monogr. V. Soc. Path. exot. (Masson, Paris 1952).
MARILL, F.-G.; HOFMAN, M., and BERTOZZI, P.: Arch. Inst. Pasteur Algér. *27:* 110 (1949).

Morocco

GAUD [1951] and BLANCHARD [1964] have summarized the schistosomiasis situation in this country. *S.haematobium* is the only human schistosome reported from Morocco. The endemic areas may be divided into two general regions, the first in the Saharan slopes of the Atlas Mountain Range and the second along the Atlantic coast.

South of the Atlas Range, endemic foci exist below altitudes of 1,200 m, where the flow of water is sufficient to maintain permanent habitats for the snail host. In this region there are four general areas of endemicity with prevalence rates as follows:

(1) West of Bani (in the south of the administrative district of Agadir) including Assa (>75%), Akka (50–75%) and Tata (25%).

(2) South-east of Agadir between the Oued Sous and the western part of the Anti-Atlas Range. There are a number of confirmed foci in this region and others may exist. Among the former are Ait Baha (>75%), Tanalt (50–75%) and Kilometer 44 (<25%).

(3) Territory of Ouarzazate along the Oued Draa. In this area foci are located at Agdz (>75%), M'hamid (<25%), Zagora (>75%), Tamegrout (50–75%), and others.

(4) Tafilalet in the southern part of the administrative region of Meknes including foci at Goulmima (50–75%), Tazouguerte (25–50%), Riche (<25%), Ksar-es-Souk (<25%), Boudenib (50–75%), and others.

In the Atlantic coastal region, there are several foci with different climatic characteristics. These are in the Gharb north of Rabat and in the region of Telata de Raisana (Jolot), which is situated inland north-east of Larache. RICO-AVELLO and ANDRES ANDRES [1946] examined urine specimens from 3,177 individuals, of whom 13.8 % were positive. The prevalence rate in various villages varied between 1 and 73 %.

In the Marrakech area the prevalence rate is between 50 and 75 % in Marrakech town and over 75 % at the main focus (Karia-ben-Aouda) in the north.

In the province of Agadir the Anezi sector is heavily infected and the disease has been found to be present along the Oued Massa [CORNU, 1969].

The molluscan intermediate hosts *B.(B.) truncatus* and *Planorbarius metidjensis* have been reported from numerous areas in Morocco. The former is the intermediate host in the greater part of the country but the latter may serve in that capacity in the north (former Spanish Morocco), although further study of this problem is necessary.

References

BLANCHARD, J.: Contribution à l'étude épidémiologique, clinique et thérapeutique de la bilharziose vésicale à *Schistosoma haematobium* au Maroc; thesis, Lyons (1964).

CORNU: in FERULLO, C., Report on assignment in the Province of Agadir. Unpublished document (1969).

GAUD, J.: Bull. Inst. Hyg. Maroc *11:* 69 (1951).

RICO-AVELLO, C. and ANDRES ANDRES, A.: Rev. San. Hig. publ. Madr. *20:* 111 (1946).

West Africa

Data from a number of West African countries are too few to warrant an accurate appraisal of the relative importance of urinary and intestinal schistosomiasis in this region. In particular, there is little published information on distribution and prevalence in such countries as Guinea, Mali, Ivory Coast, Dahomey, Niger and Gabon, and in certain other countries, statistics are markedly deficient.

Regardless of these gaps in knowledge, indications are that *S. haematobium* is by far the predominant species and is much more widely distributed than is *S. mansoni*. The former is the only species reported thus far from Mauritania, Portuguese Guinea, Niger and the Congo (Brazzaville).

Prevalence rates of both species are so disparate that it is not possible to arrive at any firm appraisal of an average rate for any country. Even in the same general locality, infection may be extremely high in certain villages and be entirely absent from others. For instance, in Senegal, where a considerable number of surveys have been undertaken, rates vary from 0 to 82%. Such variation is illustrative of the necessity for a careful evaluation of local conditions which influence the transmission pattern and render the disease of importance or non-importance in any given community.

Countries in which high prevalence rates of *S. haematobium* have been recorded, at least in some localities, include Senegal, Gambia, Mali, Portuguese Guinea, Sierra Leone, Upper Volta, Ivory Coast, Ghana, Nigeria, Cameroon and Angola.

S. mansoni has a limited distribution in West Africa. It is the predominant human schistosome in Mali and Cameroon. Especially high prevalence rates have been recorded in localities in Guinea, Gambia, Sierra Leone, Nigeria and Cameroon. The parasite is widely distributed in eastern Angola but infection rates are low and for the country as a whole the rate probably does not exceed 1%.

Mauritania

S. haematobium is the only species of human schistosome known to occur in the Islamic Republic of Mauritania. The main foci of infection are in the south and west, the northern Cercle of Adrar being almost entirely free from the disease. Infection was found in only one area, Atar, by MARILL [1961], who has conducted the most extensive investigation in the country. MARILL carried out examinations in several localities in the vicinity of Atar, including Atar, Azougui, Terjit, Toungad, Oujeft, Agminmine and Irji; of 125 individuals (99 boys and 26 girls) 50, or 40%, were positive.

In the Cercle of Inchiri, 62 boys and 5 girls were examined at Akjoujt, of whom 5, or 7.4%, were positive. In the Cercle of Trarza, 439 boys and 41 girls were examined in the localities of Rosso, Boutilimit, Méderdra, lac R-Kiz, Dieuk, and Keur-Massènes, with 49 positives or 10.2%.

In the Cercle of Brakna, urine tests were conducted on 256 boys and 58 girls in the localities of Boghé, Aleg and Aéré-M'Bar, with 77 positives or 24.5%. Villages surveyed in the Cercle of Gorgol included Kaedi, Lé-Kséiba, Rindiao, Monguel, Ouadio, Djéol and Maghama, with 106 positives in 385 individuals, or 27.5%.

RIOU [1966] reported that LE BRAS examined 505 individuals in the subdivision of M'Bout in the Cercle of Kiffa and found 231, or 45.7%, to be positive. The areas examined included M'Bout, Ouachkedi, Dieybaba, Djadjibine Chorfa, Djadjibine Gandega, Thiale and Lekseiba. *B. (B.) senegalensis* was found in 7 of 11 sites explored.

In the Valley of Karakoro, Cercle of Kiffa, LE BRAS conducted examinations on 249 school-children, of whom 207, or 83.1%, were positive for *S. haematobium*. Prevalence of infection varied between 100% at Hamoud to 11.1% at Koumoudiel.

The total number of cases of urinary schistosomiasis in the country is not known but DESCHIENS [1952] estimated the average infection rate to be 31% and GAUD [1955] believed it to be around 40%.

Molluscan intermediate hosts, *Bulinus* snails, have been collected from a number of areas. OLIVIER and BUZO [1964] stated that *S. haematobium* is apparently transmitted by *B. (B.) senegalensis*. *B. (B.) forskalii* has been found in a number of places but is probably not involved in transmission. *B. (Ph.) jousseaumei* has been reported from the Monguel area [OLIVIER and BUZO, 1964]. *B. pfeifferi* occurs in several areas even though *S. mansoni* is not present in the country.

GRÉTILLAT [1963] found *B. truncatus rohlfsi* to be the vector in the Tagant Plateau and *B. (B.) guernei* to serve in that capacity in the vicinity of Rosso in the extreme south-west.

References

DESCHIENS, R.: Le problème sanitaire des bilharzioses dans les territoires de l'Union française. Monogr. V, Soc. Path. exot. (Masson, Paris 1952).

GAUD, J.: Bull. Wld Hlth Org. *13:* 209 (1955).

GRÉTILLAT, S.: Rev. Elev. Méd. vét. Pays trop. *16:* 323 (1963).

MARILL, F.-G.: Med. trop. Madr. *21:* 373 (1961).

OLIVIER, L. J. and BUZO, Z. J.: Report on a visit to Mauritania by the Inter-regional Bilharziasis Advisory Team, 22 October–13 November 1963. WHO unpublished document, MHO/PA/135.64 (1964).

RIOU, N.: in Rapport Final de la VIe Conférence Technique de l'OCCGE, Bobo-Dioulasso, Mars 1966; vol. I, pp. 148–157. Unpublished document, (1966).

Senegal

S. haematobium is the species predominant in Senegal. It occurs in all parts of the country, with the possible exception of the Ferlo desert area [LARIVIÈRE and DIALLO, 1967]. The main endemic foci are located in the valleys of the various rivers, viz. the Senegal, the Falémé, the Saloum, the Gambia and the Casamance. Certain foci are situated in the north near the border with Mauritania.

The range of prevalence according to GAUD [1955] is 2–40% with an estimated average of 15%. According to DESCHIENS [1952] the average prevalence is 8%, and according to PFISTER [1957] it is 15%.

Infection rates vary in accordance with the region. At Dakar, the rate was 6% in 1923, and at nearby Medina it varied between 39% in 1923 and 8% in 1949. Rates in the Thiès and Kaolack areas range from 7.5 to 75%, and in Basse-Casamance from 15 to 85% [LARIVIÈRE and DIALLO, 1967].

LARIVIÈRE et al., [1958] examined numerous individuals in the Cercle of Thiès and that of Kaolack. In the subdivision of Thiès, the prevalence in three villages ranged between 7.4 and 26.9%. In the subdivision of Tivaouane (Cercle of Thiès), of three villages, infection was observed only in Makha with a rate of 1.5%. In the subdivision of M-Bour, nine villages were surveyed with infection rates varying from 0 to 65%. A total of 806 faecal examinations proved negative for S. mansoni eggs.

From four villages in the subdivision of Fatick in the Cercle of Kaolack, a total of 997 children were examined; 3.9% were positive for S. mansoni and 23% for S. haematobium. In the subdivision of Foundiougne (Cercle of Kaolack), two villages in the region of Sine showed positive urines of 75.9 and 5.35% respectively.

In the Arrondissement of Khombole, LARIVIÈRE et al. [1960] noted 20% of 115 children positive at Keur Messia Diake, 7.3% of 109 at Mandanguil Ouoloff, 7% of 129 at Bousnak-Gotte, 4% of 107 at Niangue Dakar and Djite, and 3% of 123 at Parare and Dimbe.

SARDOU [1962] reported an infection rate of 32.1% in 140 inhabitants of the village of Ngoye in the region of Diourbel.

Active transmission is also taking place around lac de Guiers in the north (3.12%); in the areas of Podor (15–20% infected), Matam (11.8%), and Bakel (22%) on the River Niger; in Eastern Senegal (Tambacounda and Kédougou); and in Haute-Casamance (Kolda) [LARIVIÈRE and DIALLO, 1967].

In Basse-Casamance, the villages of Balandine and Kartiack, north of the Casamance River, showed prevalence rates of 22 and 42% respectively. South of the river, the following rates were obtained in various villages: Nyassia 15%, Seleki 71%, M'Lomp 33%, Kodjinole 85%, and Kagnoute 82%.

In addition to endemic foci of infection with S. mansoni at Fatick and Kaolack, already mentioned, intestinal schistosomiasis occurs at Kolda and Bignona [DESCHIENS, 1952] in the Casamance River valley. GAUD [1955] reported an infection rate of 5 to 10% at Kolda in 1949. LARIVIÈRE et al. [1964] reported additional foci in the region of Kolda, the region of Kedougou and near Etiolo-Salémata-Gandjiri.

LARIVIÈRE *et al.* [1960] found 92, or 47%, of 195 children positive for *S. mansoni* in the village of Fandène-Saint-Marcel, situated 5 km from the city of Thiès, but this focus is reported to be spontaneously dying out.

A number of potential molluscan intermediate hosts of *S. haematobium* occur in Senegal. *Bulinus (Bulinus)* sp. have been reported from a number of areas. SMITHERS [1956] collected *B. (Ph.) jousseaumei* at Kolda. GRÉTILLAT [1963] noted that this species serves as an intermediate host in the upper Casamance region. LARIVIÈRE and CHARNIER [1957] found *B. (B.) forskalii* at Cap Vert. *B. (B.) senegalensis* is apparently widely distributed; however, GRÉTILLAT [1961] failed to find this species infected in an extensive survey of the Tamba Counda area where infection is apparently carried exclusively by *B. (B.) guernei*, 2 to 8% of which were found to be positive.

B. pfeifferi is the intermediate host of *S. mansoni*.

References

DESCHIENS, R.: Le problème sanitaire des bilharzioses dans les territoires de l'Union française. Monogr. V, Soc. Path. exot. (Masson, Paris 1952).
GAUD, J.: Bull. Wld Hlth Org. *13:* 209 (1955).
GAUD, J. and JAUBERTIE, R.: Ann. Parasit. *26:* 420 (1951).
GRÉTILLAT, S.: Bull. Wld Hlth Org. *25:* 459 (1961).
GRÉTILLAT, S.: Rev. Elev. Méd. vét. Pays trop. *16:* 323 (1963).
LARIVIÈRE, M.; ARETAS, R.; RABA, A., and CHARNIER, M.: Bull. méd. Afr. occid. franç. *3:* 239 (1958).
LARIVIÈRE, M. and CHARNIER, M.: Bull. Mém. Ec. nat. Méd. Pharm. (Dakar) *5:* 336 (1957).
LARIVIÈRE, M. and DIALLO, S.: Afr. méd. (Dakar) *6:* 475 (1967).
LARIVIÈRE, M.; DIALLO, S., and RANQUE, PH.: Bull. Soc. méd. Afr. noire Lang. franç. *9:* 288 (1964).
LARIVIÈRE, M.; GRÉTILLAT, S., and HOCQUET, P.: Méd. Afr. Noire, Numéro Spécial, juillet, pp. 61–68 (1963).
LARIVIÈRE, M.; LAPIERRE, J.; HOCQUET, P., and CAMERLYNCK, P.: Bull. Soc. méd. Afr. noire Lang. franç. *5:* 88 (1960).
ODEI, M. A.: J. trop. Med. Hyg. *64:* 27, 64, 88 (1961).
PFISTER, E.: in LARIVIÈRE and DIALLO, 1967 (1957).
SARDOU, R.: Bull. Soc. Path. exot. *55:* 39 (1962).
SMITHERS, S. R.: Trans. roy. Soc. trop. Med. Hyg. *50:* 354 (1956).
WRIGHT, C. A.: W. afr. med. J. *8:* 142 (1959).

Gambia

S. haematobium is the species chiefly encountered in Gambia. It is widely distributed over the Upper River Division in the eastern part of the country and along the upper and lower borders of the MacCarthy Island

Division. A limited focus occurs on the northern border of the Central Division and another limited focus in the northern part of the Western Division. A similar area is located at Kartung in the extreme south-western part of the country, where SMITHERS [1956] found a prevalence rate of 55%.

THOMAS [1947] found 6 of 39 individuals examined in the villages of Berrending, Chamen and Kebbe in the Lower Niumi District of the Western Division to be positive for *S. haematobium;* these villages are situated east of Bathurst. In the Lower Saloum District in the eastern part of the Central Division, THOMAS also located a number of infected villages (Biram Yacine, Kaur, Gange and Gimbala) where 6 positives were obtained in 29 persons examined; he believed that evidence indicated local foci at each of the above-mentioned areas in the two Divisions. In addition, THOMAS discovered many infected areas of *S. haematobium* in the MacCarthy Island and Upper River Divisions.

Prevalence rates vary considerably. DUKE and McCULLOUGH [1954] reported a combined rate of 12.4% for children and 14.2% for adults in 12 swamp villages in the Bansang area of MacCarthy Island Division. In 10 villages on the laterite plateau to the south of Bansang, the respective rates were 72.7% for children and 38.8% for adults. At Sanchabari and N'Joren (MacCarthy Island Division), the over-all rate for all ages was 50.3% in the former and 37.8% in the latter. In other villages in the MacCarthy Island Division, the rates ranged from 4 to 60.7% in children 3 to 15 years of age and 8.3 to 30.3% in adults.

S. mansoni has been reported from only one area in Gambia; the limited foci are located in the south-west portion of the Western Division. SMITHERS [1957] found 1 of 22 persons positive in Darsilami, 6 of 15 positive in Busura, and 4 of 15 positive in Keti. In Jiborah, 11 of 21 persons from 7 to 16 years of age were positive, while 19 of 21 individuals from 20 to 40 years of age were infected. These villages lie along the Allahein bolon near the Senegal border.

SMITHERS [1956] determined by animal experimentation that *B.(B.) jousseaumei, B.(B.) guernei* and *B.(B.) senegalensis* are the molluscan intermediate hosts of *S. haematobium* in Gambia. *B.(B.) forskalii* is apparently widely distributed and there is evidence that it may be involved in transmission; however, proof of this is lacking. *B.(B.) senegalensis* was found by SMITHERS to be confined to seasonal pools formed on the laterite plateau and known as laterite pools; between rainy seasons, the snail apparently survives by aestivating in the mud. *B.(B.) jousseaumei* was located in clear, cool, running water in the permanent steep-sided bolons of the Upper River Division.

B. pfeifferi is the intermediate host of *S. mansoni* in Gambia.

References

DUKE, B. O. L. and MCCULLOUGH, F. S.: Ann. trop. Med. Parasit. *48:* 287 (1954).
MCCULLOUGH, F. S. and DUKE, B. O. L.: Ann. trop. Med. Parasit. *48:* 277 (1954).
SMITHERS, S. R.: Trans roy. Soc. trop. Med. Hyg. *50:* 354 (1956).
SMITHERS, S. R.: Ann. trop. Med. Parasit. *51:* 359 (1957).
THOMAS, C. C.: The epidemiology of urinary schistosomiasis in Gambia; thesis, Cambridge (1947).

Acknowledgements

Special thanks are due to Dr F. S. MCCULLOUGH and Dr B. O. L. DUKE for supplying detailed information and to Dr C. C. THOMAS for the loan of his thesis.

Mali

Only a relatively few foci of schistosomiasis are known in the Mali Republic, although both *S. haematobium* and *S. mansoni* are widely distributed. Most of the foci are situated on the River Niger and its tributaries and in the western portion along the River Senegal and its affluents. No doubt infection is far more widespread than reports indicate. There are no recently published data.

GAUD [1955] recorded prevalence rates for *S. haematobium* from 10 communities. The highest rate was 85% in two areas at Koulikoro, based on 1942 records; the lowest rate was 2% at Bougouni (Kolondieba). In 1940, Gourma-Rarous had a rate of 75%. In the area of Kayes, 75% of the population are believed to be infected [WATSON, 1970]. GAUD [1955] estimated the average infection rate as 35% while DESCHIENS [1951] believed it to be 47%.

As with the parasites, there is little information available on the distribution of molluscan intermediate hosts. *B. (B.) forskalii* has been found in a considerable number of places but is not known to be involved in transmission. *Biomphalaria* sp. has been recorded from many areas. MANDAHL-BARTH [1957] stated that *B. (Ph.) jousseaumei* is distributed in Mali. KERVRAN [1947] recorded successful infection with *S. haematobium* of *Physopsis africana* and *B. tchadensis*. It is possible that KERVRAN was dealing with *B. (Ph.) globosus* and *B. (B.) truncatus rohlfsi*, respectively. *B. (B.) truncatus* may well be responsible for transmission of *S. haematobium* in Mali.

References

DESCHIENS, R.: Bull. Soc. Path. exot. *44:* 350 (1951).
GAUD, J.: Bull. Wld Hlth Org. *13:* 209 (1955).
KERVRAN, P.: Bull. Soc. Path. exot. *40:* 349, 364 (1947).
MANDAHL-BARTH, G.: Bull. Wld Hlth Org. *17:* 1 (1957).
WATSON, J. M.: Senegal River Valley Development. Assignment report, August 1969. WHO
   unpublished document, AFR/PHA/60 (1970).

Portuguese Guinea

S. haematobium is the only human schistosome known to be endemic
in Portuguese Guinea. All of the endemic foci are located in the northern
half of the country and extend from the Atlantic seaboard to the Guinea
border.

PINTO [1955] noted prevalence rates of 54% in the Caiomete River
Basin, 13% in the Cacheu River Basin, 34% in the Geba River Basin and
18% in part of the Corubal River Basin; the rates varied with age. In 169
persons in one village of 250, the following rates were observed: old people
0%, men 38%, women 60.7%, children 84% and infants 0%.

GILLET [1956] conducted investigations in a number of endemic areas.
At Bafata he found one child positive in 12 examined and one woman
positive in 10 examined, all examinations being conducted on members
of the Sarancule tribe. Among the Fula tribe (Peul) in the Bafata region,
one of 10 children was positive, as was one of 10 men, while none of 10
women was positive. At Nova Lamego (Gabu), the rates were higher in the
Mandinga tribe than in the Peul tribe. At Sonaco, members of the Mandinga tribe again showed higher rates than those of the Peul tribe. At
Canchungo near Texeira Pinto, high rates were encountered in the Manjaca
tribe, although again the number examined was relatively small. GILLET
stated that schistosomiasis at the time did not represent a public health
problem.

There is no doubt that the principal molluscan intermediate host is
B. (Ph.) globosus. B. (B.) senegalensis occurs in many of the endemic areas
but was not found infected under natural conditions [PINTO, 1955], although it proved to be a good host under laboratory conditions. GILLET
[1956] collected *B. pfeifferi (gaudi)* and *B. (B.) jousseaumei* in the Bafata-
Sonaco-Nova Lamego (Gabu) region.

References

GILLET, J.: Bilharziasis in Portuguese Guinea. WHO unpublished document, WHO/Bil.
   Conf./44 (1956).
PINTO, A. R.: An. Inst. Med. trop. (Lisboa) *12:* 653 (1955).

Guinea

Guinea is divided into four main geographical regions:
(1) Lower Guinea (Basse Guinée), or Guinée maritime;
(2) Middle Guinea, or Fouta Djallon;
(3) Upper Guinea (Haute Guinée);
(4) Forest Region (Guinée forestière).

Lower Guinea

Lower Guinea comprises eight administrative regions: Conakry, Boffa, Forécariah, Dubréka, Boké, Fria, Télimelé and Kindia. Its climate is monsoonal and characterized by a dry season and a wet season. The rains usually start in the first half of May and end in the first half of November, with a total annual precipitation of 3 to 4.5 m which permits the culture of one crop of rice without irrigation annually.

The coastal belt of Lower Guinea, which comprises the first five of the above-mentioned administrative regions, is a continental shelf which in recent geological times was submerged by the ocean and is traversed by the estuaries of rivers that used to flow to the ocean in well-defined valleys; it varies between 40 and 100 km in width. The land is only a few metres above sea level and there is shallow flooding of the land by the ocean twice daily except for parts protected by dykes. The flooding regime varies with the height of the tide during the usual fortnightly cycle; it also varies with the volume of fresh water descending in the rivers which reaches a peak during the rainy season in August and September. After this peak, the flow of rainwater slackens and a front of saline water gradually advances up the estuaries. The speed and salt content of this salt flood depend on the size of the river and also on the season. Salt water flows up and down the channels with the tide and ebb. The average minimum temperature is 25 ^{0}C and the maximum is 35 ^{0}C. The relative humidity is very high.

No snail hosts have up to the present been detected in the coastal belt of Lower Guinea and the cases of schistosomiasis in this belt are imported, except for some indigenous cases reported from the Forécariah and Boké administrative regions. Both these regions are on the outskirts of the coastal belt and merge into other areas known to be endemic for schistosomiasis. There is the possibility that for chemical and/or physical reasons snail hosts cannot as yet thrive in the rest of the coastal area; this may be due to the length of the dry season (about 7 months), the deep flooding which follows during the rainy season, and the marked and continuous variations of salinity and pH through the tidal movements. However, these conditions may change in some of the areas of reclamation of rice lands in this belt, where the UNDP/FAO are building dykes to prevent ocean flooding and establishing drainage canals to alleviate swamping by excess rain water.

The lowest prevalence of schistosomiasis in Guinea occurs in Lower Guinea.

Middle Guinea (or Fouta Djallon)

In Middle Guinea there is a somewhat higher rate of prevalence of schistosomiasis. This area is a plateau about 300 m above sea level, rising at some places up to 1,000 m and occupying about half of the total area of Guinea. Temperatures are lower and there is less rainfall than in Lower Guinea.

Upper Guinea

Upper Guinea is a lowland to the east of the Fouta Djallon and to the north of the Forest Region. It is near to the Sahara belt and is characterized by light rainfall and much higher temperatures. Here the rate of prevalence of schistosomiasis is much higher than in Lower Guinea and Middle Guinea.

Forest Region

The Forest Region lies north of Liberia. It is a typical West African tropical rain forest with high humidity and high temperatures. The rainfall here is heavy, but somewhat less than in Lower Guinea. This region has the highest rate of prevalence of schistosomiasis.

Insufficient data are available concerning details of the distribution and extent of schistosomiasis in the Republic of Guinea.

S. haematobium: GAUD [1955] recorded prevalence rates of 32% at Macenta (Forest Region), 40% at N'Zérékoré (Forest Region) and 30% at Kindia (Lower Guinea), all for the year 1939. DESCHIENS [1951] reported foci at Faranah (Upper Guinea), and at Kissidougou, Guékédou, Macenta, Beyla and N'Zérékoré, all in the Forest Region.

S. mansoni: MAASS and VOGEL [1930] stated that numerous cases of intestinal schistosomiasis from 32 villages in the Cercle, i. e. administrative region, of Guékédou (Forest Region) were treated in the mission hospital at Bolahun in Liberia. VOGEL [1932] examined 81 persons at Tamassadou-Digbo (Téméssadou) in the administrative region of Guékédou (Forest Region) and found 75, or 92.6%, infected. GAUD [1955] reported a prevalence rate of 68% of 1,235 persons examined at Faranah (Upper Guinea) in 1938. DESCHIENS [1951] recorded foci of *S. mansoni* at Saukaran (correctly Sankaran) near Kankan (Upper Guinea) and at Macenta (Forest Region).

More recent information was collected in 1969 by AYAD according to the hospital returns and the returns of the 'Service National des Grandes Endémies' of the Ministry of Health and Social Affairs in Guinea for the year 1967. This is shown in table VI.

It should be noted, however, that microscopic examination of urine and/or stools is only performed for cases presenting at the hospitals with clear clinical manifestations of *S. haematobium* or *S. mansoni* and that the stools are examined only by the 'direct smear' method. There have been no mass population surveys, nor even spot surveys. Such surveys, using even the routine concentration sedimentation methods would, no doubt, reveal many more positive cases.

From table VI it is evident that both *S. haematobium* and *S. mansoni* are prevalent in Guinea, with the exception of Lower Guinea, where schistosomiasis is only indigenous in the Boké and Forécariah administrative regions. The absence of *S. haematobium* cases in Boké region and of *S. mansoni* in the Tougué region for the hospital returns of 1967 is not believed to be indicative. The cases recorded in the hospitals of Conakry are most probably imported, since the hospitals of the capital are usually attended by patients converging from all over the countryside. It can also be seen from the table that *S. mansoni* is generally speaking preponderant.

Molluscan intermediate hosts: *B. (Ph.) globosus* is no doubt an intermediate host of *S. haematobium* in Guinea, although VOGEL [1932] did not find infected specimens at Tamassadou. However, he demonstrated experimentally that *B. pfeifferi* from the same place was a host of *S. mansoni*.

References

DESCHIENS, R.: Bull. Soc. Path. exot. *44:* 350 (1951).
GAUD, J.: Bull. Wld Hlth Org. *13:* 209 (1955).
MAASS, E. and VOGEL, H.: Arch. Schiffs. Tropenhyg. *34:* 564 (1930).
VOGEL, H.: Arch. Schiffs. Tropenhyg. *36:* 108 (1932).

Sierra Leone

Both *S. haematobium* and *S. mansoni* occur in Sierra Leone. Schistosomiasis is confined to the hinterland and there is no evidence of transmission of the disease in the coastal areas.

The main foci of infection with *S. haematobium* occur in the eastern

Table VI. Number of detected schistosomiasis cases in the Republic of Guinea for the year 1967

Medical regions	Urinary	Intestinal	Total	Observations
Lower Guinea				
Boké	–	40	40	
Boffa	1	1	2	imported
Dubréka	–	3	3	imported
Forécariah	12	41	53	
Fria	1	5	6	imported
Kindia	–	36	36	
Télimelé	–	–	–	
Conakry	59	43	102	imported
Total	73	169	242	
Middle Guinea (Fouta Djallon)				
Mamou	25	18	43	
Dalaba	6	1	7	
Pita	–	–	–	
Labé	17	18	35	
Tougué	11	–	11	
Mali	1	50	51	
Gaoual	9	15	24	
Koundara	195	13	208	
Total	264	115	379	
Upper Guinea				
Kankan	146	239	385	
Dabola	8	139	147	
Faranah	24	28	52	
Dinguiraye	16	553	569	
Kérouané	5	15	20	
Kouroussa	88	186	214	
Siguiri	52	22	74	
Total	339	1,182	1,461	
Forest Region				
N'Zérékoré	109	98	207	
Beyla	248	390	638	
Macenta	333	181	514	
Kissidougou	657	1,037	1,694	
Guékédou	388	3,131	3,519	
Yomou	249	66	315	
Total	1,984	4,903	6,887	
Grand Total	2,660	6,369	8,969	

part of the country, ranging from Sinkunia in the north to Naiahun in the south.

BLACKLOCK [1924] carried out examinations in 30 villages, in 12 of which infection was undoubtedly acquired locally. Of the 808 individuals examined, including children, 668 were males of whom 199, or 29.7%, were infected; of 140 females, 106, or 75.7%, were positive.

GORDON et al. [1934] found 13% of 126 persons infected at Kabala. GERBER [1952] conducted 1,855 examinations on children and adults in the Boajibu area and obtained positives in 1,222, or 65%. In the nine villages investigated, the prevalence varied between 48 and 85%.

GAUD [1955] reported an infection rate at Bo of 26% in 1915 and 13% in 1917; no mention was made of the number of persons examined.

Information based on field observations and on visits to hospitals and health centres was recently collected by ALIO [1970]. In Southern Province, S. haematobium infection is common in out-patient clinics and among pregnant women. A survey in school-children born in Bo and with no extensive travel history showed a 64.3-percent infection rate. Dr. S. D. ONAMBAMIRO of the Department of Biological Sciences, Njala University, found a 7-percent infection rate in 551 urine samples from students in the college. However, no infection was detected in several other localities and towns such as Pujehun.

In Eastern Province haematuria is common in the following areas visited: Blama, Levuma, Boajibu, Kenema, Giema, Joru, Neama, Mobai (65-percent infection rate in school-children and severe clinical cases reported by Dr. KOBBA), Pendembu, Giehun, Bandajuma and Gandorhum. At Kailahun infections in small children as well as in adults are seen almost daily at the Government medical facilities. Many infections in children as young as three years of age are seen in Manowa. In the diamond-producing district of Kono, routine examination of urine in the Government and mining company hospitals during 1968 showed an average positive rate of 43.7% for S. haematobium. The infection has been recognized for years as autochthonous in the Sebgwema area.

In Northern Province urinary schistosomiasis is now widespread in Koinadugu District and in Tonkolili District but it is still not definitely recorded from west of the Bo–Magburaka road. There has always been the possibility that for chemical or physical reasons the host snails could not live in the western part of the country; their existence only above the 152-m contour has been striking.

Intestinal schistosomiasis from S. mansoni begins to appear as an endemic disease on the upland plateau at about 800 feet (240 m) elevation. Its distribution becomes regular approximately at the 1000-foot level (300 m) [ALIO, 1970].

GORDON et al. [1934] examined 215 persons in the Kabala region, of whom 20.9% were infected; these included 11.9% of 59 adult males, 29.5% of 51 adult females and 21.1% of 95 children under 15 years of age. Stool examinations carried out at Kabala and in Kabala area revealed an average infection rate of 40 and 45% respectively among the children examined. In Kono district routine examination of stools in Government and mining company hospitals showed a 10.6-percent positive rate for S. mansoni [ALIO, 1970].

BLACKLOCK and THOMPSON [1924] showed that B.(Ph.) globosus is the molluscan intermediate host of S. haematobium in Sierra Leone. B.(B.) forskalii was collected at Kabala by GORDON et al. [1934] but is not known to serve as an intermediate host.

B. pfeifferi transmits S. mansoni. Infected snail specimens have been collected in the north, in the Kabala, Benekoro and Sinkunia foci [GORDON et al., 1934] and in the south in the Sefadu area [ALIO, 1970].

References

ALIO, I.S.: Schistosomiasis in Sierra Leone. Report on a survey, 6 April–8 May 1970. WHO unpublished document, AFR/SCHIST/18 (1970).

BLACKLOCK, D.B.: Report on an investigation into the prevalence and transmission of human schistosomiasis in Sierra Leone; in Sierra Leone, Annual Report of the Medical and Sanitary Department for the Year 1923, Freetown, appendix XI, p. 80 (1924).

BLACKLOCK, D.B. and THOMPSON, M.G.: Ann. trop. Med. Parasit. 18: 211 (1924).

GAUD, J.: Bull. Wld Hlth Org. 13: 209 (1955).

GERBER, J.H.: J. trop. med. Hyg. 55: 52, 79 (1952).

GORDON, R.M.; DAVEY, T.H., and PEASTON, H.: Ann. trop. Med. Parasit. 28: 323 (1934).

Sierra Leone: Report of the Medical and Health Services for the Year 1959, Freetown, p. 10 (1959).

Liberia

S. haematobium infection is widely distributed over the northern part of the Western and Central Provinces, although the endemic areas are not continuous. The heavily forested regions of the Western Province do not appear to offer suitable habitats for the molluscan intermediate hosts.

MILLER [1957] conducted a single urine examination on 3,429 adult male employees of two rubber companies and a mining company, and found 865, or 25%, positive for S. haematobium eggs. These individuals represented some 40 regional groups and MILLER was, therefore, able to plot distribution in accordance with the areas from which the employees came, there being no transmission in the places of employment. Cases of schistosomiasis have been reported from Monrovia and other coastal areas of Liberia but they represent infection acquired up-country.

HARLEY [1933] recorded 236 cases of schistosomiasis among 6,291 consecutive dispensary patients at the Ganta Mission, including 21 persons infected with *S. mansoni*. No doubt many of these patients came from areas relatively far removed from Ganta. At a school of Bolahun VEATCH [1946] examined 96 boys of whom 12, or 12.5 %, were infected. There were three cases of infection with *S. mansoni* but this was probably acquired elsewhere. POINDEXTER [1949] reported on a survey of the leper colony at Sanoquelle and found 16 % of the inmates infected with *S. haematobium* and 2 % with *S. mansoni*. BURCH [1953] examined children at two mission schools in the Gbanga-Suakoko area of the Central Province and found that of 41 children at Gbanga, 19, or 46.3 %, had *S. haematobium* infection and 2 of 10 were infected with *S. mansoni*. At Suakoko, 11 of 36 children were infected with *S. haematobium* and 3 of 33 with *S. mansoni*. There was evidence of transmission in both areas. BURCH also reported 3 of 24 persons infected with *S. haematobium* at Yaindawuan and 8 of 24 at Chukpuzohn.

It is apparent that *S. haematobium* is far more prevalent in Liberia than is *S. mansoni*.

In a house-to-house survey carried out in 27 communities in the Central Province of Liberia, VOGEL [1958, 1959] undertook urine and stool examinations for the detection of helminth ova. The number of excreted *Schistosoma* ova was estimated. By examining Bulinid snails collected from the same localities, an attempt was made to distinguish between villages where schistosomiasis is autochthonous or imported.

S. haematobium: Fourteen communities were proved or strongly suspected to be foci of active transmission. Out of 1,181 persons living in these 14 villages 493 (41.7 %) excreted ova of *S. haematobium*. The percentage of positives varied from 23.1 to 58.5. It was 57.2 % in the 5- to 15-year age group and 21.7 % in persons aged 36 or more. The sex distribution was almost equal.

S. mansoni: Ten out of 24 communities where stools were examined had to be considered as foci of active transmission. In these ten localities, 198 of 602 persons examined discharged eggs of *S. mansoni*. The percentage of infection ranged from 20.1 to 61.0 with an average of 32.9. There was no marked difference in the infection rate observed in the age groups between 5 and 45 years, but in contrast to the results concerning

S. haematobium there was a striking and unexplained difference between males (24.9%) and females (41.3%). The number of ova excreted was also twice as high in females than in males.

No evidence was found to indicate that schistosomiasis caused by either species is transmitted in the coastal area and in the large eastern and western regions of dense forest.

Molluscan intermediate hosts: *B. (Ph.) globosus* was found to be naturally infected with *S. haematobium* by VOGEL [1958, 1959] in 12 different bodies of water. The species of the cercariae shed was confirmed by experimental infection of primates. Depending on place and season, the percentage of naturally infected snails varied between 2.9 and 59.5.

Experimental exposure of laboratory bred snails to miracidia of *S. haematobium* from Liberian patients showed that *B. (Ph.) globosus* was highly susceptible to the infection, whereas *B. (B.) truncatus* of Egyptian origin and *B. (B.) forskalii* (probably correctly named *B. (B.) senegalensis*) which is widespread in Liberia proved to be resistant.

B. pfeifferi was shown to be the intermediate host of *S. mansoni* and 0.8 to 44% of the snails collected from six streams or ponds shed cercariae of this species.

References

BURCH, T. A.: Quarterly Report, Laboratory of Tropical Diseases, National Institutes of Health, 30 June (1953).

HARLEY, G. W.: Amer. J. trop. Med. *13:* 67 (1933).

MILLER, M. J.: Amer. J. trop. Med. Hyg. *6:* 712 (1957).

POINDEXTER, H. A.: Amer. J. trop. Med. *29:* 435 (1949).

VEATCH, E. P.: Amer. J. trop. Med. *26:* suppl., vol. 5, p. 53 (1946).

VOGEL, H.: Ann. Rep. Res. Activ. Liberian Inst. Amer. Found. trop. Med. p. 40 (1958), p. 35 (1959).

Ivory Coast

Records for the Ivory Coast are very incomplete, and apparently few inquiries have been made concerning the distribution of schistosomiasis. GAUD [1955] recorded an infection rate of 32% from 185 individuals examined for *S. haematobium* at Zuenoula in 1943. DESCHIENS [1951] mentioned foci at Bouna, Bettié and Abidjan, and recorded *S. mansoni* infection also from Abidjan. DESCHIENS thought that the foci at Abidjan probably resulted from the influx of natives from Mali, Ghana and Upper Volta. The foci of *S. haematobium* in the north are adjacent to Upper Volta and exist along affluent streams of the Black Volta. In the south, foci are located along the Comoé River and other rivers in the area. In Adzopé and

Agboville sub-prefectures infection rates in a total population of over 150,000 inhabitants averaged 25% for *S. haematobium* and 3% for *S. mansoni* [CARRIÉ, 1970]. In six villages in the same area 45,366 children, i. e. 80% of the child population up to 15 years of age, were examined; less than half this number was free of infection; 46.5% were infected with *S. haematobium*, 9.1% with *S. mansoni* and 5% with both species [PAIL-LERETS *et al.*, 1970].

GAUD [1955] estimated the average infection rate for *S. haematobium* to be 5%, but DESCHIENS [1951] placed this at 37%. For *S. mansoni*, GAUD gave an average rate of 1.6%, and DESCHIENS 0.5%. McMULLEN and FRANCOTTE [1961] estimated the number of people infected with schistosomiasis at 700,000, a figure which was confirmed by RIVES [1965].

BINDER [1957] recorded *B. (Ph.) globosus* from the environs of Gagnoa, Lacota, Divo and Agboville where the species appeared to be widespread. *B. (B.) forskalii* was found around the lagoons at Bingerville, Dabou and Toupah. The species was also located in temporary pools at Sangon-Agban and in a small lake near Toumodi.

References
BINDER, E.: Bull. Inst. franç. Afr. noire *19:* ser. A., p. 97 (1957).
CARRIÉ, J.: Méd. Afr. noire *17:* 531 (1970).
DESCHIENS, R.: Bull. Soc. Path. exot. *44:* 631 (1951).
GAUD, J.: Bull. Wld Hlth Org. *13:* 209 (1955).
McMULLEN, D.B. and FRANCOTTE, J.: Report of the preliminary survey by the Bilharziasis Advisory Team, 1960. II. Republic of the Ivory Coast. WHO unpublished document, MHO/PA/47.61 (1961).
PAILLERETS, F. DE; CARRIÉ, J.; CARRIÉ, A. L.,and PLUMEAU, R.: Méd. Afr. noire *17:* 541 (1970).
RIVES: in Rapport final de la Cinquième Conférence technique de l'OCCGE, Bobo-Dioulasso 1965, vol. 2, p. 601 (1965).

Upper Volta
Urinary schistosomiasis is widely distributed throughout the country. Intestinal schistosomiasis is more limited in extent but, since stool examinations are conducted less frequently than urine examinations, data on distribution are meagre.

MARILL [1957] believed that the whole of the Voltaic plateaux from the Niger to the Sudan comprised a vast area of endemicity for *S. haematobium* and that it is no longer justifiable to refer to individual foci in this region. GAUD [1955] gave a range of prevalence between 6 and 85% with an average of 30%. DESCHIENS [1952] believed the average to be about 46%. McMULLEN and FRANCOTTE [1962] estimated that 50% of the population, or more than 1,500,000 people, are infected at some period during their lives.

Prevalence rates of *S. haematobium* vary widely. GAUD [1955] reported rates from 11 communities with variations from 6% at Bobo-Dioulasso (Koumi) to 88% at Ouagadougou. MARILL [1957] examined 1,308 individuals in 19 communities in the vicinity of Houndé, and found 409, or 31.2%, positive.

McMULLEN and FRANCOTTE [1962] summarized available data from examinations in 15 administrative divisions and indicated villages in which less specific information was obtained. In villages in the former group, a total of 18,918 children were examined, of whom 5,500, or 29.1%, were positive; of 21,635 adults, 6,100, or 28.1%, were infected. There was little difference in prevalence rates between sexes in the adult group but a higher percentage of boys than girls were positive (57 against 27%). Of the villages surveyed, two had 100% infections, five had none, and 34 had more than 50%.

Reporting on a pilot survey undertaken to test a sedimentation technique newly developed for screening purposes, ALAUSE [1969] indicated having found the following prevalence figures: 41% of 672 inhabitants (45% of the village population) at Karankasso in the Bobo-Dioulasso Cercle; 18% of 277 people examined at Silaleba, a village more than 10 km away from Lake Bam; 40% of 295 people examined at Kourpelé at some distance from the same lake; and 37% of 470 people examined in the fishing village of Bam. The last three villages are situated in the Kongoussi area.

From the limited evidence available, it is not possible to determine areas which possess the highest prevalence rates. *S. haematobium* appears to be less extensively distributed in the eastern part of the country, but this impression may not be valid because fewer surveys have been conducted there.

As previously mentioned, valid data are inadequate concerning the distribution and extent of *S. mansoni* infection. DESCHIENS [1952] reported the parasite at Ouagadougou and Bobo-Dioulasso and estimated that 8% of the population was infected. McMULLEN and FRANCOTTE [1962] stated that the parasite has been reported from eight areas but all town reports were from hospital centres. These authors stated that scattered transmission sites may occur throughout the Black Volta and Comoé watersheds in the south-western part of the country. Foci may also be present in the lower reaches of the White Volta.

Bulinus (Physopsis) sp. and *B. (B.) forskalii* are widely distributed and the former is no doubt the chief molluscan intermediate host of *S. haematobium*. Specific determination has apparently not been made.

Biomphalaria sp. has been reported in a few areas.

References

ALAUSE, P.: in Rapport final de la Neuvième Conférence technique de l'OCCGE, Bobo-Dioulasso 1969, vol. 1, p. 58 (1969).

DESCHIENS, R.: Le problème sanitaire des bilharzioses dans les territoires de l'Union française. Monogr. V, Soc. Path. exot. (Masson, Paris 1952).

GAUD, J.: Bull. Wld Hlth Org. *13:* 209 (1955).

McMULLEN, D. B. and FRANCOTTE, J.: Bull. Wld Hlth Org. *27:* 5 (1962).

MARILL, F.-G.: Bull. Acad. nat. Méd., Paris *141:* 398 (1957).

SANSARRICQ, H.: Méd. trop. *19:* 345 (1959).

Ghana

Reasonably reliable data on the distribution and prevalence of *S. haematobium* are becoming available; systematic surveys at most villages in two thirds of the country have been completed. However, surveys in the eastern, central and western regions of the country have still to be undertaken. From the available data it is estimated that 15 to 20% of the total population (over 1,000,000 persons) have become infected with *S. haematobium* at some time in their lives but usually during childhood. Diagnosis of the infection is more rarely made in adults, but at some endemic foci high infection rates are recorded even in the older age groups [ONORI *et al.* 1963].

In the freshwater lagoons and swamps associated with the delta of the Volta River, schistosomiasis can be considered to be an occupational disease intimately allied to fishing activities and clam cultivation; the same hazard applies to the labourers who carry out weed-clearing at Owabi reservoir near Kumasi. With increasing distance from lagoon transmission sites, prevalence of the disease decreases, especially among the younger age groups (a 96-percent infection rate falling to 5% at a distance of 8 to 12 miles away), and the difference between infection rates in males and females increases [PAPERNA, 1968a; WATSON, 1970]. The prevalence of infection according to sex varies in different parts of the country [ONORI *et al.,* 1963]. In northern Ghana it is probable that *S. haematobium* infection is more common in boys than in girls due to different water-usage habits. Generally, transmission of infection is associated with such activities as washing, swimming and fishing in sites where the snail hosts occur. However, it has been frequently observed that if a pond or dam is used solely as a source of drinking water or for the washing of clothes, transmission does not then occur.

A conspicuous feature of the distribution of *S. haematobium* in Ghana is its sporadic occurrence and what can be described as 'blanket' distribution is found only in the north-east and south-east corners of the country [McCULLOUGH and ODEI, 1966]. In the central basin of the Volta drainage system endemic foci of urinary schistosomiasis are rare because, as described later, of the scarcity of the snail hosts in that area. The main factors influencing the distribution of schistosomiasis in Ghana are (a) human population density, and (b) geology with particular reference to the surface water supply; lesser factors include the extent of the primary forest, population movement, type of settlement, water body characteristics and location, water-usage habits, etc. All of these factors not only interact but in the course of time are liable to change markedly; such dynamics must be taken into consideration when control measures are being planned.

An interesting feature of *S. haematobium* in Ghana is the existence of local strains which are adapted to develop, apparently exclusively, in either *B. (Ph.) globosus* or *B. (B.) truncatus rohlfsi* [McCULLOUGH, 1959, 1962a, b]. Further elucidation of this problem is desirable.

Although *S. mansoni* is much rarer than *S. haematobium* and its distribution is sporadic, important foci occur at Tarkwa in South-West Ghana, at Wa in North-West Ghana, at several centres (Bawku, Zebilla, Navrongo, Wilaga, etc.) in the extreme north-east of the country, and at the villages of Nyive and Atikpui near Ho in the Volta region. Systematic stool surveys have been carried out in only a few areas and the total prevalence of *S. mansoni* cannot be accurately estimated at the present time. However, it is probable that less than 0.5% of the total population of Ghana harbour this parasite. The snail hosts of *S. mansoni* are far more widely distributed than the endemic foci of the disease. The factors which influence the distribution of *S. mansoni* in Ghana are similar to those described above for *S. haematobium*. In this connexion, it is worth mentioning that *Biomphalaria* spp. appear to have greater need of habitats with permanent water than do the snail hosts of *S. haematobium*.

Transmission sites: Natural water bodies and those produced by water conservation programmes are the major sources of transmission. During the 7-Year Development Plan it is expected to irrigate about 3,238 km² mainly in the eastern Accra plains and in northern Ghana [TAGOE, 1965]. Barrages have been constructed in many watercourses in Ghana; this has encouraged the breeding and survival of the snail hosts and has thus facilitated the transmission of the parasites. Examples of this type of water conservation are found at Wa. In northern Ghana, in the southern Volta region and in the Accra Plains, numerous dams have been built to conserve water during the long dry season; these are seldom protected from the point of view of schistosomiasis transmission. Nevertheless, while artificial water bodies are playing an increasing role in Ghana, transmission at the present time occurs far more commonly in the natural water sources of the country.

Molluscan intermediate hosts: Observations on the distribution of the snail hosts have been carried out regularly since 1951 [McCULLOUGH, 1956, 1957, 1962 a b; ODEI, 1964; ONORI et al., 1963].

S. haematobium is transmitted by *B. (Ph.) globosus,* which is by far the most important snail host, and is found in all the major watersheds. *B. (B.) truncatus rohlfsi* is probably the exclusive transmitter in South-East Ghana and at Tamale and Fuu in the north.

B. (B.) forskalii is very widespread and common but its role in *S. haematobium* transmission in Ghana is equivocal. If this species is subsequently established to be capable of transmitting *S. haematobium,* its significance in this respect is likely to remain of minor importance and restricted to only a few localities.

Biomphalaria spp. are widely distributed in both the forest and savannah vegetational zones.

S. mansoni is transmitted by *B. pfeifferi (gaudi)* but *B. sudanica* has also recently been recorded at several widely scattered localities in Ghana. Although the latter species can transmit the West Africa strain of *S. mansoni* its role in transmission is apparently insignificant as there is no evidence that the disease is endemic at Akuse or Nkinkasu where the snails most commonly occur. However, ONORI [1965] showed that *B. sudanica* was susceptible to infection with a local strain of *S. mansoni,* thus indicating that it may be involved in transmission.

Perhaps the most interesting feature of the distribution of the snail hosts, particularly *Biomphalaria* and *B. (Ph.) globosus,* in Ghana is their relative scarcity in the large area of the Voltaian rock series. The scarcity of the snail hosts in this area is probably associated with the long seasonal shortage of surface water, typical of the Voltaian series.

While prior to about 1950 the distribution of the snail hosts in Ghana was intimately associated with natural freshwater bodies, man-made habitats have subsequently played an increasingly important role in this respect. With the implementation of the Volta River Project, the large irrigation schemes being planned and the ever increasing number of small dams being built in the drier areas, the prospect of a markedly more widespread distribution of the snail hosts is inevitable. In particular, it will be noted that the great Volta dam lies entirely within the area of the Voltaian rock series where, formerly, the snail hosts have been rare. The ecological situation has now completely changed as a result of the filling-up of the Volta Lake and *Bulinus* spp. have become very common [PAPERNA, 1968b; OBENG, 1969].

References

McCULLOUGH, F.S.: Trans. roy. Soc. trop. Med. Hyg. *50:* 449 (1956).

McCULLOUGH, F.S.: W. afr. med. J. *6:* 98 (1957).

McCULLOUGH, F.S.: Bull. Wld Hlth Org. *20:* 75 (1959).

McCULLOUGH, F.S.: Ann. trop. Med. Parasit. *56:* 53 (1962a).

McCULLOUGH, F.S.: Bull. Wld Hlth Org. *27:* 161 (1962b).

McCULLOUGH, F.S.: Assignment report on Ghana 5 Project. WHO unpublished document, AFR/BILHARZ/12 (1965).

McCULLOUGH, F.S. and ODEI, M.A.: Schistosomiasis in Ghana: present knowledge and future prospects; in CORRADETTI Proceedings of the First International Congress of Parasitology, Rome 1964, vol. 2, p. 727 (Pergamon Press, New York/Tamburini Editore, Milano 1966).

OBENG, L.E.: in OBENG Man-made lakes: The Accra Symposium, p. 320 (Accra) (1969).

ODEI, M.A.: W. Afr. med. J. *13:* 60 (1964).

ONORI, E.: W. Afr. med. J. *14:* 3 (1965).

ONORI, E.; McCULLOUGH, F.S., and ROSEI, L.: Ann. trop. Med. Parasit. *57:* 59 (1963).

PAPERNA, I.: Ghana med. J. *7:* 210 (1968a).

PAPERNA, I.: Ghana J. Sci. *8:* 30 (1968b).

TAGOE, C.E.: Irrigation and land reclamation in Ghana. Paper read at Symposium on Bilharziasis in Ghana, Accra, 15–16 March 1965; cited by McCULLOUGH, 1965 (1965).

WATSON, J.: Asutsuare Pilot Irrigation Development Scheme. Health Component. Assignment Report, July 1970. WHO unpublished document (1970).

Togo

Both *S. haematobium* and *S. mansoni* are endemic although the former predominates. Data are limited but schistosomiasis is no doubt far more widely distributed than records indicate.

GAUD [1955] mentioned prevalence rates for *S. haematobium* varying between 4 and 80%. The highest rate was at Agomé on Lake Togo. GAUD estimated an average infection rate for the country of 5%, while DESCHIENS [1951] put the figure at 4%.

McMULLEN and BUZO [1960] cite specific surveys in school-children in certain areas. At Kandé the rate was 31%; at Tchitchao 44.7% with haematuria, and at Avévé 30.7%. These authors noted that BARADAT [1952] conducted surveys in the Anecho District and that AMORIN [1958] included the disease in a survey of hospital and public health reports from 1934 to 1954. However, hospital data are not usually helpful in determining distribution of a disease since in rural Africa patients frequently travel long distances to seek medical treatment. Neither of the above reports has been published.

McMullen and Buzo [1960] believed that transmission takes place in each of the 10 districts of the country but that there appear to be two general areas where the prevalence is relatively high. One of these is in the southern part of the country in the Districts of Tsévié and Anecho in the marshy areas or in the vicinity of slow-moving streams that form the drainage systems of the Mono, Haho and Sio Rivers. The other principal focus is in the vicinity of Lama-Kara, Pagouda and Niamtougou, in the upper reaches of the Kara and Koumaga River watersheds. Tibou, Kousmondé, Kolowaré, Koussoumtou, Fasoa and some villages in the Klouto District appear to be transmission sites of secondary importance.

There is little evidence concerning the distribution of *S. mansoni* in Togo. It has been reported from near Agomé and at Sokoda. McMullen and Buzo [1960] stated that the species is found only in the northern half of the country.

Little is known concerning the species of molluscan intermediate hosts responsible for transmission in Togo; *Bulinus (Ph.)* sp. is said to be rather generally distributed and *B. (B.) forskalii* also occurs. McMullen and Buzo [1960] indicated that *Biomphalaria* sp. is found only in the northern half of the country.

References

Amorin, J.: Panorama de l'évolution de la pathologie au Togo sous tutelle française de 1934 à 1954; Doctoral thesis; cited by McMullen and Buzo, 1960 (1958).
Baradat, J.: Enquête sur la bilharziose dans le cercle d'Anecho. Unpublished document (1952).
Deschiens, R.: Bull. Soc. Path. exot. *44:* 350 (1951).
Gaud, J.: Bull. Wld Hlth Org. *13:* 209 (1955).
McMullen, D.B. and Buzo, Z.J.: Report of the preliminary survey by the Bilharziasis Advisory Team, 1959. V. Togo. WHO unpublished document, MHO/PA/55.60 (1960).

Dahomey

Published information concerning schistosomiasis in the Republic of Dahomey is extremely limited.

In a survey undertaken to assess the health aspects of an irrigation scheme for agricultural development in the valley of the Ouémé River, more than 80% of the school-children examined were found to be infected [MICHEJDA, 1970].

GAUD [1955] reported *S. haematobium* prevalence rates of 4% at Porto Novo (Attaké), 8% at Porto Novo (Bekon), 60% at Savalou (Agouagon), 8% at Parakou and 25% at Abomey. The parasite has also been reported from Cotonou [DESCHIENS, 1951]. The same author indicated that the average rate for the country was 27%.

DESCHIENS [1951] noted foci of *S. mansoni* at Savalou and Cotonou, and estimated the average prevalence rate for the country at 0.2%.

No systematic surveys on the distribution of molluscan intermediate hosts have apparently been conducted. GAUD [1955] recorded *B. (B.) forskalii* from Ouidah and Porto Novo and MANDAHL-BARTH [1957] also noted this species from Porto Novo. DESCHIENS [1951] mentioned *B. (Ph.) africanus* and *B. dybowski (B. truncatus)* as intermediate hosts of *S. haematobium* and *B. pfeifferi* as the host of *S. mansoni*.

References

DESCHIENS, R.: Bull. Soc. Path. exot. *44:* 350, 631 (1951).
GAUD, J.: Bull. Wld Hlth Org. *13:* 209 (1955).
MANDAHL-BARTH, G.: Bull. Wld Hlth Org. *17:* 1 (1957).
MICHEJDA, J.: Mission interdisciplinaire du PNUD pour le développement intégré du bassin du fleuve Niger. Problèmes de santé publique. Rapport. WHO unpublished document (1970).

Niger

There is a paucity of information concerning schistosomiasis in the Niger Republic. No recent data are available. GAUD [1955] noted prevalence rates for *S. haematobium* of 40 and 60% in Zinder and adjacent areas and a rate of 33% at Tanout. DESCHIENS [1951] reported additional foci at Tillabery, Niamey, Dasso, Birni-N'Konni and N'Guigmi. According to CHAMORIN [1965] eggs of *S. haematobium* were found in 44.61% of 13,857 urine examinations made in 1964 in the Tillabery Cercle; 68% of the persons infected were school-children from 6 to 12 years of age. In the Magaria Cercle 21.12% of 1,008 urine samples were found to be positive and at Tessahoua the proportion was 25.04% of 1,174 individuals. Of 1,420 urine samples taken from nomad people 11.26% were positive. Prevalence is highest among populations along the River Niger (44.61%). *S. mansoni* has not been reported from Niger.

B. (Ph.) globosus has been found at a location near the Nigerian border east of Maradi and *B. (B.) forskalii* and *Bulinus (B.)* spp. near Zinder.

WRIGHT [1959] reported *B.(B.) senegalensis* from Dungas, south-east of Zinder.

References

CHAMORIN: in Rapport final de la Cinquième Conférence technique de l'OCCGE, Bobo-Dioulasso 1965, vol. 2, p. 609 (1965).
DESCHIENS, R.: Bull. Soc. Path. exot. *44:* 350 (1951).
GAUD, J.: Bull. Wld Hlth Org. *13:* 209 (1955).
WRIGHT, C. A.: W. afr. med. J. *8:* 142 (1959).

Nigeria

Both *S. haematobium* and *S. mansoni* are prevalent in Nigeria, although the former species is more widely distributed. The best source of information about the general distribution of schistosomiasis in the country is COWPER'S review [1963] from which most of the following data are taken. No doubt there are in existence many foci which have remained undetected or unrecorded.

S. haematobium: This parasite is endemic throughout the Northern Region. Heavy infection rates are recorded in the area extending from Katsina, Kano, Kankija, Zaria and Kaduna to the western frontier in the region of Birnin, Kebbi and Argungu. In parts of the area infection rates of over 90% have been found. In a study of 4,574 males in Zaria, BLAIR [1956] showed an over-all prevalence rate of 32%, with the highest rate in young teenagers. The north is probably the most heavily infected area in Nigeria, followed in turn by the south-western region. Other parts of the Northern Region in which high or fairly high rates have been found include the Plateau area, the Zinna-Yola-Biu area, the Maiduguri-Potiskum area, the Wulgo region of the Lake Chad basin, the riverine area along the Niger from Wawa to Pategi, and Bida. In the latter area, which is the present site of Kainji Dam, the infection rate of *S. haematobium* varies from 3% at Wawa to 87% in children at Bacita.

Urinary schistosomiasis is almost certainly universal throughout the Western Region, with high or very high incidence in three areas. The first extends from the coast at Badagry and Epe north to the Oyo-Oshogbo-Iseyin region, with especially high figures in and near Ibadan, Abeokuta, Epe and Ijebu-Ode. A second heavily infected area centres around Ondo, and extends north to Addo-Ekiti and south to Okitipupa. The third area is in the south-eastern part in the creeks and delta country, as well as further inland; here it extends from Benin to Burutu on the coast. In the Western Region, the coastal belt is almost free from infection, which tends to increase as one proceeds inland. OLDENBURG [1942] found an infection rate of up to 54% in school-children at Abeokuta. COWPER and WOODWARD [1961] found that in routine examinations on in-patients at University College Hospital, Ibadan, 3.1% of 8,662 individuals were positive. In the same town, 91% of 78 school-children were found to be infected, and intravenous pyelography revealed severe lesions of the urinary tract in a significant percentage of children examined [GILLES et al., 1965a]. Still in Ibadan, S. haematobium eggs were found in 3.3 to 58.8% of 3,000 children from 13 schools, and 17.4% of 279 preschool-children; the earliest age of infection was two years [SIEGAL, 1968]. At Epe, OKPALA [1961] showed that up to 90.9% of 1,325 school-children were infected, and GILLES et al. [1965b] found 50% of 94 boatmen infected.

The savannah area southwest of the confluence of Rivers Niger and Benue is endemic for S. haematobium [ELLIS et al., 1968].

S. haematobium is less common in the Eastern Region than elsewhere. It is more prevalent in Ogoja Province than in other parts of the region; another area of endemicity is located around Owerri, where OLDENBURG [1942] reported infection rates of up to 30%.

S. mansoni: In the Northern Region, intestinal schistosomiasis is almost as widespread as the urinary form but is less frequently recorded because of greater difficulties in diagnosis. In the Niger River area in Ilorin Province over-all figures up to 78% were recorded in the Share-Pategi region and 9.4% at Wawa. Significantly, the use of concentration techniques raised the figure from 2 to 9.4% in the Wawa district and from 30 to 78% in the Share district. The approximate area from Garagini to Pategi is the most heavily infected zone of the Northern Region. On the eastern escarpment of the Plateau only low prevalence rates have been recorded. In the north, RAMSAY [1934, 1935] reported the highest prevalence rate at Yola. Figures of over 20% have been recorded from Bida, Sokoto, Jos and Bauchi.

S. mansoni is encountered less frequently in the Western Region, although centres of endemicity exist around Ibadan, Epe, Akure and Ado-Ekiti. BLAIR [1956] recorded a rate of 2% at Epe.

According to COWPER [1963] there are no records of the occurrence of S. mansoni in the Eastern Region.

Schistosomiasis in Nigeria is likely to increase, with two major factors contributing to this spread. Firstly, the construction of the Kainji dam and the creation of a man-made lake along with other smaller water impoundment projects in the country will provide excellent habitats and breeding sites for the snail intermediate hosts. Secondly, the increased mobility of the people from regions in the east will unfortunately aid in spreading schistosomiasis in areas formerly free from the disease.

A great variety of vertebrates dissected for *S. haematobium* and *S. mansoni* infections proved negative in Ibadan. Pigs infected with *S. haematobium* cercariae did not yield any adult worms [HIRA, 1970].

Molluscan intermediate hosts: As in other areas of West Africa, there are apparently two distinct strains of *S. haematobium,* one transmitted by *B.(Ph.) globosus* and the other by *B.(B.) truncatus rohlfsi.* The former species is without doubt the most common host in Nigeria. According to COWPER [1963], both of these species have never been infected with *S. haematobium* miracidia from the same specimen of urine. *B.(B.) truncatus rohlfsi* has been recorded from Ibadan, Epe and Akura in the western region and from the Wulgo area in the northern region.

B.(B.) senegalensis, a potential host in West Africa, has been reported by WRIGHT [1959] from Katsina, although only on the basis of a single dead shell.

B.(B.) forskalii, also a potential host of *S. haematobium,* has been recorded from a number of areas in Nigeria, but is not actually known to be involved in the transmission of the disease. However, ODEI [1961] mentions a WHO report of 1953 incriminating it as an intermediate host at Tudun Wada near Zaria. Confirmation of this role for the species in Nigeria is required.

There are many records of unidentified *Bulinus* spp. from various parts of Nigeria. COWPER [1963] believed that the majority probably represented *B.(Ph.) globosus.*

In Nigeria *S. mansoni* is transmitted by *B. pfeifferi.*

Recently, the WHO Schistosomiasis Research Team based in Ibadan discovered near this town the presence of yet another snail intermediate host, *B. camerunensis,* which was formerly known to exist only in the Congo and Cameroon.

References

BLAIR, D. M.: Bull. Wld Hlth Org. *15:* 203 (1956).

COWPER, S. G.: Ann. trop. Med. Parasit. *57:* 307 (1963).

COWPER, S. G. and WOODWARD, S. F.: W. afr. med. J. *10:* 366 (1961).

ELLIS, C. R., jr.; LONG, S., and FRIEDLAND, G.: W. afr. med. J. *17:* 21 (1968).

GILLES, H. M.; LUCAS, A.; ADENIYI-JONES, C.; LINDNER, R.; ANAND, S. V.; BRABAND, H.; COCKSHOTT, W. P.; COWPER, S. G.; MULLER, R. L.; HIRA, P. R., and WILSON, A. M. M.: Ann. trop. Med. Parasit. *59:* 441 (1965a).

GILLES, H. M.; LUCAS, A.; LINDNER, R.; COCKSHOTT, W. P.; ANAND, S. V.; IKEME, A., and COWPER, S. G.: Ann. trop. Med. Parasit. *59:* 451 (1965b).

HIRA, P. R.: W. afr. med. J. *19:* 57 (1970).
ODEI, M. A.: J. trop. med. Hyg. *64:* 27 (1961).
OKPALA, I.: W. afr. med. J. *10:* 402 (1961).
OLDENBURG, E.: Dtsch. tropenmed. Z. *46:* 193 (1942).
RAMSAY, G. W. ST. C.: W. afr. med. J. *8:* 2 (1934).
RAMSAY, G. W. ST. C.: W. afr. med. J. *8:* 217 (1935).
SIEGAL, F. M.: Amer. J. trop. Med. Hyg. *17:* 737 (1968).
WRIGHT, C. A.: W. afr. med. J. *8:* 142 (1959).

Cameroon

Most of the information given below is derived from the reviews by
DESCHIENS *et al.* [1968] and MBARGA [1970]. *S. haematobium, S. mansoni*
and *S. intercalatum* are probably more widely distributed than available
data indicate.

S. haematobium is found all over North Cameroon from Lake Chad to
the northern slopes of the Adamaoua plateau [MOUCHET and DELAS, 1960].
Prevalence rates of 90 to 98% have been recorded on the flood plains of
the Logone River and in the Mayo-Danai. GAUD [1955] reported 4%
positive of 57 persons at Goulfei, 8% of 40 at Maltam, and 13% of 59 at
Kousseri. AZEVEDO [1956] noted that the areas of highest prevalence were
around Yagoua (98%), Maroua and Mokolo (50%). Another important
area appears to lie between Wulgo and Lake Chad, a district in which
extensive irrigation is carried out [AZEVEDO, 1958]. GAUD [1955] estimated
the prevalence of *S. haematobium* in northern Cameroon to average 15%
of a population of 195,000 and DESCHIENS *et al.* [1968] at 15 to 20%.

Secondary foci created as a result of temporary or permanent settling
of infected people coming from the northern endemic areas are to be found
in Ngaoundéré, Bafia on the M'Bam River (over 60% prevalence) and
Bertoua. Other autochthonous foci, some of which have long been known,
are situated in the areas of the Barombi-Mbo Lake (near Kumba, over 80%
prevalence), the Barombi-Kotto Lake (45 to 95% prevalence) [DUKE,
1970], Kotto Strangers, and Barombi-Kotto New Town in West Cameroon
(99 and 76% prevalence) [ZAHRA, 1953], the Mungo focus (10% prevalence at Njombe) [CASANOVA, 1967], the Kribi focus and the foci in the
Lom, Djerem and Kadei (over 50% prevalence) river valleys in the east.

S. mansoni is well distributed in Cameroon. In the north GUYON'S
report [1965] noted high prevalence of *S. mansoni* at Fort Foureau,
Maroua, Yagoua and Guider. This species is often associated with *S.
haematobium* in Diamare department and is frequently observed in the
north-western mountainous areas [MOUCHET and DELAS, 1960] where

prevalence reaches 30% at Godola. This infection is predominant on the Adamaoua plateau – Ngaounderé town 6%, Dourou plain 26%, Meiganga 16%, Tibati 5%, Tignéré 6% [OLIVIER and BUZO, 1964]. This large focus extends toward the south into the department of M'Bam.

In the southern parts of Central Cameroon, the disease is endemic in certain town areas. GARIOU et al. [1961] believed that the establishment of fish ponds in the vicinity (now included in the town) of Yaoundé was followed by the introduction of S. mansoni. This was confirmed later when 54 to 74% prevalence rates were recorded in the area [DELAS et al., 1968; NGALLE-EDIMO et al., 1970].

S. mansoni foci also occur in the west and south, in particular at Ebolowa in Ntem department as well as in Kribi and Mungo.

In recent years, several foci of S. intercalatum have been discovered in the forest and savannah zones in the south and south-west of the country, e.g. Edéa in Sanaga Maritime; Eséka in Nyong and Kélé; Obala, M'Balmayo and Yaoundé in Nyong and Sanaga; Bokito in M'Bam; and Penja in Mungo. Infection rates range from 15 to 25% [MBARGA, 1970]. Cases have also been found in Garoua, Benue Department and at Maroua in Diamare in the north [DESCHIENS and DELAS, 1969]. According to MBARGA, 121,917 new cases have been detected in the country in the course of survey work from 1960 to 1969 inclusive.

In North Cameroon S. haematobium is transmitted by B. truncatus, B. globosus and B. africanus [LANDON, 1960; DESCHIENS et al., 1968]. B. truncatus occurs in Central Cameroon and B. truncatus rohlfsi in West and South Cameroon. WRIGHT [1965] demonstrated that B. (B.) truncatus rohlfsi is the intermediate host in the Barombi lakes region, as is B. (B.) camerunensis in Barombi Kotto Lake [DUKE, 1970].

B. pfeifferi is an intermediate host in the Adamaoua and was collected from Lake Wum in western Cameroon by WRIGHT [1965], although S. mansoni is apparently not endemic in the area. B. camerunensis is commonly encountered in the Adamaoua and in Central and South Cameroon.

To date the only species identified as host of S. intercalatum in Cameroon is B. (P.) forskalii.

References

AZEVEDO, J. FRAGA DE: Rapport sur les bilharzioses humaines au Cameroun français. WHO unpublished document, WHO/BIL.CONF/49 (1956).

AZEVEDO, J. FRAGA DE: Bull. Wld Hlth Org. *18:* 1052 (1958).

CASANOVA, B.: Enquête sur la bilharziose à Njombe. Rapport du Service des grandes endémies (SGE) (1967).

DELAS, A.; DESCHIENS, R.; NGALLE-EDIMO, S., and POIRIER, A.: Bull. Soc. Path. exot. *61:* 625 (1968).

DESCHIENS, R. and DELAS, A. E.: Trans. roy. Soc. trop. Med. Hyg. *63:* suppl., vol. 57 (1969).

DESCHIENS, R.; DELAS, A.; NGALLE-EDIMO, S., and POIRIER, A.: Bull. Soc. Path. exot. *61:* 772 (1968).

DESCHIENS, R.; DELAS, A.; NGALLE-EDIMO, S., and POIRIER, A.: Bull. Wld Hlth Org. *40:* 893 (1969).

DUKE, B.O.L.: In Rapport final de la Ve Conférence technique de l'oceac, Yaoundé, 1970, vol. 2, p. 403 (1970).

GARIOU, J.; GAMET, A., and LANDON, A.: Bull. Soc. Path. exot. *54:* 1053 (1961).

GAUD, J.: Bull. Wld Hlth Org. *13:* 209 (1955).

GUYON: in Rapport final de la Première Conférence technique de l'OCCGEAC, Yaoundé 1965, vol. 1, p. 133 (1965).

LANDON, A.: Aperçus sur la bilharziose au Cameroun; in Rapport de l'Institut Pasteur du Cameroun (1960).

MBARGA, J.R.: Les bilharzioses humaines au Cameroun. Document (1970).

MOUCHET et DELAS, A.: Enquêtes préliminaires sur les bilharzioses dans le Nord Cameroun. Rapport SIIMP, ORSTOM (1960).

OLIVIER, L.J. and BUZO, Z.J.: Report on bilharziasis in Cameroon, based on a visit by the Inter-regional Bilharziasis Advisory Team, 3–8 June 1964. WHO unpublished document, PA/13.65 (1964).

WRIGHT, C.A.: Bull. Brit. Mus. (nat. Hist.) Zool. *13:* 75 (1965).

ZAHRA, A.: W. afr. med. J. *2:* 26 (1953).

Gabon

Schistosomiasis in Gabon is known from only a few localities and in many of these transmission appears to be at a low level. However, very few investigations have been conducted and additional search may disclose new foci. This country is characterized by virgin equatorial forest which appears to be inimical to snail intermediate hosts. Nevertheless, schistosomiasis cases are reported from all medical sectors [GATEFF *et al.,* 1970].

Several foci of *S. haematobium* have recently been discovered, namely in the N'Dende area whose epicentre is situated at Monkoro near the Congo border; in Nyanga (Doussala); at Palmaveas (Moyen Ogooué) and along the M'binie River [GILLES, 1970].

S. intercalatum cases have been reported from Libreville, Lambaréné and N'Djole. LALOUEL [1954] stated that 30 cases were diagnosed in 1953 at Libreville and indicated that the endemic focus was near the hospital. GAUD and JAUBERTIE [1951] recorded a substantial number of cases of *S. mansoni* from Kouilou, most of which apparently originated in the interior and were treated at Pointe-Noire; the same authors mention one case at Pool and three at Likouala-Mossaka. BECQUET [1967] reported Libreville and the Ogooué region as the principal foci of *S. intercalatum*

in Gabon. DESCHIENS and POIRIER [1967] found an infection rate of 18 %
of *S. intercalatum* in 561 adults at Libreville, rates of 7 to 15 % in school-
children between the ages of 6 and 10 years, and rates of 6 to 23 % in
those between the ages of 10 and 15 years. According to GILLES [1970],
cases have been reported to occur in all medical sectors, and in 1969,
4.6 % positives were found in 29,220 stool examinations performed at the
National Laboratory.

DESCHIENS [1952] stated that foci of *S. mansoni* exist at Lambaréné
and N'Djole with an additional focus at Oyem. Confirmatory evidence is
needed concerning the occurrence of *S. mansoni* in Gabon.

Little is known regarding molluscan intermediate hosts. *Biomphalaria*
spp. have been reported from N'Djole and *B. pfeifferi* from the Ogooué
Basin. *B. (Ph.) globosus* and *B. (B.) forskalii* have been found in the same
general area. The latter species is the intermediate host snail of *S. intercalatum*.

References

BECQUET, R.: Ann. Soc. belge Med. trop. *47:* 35 (1967).
DESCHIENS, R.: Le problème sanitaire des bilharzioses dans les territoires de l'Union fran-
    çaise. Monogr. V, Soc. Path. exot. (Masson, Paris 1952).
DESCHIENS, R. and POIRIER, A.: Bull. Soc. Path. exot. *60:* 228 (1967).
GATEFF, C.; LEMARINIER, G.; LABUSQUIÈRE, R., and NEBOUT, M.: Epidemiological impor-
    tance of bilharziasis within Member States of OCED. OAU Symposium on Schistoso-
    miasis, Addis Ababa 1970. Document CS/17 (I) (1970).
GAUD, J. and JAUBERTIE, R.: Ann. Parasit. *26:* 420 (1951).
GILLES: in Rapport final de la Cinquième Conférence technique de l'OCEAC, Yaoundé
    1970, vol. 1, p. 28 (1970).
LALOUEL, J.: Bull. Soc. Path. exot. *47:* 531 (1954).
World Health Organization (1956): Bilharziasis surveys in Africa by WHO Consultants
    (1950–1956). WHO unpublished document, WHO/Bil. Conf./51 (1956).

Congo (Brazzaville)

Schistosomiasis has been reported from only a few localities, in many
of which transmission is apparently low. Only a small number of investigations have been made and possibly additional foci may yet be discovered.

Main foci of *S. haematobium* infection occur in the southern part of
the country although two foci are found near Kibangou, which is situated
further north, with two additional suspected areas nearby. McCULLOUGH
[1964] is of the opinion that urinary schistosomiasis was not endemic in the
country prior to the First World War, or, even previous to the construction
in 1923 of the rail line between Pointe-Noire and Brazzaville. The disease is
believed to have been introduced by troops recruited from Chad, the

Central African Republic and Senegal, and transmitted at military posts at Loudima and Dolisie.

Foci at Jacob, Dolisie, Loudima Gare and Kibangou show prevalence rates higher than 50% in the local school-children. The infection exists in the Prefecture of Kouilou in the extreme south-west. GUYON [1965] reported a prevalence rate of over 50% at Kayes.

Other areas are under suspicion as foci of urinary schistosomiasis DOLL [1960] reported on a survey of 2,774 individuals of a population of 15,896 in the Sub-Prefecture of Mossendjo (Prefecture of la Nyanga-Louesse) north of Dolisie. Fifteen cases of the disease were encountered but evidence indicated that infection was probably acquired elsewhere, although this was entirely ruled out in two cases. Other suspected foci are in villages situated on the shore of Lake Nanga in the Sub-Prefecture of Madingo-Kayes.

In studies in the Sub-Prefecture of Pointe Noire involving 6,739 children and adults, 62 were found to be positive for *S. haematobium;* positive children in schools at Pointe-Noire were thought to have been exposed elsewhere. Two new foci were discovered, however, one at N'Goyo (5 or 6 km from Pointe-Noire on the road to Cabinda) and the other at Holle near the border of the sub-prefecture on the road to Dolisie.

According to AZEVEDO [1956], GAUD estimated an average prevalence rate of infection with *S. mansoni* of 0.3% in Chad and former Moyen-Congo; however, in the latter country, intestinal schistosomiasis is extremely rare. LAMY [1953] noted that cases of both types of schistosomiasis treated at Brazzaville came from other countries and that none was autochthonous. McCULLOUGH [1964] indicated that there is some evidence for foci of infection at Dolisie where he found *B. camerunensis* in streams. Other foci possibly exist but there is no concrete evidence to support this at present.

McCULLOUGH [1964] reported finding *B.(Ph.) jousseaumei* in the Duenzé stream at Brazzaville, where *S. haematobium* is not known to be endemic. McCULLOUGH also recovered *B.(B.) truncatus* from the Pinaré stream at Dolisie. The form represented a new sub-species. The snail was recovered at Loudima Gare and is undoubtedly the intermediate host, at least in the southern part of the country. *B.(B.) forskalii* is widely distributed in the Kouilou and Loémé watersheds. According to McCULLOUGH [1964] MANDAHL-BARTH believes that all collections of the species in the Congo Republic belong to the short-spired form originally described as

B. schmidtii Dunker. The role of the species as a transmitter is *sub judice*. McCULLOUGH found a single specimen of *B.(Ph.) globosus* in Lake Cayo.

References

AZEVEDO, J. FRAGA DE: Rapport sur les bilharzioses humaines en Afrique Equatoriale Française. WHO unpublished document, WHO/Bil.Conf./48 (1956).
DOLL, A.: Résultat d'une enquête sur la bilharziose vésicale effectuée par les équipes mobiles
du Service des Grandes Endémies dans la Sous-Préfecture de Mossendjo (Préfecture
de la Nyanga-Louesse) du 28 juillet–14 septembre 1960. Unpublished document
(1960).
GUYON: Les Bilharzioses; in Rapport final de la première Conférence technique de
l'OCCGEAC, Yaoundé 1965, vol. 1, p. 133 (1965).
LAMY, L.: Bull. Soc. Path. exot. *46:* 700 (1953).
McCULLOUGH, F.S.: Bull. Wld Hlth Org. *30:* 375 (1964).

Angola

Both *S. haematobium* and *S. mansoni* occur in Angola although the former is much more widely distributed.

SARMENTO [1944] designated the main endemic foci of *S. haematobium* based on hospital and treatment centre reports. These included areas in Loanda, Benguela, Hiula, Malange and Bié provinces or districts. Subsequent investigations have confirmed the existence of the parasite in these areas. On similar data FERREIRA [1953] indicated the principal foci to be Cabinda, Ambriz, Catete, Malange, Chibia, Ganguelas and Humbe.

In the northern districts of Zaire and Uige, *S. haematobium* is limited in extent. Although foci have been reported on the Congo border, JANZ and CARVALHO [1957] believed that these foci no longer existed; they also stated that Cabinda was free from infection.

MESQUITA [1952] conducted examinations in the Zaire and Luanda Districts with prevalence rates varying between 16% at Ambriz to 61% at Dande. In the Malange area the rate was 65% and at Duque de Bragança it was 31%.

In the Cuanza Norte District, CASACA and CARVALHO [1955] conducted 500 examinations in the region of Vila Salazar and found infection rates of 46% in individuals up to 15 years of age, and 17.6% in those above 15 years.

FERREIRA and GOMES [1959] stated also that the old foci in Cabinda no longer existed and they surveyed various areas in the Malange District, confirming the findings of MESQUITA [1952]. In the Bondo and Bângola area the rates varied between 81 and 34% of the population at Xa Muteda to 53.9 and 11.5% of the population at Xandel. In the vicinity of Malange, the District capital, 6,575 persons, or 12.8% of the population, were examined, of whom 56.3% were positive. In the Duque de Bragança area, 13% of the population were examined with a prevalence rate of 47%. In the Songo area near Nova Gaia in the Malange District, FERREIRA and GOMES found 31.7% of 3,313 individuals infected. In all, these workers conducted a total of 27,577 examinations on 15% of the population of 182,136 in four circumscriptions and 15 administrative posts in the Malange District. The over-all prevalence rate was 43%, thus signifying that this District is an important endemic area.

The arid and semi-arid coastal region and the south are free from the infection for the most part. The endemic areas in the Luanda District are an exception. Here water usage is mainly concerned with irrigation and small lakes which are favourable habitats for *B.(Ph.) globosus* [WRIGHT, 1963]. It is possible that the foci at Lobito, Benguela and in the south-western district of Moçamedes refer to imported cases.

S.haematobium is highly endemic in the central plateau. CARVALHO [1959] examined 866 persons from numerous villages in the Ganguelas area of Huila District and observed rates of 33.3 to 86.6%. MESQUITA [1952] found 66% of 150 individuals in this area to be positive. The rate at Lubando was 30% and that at Chibia 34%.

In the Mulonda area on the Cunene River in Huila District, CAM-BOURNAC and CASACA [1956] obtained a rate of 12.9% in 200 individuals under 15 years of age and a rate of 11% in 800 over 15 years. CAMBOURNAC et al. [1956] noted an infection rate of 13.8% in 500 individuals in the Capelongo and Matala areas of Huila District, and JANZ and CARVALHO [1956] obtained a rate of 42.8% at Galangue in this district.

The eastern part of the Benguela District is also an endemic area. MESQUITA [1952] noted rates of 25% at Bailundo, 34% at Quibala and 34% at Libolo. JANZ and CARVALHO [1956] obtained a rate of 39.3% from 1,002 persons at Ganda.

The Cuchi area in Bié District is apparently a heavy endemic area; JANZ and CARVALHO [1956] found 54.1% of 109 persons infected and CAMBOURNAC et al. [1955] obtained a rate of 42.3% at Cuchi.

Menogue, in Cuando Cubango District in the south, appears to be an important focus. Here JANZ and CARVALHO [1956] noted an infection rate of 50% in 82 individuals.

S.haematobium is generally distributed in Angola with a few exceptions. These include Zaire and Uige Districts in the north, Cabinda, the narrow arid and semi-arid coastal strip, the south-eastern portion of

Cuando Cubango District in the south-east, nearly all of Lunda District in the north-east and the southern part of Moxico District in the east.

The most heavily infected areas appear to be Catet and Dande in Luanda District, Malange in Malange District, Cuchi in Bié District, Menongue in Cuando Cubango District and the Ganguelas area in Huila District.

AZEVEDO [undated] gave a list of schistosomiasis cases for the years 1951–1955, as registered by the health services. The District of Luanda (outside the town) had the largest number, followed in order by Benguela, Huila, Cuanza Sul and Malange. The District of Benguela contains two important towns, Benguela and Lobito. It is possible that treatment centres in these towns drew many patients from the interior.

S. mansoni is almost entirely confined to the eastern part of Angola in the districts of Lunda, Moxico and Cuando Cubango. According to AZEVEDO [1964] there is a focus at Sautar in Malange District and foci at Cuembe, Umpulo and V. General Machado in Bié District.

JANZ and CARVALHO [1957] conducted stool examinations on 2,016 individuals in the Alto Zambeze region of Moxico District. Of these, 1.1% were positive for *S. mansoni*. Infection rates varied between 0.4% at Macondo and 2.6% at Cazambo.

FERREIRA and GOMES [1959] failed to find any positives in 3,227 examinations in the Bondo and Bângala areas in Malange District.

Molluscan intermediate hosts: JANZ and CARVALHO [1956] experimentally infected both *B.(Ph.) globosus* and *B.(Ph.) africanus* with *S. haematobium*. *B.(B.) forskalii* also became infected but did not shed cercariae.

WRIGHT [1963] has published extensive studies on the freshwater gastropod mollusca of Angola and has reviewed the schistosome-intermediate host situation. He points out the enormous numbers of *B.(Ph.) globosus* in the lakes in the Catete region near the Cuanza and Bengo Rivers in the Cuanza Norte District and the consequent abundant opportunities for human exposure. WRIGHT also found *B.(B.) truncatus rohlfsi* in two of the lakes and successfully infected the specimens with *S. haematobium* strains from Cairo and Khartoum.

In the southern plateau region, WRIGHT [1963] found *B.(Ph.) africanus* to be widely distributed in the Huila District where it undoubtedly serves as an intermediate host. He emphasized a significant point in the epidemiology of *S. haematobium* in the region; the fear of crocodiles on the part of the inhabitants apparently prevents them from using the snail-free rivers for bathing and induces them to resort to small streams and pools in which *B.(Ph.) africanus* is nearly always present, often in large numbers.

According to WRIGHT [1963] *B.(B.) crystallinus* may be involved in the transmission of *S. haematobium* in the Rio Moembege area. CASACA and CARVALHO [1955] refer to *Physa* spp. which they found infected from the river in the region of Vila Salazar. Because of the frequency of *B.(B.) crystallinus,* the absence or limited occurrence of other intermediate hosts and the high prevalence rates in the human population, WRIGHT believes that the species may be the local intermediate host.

B. angolensis was collected by WRIGHT in several places in Huila District and near Malange. Apparently, the taxonomic status of this form is at present debatable, since it appears to demonstrate characteristics of both the *truncatus* group and the *tropicus* group. It is not believed to be involved in transmission.

B. pfeifferi is the intermediate host of *S. mansoni* in Angola. It is widely distributed and occurs in areas from which the parasite itself has not been recorded.

References

AZEVEDO, J. FRAGA DE: Permanent Inter-African Bureau for Tsetse and Trypanosomiases, Leopoldville. Publ. No. 2/T (undated).

AZEVEDO, J. FRAGA DE: O homen nos trópicos aspectos bioecológicos. Estudos, Ensaios e Documentos No. 114 (Junta de Investigações do Ultramar, Lisbon) (1964).

CAMBOURNAC, F.J.C. and CASACA, V.R.: An. Inst. Med. trop., Lisboa *13:* 17 (1956).

CAMBOURNAC, F.J.C.; GÂNDARA, A.F., and CASACA, V.R.: An. Inst. Med. trop., Lisboa *13:* 5 (1956).

CAMBOURNAC, F.J.C.; GÂNDARA, A.F., and PENA, A.J.: An. Inst. Med. trop., Lisboa *12:* 549 (1955).

CARVALHO, R.G. DE: An. Inst. Med. trop., Lisboa *16:* 433 (1959).

CASACA, V.R. and CARVALHO, A.M. DE: An. Inst. Med. trop., Lisboa *12:* 575 (1955).

FERREIRA, E.G.: An. Inst. Med. trop., Lisboa *10:* 1739 (1953).

FERREIRA, E.G. and GOMES, J.A.: An. Inst. Med. trop., Lisboa *16:* 407 (1959).

JANZ, G.J. and CARVALHO, A.M. DE: An. Inst. Med. trop., Lisboa *13:* 597 (1956).

JANZ, G.J. and CARVALHO, A.M. DE: An. Inst. Med. trop., Lisboa *14:* 377 (1957).

MESQUITA, B. DE: An. Inst. Med. trop., Lisboa *9:* 1185 (1952).

SARMENTO, A.: An. Inst. Med. trop., Lisboa *1:* 375 (1944).

WRIGHT, C.A.: Bull. brit. Mus. (nat. Hist.) Zool. *10:* 447 (1963).

Central Africa

Both *S. haematobium* and *S. mansoni* occur in the countries listed here as comprising Central Africa. In addition, *S. intercalatum,* another human species, is endemic in certain parts of Zaire, ex-Congo (Kinshasa). Unlike North and West Africa, *S. mansoni* appears to be the dominant species in Central Africa.

In Chad, the two major species are fairly well distributed, although *S. haematobium* is found in the north where, apparently, *S. mansoni* does not exist. Prevalence rates of *S. haematobium* are high, especially in the south-west. Elsewhere, *S. mansoni* is common, although infection rates appear to be low with the possible exception of the Fort Archambault region, where prevalence rates are from 5 to 15%.

In central Sudan, urinary schistosomiasis occurs along a broad belt from the east to the west, as well as along the Blue and White Niles below Khartoum and the main Nile in the north. Prevalence rates are moderate and seldom exceed 50%, probably averaging 25% or less. Intestinal schistosomiasis in Sudan is mainly centred in Equatoria Province in the south, in the Gezira area, and along the White Nile south of Khartoum where the infection rate is extremely high.

In the Central African Republic, *S. haematobium* is not as widely distributed as *S. mansoni,* infection is, however, high in many localities reaching 86% in some, but *S. mansoni* presents the greater health problem with more clinical cases reported; prevalence rates are generally high, amounting to 34% in some villages.

S. mansoni is by far the most predominant species in Zaire. The parasite occurs along the northern and eastern portions of the country and is well distributed in Katanga in the south-east. Some small isolated foci are found around Kasai and in the south-west. A high percentage of the population is infected and in some places rates of 60 to 70% have been reported. *S. haematobium* has a very limited distribution and is found mainly in the south-east. The prevalence rate is fairly high and usually varies between 50 and 60%. *S. intercalatum* occurs along the Congo-Luabala River from Kongolo in the south to Valerina on the north. No current data are available on the extent of infection with this parasite but prevalence rates revealed by former surveys were of a moderate degree.

S. mansoni is the only species endemic in Rwanda and Burundi, where it occurs in the western portion.

In Uganda, there are small endemic areas of *S. haematobium* with prevalence rates varying between 15 and 25%. *S. mansoni* is more widespread, the average rate being around 31% in the West Nile district.

According to current data, schistosomiasis occurs most frequently in the Northern Province of Zambia. Scattered foci are found in the central and western parts of the country and along the Zambezi River. Both species appear to be fairly uniformly distributed. *S. haematobium* infection rates are generally low, although the rate is high at Matanda and along the Luapula River in the north. Here also, *S. mansoni* rates are high and in some villages in the northern province 60 % of the inhabitants are infected.

Chad

Urinary and intestinal schistosomiasis are endemic in all the Chad Basin areas. The most important hyperendemic foci are situated around the lake and in the valleys of its affluents. However, both forms have been reported from Abeché in the north-east. According to GUYON [1965], nowhere are less than 10 % of the children found infected with *S. haematobium,* prevalence in this age group being usually higher (20–50 %). Intestinal schistosomiasis occurs also north of 12 ° latitude and, contrary to the urinary disease, its prevalence increases towards the south. The desert areas of the far north are apparently free from infection except for a focus near Faya-Largeau.

GAUD [1955] stated that the prevalence of *S. haematobium* in various areas ranged from 16 to 87 %, with an average of 30 %. DESCHIENS [1951] placed the average rate at 43 % and WATSON [1970] at 27 %. GUYON [1965] indicated that the rate in Bousso, Fianga, Kelo and Kyabé was higher than 50 %. In many other areas the prevalence ranged between 25 and 50 %.

RANQUE and RIOUX [1963] reported that 77.5 % of 214 children in the oasis of Faya-Largeau in the Borkou-Tibesti region of North Chad had haematuria.

It is evident that urinary schistosomiasis is common in the south-western areas of the country, particularly in Chari-Baguirmi and Logone [GATEFF *et al.,* 1970]. Compared with endemic areas in many other countries, the prevalence rates are fairly high and transmission must be taking place with great frequency.

Three percent of the population of the country is estimated to be infected with *S. mansoni* [WATSON, 1970]. In the Fort Archambault region infection rates of 5 to over 15 % have been obtained [GUYON, 1965]. Notorious foci are found at many places in the valleys of the Chari and Logone rivers and of their tributaries.

Two cases of *S. intercalatum* infection have been reported from the Mayo-Kebbi area north of Pala [BECQUET *et al.,* 1970].

As part of a multipurpose survey, BUCK *et al.* [1968] carried out a schistosomiasis investigation in five communities, viz. Djimtilo situated north of the Chari River at Lake Chad, Ouli Bangala in the southernmost part of the country, Ouarai in the south central part south-east of Koumra, Boum Khéhia on the northern shore of Lake Iro, and in the town of Farga-Largeau, a northern oasis. Infection rates as determined by parasitological and serological (side-flocculation and complement fixation tests) examinations were as shown in table VII.

Table VII

	S. haema-tobium %	S. mansoni %	Side-flocculation test, %	Complement fixation test, %
Djimtilo	26	0.8	62	47.4
Ouli Bangala	7	44	76	38
Ouarai	32	–	81	61
Boum Khéhia	–	0.8	40	–
Farga-Largeau	1.5	–	33	9

The following snail species have been incriminated as intermediate hosts: *B. truncatus rohlfsi, B. (B.) forskalii* and *B. jousseaumei*. AMBERSON and SCHWARZ [1953] summarized old records which included *B. (B.) senegalensis* and *B. (B.) truncatus* from Lake Chad. However, there are no recent reports of these species from this location. WRIGHT [1959] reported *B. (B.) senegalensis* from Moussoro although MANDAHL-BARTH [1965] thinks that the record must be viewed with some reservation.

At the *S. haematobium* focus at Faya in North Chad, RANQUE and RIOUX [1963] found infection with this species in 0.4% of 1,022 specimens of *B. (B.) truncatus*. None of 495 specimens of *Biomphalaria pfeifferi* was infected.

B. sudanica is present in Chad and *B. pfeifferi* has been noted from several areas.

References
AMBERSON, J. M. and SCHWARZ, E.: Trans. roy. Soc. trop. Med. Hyg. *47:* 451 (1953).
BECQUET, R.; SAOUT, J., and PASCAL, J. M.: Bull. Soc. Path. exot. *63:* 343 (1970).
BUCK, A. A.; ANDERSON, R. I.; SASAKI, T. T.; KAWATA, K., and HITCHCOCK, J. C., jr.: Diseases and infections in the Republic of Tchad. Geographic Epidemiology Unit, The Johns Hopkins University, Baltimore, p. 409 (1968).

DESCHIENS, R.: Bull. Soc. Path. exot. *44:* 350 (1951).
GATEFF, C.; LEMARINIER, G.; LABUSQUIÈRE, R., and NEBOUT, M.: Epidemiological impor-
    tance of bilharziasis within Member States of OCED. OAU Symposium on Schistoso-
    miasis, Addis Ababa 1970. Document CS/17 (I) (1970).
GAUD, J.: Bull. Wld Hlth Org. *13:* 209 (1955).
GUYON: Les bilharzioses; in Rapport final de la première Conférence technique de
    l'OCCGEAC, Yaoundé 1965, vol. *1*, p.133 (1965).
MANDAHL-BARTH, G.: Bull. Wld Hlth Org. *33:* 33 (1965).
RANQUE, J. and RIOUX, J. A.: Méd. Afr. noire *10:* 287 (1963).
WRIGHT, C. A.: W. afr. med. J. *8:* 142 (1959).

Sudan

S. haematobium and *S. mansoni* are both present in Sudan. Schistosomiasis has been reported from all of the 9 provinces. AYAD [1956]
collected data concerning urine and stool examinations in 1949: 270,638
urine specimens were examined and 22,031, or 8.1%, were positive; of
163,140 faecal examinations, 8,861, or 5.4%, were positive. On the basis
of these figures, which are no doubt extremely conservative, MCMULLEN
and BUZO [1959] estimated that in Sudan, 830,000 persons were infected
with *S. haematobium* and 554,000 with *S. mansoni*.

Not many sustained surveys have been made and accurate distribution
data are only available in a few areas. Prevalence rates cannot usually be
evaluated satisfactorily and existing records may not provide a completely
reliable index because of the heavy migratory labour, the seasonal tribal
movements and other human traffic between West and Central Africa
and Sudan.

The arid northern and Red Sea deserts are apparently free from
schistosomiasis. A practically non-endemic zone, extending across the
country between the latitudes 12°N and 8°N, separates a northern steppe-
belt of mixed, but predominantely urinary, infection from a southern zone
of endemicity where intestinal schistosomiasis prevails in the savannah
and forest plateau, which is topographically and ethnographically homogeneous with the bordering regions of Uganda and Congo (Kinshasa).
This non-endemic belt, where schistosomiasis is rare except along the
infiltration line of the Nile, is believed to be more or less free from the
disease, because it is sparsely populated and lies outside the main transit
routes, the high Ethiopian massif and the papyrus swamps forming an
effective barrier to population movements.

Unfortunately, the Annual Report of the Medical Services does not
enumerate the two species of parasites separately. In the 1961-1962 report,
the largest number of reported cases came from Blue Nile Province

followed by Darfur Province. The reported incidence in the years 1952-1953 to 1961-1962 rose from 29,286 to 57,218 cases. There is, of course, no means of knowing whether the increase is real or whether the result is due to better reporting.

S.haematobium is found throughout a broad belt of Central Sudan from Darfur Province in the west to the Ethiopian border in the east. Above this belt, the disease follows the main Nile to the border of the United Arab Republic. In the 1949 figures cited by AYAD [1956] the highest prevalence was in Kordofan Province (22.8%), followed by 17.8% in Darfur Province directly to the west. High prevalence rates are recorded along the Blue and White Nile below Khartoum. FAROOQ [1961] showed that the largest numbers of cases of schistosomiasis for 1956-1957 were reported from Blue Nile Province, followed by Kordofan Province.

In the Gezira irrigation area along the Blue Nile south of Khartoum, S.haematobium rates have apparently decreased over a period of years. This decrease is probably associated with control measures which have been in effect for several decades. FAROOQ [1961] gives the following data concerning infections among 7-year-old new entrants to 19 schools in the area for 1957–1960.

	1957	1958	1959	1960
Number examined	902	936	979	897
Number infected	256	132	45	30
Percentage infected	28.3	14.1	4.6	3.3

FAROOQ noted, however, that no separate figures were given for S.haematobium and S.mansoni and that at least eight of the schools examined were included among the 90 villages under intensive treatment. Thus, the children who were examined would have received treatment, in some cases more than once.

Records of urine examinations in the Gezira area over the period 1951–1960 indicate a reduction of the infection rate of S.haematobium from 4.1 to 1.0% in children, and a reduction in both children and adults from 2.5 to 0.9%. However, as FAROOQ has pointed out, the data are not strictly comparable because of varying factors.

The tabulation for the Gezira area in the 1961-1962 medical report does not agree with the above. The figures show a reduction of S.haema-

tobium prevalence in children from 2.9 % in 1957-1958 to 1.4 % in 1961-1962, and in adults a reduction from 1.7 to 1.2 % in the same period.

During recent years, there has been a considerable increase in schistosomiasis in Northern Province because of the installation of numerous pump irrigation schemes along the Nile. Prevalence rates in school-children are reported to range between 5 and 40 %.

The number of new cases treated during 1959-1960 in the six districts of Northern Province were as follows:

Halfa	2,536
Dongola	45
Merowe	769
Berber	79
Atbara	1,395
Schendi	106

That part of the Annual Report of the Medical Services for 1961-1962 concerning medical examination of school-children shows that 2.9 % of 137,870 from the nine provinces were positive for schistosomiasis. The highest infection rate (12 %) was in Darfur Province, followed by Kordofan Province (7.5 %) and Northern Province (4.5 %). Here again, no distinction is made between the species.

Urinary schistosomiasis has apparently increased in Khartoum Province because of pump irrigation. MALEK [1960] found 23.2 % of 439 schoolboys, 6 to 12 years of age, infected at Shambat, 9.46 km north of Khartoum. Only 3 of 395 girls were positive.

S. haematobium extends into Kassala Province in the east. AYAD [1956] found 6 positives in 50 children examined at the Kassala intermediate school.

AYAD [1956] came to the conclusion that *S. haematobium* was not endemic in Equatoria Province in the extreme south. However, *Bulinus* snails have been recorded from the Province and changing methods of agriculture may be conducive to the establishment of the parasite.

In Bahr el Ghazal Province in Western Sudan, *S. haematobium* is probably not endemic, although a low infection rate was recorded in 1949. The cases may have been imported. Further information is needed.

In Darfur Province, prevalence of *S. haematobium* (which predominates everywhere except in the mountains) is reported to be high, reaching

90% [WATSON and LINDQUIST, 1967]. Between 1941 and 1947, infection rates in the Nyala and El Fasher districts, east of Jebel Marra, ranged from 20 to 40%, in the Geneina district of Jebel Marra, from 11 to 15%, and localities in the north and south of the Province varied between 0 and 9%.

In the Nuba Mountains of southern Kordofan Province, prevalence rates in the 1940s ranged generally between 35 and 47%. At El Obeid, 9 to 20% of school-children were positive.

S. mansoni is not as extensively distributed as is *S. haematobium*. Highest prevalence rates are found in Equatoria Province. In 1951, 4.3% of 2,486 school-children and 7.8% of 53,162 hospital patients were infected. At Meridi, 30.6% of 147 children were positive. Among hospital patients, highest infection rates were found in those from Yambio, Meridi, Tembura and Yei. AYAD [1956] recorded a rate of 51% in 39 school-children at Juba. A severe form of *S. mansoni* infection with extensive visceral involvement has been reported from the south of Bor district in Upper Nile Province [EL-AMIN, 1970].

S. mansoni is found in Darfur Province in the west but apparently it has low endemicity and is limited to a few districts in the Jebel Marra massif. The parasite may be present in Kordofan Province but AYAD [1956] believed reports to be doubtful. MALEK [1960] indicated that it was not present in Khartoum Province.

One of the most heavily infected areas of *S. mansoni* occurs along the White Nile south of Khartoum where prevalence rates ranging from 60 to 90% have been recorded. This area extends from about 48 km south of Khartoum to approximately 160 km north of Malakal. Some manifestations of the disease, mainly hepatosplenomegaly and ascites, are prevalent among patients in this area.

The Gezira area is also endemic for intestinal schistosomiasis. FAROOQ [1961] collected data which indicated a decrease in prevalence rates in children and adults from 11.0% in 1951-1952 to 4.1% in 1959-1960 but, as the examinations were conducted under varying conditions, the actual decrease may not have been as marked. In the 1961-1962 Report of the Medical Services, the reduction of *S. mansoni* infection in children was from 5.1% in 1957-1958 to 4.2% in 1961-1962. In adults, the rate decreased during this period from 6.8 to 4.6%.

In Northern Province *S. mansoni*, like *S. haematobium*, has spread with the increasing introduction of irrigation along the main Nile. There are no recent data available on prevalence rates. The snail host for

S. mansoni is known to occur in the Zeidab agricultural scheme at the confluence of the Atbara River with the Nile.

Molluscan intermediate hosts: MALEK [1959] has reported on natural and experimental infection of various species of snails with *S. haematobium* and has reviewed [1958, 1966] the role of the several species in the transmission of the disease in Sudan.

The main snails involved in the transmission of urinary schistosomiasis are *B. (B.) truncatus (truncatus)* and *B. (Ph.) globosus*. Certain strains of *B. (B.) ugandae* were found by MALEK to be susceptible to infection with *S. haematobium* and the species could serve as a poor transmitter in some parts of the country. *B. (B.) forskalii* is found in various parts of Sudan but its role in transmission has not been substantiated. MANDAHL-BARTH [1957] reported *B. (B.) truncatus rohlfsi* from Jebel Marra.

B. (B.) truncatus is found in northern and central Sudan, and in Darfur, Kordofan and Bahr el Ghazal Provinces, although it is rare in the last-named province. *B. (Ph.) globosus* occurs in southern Equatoria Province.

B. pfeifferi and *B. sudanica* serve as intermediate hosts of *S. mansoni*. *B. pfeifferi* occurs mainly in Blue Nile and White Nile Provinces, but is also found in Bahr el Ghazal and Upper Nile Provinces and in some agricultural schemes in Khartoum and Northern Provinces. The *gaudi* variety is found in the Jebel Marra area of Darfur Province. *B. sudanica* is common in Bahr el Ghazal and Upper Nile Provinces, and occurs on papyrus islands in the White Nile south of Kosti.

References

AYAD, N.: Bull. Wld Hlth Org. *14:* 1 (1956).

EL-AMIN ABDALLA, R.: Schistosomiasis in Bor District. A clinico-pathological study. Preliminary report. OAU Symposium on Schistosomiasis, Addis Ababa 1970. Document CS/44 (I) (1970).

FAROOQ, M.: Report on a visit to the Sudan, 26 December 1960–11 January 1961. WHO unpublished document, EM/BIL/18 (1961).

MCMULLEN, D. B. and BUZO, Z. J.: Report of the preliminary survey by the Bilharziasis Advisory Team, 1959. I. Sudan. WHO unpublished document, MHO/PA/169.59 (1959).

MALEK, E. A.: Bull. Wld Hlth Org. *18:* 691 (1958).

MALEK, E. A.: in Proceedings of the Sixth International Congresses of Tropical Medicine and Malaria, Lisbon 1958, vol. 2, p. 43 (1959).

MALEK, E. A.: J. Parasit. *46:* 111 (1960).

MALEK, E. A.: Alhakeem, No. 20, p. 26 (1966).

MANDAHL-BARTH, G.: Bull. Wld Hlth Org. *17:* 1 (1957).

Republic of the Sudan: Report of the Medical Services, Ministry of Health, for the Year 1961–1962 (1964).

WATSON, J. M. and LINDQUIST, K. H. L.: Assignment report. Health implications of the Jebel Marra area land and water resources development project. WHO unpublished document PD/67.14 (1967).

Central African Republic

Both *S. haematobium* and *S. mansoni* are endemic but the latter is more generally distributed and constitutes a greater problem. A report by BRYGOO [1964] provides detailed information relating to schistosomiasis in the Central African Republic.

From data collected by the Service des Grandes Endémies, giving prevalence rates and the year of survey, it would appear that the principal endemic foci of *S. haematobium* are as follows: Birao (57%, 1962) and N'Dele (86%, 1960) in the north-east, Paoua (25%, 1963) in the north-west and M'Baiki (80%, 1962) in the south. GAUD [1955] reported prevalence rates for Oubangui Shari ranging from 4 to 64% in seven localities, while DESCHIENS [1952] indicated an average rate of 22%.

According to BRYGOO [1964] the number of cases of intestinal schistosomiasis caused by *S. mansoni* reported annually in the Central African Republic has been consistently far in excess of that of urinary schistosomiasis. In fact, the former is second to malaria from the viewpoint of recorded morbidity. It is possible that the difference may be explained, in part, by the fact that many of the reports are based on clinical diagnosis without resort to faecal examination. According to GUYON [1965], the infection occurs throughout the country, with the possible exception of Berberati sub-prefecture, and the country may be divided into three zones regarding the prevalence of *S. mansoni:*

(a) a zone in the south-west consisting of the Prefectures of Lobaye, Haute Sangha and Bouar-Baboua, where the endemicity is slight, not exceeding 5%;

(b) a zone in the north-west in the Prefectures of Ouham Pende and Ouham, where infection is maximal, varying between 13 and 34%;

(c) the remainder of the country where the rate varies between 1 and 19%. The intestinal form is, however, spreading in the central parts of the country where one-third of the population is infected [GATEFF *et al.*, 1970].

SAUGRAIN [1967] reported prevalence rates of 11.4% in 174,674 faecal examinations for *S. mansoni* and 5.8% in 18,230 urine examinations for *S. haematobium* in 39 localities.

B. (Ph.) globosus is the molluscan intermediate host for *S. haematobium*. *B. (B.) forskalii* is present but is not known to be involved in transmission.

B. pfeifferi is the principal host of *S. mansoni* but *B. sudanica* is present and must be regarded as a potential host.

Snail species involved in the transmission of schistosomiasis in the Central African Republic have been reviewed by SAUGRAIN [1968].

References

BRYGOO, E. R.: Rapport sur une brève enquête concernant les bilharzioses en République Centrafricaine, 18 janvier–20 février 1964. WHO unpublished document, AFR/BILH/11 (1964).

DESCHIENS, R.: Le problème sanitaire des bilharzioses dans les territoires de l'Union française. Monogr. V, Soc. Path. exot. (Masson, Paris 1952).

GATEFF, C.; LEMARINIER, G.; LABUSQUIÈRE, R., and NEBOUT, M.: Epidemiological importance of bilharziasis within Member States of OCED. OAU Symposium on Schistosomiasis, Addis Ababa 1970. Document CS/17 (I) (1970).

GAUD, J.: Bull. Wld Hlth Org. *13:* 209 (1955).

GUYON: in Rapport final de la Première Conférence technique de l'OCCGEAC, Yaoundé 1965, vol. 2, p. 133 (1965).

SAUGRAIN, J.: Méd. trop. *27:* 156 (1967).

SAUGRAIN, J.: Bull. Soc. Path. exot. *61:* 44 (1968).

Zaire, Rwanda and Burundi

Three types of human schistosomiasis exist at present in Zaire. In order of importance these are: intestinal schistosomiasis caused by *S. mansoni,* urinary schistosomiasis caused by *S. haematobium,* and intestinal schistosomiasis caused by *S. intercalatum.* Only *S. mansoni* has been found in Rwanda and Burundi.

S. mansoni probably existed in these countries before the explorations of the 19th century as the first cases of intestinal schistosomiasis were detected by FIRKET [1897] in Congolese soldiers staying in Belgium at the time of the Universal Exposition in 1897. The 1900—1905 report of the Leopoldville Laboratory, directed by A. BRODEN, mentions four cases of intestinal schistosomiasis with bloody diarrhoea. In subsequent reports the numbers mount rapidly, with year 1933 as the only exception:

Year	Cases	Deaths
1923	433	14
1933	358	20
1950	8,744	36
1953	33,358	127
1958	49,045	67

This great progressive increase since 1923 is due to more extensive medical screening as well as to the spread of the disease. The endemicity is characterized generally by a large proportion of relatively well tolerated schistosomiasis infection with only a very low mortality rate.

The first epidemic was noted by A. N. DUREN in 1923 among students of the Lemfu Mission (ex-Lower Congo). Forty subjects among 82 examined had overt symptoms or were carriers [DUREN, 1942].

S. mansoni distribution is roughly accorded to four large geographical regions:

(1) northern and north-eastern region; northern Ubangi (Banzyville), Uele, Kibali-Ituri, Lake Albert;

(2) eastern region; foci on Lake Edward, Lake Kivu and Lake Tanganyika;

(3) south-eastern and southern region; Katanga and Kasai;

(4) western region; includes the small focus of Buku-Bandu near Tshela and especially that of Kimpese.

This distribution is obviously approximate because in the large foci, which are in constant growth, the infection often exceeds the geographical limits described above. Thus, the Katanga epidemic ascends the River Lualaba to Kasongo while the focus of Ituri spreads southward to Butembo, a station at an altitude of 1,800 m where infected planorbes *(B. pfeifferi)* have been collected.

Extensive zones are free from intestinal schistosomiasis: Kwango in the south, Congo-Ubangi in the north (with the exception of a narrow band along the Banzyville frontier) and, in the centre, the regions of Lake Leopold II, Tshuapa, and Sanuru north of the 5th Parallel south. The valley of the Lualaba River from Kasongo to Kisangani (Stanleyville) is also free due to the absence of snail hosts. The Kisangani region is uninfected, with the possible exception of the town itself where planorbes were found several years ago by LASSANCE [1958].

Briefly, in Zaire, two very important zones of intestinal schistosomiasis exist: Ituri-Uele and Kasai-Katanga, united in the east by the secondary foci of Lakes Edward, Kivu and Tanganyika. These zones are probably the two most ancient localizations of *S. mansoni*. In fact, from 1922 the reports of the 'Direction générale des Services médicaux' indicate that the greatest number of cases occurs in the Eastern Province and in the Province of Katanga which, under the old administrative division, included Kasai and Lower Katanga. Originating from these two ancient foci, the endemicity has progressed slowly, allied to the population movements resulting from economic development, and spreading along the main paths of communication wherever there is commercial exchange. Thus, when the industry of Upper Katanga recruited part of its workers in the schistosomiasis area of Kasai, the disease was introduced to the region. In support of this thesis advanced by RODHAIN, there are figures giving the percentage of stool specimens positive for schistosomiasis among the recruits coming from Rwanda, Burundi, Rhodesia and Lomami-Kasai:

Year	Rwanda-Burundi %	Rhodesia %	Lomami-Kasai %
1930	0.65	3.35	13.10
1931	0.5	0.48	12.04
1932	1.61	3.57	18.18
1933	0	6.84	15.20

PARENT and VERDRUGGEN, 1952.

A supporting argument that these foci are very old is that of all the customary areas infected by *S. mansoni*, those of Ituri and Kasai show the highest rates of infection. In the territory of Faradje (Haut Ituri), the proportion of intestinal schistosomiasis due to *S. mansoni* varies from 70 to almost 100% [LEGRAND and CATRYSSE, 1952]. The rates are more than 50% in the Tshilenge region [JANSSENS, 1951].

To the west, the endemicity is stationary and mainly confined to the region of Kimpese where the infection could well have been introduced by the foreign workers recruited for the construction of the Matadi–Leopoldville railroad.

The final observation to be made with reference to *S. mansoni* is that in Zaire, man is the only reservoir of the parasite. Although many species of rodent, both wild and domestic, have been infected experimentally, the natural infection which is very slight, is found only in a few foci and always in a small proportion of specimens: Albertville (1.6–4%); Irumu (one rodent). In other regions or localities, Bunia, Lake Albert, Lake Kivu, Kasongo, the rodents have been shown to be negative [SCHWETZ, 1953a, b; 1954, 1955, 1956, GILLET, 1953]. Monkeys have never been found to be carriers of *S. mansoni*.

In Rwanda and Burundi *S. mansoni* infection is rapidly spreading, especially on the shores of Lake Kivu as well as in the Ruzizi plain where prevalence reaches up to 65%.

S. *haematobium* was probably imported into Zaire. The establishment of this parasite, which comes from the neighbouring countries, occurred insidiously in Katanga. It was only in 1925 that the 'Direction générale des Services médicaux' first mentioned urinary schistosomiasis in Zaire and more especially in Katanga, 38 cases. From then on, the infection moved progressively toward the north following the Luapulato River to the east and the Lualaba River to the west. The extreme southeasterly point of Upper Katanga, the first region to be affected by urinary schistosomiasis, is also the major area affected and the urinary form clearly predominates over the intestinal form. However, moving northward, the prevalence of *S. haematobium* steadily declines whilst *S. mansoni* becomes progressively more important. This situation is shown by the figures of morbidity given in table VIII by different centres on a line from south to north along the Luapula and along Lake Mwero to Pweto.

Table VIII

Hospital or dispensary	All causes		Schistosomiasis			
	cases	deaths	urinary		intestinal	
			cases	deaths	cases	deaths
Kakielo	2,999	29	331	1	28	–
Tela	870	–	23	–	11	–
Kiniama	13,426	–	143	–	131	–
Kasenga	16,136	–	52	–	24	–
Chibambo	5,439	–	398	–	51	–
Kilwa	10,452	–	87	–	17	–
Lukonzolwa	4,312	41	5	–	878	1
Luanza	5,194	22	129	–	727	1
Pweto	6,582	23	45	–	151	2

GILLET and WOLFS, 1954.

The same phenomenon is observed in following the western limit of the focus starting from Upper Katanga. At Sakania, urinary schistosomiasis is more common than the intestinal form [SCHWETZ, 1953b]. At Lubumbashi (Elizabethville), there is a similar situation: 58.9% urinary schistosomiasis among children [DRESSE, 1951] and 15.08% intestinal schistosomiasis for the same age group [DELVILLE and DRESSE, 1951]. In the Lufira lake area 12.1% of 3,019 persons examined were infected with

S. haematobium, 6.3% with *S. mansoni* and 1.4% with both species [RIPERT *et al.,* 1969]. Further north, in the Lualaba valley, the proportions are reversed: at Mulongo on Lake Kabumba (to the east of Mwanza), there were four cases of urinary schistosomiasis and 811 cases of intestinal schistosomiasis out of 10,795 cases treated; at Muyumba the figures are respectively 63 and 314 cases out of 3,657 patients treated [GILLET and WOLFS, 1954]. However, in the region of Kongolo, *S. haematobium* again predominates due to the great abundance of *B. (Ph.) globosus* and the rarity of planorbes: 69.4% urinary schistosomiasis and 13.6% intestinal schistosomiasis.

Finally, Kasongo and Kibombo being unaffected, *S. haematobium* is again found at Kindu which is at present the northern limit of its spread from Katanga.

A very small focus has been reported at Bosobolo, in the northern part of Equateur Province. It is probable that the infection was introduced there from the north.

The focus in Moyen Congo is situated on both sides of the Congo River downstream from Luozi but its extension is rather limited.

In Bas-Congo urinary schistosomiasis is located in two foci of little importance; the village of Buku-Dundji and the Island of Mateba. The former locality lies near the enclave of Cabinda where urinary schistosomiasis and the presence of *B. (Ph.) globosus* have been reported. This focus is mentioned merely for information; 46 cases occurred in 1939 but only one case in 1951 and the focus has probably disappeared by now. Another focus situated on the island of Mateba, several kilometers downstream from Boma, is also unimportant; the cattle raised since 1894 on this island harbour *S. bovis.* The two parasites live side by side in their respective hosts [GILLET, 1950].

S. intercalatum has been discovered in foci distributed along the River Congo, Lualaba from Yalikina (at the mouth of the Lomami) downstream, to Kongolo upstream with intermediate points at Yakusu, Kisangani (Stanleyville) and Ponthierville. The parasite provokes an intestinal schistosomiasis (usually) with associated symptoms; the urines are rarely positive and the eggs eliminated have a long terminal spine. This long terminal spine combined with the lozenge-shape of the eggs, gives them a strong resemblance to those of *S. mattheei.* The morphology of the adult worms is also similar and experimentation shows the infectivity of the two species to be comparable. Sheep can be infected equally well by *S. mattheei* and *S. intercalatum,* yet they are resistant to *S. haematobium.* The resemblance between the two species is, therefore, very strong. This explains the hypothesis put forward by SCHWETZ [1951a] according to which *S. intercalatum* could be an adaption to man of *S. mattheei*. An unsuccessful search has been made for natural infection of sheep and goats at Yakusu [FISHER, 1934] and of sheep only at Kisangani (Stanleyville).

Some animal schistosomiasis unconnected with the pathology of the human disease has been found: *S. bovis* in the bovines of Katanga [VAN DEN BERGHE, 1936], on Mateba Island [GILLET, 1950], of Ituri [FAIN, 1951], and in two antelopes *(Limnotragus spekei)* in Rwanda [VAN DEN BERGHE, 1936]; *S. rodhaini* in the wild rodents at Sakania, Lubumbashi (Elizabethville), and Albertville [SCHWETZ, 1950, 1951b, 1952a, b, c; STIJNS, 1952], on the shores of Lake Kivu [GILLET, 1960] as well as in canines of Astrida, Rwanda [DERAMEE et al., 1953].

Man is subject, though very rarely, to an asymptomatic intestinal infection by these two species. This has been observed only in Zaire, in Rwanda and in Uganda [BERRIE and GOODMAN, 1962]. The parasite is recognized by the typical aspect of the mature eggs; the terminal spine is bent in the opposite direction to the elongated rounded further extremity.

All the large planorbes *(B. pfeifferi, B. smithi, B. stanleyi* and *B. sudanica)* are intermediate hosts of *S. mansoni* [VAN DEN BERGHE, 1936; COURTOIS and WANSON, 1949; SCHWETZ, 1949, 1950, 1953b; CRIDLAND, 1957] while *B. pfeifferi* and *B. sudanica* are hosts also for *S. rodhaini* [STIJNS, 1952; SCHWETZ, 1952]. *B. smithi* is found only in Lake Edward while *B. stanleyi* is known only in Lake Albert. The other two species have a broader but apparently more irregular distribution. *B. pfeifferi* is much more common than *B. sudanica* and is the most important intermediate host of *S. mansoni* in Zaire. These planorbes are numerous in some regions (Great Lakes, Ituri, Uele, Katanga, Kasai) but much less numerous in others (Bas-Congo) and are even absent in extensive areas. Although in the past few years *B. pfeifferi* has been found at Kisangani (Stanleyville) [LASSANCE, 1958], planorbes are not found in the hinterland of this locality, probably not until the Lindi River, and there are probably none in the Lualaba valley from Kisangani up-river to Kibombo-Kasongo. A pH from 6.2 to 9.2 is tolerated by these snails, so it is not a factor in determining their presence or absence.

The role of *B. (Ph.) globosus* in the transmission of *S. haematobium* in Zaire has been established experimentally by GILLET [1949]; it is also the host of *S. intercalatum*. FISHER [1934] has actually transmitted the latter parasite to the mouse and one sheep from *B. (Ph.) globosus* found naturally infected. SCHWETZ [1951a] and GILLET [1954] succeeded in establishing the experimental cycle. *B.(Ph.) globosus* is very abundant in eastern Zaire from north to south, but it is found more rarely in the regions of Lubilash (Kasai) and the Bas-Congo, although these areas have been thoroughly searched. The distribution area of *B.(Ph.) globosus* is far larger than the endemic zone of *S. haematobium* which is located principally around Katanga. The region of the great lakes (Tanganyika, Kivu, Edward, Albert) seems to be at present free from urinary schistosomiasis. The regions of Kisangani (Stanleyville), the north-east (Uele, Ituri), Rwanda and Burundi are also unaffected.

Bulinus spp., *sensu stricto,* are quite common in the great lakes and in several of the small eastern lakes (Monkoto region). The role of *B.(B.) coulboisi* in the transmission of *S. haematobium* in Zaire is not yet proven. *B.(B.) forskalii* is widespread in Zaire, but attempts to transmit *S. haematobium* experimentally through it have failed [GILLET, 1949].

References

BERGHE, L. VAN DEN: Bull. Soc. Path. exot. *29:* 41 (1936).

BERRIE, A.D. and GOODMAN, J.D.: Ann. trop. Med. Parasit. *56:* 297 (1962).

COURTOIS, G. and WANSON, M.: Ann. Soc. belge Méd. trop. *29:* 447 (1949).

CRIDLAND, C.C.: J. trop. Med. Hyg. *60:* 18 (1957).

DERAMÉE, O.; THIENPONT, D.; FAIN, A., and JADIN, J.: Ann. Soc. belge Méd. trop. *33:* 207 (1953).

DRESSE, A.: Ann. Soc. belge Méd. trop. *31:* 523 (1951).

DUREN, A.: Ann. Soc. belge Méd. trop. *22:* 253 (1942).

FAIN, A.: Ann. Soc. belge Méd. trop. *31:* 149 (1951).

FIRKET, CH.: Bull. Acad. roy. Méd. Belg. *11:* 451 (1897).

FISHER, A.C.: Trans. roy. Soc. trop. Med. Hyg. *28:* 277 (1934).

GILLET, J.: Ann. Soc. belge Méd. trop. *29:* 457 (1949).

GILLET, J.: Ann. Soc. belge Méd. trop. *30:* 195 (1950).

GILLET, J.: Bull. Inst. roy. colon. belge *24:* 1323 (1953).

GILLET, J.: Carte nosologique de l'Atlas général du Congo, index No. 622, Institut Royal colonial belge (1954).

GILLET, J.: Ann. Soc. belge Méd. trop. *40:* 639 (1960).

GILLET, J. and WOLFS, J.: Bull. Wld Hlth Org. *10:* 315 (1954).

JANSSENS, P.: Ann. Soc. belge Méd. trop. *31:* 441 (1951).

LASSANCE, M.: Ann. Soc. belge Méd. trop. *38:* 953 (1958).

LEGRAND and CATRYSSE: Personal communication to Dr. J. GILLET (1952).

PARENT, M. and VERBRUGGEN, J.: Ann. Soc. belge Méd. trop. *32:* 255 (1952).

RIPERT, C.; CARTERET, P., and GAYTE, M.J.: Bull. Soc. Path. exot. *62:* 571 (1969).

SCHWETZ, J.: Ann. Soc. belge Méd. trop. *29:* 67 (1949).

SCHWETZ, J.: Ann. Soc. belge Méd. trop. *30:* 585 (1950).

SCHWETZ, J.: C. R. Soc. Biol., Paris *145:* 1257 (1951a).

Schwetz, J.: Ann. Soc. belge Méd. trop. *31:* 93 (1951b).
Schwetz, J.: Ann. Parasit. hum. comp. *27:* 578 (1952a).
Schwetz, J.: Ann. Soc. belge Méd. trop. *32:* 473 (1952b).
Schwetz, J.: Ann. Soc. belge Méd. trop. *32:* 673 (1952c).
Schwetz, J.: Bull. Inst. roy. colon. belge *24:* 1453 (1953a).
Schwetz, J.: Ann. Soc. belge Méd. trop. *33:* 67 (1953b).
Schwetz, J.: Trans. roy. Soc. trop. Med. Hyg. *48:* 89 (1954).
Schwetz, J.: Bull. Soc. Path. exot. *48:* 182 (1955).
Schwetz, J.: Ann. Soc. belge Méd. trop. *36:* 845 (1956).
Stijns, J.: Ann. Parasit. hum. comp. *27:* 385 (1952).
World Health Organization: African Conference on Bilharziasis, Brazzaville 1956. Report
    Wld Hlth Org. techn. Rep. Ser. *139* (1957).
World Health Organization: Second African Conference on Bilharziasis (WHO/CCTA).
    Lourenço Marques 1960. Report. Wld Hlth Org. techn. Rep. Ser. *204* (1960).
World Health Organization: Snail Control in the Prevention of Bilharziasis. Wld Hlth Org.
    Monogr. Ser. No. 50 (1965).

Uganda

Both *S. haematobium* and *S. mansoni* occur in Uganda but the latter is by far the more predominant species.

The main endemic focus of infection with *S. haematobium* is situated in the Lango area north of Lake Kioga, although Blair [1956] noted that the parasite occurred in many places south of the lake. A series of surveys made in Lango District showed that the infection occurs in people living along three shallow river valleys draining towards the Nile, and possibly in other foci [Bradley *et al.,* 1967]. In the Lango District, 25% of children aged 5 years and 50% of those aged from 10 to 14 years were found to have *S. haematobium* infections. Apparently, infections with this parasite are common in the vicinity of Lira. In the Adyeda sub-district, 144 of 653 persons were positive as were 40 of 586 persons in the neighbouring Anyeke sub-district; the prevalence rates appeared to be as high in adults as in children [Blair, 1956]. Schwetz [1951a] mentioned foci at Aloro and Ayer.

Rosanelli [1960] conducted surveys on children in the village of Odek and children and adults in the village of Dino, both in the Acholi District. Prevalence rates for *S. haematobium* were 17.0 and 16.5% respectively. Urinary schistosomiasis was absent at Awere on the Aswa River. *S. mansoni* was not encountered at any of these three places.

In 1953, the parasite was present in about 8% of children examined at Jinja in Busoga Province, east of the Victoria Nile [Blair, 1956].

The chief endemic area for *S. mansoni* infection is in north-western Uganda comprising the West Nile District and extending south-easterly to beyond Gulu. NELSON [1959] estimated that at least 100,000 of a total population of 340,000 in this district were infected; the highest rate was in children aged from 5 to 15 years. NELSON [1958a] examined a single stool specimen from each of a total of 7,064 persons in the major political divisions of the West Nile District and found 927, or 13.1%, infected; he estimated the probable mean prevalence rate to be 31%. NELSON [1958b, c] reported on other foci in this district. A recent sample survey in Jonam County, West Nile District, showed that 90% of 179 people were infected with S. mansoni. The mean egg output was about 1,000/g from the age of 10 in males and half this amount in females [ONGOM, 1969].

Another focus of S. mansoni is located around Mbale and Tesa, south of Lake Salisbury in the eastern part of the country [BLAIR, 1956]. SCHWETZ [1951b] discovered an endemic area in the south-west around Lake Bunyoni in the Kigesi District.

In Lango District, S. mansoni is confined mainly to the Aswa River system which flows northwards to join the Nile downstream of the West Nile District [BRADLEY et al., 1967]. Low grade S. mansoni infection has been found along the northern shores of Lake Victoria [BRADLEY, 1968] and BARNLEY and PRENTICE showed that 14% of immigrants living in Kampala and Entebbe, with a definite history of sailing and swimming in Lake Victoria, had S. mansoni infection. There is strong evidence that transmission occurs through B. choanomphala which has been collected at a depth of 2 to 3 m about 20 to 30 m from the shore [PRENTICE et al., 1970].

The following are molluscan intermediate hosts and potential hosts of S. haematobium and S. mansoni reported from Uganda:

For S. haematobium	Bulinus (B.) truncatus truncatus
	B. (B.) truncatus trigonus
	B. (B.) coulboisi
	B. (B.) forskalii
	B. (Ph.) globosus
	B. (Ph.) nasutus productus
	B. (Ph.) ugandae
	B. (Ph.) africanus ovoideus
For S. mansoni	Biomphalaria pfeifferi
	B. choanomphala
	B. smithi
	B. sudanica
	B. stanleyi

Of those potential hosts of *S. haematobium*, CRIDLAND [1955] was able to obtain experimental infections in *B. (Ph.) globosus* and *B. (Ph.) nasutus productus*. Negative results were obtained with other species. CRIDLAND [1957] believed that the only species involved in transmission in Uganda was *B. (Ph.) globosus*. BERRIE [1964] indicated that *B. (Ph.) ugandae* is a host of *S. bovis* but could not be infected with a strain of *S. haematobium* from Mwanza, Tanzania. MANDAHL-BARTH [1957] reported *B. (B.) truncatus truncatus* from Buyende, the only record in Uganda.

CRIDLAND [1955] reported experimental infections with *S. mansoni* in *B. pfeifferi*, *B. sudanica* and *B. choanomphala;* later [1957] he successfully infected *B. smithi* and *B. stanleyi*. *B. choanomphala* is implicated in the transmission of *S. mansoni* on the northern shores of Lake Victoria [PRENTICE *et al.*, 1970].

References

BERRIE, A. D.: Ann. trop. Med. Parasit. *58:* 457 (1964).
BLAIR, D. M.: Bull. Wld Hlth Org. *15:* 203 (1956).
BRADLEY, D. J.: E. afr. med. J. *45:* 254 (1968).
BRADLEY, D. J.; STURROCK, R. F., and WILLIAMS, P. N.: E. afr. med. J. *44:* 193 (1967).
CRIDLAND, C. C.: J. trop. med. Hyg. *58:* 1 (1955).
CRIDLAND, C. C.: J. trop. med. Hyg. *60:* 18 (1957).
MANDAHL-BARTH, G.: Bull. Wld Hlth Org. *17:* 1 (1957).
NELSON, G. S.: E. afr. med. J. *35:* 311 (1958a).
NELSON, G. S.: E. afr. med. J. *35:* 543 (1958b).
NELSON, G. S.: E. afr. med. J. *35:* 581 (1958c).
NELSON, G. S.: E. afr. med. J. *36:* 29 (1959).
ONGOM, V. L.: *Schistosoma mansoni* infection in a Jonam village; Makerere University College Medical School, Diss. (1969).
PRENTICE, M. A.; PANESAR, T. S., and COLES, G. C.: Ann. trop. Med. Parasit. *64:* 339 (1970).
ROSANELLI, J. D.: E. afr. med. J. *37:* 113 (1960).
SCHWETZ, J.: Trans. roy. Soc. trop. Med. Hyg. *44:* 501 (1951a).
SCHWETZ, J.: Trans. roy. Soc. trop. Med. Hyg. *44:* 515 (1951b).

Zambia

S. haematobium and *S. mansoni* are both present in Zambia. Two major surveys have been conducted in this country, in the Northern and Luapula Provinces, but data on distribution and prevalence are minimal for the remainder of the country.

BUCKLEY [1946] examined 2,617 persons in various localities in the Chambezi-Luapula area and found 14.7% positive for *S. haematobium*. Prevalence rates ranged between 0 and 62%. Rates of 25 to 60% were found near the southern end of Lake Tanganyika and the area of the Luapula River.

McCULLOUGH and FRIIS-HANSEN [1961] reported an infection rate approaching 100% at Matanda with a high prevalence, even in adults. At Fort Rosebery the rate did not exceed 30% in school-children and at Shikamushile it was around 9%.

Information on other foci of *S. haematobium* based largely on annual public health reports, has been summarized by EDGE [1937, 1939, 1940, 1946] and by BLAIR [1956]. BLAIR [1959] reported on urine and faecal surveys carried out on African populations living on the north bank of the Zambezi River upstream from Kariba because of the resettlement of these populations as the result of flooding of Lake Kariba. Of 10,633 individuals examined only 681, or 6.8%, were positive. Prevalence rates varied between 2.3 and 8.8%.

On Lake Kariba, prevalence rates of 4 to 56% have been recorded in the Siavonga area where high infection in school-children (69%) indicates the presence of active foci of transmission [HIRA, 1969].

BUCKLEY [1946] reported a rate of 6.99% of positive *S. mansoni* infection in 2,575 Africans in the Chambezi-Luapula area. The rate at Mamkola was 61%, at Luena Wantipa near Lake Mweru it was 34%, and at Kafulwe at the lake it was 42%. On the other hand, McCULLOUGH and FRIIS-HANSEN [1961] observed only three cases of *S. mansoni* in the area surveyed by them; two of the cases were at Matanda and one was at Fort Rosebery. However, they emphasized the danger of spread in the area because of the presence of potential snail hosts belonging to the genus *Biomphalaria*.

BLAIR [1959] noted a variable prevalence of *S. mansoni* in the population north of the Zambezi River, as mentioned above. The over-all rate in the 10,633 persons was 2.4% but ranged from negative findings in many places to 16.2% in 1,278 individuals in one location.

In the Mankoya District of Barotse Province, stool and urine specimens were taken from 436 patients picked at random among people attending the out-patient department of Luampa hospital in June-July 1968. Only one patient had both *S. mansoni* and *S. haematobium*. The over-all prevalence of *S. mansoni* was 57.6% (60% in boys and girls up to 15 years of age, 65% in women and 43% in men) [HENDERSON, 1969].

Focal transmission of *S. mansoni* has also been found to occur at Lake Kariba, in the Siavonga area where prevalence rates range between 0 and 17% in the general population, and average 15.6% in school-children 5 to 14 years old [HIRA, 1969, 1970].

B. (Ph.) globosus and *B. (Ph.) africanus* have been reported from various areas and are probably responsible for transmission of *S. haematobium*. The chief intermediate host remains to be determined. *B.(B.) forskalii* has been recorded from the northern districts.

B. pfeifferi is no doubt responsible for transmitting *S. mansoni*. *B. angulosa* has been found north-west of Mpika.

References

BLAIR, D. M.: Bull. Wld Hlth Org. *15:* 203 (1956).
BLAIR, D. M.: Report on bilharziasis, Federation of Rhodesia and Nyasaland for the year 1958. Permanent Inter-African Bureau for Tsetse and Trypanosomiasis, Publ. No. 12/0 (1959).
BUCKLEY, J. J. C.: J. Helminth. *21:* 111 (1946).
EDGE, P. G.: Trop. Dis. Bull. *34:* suppl. (1937).
EDGE, P. G.: Trop. Dis. Bull. *36:* suppl. (1939).
EDGE, P. G.: Trop. Dis. Bull. *37:* suppl. (1940).
EDGE, P. G.: Trop. Dis. Bull. *43:* suppl. (1946).
HENDERSON, A. C.: Med. J. Zambia *2:* 167 (1969).
HIRA, P. R.: Nature, Lond. *224:* 670 (1969).
HIRA, P. R.: Trop. geogr. Med. *22:* 323, 335 (1970).
McCULLOUGH, F. and FRIIS-HANSEN, B.: Bull. Wld Hlth Org. *24:* 213 (1961).

East Africa

Some countries of East Africa have been well surveyed for schistosomiasis but more information is needed concerning the distribution of the disease in Ethiopia and Somalia and possibly in Malawi.

Other than Somalia, where only *S. haematobium* has been recorded, the two major human species are well distributed, although in some countries many regions are free from infection.

In Ethiopia, *S. haematobium* infection is apparently more scattered than is that of *S. mansoni,* which for the most part seems to be more common in the north. However, records of urinary schistosomiasis are extremely meagre and certain reports are unreliable. There are few data available on prevalence rates. Certain areas show high rates (up to 60%) of *S. mansoni,* although the rates are usually lower than this figure. At the present time, intestinal schistosomiasis seems to be the greater problem.

In Somalia, *S. haematobium* is mainly confined to the valleys of the Webi Shebeli and Juba Rivers. Certain villages are reported to be highly infected but the rate in most areas appears to be approximately 25%.

In Kenya, schistosomiasis is confined to the central and southern areas. S. haematobium occurs along the coast and up the Tana River valley, as well as in several inland foci. S. mansoni is found around Taveta, Kitui, Machakos, Thika and in the Kano Plain in western Kenya. Few data are available on prevalence rates of either parasite.

In Tanzania, the eastern and southern provinces have not been adequately surveyed. S. haematobium is heavily endemic in Tanga Province in the north-east, where S. mansoni does not occur, and extends over considerable territory in Lake Province in the north-west. S. mansoni is prevalent in the Lake Victoria area. Both parasites are found in the southern highlands, as well as in scattered foci elsewhere. Prevalence rates of S. haematobium in Tanga Province are very high in most places; they tend to be lower in Lake Province where S. mansoni rates are elevated in many localities.

In Malawi, S. haematobium is prevalent along the shore and inland from Lake Nyasa as well as all through the valley of the Shire and its tributaries in the south. Prevalence rates are usually 50% or higher. S. mansoni is found in a number of areas, especially around Karonga in the north and Port Herald in the extreme south. No recent data are available on prevalence rates but surveys conducted several decades ago indicated very heavy infection in many localities.

S. haematobium is distributed throughout Mozambique. Prevalence rates in the various districts range on average from 45 to 67%. S. mansoni occurs in all districts with the exception of Cabo Delgado in the north-east. In the infected districts, average prevalence rates vary from 5 to 18%.

Ethiopia

Both S. mansoni and S. haematobium infections are endemic in Ethiopia. The former is found mainly in the highland areas but has also been reported to occur in the Lower Awash Valley. The latter is restricted to the warm and arid lowlands such as the Middle and Lower Awash Valley [LEMMA, 1969]. The problem of schistosomiasis in Ethiopia is relatively new and, so far, only a limited number of surveys have been carried out.

Early reports were summarized by AYAD [1956] who also conducted a few surveys and made snail collections in the more accessible areas.

AYAD found a few individuals infected with S. mansoni in Asmara, Decamere, Ma'araba, Saganeiti and Adi Ugri in Eritrea. In the Nutrition Survey [1959] 6.9% of 29 persons examined in the Asmara area were positive, as were a few individuals at Tessenei. At Bahrdar in Gojjan

Province, AYAD [1956] examined 17 pupils and staff members of the elementary school, of whom 10 were positive, as were 12 of 22 men and officers in a military camp at the same place. AYAD also obtained one positive result in 16 patients at Harar hospitals. In the Nutrition Survey [1959], the following prevalence rates were encountered in other areas: Gondar, 9.4% of 53 persons; and Harar, 9.5% of 21 persons.

CHANG [1960] conducted a survey in Gorgora north of Lake Tana. In an elementary school 22.8% of 202 pupils were positive, as were 5% of persons in a military camp and 1.5% of polyclinic patients. No *S. haematobium* cases were encountered. In Gorgora, BUCK *et al.* [1964a] reported a prevalence rate of 37.5% in 100 villagers ranging in age from 3 to 50 years.

KUBASTA [1964] conducted a survey in Harar Province. A total of 1,845 hospital in-patients were examined, of whom 244, or 13.2%, were positive for *S. mansoni*. The majority were believed to have become infected in the vicinity of Harar; 8 positive individuals were from Yemen. An examination of 152 school-children revealed 108 positives. *S. haematobium* was not encountered in 4,548 persons examined in Harar, except one who became infected in Egypt.

BUCK *et al.* [1964b] and LEMMA [1964] showed that intestinal schistosomiasis is also highly endemic in Tigre Province, particularly in the town of Adwa where 80.7% of 820 individuals were found to be positive on skin test and 61.4% of 459 persons harboured *S. mansoni* eggs. A recent 10-percent statistically random sample of the town population (roughly 17,000) showed a prevalence rate of 63.5% *S. mansoni* infection [DUNCAN, 1970].

In another survey LEMMA *et al.* [1968] did not find any schistosomiasis in Addis Ababa or Dobre Zeit.

S. mansoni is believed to be endemic along the Gogeb River near Jimma and around Lake Lagano and Lake Zwai, south of Addis Ababa. However, the 'Institut Pasteur' concluded that Lake Lagano was free from infection. The other areas are suspect but there are no conclusive data [OLIVER and BUZO, 1964]. A reported focus lies in the far western tip of Ilubaba Province near the Sudan border but this has not been confirmed.

Foci of *S. haematobium* have been reported from northern Bagemder Province and near Gondar and Lake Tana in the same Province, as well as from northern Wallo Province. Two questionable records are from central Harar Province. A reported focus is located at Asosa in Wallaga Province, but this also needs confirmation.

The first conclusive evidence of the occurrence of urinary schisto-somiasis in the Awash Valley was provided by RUSSELL [1958] who recognized 277 clinical cases of S. haematobium: 274 of these were from the Gewani district and three from the Awash district. Urine specimens from 189 adult Danakil tribesmen at Gewani revealed that 91, or 48.1 %, had eggs of S. haematobium. Gewani is located in the middle Awash River Valley in north-western Harar Province.

Since the Imperial Ethiopian Government, with the assistance of the UNDP Special Fund and FAO, has started a project to develop over 1,500 km² of irrigated land in the Awash Valley, a survey was initiated in 1965 to determine the prevalence of schistosomiasis in different parts of the valley. The results of urine and stool examinations were as shown in table IX.

Table IX

	S. mansoni		S. haematobium	
	number examined	%	number examined	%
Lower Awash Valley				
Dubti	95	2.1	104	0
Assayta	116	5.2	144	3.5
Hadeleguera	0	0	10	40
Barga	99	1	112	0
Middle Awash Valley				
Awash station	120	2.5	188	0
Melka Werer	–[1]	–	47	21.3
Angelele	–	–	36	58.3
Cortume	–	–	38	67.9
Hertale	–	–	51	41.2
Gewani	–	–	272	60.7
Upper Awash Valley				
Melka Kontoure	46	0	47	0
Koka Village	30	3	30	3
Wonji and Shoa (HVA sugar estates)	526 (47)[2]	10 (60.0)	320	0

1 Stool samples not obtainable.
2 Adult male labourers, selected for their close association with irrigation canals and irrigation water.

According to this survey [LEMMA, 1969], *S. haematobium* has been found to be well established in varying degrees of prevalence in the Middle and Lower Awash Valley but not in the Upper Valley, into which it may, however, spread. *S. mansoni* occurs in the Lower and Upper Awash Valley. There is enough evidence to indicate that both infections have been recently introduced into the Awash Valley.

AYAD [1956] was able to make limited surveys of molluscan intermediate hosts but the most comprehensive investigation was conducted by BROWN [1964, 1965]. The available data cover only a small portion of the country and no doubt potential snail hosts are far more widely distributed than is known at present.

The main intermediate host for *S. mansoni* is *B. pfeifferi ruepelli* which has a broad distribution on the Ethiopian Plateau up to 2,600 m elevation, but is rare in the north-east and south-east lowlands [BROWN, 1964, 1965]. *B. sudanica* occurs in certain lakes of the southern Rift Valley but confirmation of this species as a host is still needed. All four groups of *Bulinus*, the carriers of *S. haematobium,* are present. Of these, *B. (B.) sericinus,* a suspected vector of the 'North African strain' of *S. haematobium,* which is also recorded from Yemen and Southern Yemen, occurs over a broad range of the plateau up to 2,900 m elevation. The role of *B. (Ph.) abyssinicus* in the transmission of *S. haematobium* in the Middle and Lower Awash Valley has been confirmed in field and experimental investigations [LO, 1970a, b].

References

AYAD, N.: Bull. Wld Hlth Org. *14:* 1 (1956).
BROWN, D.S.: Bull. brit. Mus. (nat. hist.) Zool. *12:* 37 (1964).
BROWN, D.S.: Ethiop. med. J. *2:* 250 (1965).
BUCK, A.A.; SADUN, E.H.; ANDERSON, R.I., and SHAFFA, E.: Amer. J. Hyg. *80:* 75 (1964a).
BUCK, A.A.; SPRUYT, D.J.; WADE, M.K.; DERESSA, A., and FEYSSA, E.: Ethiop. med. J. *3:* 93 (1964b).
CHANG, W.P.: Ethiop. med. J. *1:* 9 (1962).
DUNCAN, J.: A brief description of schistosomiasis in Ethiopia. OAU Symposium on Schistosomiasis, Addis Ababa 1970. Document CS/15 (I) (1970).
KUBASTA, M.: Ethiop. med. J. *2:* 260 (1964).
LEMMA, A.: Ethiop. med. J. *3:* 84 (1964).
LEMMA, A.: Ethiop. med. J. *7:* 147 (1969).
LEMMA, A.; DEMISSE, M., and MEZENGIA, B.: Ethiop. med. J. *6:* 61 (1968).
LO, CHIN-TSON: Snail intermediate hosts of *S. haematobium* in Ethiopia. OAU Symposium on Schistosomiasis, Addis Ababa 1970. Document CS/30 (I) (1970a).
LO, CHIN-TSON: Experimental exposure of *Bulinus* spp. to miracidia of *Schistosoma haema-*

tobium from Ethiopia. OAU Symposium on Schistosomiasis, Addis Ababa 1970. Document CS/29 (I) (1970b).

Nutrition Survey, Ethiopia: A report by the Interdepartmental Committee on Nutrition for National Defense, Department of Defense, Washington D.C. (1959).

OLIVIER, L.J. and BUZO, Z.J: Bilharzia in Ethiopia. Report on a visit to Ethiopia by the Inter-regional Bilharziasis Advisory Team, 4–21 February 1964. WHO unpublished document, PA/231.64 (1964).

RUSSELL, H.B.L.: The Pilot Mobile Health Team, Ethiopia. Final report. WHO unpublished document, EM/PHA/62 (1958).

Somalia

S.haematobium is the only species known to be present. Infection is confined mostly to the southern part of the country mainly along the Webi Shebeli and Juba Rivers, but DECLINA *et al.* [1933] found numerous cases at Oddur situated in the higher terrain between the two rivers, and ROSSI [1939] reported the disease from Tohen in the extreme north-east.

AYAD [1956] found positive cases at Villaggio Duca degli Abruzzi and Genale in the Webi Shebeli Valley and at Gelib and Urufle in the Juba Valley. NAGATY [1963] examined 1,254 individuals of less than 5 to more than 20 years of age from numerous schools in South Somalia; of these, 320, or 25.5%, were positive for *S.haematobium* (27.4% of 1,024 males, and 17.0% of 230 females). The highest infection rate was found in the age group 10 to 14 years, in which 31.2% of the males and 22.7% of the females were positive. No positive cases were encountered at El Bur and Galkojo north of the Webi Shebeli. In two places in the highlands between the two main rivers, 94 persons at Baidoa were negative but one of 75 at Burakaba was positive. Although the disease had previously been reported at Bardera in the upper Juba Valley, 75 individuals examined by NAGATY were negative. At Malabel on the upper Madagoi River, NAGATY reported 2 of 6 school-children positive.

BARUFFA [1962] examined 137 Villabruzzi schoolboys 5 to 17 years of age, of whom 79, or 57%, were positive. A prevalence rate of 97.0% was obtained in the examination of 167 persons living in an irrigated area on the outskirts of the village.

In connexion with a water control and management project on the Shebeli River, stool examinations were performed in Balad, Afgoi-Mordele and Giohar districts and at Genale. Prevalence averaged 47.5% of 999 people examined [AARFA, 1969].

In 1960, 1961 and 1962, the numbers of cases referred to hospitals and ambulatory clinics were 8,769, 7,883 and 8,587 respectively, and no cases were reported from the north [WHO, 1965].

In summary, most recently available evidence would indicate that *S. haematobium* is distributed in the middle and southern portions of the Webi Shebeli Valley and in the southern part of the Juba River Valley. LIPPARONI [1950] stated that the endemic area in the Webi Shebeli Valley extended 80 km from Mahaddei Uen to Balad and was 40 to 50 km wide. It would appear that the area extends further than indicated by LIPPARONI, as NAGATY detected infection at Merca some 80 km south of Balad. Possible foci exist in the highlands between these two river valleys. There is no recent information on the reported focus at Tohen in the extreme north-east.

Few data are available on the distribution of *B. (Ph.) abyssinicus,* the molluscan intermediate host of *S. haematobium.* Distribution is undoubtedly far more extensive than indicated by published records. AYAD [1956] found *B. (B.) forskalii* at Villaggio Duca degli Abruzzi and at Audegle, west of Mogadishu. There is no present evidence to incriminate this species as an intermediate host in the Somalia Republic. AYAD collected *B. pfeifferi* in three areas north of Hargeisa in former British Somaliland but no cases of *S. mansoni* were encountered.

References

ARFAA, F.: Water control and management, Shebelli River, Somalia. I. Epidemiological survey of parasitic diseases. WHO unpublished document, EM/PD/2 (1969).
AYAD, N.: Bull. Wld Hlth Org. *14:* 1 (1956).
BARUFFA, G.: Trans. roy. Soc. trop. Med. Hyg. *56:* 143 (1962).
DECLINA, C.; TEDESCHI, C., and RUFFINO, P.: G. ital. Mal. esot. *7:* 169 (1933).
LIPPARONI, E.: Arch. ital. Sci. med. trop. *31:* 769 (1950).
NAGATY, H.F.: A survey of bilharziasis and other parasitic infections in Somalia. WHO unpublished document, EM/BIL/27 (1963).
ROSSI, G.: G. ital. Clin. trop. *8:* 3 (1939).
WHO: Advisory Health Planning Team. Report; in AARFA, F., 1969 (1965).

Kenya

It has been estimated [McMULLEN and RAINEY, 1959] that one million persons in a population of 6,000,000 have schistosomiasis in Kenya. Both *S. haematobium* and *S. mansoni* are endemic.

S. haematobium occurs in the coastal areas and northward along the Tana River. A focus is found on the Galana River, one in the vicinity of Nairobi, one south-east of Mwea-Taberre and another south of Kisumu. In addition, *S. haematobium* occurs, together with *S. mansoni,* around Taveta. Kitui, Machakos, Thika and in the Kano Plain in western Kenya.

There are few data on the extent of infection in the various endemic areas. DOWDESWELL [1938] surveyed an area along the north shore of Kavirondo Gulf and found 88 of 123 persons infected.

HEISCH [1948] failed to find *S. haematobium* infection in Mata and Kitogoro in the Taveta area.

Positive *S. mansoni* infection was noted by HEISCH [1948] in 4 of 50 persons examined at Mata and 6 of 38 at Kitogoro.

ROBERTS [1949] reported on the results of routine diagnostic tests in the Nairobi area from 1938 to 1944. *S. mansoni* infection was found to be positive in 222 of 33,166 Europeans, 965 of 40,503 Africans and 65 of 5,309 Asians.

TEESDALE and NELSON [1958] indicated that *B. pfeifferi* is the molluscan intermediate host of *S. mansoni; B. sudanica* is the intermediate host around Kisumu. TEESDALE [1962] believed that *B. (Ph.) globosus* is probably the host of *S. haematobium* in the coastal region. Around Kitui, *B. (Ph.) africanus ovoideus* may serve in that capacity as well as in the Nairobi-Makuyu area. *B. (Ph.) nasutus* is also found in the Kitui area. *B. (B.) forskalii* is widespread in Kenya and is suspected of playing a role in transmission of *S. haematobium* in certain parts of the country [TEESDALE, 1962]. *B. (Ph.) ugandae* and *B. (Ph.) nasutus productus* have been found in the Kavirondo Gulf region, as has *B. (B.) truncatus trigonus*. The status of these species in transmission in this locality has not been determined, although DOWDESWELL [1938] believed that *B. (Ph.) nasutus* probably constituted the chief intermediate host in the region.

References

DOWDESWELL, R. M.: Trans. roy. Soc. trop. Med. Hyg. *31:* 673 (1938).

HEISCH, R. B.: E. afr. med. J. *25:* 78 (1948).

MCCLELLAND, W. F. J. and JORDAN, P.: Ann. trop. Med. Parasit. *56:* 396 (1962).

MCMULLEN, D. B. and RAINEY, M. B.: Report in the preliminary survey by the Bilharziasis Advisory Team, 1958. III. Kenya. WHO unpublished document, MHO/PA/18.59 Add. 2 (1959).

ROBERTS, J. I.: J. trop. Med. Hyg. *52:* 49 (1949).

TEESDALE, C.: Bull. Wld Hlth Org. *27:* 759 (1962).

TEESDALE, C. and NELSON, G. S.: E. afr. med. J. *35:* 427 (1958).

Tanzania

Prevalence rates of *S. haematobium* and *S. mansoni* in primary schoolchildren in many parts of Tanzania have been determined by workers at the East African Institute for Medical Research. Annual reports from 1957 onwards give the details of their findings.

S. *haematobium* is very widespread and high prevalence rates (80%) or more) are common in the south and to the south-east of Lake Victoria. Similar rates are found in parts of Pemba and Zanzibar. In the Tanga area the prevalence of active infection was found to be 38% of 2,270 children examined [BAILEY and DAVIS, 1970]. Elsewhere lower prevalence rates are shown but to the west of Lake Victoria and to the north-east of Lake Tanganyika, in the highland areas around Mbulu and Mount Kilimanjaro, no transmission occurs.

The possible influence of irrigation on the transmission of this infection has been discussed recently by WEBBE and JORDAN [1966]. It is thought that the greatest danger will be in any schemes developed in the low-lying coastal areas.

S. *mansoni* is generally less widespread than S. *haematobium,* though foci with high prevalence rates (50% and above) have been found in such places as Songea, Kasulu and Mwanza. A two-year survey of 160 primary school-children in Mwanza revealed an increase in the infection rate from 33.1% in 1965 to 45.6% in 1966 [PURNELL, 1967]. The infection is widespread, however, on the islands and around the shore of Lake Victoria, and high prevalence rates have been found there. In other areas of the country, prevalence is lower and in the coastal area and on Zanzibar there appears to be no transmission. The possibility of this being due to the effect of high temperatures in these areas has been investigated [STURROCK, 1966b].

An irrigation scheme established on the edge of the coastal plain in the Kilombero Valley has not yet become infested with snail hosts but the possibility of this happening in man-made canals cannot be excluded [STURROCK, 1965b].

The influence of irrigation on the prevalence of S. *mansoni* in other schemes has been shown by STURROCK [1965b] who found an increase in prevalence from 14.5 to 28.9% over a 3-year period in a newly developed scheme near Mbeya in the south of Tanzania. CROSSLAND [1963] investigated transmission, and controlled it, in a further scheme at Arusha Chini (near Moshi).

The apparent absence of schistosomiasis, both S. *haematobium* and S. *mansoni,* from inland waters to the west of Lake Victoria was investigated by MCCLELLAND and JORDAN [1962] who found that the inland waters there had a very low conductivity and this, directly or indirectly, appeared to be inimical to the snails. Conductivity of the water of Lake Victoria, however, was high and infected B. *choanomphala choanomphala* were found.

The molluscan fauna appears to be extremely varied and there are a number of actual and potential intermediate hosts of the human schistosomes. Considerable experimental work has been conducted in an effort to elucidate the varying susceptibility of various snails to schistosome infection and to determine those species chiefly responsible for transmission of schistosomiasis.

As far as *S. haematobium* is concerned, the following are possibly involved in transmission: *B.(Ph.) globosus, B.(Ph.) africanus africanus, B.(Ph.) africanus ovoideus, B.(Ph.) nasutus nasutus, B.(Ph.) nasutus productus, B.(Ph.) ugandae, B.(B.) truncatus trigonus, B.(B.) forskalii* and *B.(B.) coulboisi.*

B.(Ph.) globosus appears to be widely distributed. It was thought by MOZLEY [1939] to be the chief host in the east and in Zanzibar and Pemba. It has been recorded from various other sections of the country. WEBBE [1963] regarded it as a more efficient intermediate host than *B.(Ph.) nasutus nasutus*. MACLEAN *et al.* [1958] believed *B.(Ph.) globosus* to be the chief host in the Tanga District.

B.(Ph.) nasutus nasutus occurs in many sections of the country and is no doubt involved in transmission depending on local conditions.

B.(Ph.) nasutus productus, according to WEBBE [1962], is the principal intermediate host in the Usagara area south of Mwanza.

B.(Ph.) africanus ovoideus was experimentally infected with *S. haematobium* by TEESDALE and NELSON [1958]. This species occurs both in the coastal plain and inland, usually in temporary streams, swamps and dams.

B.(Ph.) africanus africanus is present in the southern highland area. Its exact role in transmission needs to be defined. STURROCK [1964] found it along the Little Ruaha River near Iringa, where there is a low incidence of schistosomiasis in the local population.

B.(Ph.) ugandae is capable of carrying *S. haematobium* [MALEK, 1959]. However, BERRIE [1964] could not infect a strain from Entebbe, Uganda, with a strain of *S. haematobium* from Mwanza. It is probably not materially involved in transmission, if at all.

B.(B.) truncatus trigonus has been reported from Kyoka, near Lake Victoria. Its status as a host is not clear.

B.(B.) coulboisi occurs in many areas in Tanzania but it is not believed to transmit *S. haematobium*.

B.(B.) forskalii is also widespread and TEESDALE [1962] believed that it may act as an intermediate host in Kenya. However, WEBBE [1960a] failed to find schistosome infection in some 5,000 specimens examined.

S. mansoni intermediate hosts of the *Biomphalaria* spp. present in Tanzania, include the following:

B. choanomphala is present in Lake Victoria where it is responsible for local transmission.

B. sudanica is found in dams, in permanent and seasonal water-courses and in seepages around the southern shores of Lake Victoria and near Arusha. It is probably a host in some areas.

B. angulosa was recently discovered by STURROCK [1965a] in a colony in a swamp at Kalenga near Iringa. It proved very susceptible to infection by *S. mansoni*.

B. pfeifferi occurs in many parts of Tanzania but apparently is absent along the coast. The species is an efficient host of *S. mansoni*.

KINOTI [1964] exposed various local snails to *S. bovis* from Tanzania and *S. mattheei* from South Africa. Both species developed well in *B. (Ph.) africanus ovoideus,* but *B. (Ph.) globosus* was only slightly susceptible to either. *S. bovis* developed also in *B. (Ph.) africanus africanus* and in *B. (B.) forskalii.*

STURROCK [1965b] has mapped molluscan intermediate host distribution in Tanzania.

References

BAILEY, D. R. and DAVIS, A.: E. afr. med. J. *47:* 106 (1970).
BERRIE, A. D.: Ann. trop. Med. Parasit. *58:* 457 (1964).
CROSSLAND, N. B.: Bull. Wld Hlth Org. *29:* 515 (1963).
East African Common Services Organization, Nairobi: East African Institute for Medical Research. Annual Reports.
JORDAN, P.: Bull. Wld Hlth Org. *25:* 695 (1961).
KINOTI, G.: Bull. Wld Hlth Org. *31:* 815 (1964).
MACLEAN, G.; WEBBE, G., and MSANGI, A. S.: E. afr. med. J. *35:* 7 (1958).
MALEK, E. A.: in Proceedings of the Sixth International Congresses on Tropical Medicine and Malaria, Lisbon 1958, vol. 2, p. 43 (1959).
MCCLELLAND, W. F. J. and JORDAN, P.: Ann. trop. Med. Parasit. *56:* 396 (1962).
MOZLEY, A.: Trans. roy. Soc., Edinb. *59:* 687 (1939).
PURNELL, R. E.: E. afr. med. J. *44:* 31 (1967).
STURROCK, R. F.: Nature, Lond. *202:* 1356 (1964).
STURROCK, R. F.: Ann. trop. Med. Parasit. *59:* 1 (1965a).
STURROCK, R. F.: Bull. Wld Hlth Org. *32:* 225 (1965b).
STURROCK, R. F.: E. afr. med. J. *43:* 1 (1966a).
STURROCK, R. F.: Bull. Wld Hlth Org. *34:* 277 (1966b).
TEESDALE, C.: Bull. Wld Hlth Org. *27:* 759 (1962).
TEESDALE, C. and NELSON, G. S.: E. afr. med. J. *35:* 427 (1958).
WEBBE, G.: J. trop. med. Hyg. *62:* 37 (1959).

WEBBE, G.: in East Africa High Commission, East African Institute for Medical Research, Report 1959–60, p. 26 (1960a).
WEBBE, G.: Ann. trop. Med. Parasit. *54:* 54 (1960b).
WEBBE, G.: Bull. Wld Hlth Org. *27:* 59 (1962).
WEBBE, G.: E. afr. med. J. *40:* 235 (1963).
WEBBE, G. and JORDAN, P.: Trans. roy. Soc. trop. Med. Hyg. *60:* 279 (1966).
WEBBE, G. and MSANGI, A. S.: Ann. trop. Med. Parasit. *52:* 302 (1958).

Malawi

Schistosomiasis is found in most areas in the country and is probably more widespread than indicated by published reports. The mountainous areas are least affected.

S. haematobium is prevalent along the Malawian shore of Lake Nyasa, in the northern part of the country and all through the valley of the Shire River and its tributaries. Most of the available data relevant to prevalence rates are contained in past medical reports which have been summarized by BLAIR [1956]. In 1930 and 1931, 263 of 322 urine specimens were positive at Kota Kota. In the latter year 80% of 400 persons in the Lower Shire River Valley were positive. In 1935, 74 of 158 urine examinations of the inhabitants of an island in Lake Chilwa were positive.

RANSFORD [1948] reported on the disease in the Kota Kota District, an area of 6,263 km² extending up the western shore of Lake Nyasa for nearly 160 km and 72 km broad at its widest point. During the period 1935 to 1944, 9,861 urine examinations were conducted on patients attending the Kota Kota hospital, of which 5,189, or 53%, were positive for *S. haematobium*.

RANSFORD examined 1,857 children between 6 and 12 years of age in various villages of the District and found 51% to be positive for *S. haematobium*. In 1,519 consecutive examinations, 58% of the boys and 49% of the girls were infected. The highest prevalence rates were noted along the shores of Lake Nyasa. In Kota Kota, 81% of the children were infected with *S. haematobium*.

MACLEAN and HAY [1954] recorded an infection rate of 22% in 3,600 inhabitants of Likoma Island in Lake Nyasa.

In Chiradzulu District, a 61-percent infection rate was found in a secondary school population of 140 boys and girls [BIJL and GARGAN, 1969].

S. mansoni is highly prevalent in certain localities, especially around Karonga in the north and Port Herald in the extreme south [BLAIR, 1956]. In 1913, 32% of 522 persons examined at Karonga were positive and in

1931, 80% of 204 were positive. In 1930 and 1931, 0.7% of 526 at Kota Kota were found to be infected; RANSFORD [1948] recorded a rate of 7% at Kota Kota in 1935 but indicated a decline to 1% in 1944. In 1931, the prevalence rate on the Lower Shire River was 20% and in 1932, it was 29.4% at Cholo in the southern part of the Shire Highlands. In 1935, *S. mansoni* was found in 13 of 166 persons examined on an island in Lake Chilwa.

RANSFORD [1948] demonstrated experimentally that *B. (Ph.) globosus* is an intermediate host of *S. haematobium. B. (B.) africanus* is present in the country and may be involved. *B. (B.) forskalii* which has also been found is probably not of importance.

S. mansoni is probably transmitted by *B. pfeifferi. B. sudanica* is also present but its role as a host has not been determined.

References

BIJL, A. C. M. and GARGAN, T.: Malawi med. Bull. *3:* 13 (1969).
BLAIR, D. M.: Bull. Wld Hlth Org. *15:* 203 (1956).
MacLEAN, G. and HAY, U.: Ann. trop. Med. Parasit. *48:* 21 (1954).
RANSFORD, O. N.: Trans. roy. Soc. trop. Med. Hyg. *41:* 617 (1948).

Mozambique

Schistosomiasis has long been known in Mozambique but it is only in recent years that adequate studies have been conducted to determine its distribution and prevalence. Beginning in 1952 with the investigations of BEUCHAT in the Gaza and Baixo-Limpopo areas, an increasing amount of information has become available.

Table X summarizes the data by districts and gives the average, high, and low prevalence rates for *S. haematobium* and *S. mansoni*.

S. haematobium is distributed over the entire country. The highest average infection rate, 81.88%, was found in the Zambézia District closely followed by Moçambique with 80.91%. The Districts of Niassi and Cabo Delgado had respective rates of 70.53 and 67.83%. These four districts are in the northern part of the country. The district with the lowest rate for *S. haematobium* was Tete with 45.67%. MORAIS [1959a] noted that a total of 15,279 Africans between the ages of 3 and 24 years showed a prevalence rate of 66.17%. The rate in males was 62.7% and that in females 70.91%. The highest rate (69.2%) was encountered in the age group 11 to 15 years.

S. mansoni was encountered in all districts of Mozambique with the exception of Cabo Delgado in the north-east. According to MORAIS

Table X. Mozambique schistosomiasis prevalence rates

District	Prevalence rates percentage						author
	S. haematobium			S. mansoni			
	average	high	low	average	high	low	
Cabo Delgado	67.83	92.0	8.3	0	0	0	Morais, 1957b
Niassi	70.53	91.0	54.0	5.78	17.0	2.0	Morais, 1957a
Moçambique	80.91	98.3	40.0	6.42	40.0	0	Morais, 1957c
Zambézia	81.88	95.3	65.8	9.66	27.5	0	Morais, 1956
Tete	45.67	71.4	20.0	17.94	24.5	0	Morais, 1956
Manica and Sofala	64.4	92.0	51.0	9.29	23.7	0	Azevedo et al., 1957
Inhambane	60–70	78.5	39.4	11.85	34.4	0	Azevedo, 1964
Gaza	60–70	88.9	34.4	11.85	34.4	0	Azevedo et al., 1954
Lourenço Marques	50–55	58.5	23.4	11.85	34.4	0	Morais, 1956

[1959a], a total of 8,841 examinations had been conducted in individuals ranging in age from 3 to 25 years. Of these, 9.33% were infected; the infection rate in males was 10.07% and in females 8.1%. The age group demonstrating the highest prevalence rate (13.1%) was that from 16 to 20 years.

The Tete District had the highest average infection rate (17.94%). This was the district with the lowest rate of S. haematobium. S. mansoni was also encountered frequently in the Zambézia District in the north and in the District of Manica and Sofala in the central part of the country. In the Sul do Save area in the south, consisting of the districts of Inhambane, Gaza and Lourenço Marques, the rate was 11.85%. Therefore, intestinal schistosomiasis would appear to be irregularly distributed. Even within various districts, the distribution is patchy, with relatively high rates in some localities and low rates in others.

Detailed observations on the distribution and biology of schistosome intermediate hosts in Mozambique have been published by Azevedo et al. [1961]. B.(Ph.) globosus and B.(Ph.) africanus are involved in the transmission of S. haematobium. B.(B.) forskalii occurs in many parts of Mozambique. Morais [1959b] doubted that it was a factor in transmission, although the species was subject to laboratory infection with S. haematobium.

B. pfeifferi is the intermediate host of *S. mansoni*. Apparently it is found in most of the country but was not encountered in the District of Cabo Delgado [SOEIRO and MORAIS, 1956].

References

AZEVEDO, J. FRAGA DE: O homen nos trópicos. Aspectos bioecologicos. Junta de Investigações do Ultramar, Estudos Ensaios e Documentos, Lisbon, No. 114 (1964).

AZEVEDO, J. FRAGA DE; COLACO, A. T. F., and COSTA FARO, M. M. DA: An. Inst. Med. trop., Lisboa *11:* 5 (1954).

AZEVEDO, J. FRAGA DE; COSTA FARO, M. M. DA; MORAIS, T. DE, and ALMEIDA DIAS, J. A. P. DE: An. Inst. Med. trop., Lisboa *14:* 5 (1957).

AZEVEDO, J. FRAGA DE; MEDEIROS, L. DO C. M. DE; COSTA FARO, M. M. DA; LOURDES XAVIER, M. DE; GANDARA, A. F., and MORAIS, T. DE: Fresh water mollusks of the Portuguese overseas provinces. III. Mollusks of Mozambique. Junta de Investigações do Ultramar, Estudos Ensaios e Documentos, No. 88 (1961).

BEUCHAT, A.: An. Inst. Med. trop., Lisboa *9:* 1081 (1952).

MORAIS, T. DE: An. Inst. Med. trop., Lisboa *13:* 69 (1956).

MORAIS, T. DE: An. Inst. Med. trop., Lisboa *14:* 145 (1957a).

MORAIS, T. DE: An. Inst. Med. trop., Lisboa *14:* 455 (1957b).

MORAIS, T. DE: An. Inst. Med. trop., Lisboa *14:* 461 (1957c).

MORAIS, T. DE: An. Inst. Med. trop., Lisboa *16:* 179 (1959a).

MORAIS, T. DE: An. Inst. Med. trop., Lisboa *16:* 187 (1959b).

SOEIRO, A. and MORAIS, T. DE: An. Inst. Med. trop., Lisboa *13:* 671 (1956).

South Africa

S. haematobium and *S. mansoni* are prevalent in parts of South Africa. In addition, *S. mattheei* has been reported from man in Rhodesia and the Republic of South Africa.

Throughout Rhodesia, both of the common species are prevalent with the exception of a limited area in the cold highlands near the eastern border. No general surveys have been conducted but it has been estimated that 80% of the African population harbours *S. haematobium*. For the most part, high prevalence rates of *S. mansoni* have been observed in localities which have been surveyed.

In the Republic of South Africa, *S. haematobium* is endemic in Transvaal except in the eastern highveld and the area south of the Witwatersrand. The parasite also occurs in the middleveld and lowveld of Swaziland, most of Natal east of the Drakensberg and the coastal areas of Eastern Cape Province as far south as Humansdorp. Recently, endemic foci have been discovered along the Okavango River in Botswana (Bechuanaland) and the

Caprivi Strip. Prevalence rates are high in Transvaal but low in eastern Cape Province.

S. mansoni is more limited in extent. It is found in eastern Transvaal with a few scattered foci in the central portion, in the lowveld of Swaziland and the coastal area of Natal as far south as Durban. The parasite also occurs near the Okavango Swamps and along the Okavango River in Botswana. High prevalence rates have been observed in parts of Transvaal where the parasite seems to be on the increase in some irrigation schemes.

Rhodesia

S. haematobium and *S. mansoni* are both prevalent throughout Rhodesia, with one exception: in the cold highlands of the eastern border of the country there are limited areas where no transmission takes place. McMULLEN *et al.* [1961] estimated that about 80% of the African population is infected with *S. haematobium*. Meagre data indicate that possibly 10 to 30% of the European and Asiatic population carries this parasite. *S. mansoni* is probably more common than currently available data indicate, and has become increasingly so because of the development of irrigation schemes during recent years.

Despite the fact that both species of schistosomes are found virtually throughout Rhodesia it is possible to divide the country into four categories according to the prevalence and intensity of infections in the human population. These categories are:

(1) The high altitude area (over 1,068 m above sea level) of the north-eastern area of Rhodesia. In this area the warm summer temperatures, the extent of the natural water bodies and the density of the human population give rise to conditions under which transmission of both *S. mansoni* and *S. haematobium* infections take place during the summer, but cold winter temperatures are sufficient to depress, or even prevent, transmission. Under these circumstances, as illustrated later by the Arcturus Mine, the Iron Duke Mine and the Alask Mine, prevalence of *S. haematobium* infections reaches a fairly high level in children but falls to a very low figure in adults. *S. mansoni* infections are less frequent but, nevertheless, approximately half the population will show these infections at some stage in their lives.

(2) The high altitude areas of the south-western part of Rhodesia. In these dry, arid areas the scarcity of water, low density of human population and the very cold winter conditions do not allow a high level of transmission at any time of the year. Again, transmission appears to be seasonal, but even during summer it is limited.

(3) To the south-east and north-east of the country in the valleys of the Sabi, Lundi and Limpopo Rivers in the south, and of the Zambesi River in the north, are the so-called 'lowveld' areas of Rhodesia. In these areas there is little open water except for large rivers. The very low human density and the scarcity of water prevents any, other than very limited. transmission unless dams or weirs are constructed.

(4) In the lowveld areas of the country a widescale development of irrigated area, primarily for the production of sugar cane, is at present taking place. In such irrigation projects the perennially high temperatures, peak permanence of the water bodies, and the dense concentration of the human population give rise to hyperendemic conditions of transmission of both *S. haematobium* and *S. mansoni*. Under these conditions virtually all the people sooner or later show infections of both species. Prevalence is particularly high in children, but the tendency for the prevalence rate to decrease with advancing age is less marked, due to the intense infections to which the people are exposed.

S. haematobium: BLACKIE [1932] conducted surveys of indigenous peoples in seven districts of Rhodesia for both *S. haematobium* and *S. mansoni*. Infection rates for *S. haematobium* were as follows: Sebungwe 9.6%, Darwin 21.8%, Umtali 20%, Melsetter 15.8%, Bikita and Ndanga, etc. 26.9% and Wankie 21.7%.

In 1954, a survey was conducted on hospital patients at Karoi in the northern part of the country. A total of 759 patients came from Rhodesia; 285, or 37.5%, of these had *S. haematobium* or *S. mansoni* infections [BLAIR, 1956].

BENNIER and BLAIR [1955] surveyed 10,019 children in 39 government schools in Salisbury and within a radius of 80 km thereof; 4.2% of European children were infected. A total of 5,529 African children over 5 years of age in rural areas had an infection rate of 51.2%, while 33.9% of 888 in urban areas showed *S. haematobium*.

BLAIR [1956] has recorded prevalence rates of *S. haematobium* in certain African reserves. In a reserve in Northern Mashonaland, 53.2% of 5,086 adult males and 56.0% of 4,987 males 1 to 16 years of age, were positive. In the Chiweshe Reserve, 218 of 239 males and 218 of 242 females in the 6- to 10-year age group were infected; in Mtoko, 433 of 650 males and 432 of 498 females in this age group were positive as were 113 of 150 males and 229 of 250 females in the age group 11 to 16 years. In eight African reserves, with a total population of over 200,000, the lowest infection rate in the 6- to 10-year age group and also the lowest rate in the 11- to

16-year age group was found in the Chindamora Reserve. In all other areas, the rates were over 50% and actually reached 100% in the 11- to 16-year age group in several reserves; in one reserve this percentage applied even to the age group of 6 to 10 years.

S. mansoni: The survey by BLACKIE [1932] in seven districts of Rhodesia, showed prevalence rates for *S. mansoni* as follows: Sebungwe 1.8%, Darwin 9.2%, Umtali 3.5%, Melsetter 16.6%, Bikita, Ndanga, etc., no report, Wankie 6.6%.

BARRETT *et al.* [1964] gave data concerning faecal examinations at various places during the years 1953 to 1963, including Salisbury, Umtali, Bulawayo and Gwelo. The patients were divided into two categories: (1) European, Coloured and Asian (ECA) and (2) African (Afr.). The following infection rates were obtained from patients for the four localities for the years named:

Year	Category	Infection rate, %
1953–1957	ECA	0.6
	Afr.	3.9
1958–1962	ECA	3.4
	Afr.	6.2
1963	ECA	1.4
	Afr.	5.4
Totals		
1953–1963	ECA	1.9
	Afr.	5.4

Little specific information exists concerning distribution and prevalence rates of *S. haematobium* and *S. mansoni* for many parts of Rhodesia. Due to limited staffs, health authorities have chosen to concentrate on a few areas. Data from some of these localities have been supplied by CLARKE [1966] (table XI).

Children in the age group 4 to 12 years apparently contribute most to the transmission of urinary schistosomiasis, since it was found that children from this group showed the highest prevalence rate and passed the greatest number of eggs [BARRETT *et al.*, 1964].

The relatively high prevalence rates for *S. mansoni* in some of the sites mentioned in table XI would seem to emphasize the importance of

Table XI

Locality	S.haematobium		S.mansoni	
	number examined	positive %	number examined	positive %
Chipoli Irrigation Estate	335	84	318	70
Triangle and Hippo Valley Sugar Estates	722	83	722	14
Premier Citrus Estate	458	29	445	18
Golden Valley Mine	466	14	434	10
Mazoe Citrus Estates	251	51	251	39
Bikita Minerals Lithium Mine	427	40	368	6
Turk Gold Mine	463	11	428	4
Arcturus Mine	464	34	462	19
Nyanaropa Irrigation Settlement	368	9	377	18
Trojan Mine	147	27	145	17
Alaska Mine	365	32	361	21
Chirundu Sugar Estates	383	30	406	14
Karoi TMB	287	60	291	20
Iron Duke Mine	328	52	199	56
RAN Gold Mine	284	18	274	21

intestinal schistosomiasis in Rhodesia. Egg-counts were not performed on faecal specimens in the surveys. However, in the majority of instances, the highest infection rates were encountered in the 4- to 15-year age groups although some exceptions were noted.

S.mattheei: The extent of human infection with this parasite is not known. In a limited survey of cattle slaughtered at Salisbury, 90% were found to have *S.mattheei* [McMULLEN *et al.,* 1961]. BLACKIE [1932] diagnosed 10 cases in man; in eight of these, diagnosis was based on the size and morphology of the egg and in the other two, the adult worms were recovered at autopsy. Infections with the parasite are not uncommon, since BLAIR [1956] mentioned its recognition in several surveys of European and African children and adults.

Molluscan intermediate hosts: BLACKIE [1932] demonstrated *B.(Ph.) globosus* to be the intermediate host of *S.haematobium* and *S.mattheei,* and *B.pfeifferi* to serve in that capacity for *S.mansoni.* These snails are widely distributed except in the arid zone in the south where they are only sparsely located. The species are apparently absent from a small area in the highlands of eastern Rhodesia near the Mozambique border.

B.(B.) africanus africanus and *B.(B.) forskalii* have been reported from the Salisbury area; the former species is very rare in Rhodesia, but the latter is quite common.

References

BARRETT, P. D.; BLAIR, D. M.; CLARKE, V. DE V., and GARNETT, P. A.: Epidemiological surveys. WHO unpublished document, BILH/Exp.Com.3/INF. 7 (1964).

BENNIER, I. and BLAIR, D. M.: Trans. roy. Soc. trop. Med. Hyg. *49:* 424 (1955).

BLACKIE, W. K.: A helminthological survey of Southern Rhodesia. Memoir Series of the London School of Hygiene and Tropical Medicine, No. 5 (1932).

BLAIR, D. M.: Bull. Wld Hlth Org. *15:* 203 (1956).

CLARKE, V. DE V.: Personal commun. (1966).

McMULLEN, D. B.; BUZO, Z. J., and HAIRSTON, N. G.: Preliminary report by the WHO Bilharziasis Advisory Team on a visit to Southern Rhodesia, 13 May–22 June 1961. WHO unpublished document, S. 515 (61) (1961).

OLIVIER, L. J.; McMULLEN, D. B.; BUZO, Z. J.; McCULLOUGH, F.; GRAM, A. L., and JOBIN, W. R.: Report on a visit of the WHO Inter-regional Bilharziasis Advisory Team to Southern Rhodesia, June-August 1963. WHO unpublished document, MHO/PA/127.64 (1964).

Republic of South Africa, Botswana, Swaziland, Lesotho and Namibia

The endemic area of *S. haematobium* extends from the north and southward across the Limpopo River into South Africa, and includes all of the Transvaal except the eastern highveld and the area to the south of the Witwatersrand, the middleveld and lowveld of Swaziland, most of Natal east of the Drakensberg escarpment and the coastal areas of eastern Cape Province to as far south as Humansdorp about 80 km west of Port Elizabeth.

The endemic area of *S. mansoni* in South Africa is not as extensive as that of *S. haematobium* and includes the area of the Transvaal east of the Drakensberg escarpment and north of the Zoutpansberg with a few scattered foci in the central Transvaal, the lowveld of Swaziland and the coastal area of Natal to as far south as Durban.

As far as is known, there have been no recent extensions of either *S. haematobium* or *S. mansoni* endemic areas in the Republic of South Africa.

In the Transvaal, human infection rates remain high on the eastern side of the Drakensberg where about 80% of the population under 30 years of age are infected. Infections of *S. haematobium* in the western and central Transvaal vary from 20 to 80%.

In Swaziland no new endemic areas have been reported but an increase in the prevalence rates of *S. mansoni* infections has been noted in communities on irrigation schemes in the lowveld area:

Mhlume Irrigation Scheme	25–56%	1959–1962
Ngonini Irrigation Scheme	34–73%	1958/59–1963
Big Bend Irrigation Scheme	15–50%	1958–1962

The increase of infection probably results from the living conditions on these schemes where almost all villages and houses have been built above and in close proximity to canals, dams, or seepage streams which are the sole water supply for domestic use.

The low prevalence rates of *S. haematobium*, ±20% in the south-western endemic area of eastern Cape Province, appear to have been still further reduced, probably due to improved living conditions and to resiting of the townships away from infected streams, as was done at Uitenhage, and to the effect of treatment campaigns such as were undertaken at King Williamstown.

In a 1965 survey of the northern areas of Namibia (South West Africa) and Botswana (Bechuanaland), clear evidence of an extension of *S. mansoni* infection was found at Maun on the south-east edge of the Okavango Swamps in Ngamiland, Botswana. On previous surveys both *Biomphalaria* spp. and *Bulinus (Ph.)* spp. were found in this area but no human infections were detected by DE MEILLON (1956) on the examination of urine specimens in 1949, by PITCHFORD who examined rectal snips from a representative sample of the population in 1956, or by the Bechuanaland Health Authorities. In the 1965 survey, 13% of 69 children in a school at Maun were found to be infected with *S. mansoni*. In this survey, too, a high endemicity of *S. mansoni* and *S. haematobium* was found in the inhabitants along the Okavango River in Botswana and the Caprivi Strip. This area, as far as is known, had not been surveyed previously but cases of schistosomiasis have been reported.

In the Orange Free State no confirmed locally acquired cases have so far been reported, although large numbers of infected African labourers come from tropical Africa every year to work in the gold mines of this region. No autochthonous cases have been reported from Lesotho (Basutoland).

The distribution of *S. mattheei* in cattle and sheep in South Africa is similar to the distribution of *S. haematobium* and may in some areas be slightly more extensive.

A serious epizootic of *S. mattheei* in stock occurred in the Pietersburg area of the northern Transvaal in 1965 and similar epizootics occurred in Zululand and northern Natal in 1961 and 1964. Fencing and the provision of proper watering facilities has brought the infection under control and one area, severely infected in 1961, was apparently free from the danger of infection in 1965. In the Humansdorp area, where in 1929 there had been heavy losses of sheep and the prototype was discovered, *S.mattheei* infection has also been greatly diminished by the provision of fencing and proper watering facilities. Human infections with *S.mattheei* have been found throughout the endemic region and in the Komati River area near Komatipoort up to 40% of the children have been found to have this infection.

In the Kruger National Park there is a low incidence of *S.mattheei* infection in several species of wild game including impala, wildebeest and zebra. A high proportion of the hippopotami in the Letaba River were found to be heavily infected with *Schistosoma* spp. by workers from Onderstepoort in 1964. The sites of the adult and egg deposition suggest that the hippopotami are not the true definitive hosts of this schistosome which has yet to be identified.

Bulinus (Ph.) spp. occur over most of the Transvaal from the Limpopo River southward, and their range may extend westward into the few small streams of the arid regions of northern Cape Province. Foci of these snails have also recently been found in the tributaries of the Vaal River south of the Witwatersrand and in the south-western Transvaal but not in the Vaal River itself. Whether these represent a recent extension of distribution is not known.

In Swaziland the sub-genus *Physopsis* occurs throughout the middleveld and lowveld. A recent survey of Natal [BROWN, 1966] showed *B. (Ph.) africanus* to be present up to an altitude of approximately 1,250 m in the area east of the Drakensberg escarpment, whereas *B. (Ph.) globosus* was found to be restricted to the warmer low altitude area in the north-east. From this result it appears likely that the sub-genus is represented by only *B. (Ph.) africanus* in the southward extension of range in eastern Cape Province to Uitenhage and Humansdorp [VAN EEDEN *et al.*, 1965].

B.pfeifferi is somewhat less widely distributed than *B. (Physopsis)* spp. in Transvaal and Natal. It has a continuous distribution east of the Drakensberg escarpment, through the lowveld of Swaziland and the coastal area of Natal to as far south as the Umzinto District approximately 64 km south of Durban [VAN EEDEN *et al.*, 1965]. One focus has been found in the coastal area of eastern Cape Province.

Surveys of the Fish and Sundays Rivers' valleys during 1964 did not reveal the presence of either of the snail intermediate hosts. Surveys of the north-western Cape areas along the Orange River showed that this area was also free from snail intermediate hosts although several other species of snails were found.

B.pfeifferi is the host of *S.mansoni* while both *B. (Ph.) globosus* and *B. (Ph.) africanus* are involved in the transmission of *S.haematobium*.

It has been demonstrated (tables XII–XV) that in South Africa transmission of *S.mansoni* and *S.mattheei* from snails is largely seasonal, from
about mid-September to the end of January. This fact appears to be influenced
by the definitive host population density. Transmission of *S.haematobium* is
almost certainly seasonal from October until the middle of March.

Tables XVI, XVII and XVIII show the results of exposing snails to
miracidia of *S.mansoni*, *S.mattheei* and *S.haematobium* and keeping them
under outside conditions from 1961 to mid 1965.

Under outside conditions at Nelspruit, it was found that the incubation
period in snails varied greatly from summer to winter:

	Winter, weeks	Summer, weeks
S. mansoni	20–21	4–5
S. mattheei	19–20	4–5
S. haematobium	24–30	5–6

The majority of snails exposed in winter to *S.mansoni*, *S.haematobium*
and *S.mattheei* started to shed cercariae almost simultaneously during the
spring in September or October. This was reflected in the results of field observations using immersed rodents for the detection of infection. These studies
showed that the start of transmission or a pronounced increase of *S.mansoni*
and *S.mattheei* occurred in September or October of every year; the field
picture of *S.haematobium* is not yet clear. No correlation between the length
of the incubation period and the number of snails eventually shedding cercariae is apparent, except that there appears to be some reduction in their
number when the incubation period of *S.haematobium* is excessively long.

Long periods of high temperature caused a high mortality of *Biomphalaria*
spp. and, as a result, a shortening of the shedding period during the hot
weather of late spring or summer. The low temperatures of winter caused a
cessation of shedding of *S.haematobium* and, to a lesser extent, of *S.mansoni*
and *S.mattheei*. Shedding was resumed from these snails with the coming of
the warmer weather of spring. In outside conditions at Nelspruit temperatures
seemed to play little part in determining the proportion of snails shedding
S.mattheei and *S.mansoni* cercariae. Snails exposed to infection in the late
summer showed the longest shedding period of *S.mattheei*. In the case of
S.mansoni, snails exposed in the late summer had a short incubation period
followed by high infection rates and a relatively long period of from 5 to 8
months before they died.

Table XII. Pattern of *S. mattheei* transmission in the field

Month	Dense cattle population			Scanty cattle population		
	number of rodents	number of worms	worms/ rodents	number of rodents	number of worms	worms/ rodents
January	164	272	1.6	194	117	0.6
February	176	467	2.6	158	240	1.5
March	207	117	0.5	161	172	1.0
April	264	64	0.2	142	7	0.04
May	157	38	0.2	182	11	0.05
June	173	26	0.1	167	0	0
July	162	85	0.5	185	0	0
August	175	53	0.3	117	0	0
September	195	205	1.0	137	17	0.1
October	209	487	2.3	146	38	0.2
November	181	381	2.1	183	16	0.08
December	181	532	2.9	113	37	0.3

Table XIII. Pattern of *S. mansoni* transmission in the field

Month	Dense human population			Scattered or casual human population		
	number of rodents	number of worms	worms/ rodents	number of rodents	number of worms	worms/ rodents
January	284	290	1.0	416	357	0.8
February	236	91	0.4	383	176	0.4
March	241	220	0.9	393	20	0.05
April	319	691	2.1	434	28	0.06
May	338	363	1.0	355	10	0.02
June	329	413	1.2	345	11	0.03
July	200	397	1.9	313	5	0.01
August	147	307	2.0	302	6	0.02
September	211	1654	8.0	392	136	0.3
October	228	2156	9.4	420	221	0.5
November	233	628	2.7	374	335	0.8
December	181	183	1.0	325	1075	3.3

Table XIV. Total S. mattheei transmission

Month	Number of rodents	Number of adult worms	Worms/rodents
January	358	389	1.0
February	334	707	2.1
March	368	289	0.7
April	406	71	0.1
May	339	49	0.1
June	340	26	0.07
July	347	85	0.2
August	292	53	0.2
September	332	222	0.6
October	355	525	1.5
November	364	397	1.0
December	294	569	1.9

Table XV. Total S. mansoni transmission

Month	Number of rodents	Number of adult worms	Worms/rodents
January	700	647	0.9
February	619	267	0.4
March	634	240	0.3
April	753	719	0.9
May	693	373	0.5
June	674	424	0.6
July	513	402	0.7
August	449	313	0.7
September	603	1820	3.0
October	648	2377	3.6
November	607	963	1.5
December	506	1258	2.4

Neither *S. mattheei* nor *S. haematobium* were lethal to *Bulinus* spp. exposed to five miracidia respectively. The same is probably true of *S. mansoni*.

When the population of the definitive host is dense, transmission of both *S. mansoni* and *S. haematobium* may extend throughout the year but shows a marked increase in September or October. When the definitive hosts are

Table XVI. S. Mattheei: data of snails exposed and kept under outside laboratory conditions at Nelspruit

1	2	3		4		5	6	7
Month exposed	Number exposed	Maximum shedding	%	Number of snails of whole groups dead before shedding	%	Length of incubation period days	Average length shedding weeks	Average length of life from exposure (days), excl. col. 4
January	204	98	48	0		38	7.4	89
February	248	117	47	0		42	11.6	124
March	264	127	48	0		53	13.8	149
April	150	48	32	30	20	110	9.7	177
May	150	41	27	30	20	127	8.5	186
June	180	95	52	0		100	8.1	156
July	150	80	53	0		86	7.2	136
August	167	96	57	0		65	5.3	102
September	112	65	58	0		54	7.3	105
October	240	112	47	0		53	7.7	106
November	261	149	57	0		44	6.8	91
December	200	93	46	30	15	40	5.7	79

present in small or moderate numbers, *S. mansoni* transmission occurs during the summer months only, beginning about the middle of September and continuing until the end of January. Transmission of *S. mattheei* under these conditions is unpredictable. It appears almost certain that the transmission picture of *S. haematobium* is similar to that of *S. mansoni*, allowing for the different epidemiological characteristics of the two diseases. In streams that interrupt flowing water, little or no transmission of *S. mansoni* or *S. mattheei* occurs more than 800 m downstream from the point at which pollution by the definitive hosts originates.

Casual movements of human beings from non-endemic areas into endemic areas from 1.6 to 16 km apart have not resulted in infection rates greater than about 10% for either *S. mansoni* or *S. haematobium* in the 5- to 19-year age group.

In a recent study it was shown that casual transference of human beings did not result in high infection rates. On the other hand, the migration of labourers from moderately endemic areas to highly endemic areas resulted, after one year, in infection rates as high as in the local permanent population.

The resettlement of Bantu populations on irrigation schemes without provision of safe water for drinking, washing and swimming has resulted, in several instances, in a fairly rapid increase in schistosomiasis in the newly settled areas; for example, in the Swaziland irrigation schemes, already mentioned.

In South Africa, irrigation is commonly by means of canals receiving water from pumps or weirs, or taken from rivers into storage dams and from there by canals to the fields. Storage dams are an essential water conservation measure. The policy of the State Department is to protect primary canals with storm water drains and fences, to cement-line all canals and to prohibit any habitation within 30 m of, or above, the main canals. Swimming and washing in the storage dams is prohibited. The application of these policies has resulted in a low incidence of schistosomiasis as, for example, in one irrigation scheme established about 30 years ago where the infection rate of *S. mansoni* has remained below 5% and that of *S. haematobium* below 20%. Unfortunately, the majority of the irrigation schemes in the schistosomiasis endemic area are privately owned and do not conform to these requirements. Villages are often established above canals and the storage dams are constantly used by the inhabitants for washing and swimming. The canals are not fenced, nor are they protected by storm water drains, and the natural waters in the area are not protected from human contacts. In these circumstances the infection rate is extremely high. In contrast, in some private irrigation schemes where the

Table XVII. S. haematobium: data of snails exposed and kept under outside laboratory conditions at Nelspruit

1	2	3		4		5	6	7
Month exposed	Number exposed	Maximum shedding	%	Number of snails of whole groups dead before shedding	%	Length of incubation period days	Average length shedding weeks	Average length of life from exposure (days), excl. col. 4
January	101	30	29	0		46	10.6	120
February	270	60	22	30	11	49	7.6	102
March (early)	120	50	41	0		58	5.3	95
March (late)	90	13	14	0		183	2.7	201
April	205	50	24	0		159	4.3	189
May	336	68	20	80	23	149	8.8	210
June	156	24	15	30	18	131	6.8	178
July	90	12	13	30	33	85	5.0	120
August	157	25	15	30	18	77	5.1	112
September	140	49	35	0		67	6.8	114
October	330	153	46	0		55	7.5	107
November	263	99	37	0		46	6.2	89
December	180	71	39	0		44	5.5	82

Table XVIII. S. mansoni: data of snails exposed and kept under outside laboratory conditions at Nelspruit

1	2	3		4		5	6	7
Month exposed	Number exposed	Maximum shedding	%	Number of snails of whole groups dead before shedding	%	Length of incubation period days	Average length shedding weeks	Average length of life from exposure (days), excl. col. 4
January	204	60	29	90	44	35	3.0	56
February	415	61	14	150	36	41	11.4	120
March	300	49	16	120	40	47	11.7	128
April	329	43	13	30	9	121	9.2	185
May	266	44	16	30	11	127	8.4	185
June	330	100	30	30	9	109	9.7	176
July	150	44	29	0		82	12.6	170
August	180	52	28	0		69	5.6	108
September	187	90	48	0		56	5.4	93
October	302	95	31	30	9	49	6.7	95
November	315	9	3	233	73	42	2.6	60
December	210	26	12	150	71	36	4.0	64

water in the immediate vicinity of human habitation has been protected from human access and where safe water has been provided for all purposes, including swimming, the infection rate of both *S. mansoni* and *S. haematobium* in children under 5 years of age has been reduced from about 40% to 20 and 15% respectively in a 5-year period of observation.

References

In the preparation of this section the following articles, as well as certain unpublished data, have been used.

Brown, D. S.: Ann. Natal Mus. *18:* 401 (1966).

Eeden, J. A. van; Brown, D. S., and Oberholzer, G.: Ann. trop. Med. Parasit. *59:* 413 (1965).

Gauldie, R. D.: Internal report on bilharzia in Swaziland. The Health Office, Manzini, Swaziland. Unpublished document (1965).

Le Roux, P. L.: in Union of South Africa, 15th Annual Report of the Director of Veterinary Services, Pretoria, pp. 347–438 (1929).

Meillon, B. de: Med. Klin. *51:* 670 (1956).

Pitchford, R. J.: Bull. Wld Hlth Org. *18:* 735, 1050 (1956).

Pitchford, R. J. and Geldenhuys, P. J.: S. afr. J. Lab. clin. Med. *6:* 237 (1960).

Pitchford, R. J. and Visser, P. S.: Trans. roy. Soc. trop. Med. Hyg. *56:* 294 (1962).

Pitchford, R. J. and Visser, P. S.: Bull. Wld Hlth Org. *32:* 83 (1965).

Strydom, H. F.: J. S. afr. vet. med. Ass. *34:* 69 (1963).

Schistosomes and Intermediate Hosts in Madagascar and the Mascarene Islands

Schistosomiasis is endemic in two islands which are situated in the Indian Ocean off the coast of Africa. *S. haematobium* and *S. mansoni* are found in Madagascar while only the former is endemic in Mauritius.

Madagascar

Detailed information is available concerning the distribution of *S. haematobium* and *S. mansoni* through the extensive review by Brygoo [1969]. This review summarizes past data and brings the findings of the 'Groupes mobiles d'Hygiène', in co-operation with the Director General of Public Health and the Pasteur Institute of Madagascar up to date (1968).

Of the 706 cantons in the six provinces, 455 have been surveyed for *S. haematobium* and 438 for *S. mansoni* infections. Of these, 120 were found to be infected with *S. haematobium* and 201 with *S. mansoni*. The distribution of both forms of the disease is now fairly well known. *S. haematobium* is prevalent on the west coast, starting in the south-west portion of Diégo-Suarez Province, in the north, down into the northern part of Tuléar Province, in the south; two foci are, however, known on the east coast of Diégo-Suarez Province. *S. mansoni* is found in isolated foci in the north of Tamatave Province and in the south-eastern part of Majunga Province but affects a broad area extending over the south of Tamatave Province, the south-east of Tananarive Province, the whole of Fianarantsoa and the south of Tuléar. In the infected provinces, the disease is unevenly distributed and prevalence rates vary widely, depending on local transmission patterns.

Majunga Province (92 cantons)

S. haematobium was found to be endemic in 65 of 77 cantons surveyed in this north-western province. The general prevalence rate was over 50%. The rates in the various sub-prefectures varied between 6 and 88%. Intestinal schistosomiasis occurs only in isolated foci in the south-eastern portion in the foothills of the plateau, but four sub-prefectures in the south-west remain to be surveyed. *S. mansoni* infection has been found in eight of 49 cantons in three sub-prefectures. Very low rates were observed in two, but the rate at Maevatanana was 15%.

Tuléar Province (112 cantons)

This western province has been well surveyed. *S. haematobium* was encountered in 45 of 106 cantons investigated. Prevalence rates ranged from 7 to over 60%, the highest rates occurring in the sub-prefectures of Morondava and Miandrivazo. Of 74 cantons where examinations for *S. mansoni* were conducted, infection was found in 38. Prevalence rates varied between 4 and 59%, the highest rates being encountered in the south. The parasite is apparently absent in the northern part of the province and is mainly distributed in the south where *S. haematobium* is absent. However, the northern and western portions have been inadequately surveyed.

Diégo-Suarez Province (58 cantons)

In this far northern province, *S. haematobium* was encountered in 12 of 40 cantons surveyed for that disease. Apparently the parasite is not highly endemic as infection rates, where available, were under 20%. This province appears to be free from *S. mansoni* infection.

Tananarive Province (146 cantons)

Surveys in this centrally located province have been carried out in 20 cantons for *S.haematobium* and in 30 cantons for *S.mansoni*. No urinary schistosomiasis has been encountered, and only one focus of *S.mansoni* has been found in the sub-prefecture of Antsirabe in the south-east where the prevalence rate did not exceed 0.1%.

Fianarantsoa Province (180 cantons)

Of 161 cantons surveyed for *S.mansoni*, infection was discovered in 123. Prevalence rates varied widely even in the same sub-prefectures; up to 100% in Midongy-du-Sud, up to 90% in Nosy-Varika and Mananjary, up to 80% in Ambalavao and Ihosy, up to 70% in Ivohibe and up to 40% in Vondrozo. Hence, the north-eastern and south-central parts of the province constitute the most heavily infected areas.

Tamatave Province (118 cantons)

S.mansoni has been reported from 27 of 84 cantons surveyed for that disease. The southern focus is an extension of the focus situated to the north of the Mananjary. Other foci are located in Tamatave sub-prefecture in the central portion and Mananara sub-prefecture in the north. Prevalence rates in Vatomandry were between 10 and 41%, in Manhanoro 13 to 48% and in Marolambo 2 to 25%. No urinary schistosomiasis has been encountered in the 91 cantons surveyed.

B.pfeifferi is the molluscan intermediate host of *S.mansoni*. That for *S.haematobium* has been in doubt. *B.(B.)forskalii* is distributed in most parts of the Island except in the highlands and has been suspected as a host of *S.haematobium*, but proof is lacking. *B.(B.) liratus* has been thought to be involved but the possibility seems remote since this species belongs to the *tropicus* group. *B.(B.) bavayi*, a species closely related to *B.(B.)forskalii*, is a potential host [MANDAHL-BARTH, 1965]. BRYGOO [1966] has recently reported that the intermediate host of *S.haematobium* is a species of snail which MANDAHL-BARTH has determined to be *B.obtusispirus*. This species, formerly confused with *B.(B.) liratus*, has been found infected in nature and has been susceptible to laboratory infection.

References

BRYGOO, E. R.: Les bilharzioses humaines à Madagascar, Tananarive; 2nd ed. (1969).
BRYGOO, E. R.: Personal commun. (1966).
MANDAHL-BARTH, G.: Bull. Wld Hlth Org. *33:* 33 (1965).

Mauritius

S. haematobium is the only human schistosome known to be present in Mauritius. Infection occurs over large areas of the island and in the belt in Grand Port-Savanne, the southern provinces. GAUD [1961] estimated that 27,000 individuals in a population of some 600,000 were carrying *S. haematobium*. MCMULLEN and BUZO [1960] thought the figure to be approximately 35,000.

COWPER [1953] surveyed children in 50 schools between 1951 and 1953; 10 of the schools were in Port Louis and 40 were spread throughout all other areas. A total of 7,318, or 32%, of the 22,948 children on the school rolls were examined, of whom 9.2% were infected. The ratio of positive males to females was 1.9 to 1. The highest prevalence rate (49%) was encountered in the age group 6 to 10 years, although the group 11 to 15 years had a rate of 44%; in the group over 15 years of age, the rate was only 3%. The rate in two schools was above 50%, above 25% in eight and above 10% in 15. No significant seasonal incidence in cases recorded in routine laboratory examinations was noted but there is some evidence that transmission corresponds with the hot, wet season which occurs from December to April.

GAUD [1961], who conducted investigations on the island in 1959, presented some evidence to indicate that the disease was decreasing. Taking the average of medical statistics from 1949 to 1953 and comparing them with those for the years 1954 to 1958, he found that the number of cases diagnosed decreased from 426 to 344, the number of hospitalizations for schistosomiasis from 83 to 42 and the percentage of positive urines from 9.8 to 6.3. GAUD also found that there had been a reduction in the infection rate in two schools and a slight increase in two others, as compared with the findings of COWPER [1953]. The greatest decrease was noted in the Ste-Croix (Père Laval) school in the northern part of Port Louis, a decrease from 62.8 to 25.2%.

More recent data, however, would belie the impression that any reduction has occurred in the amount of schistosomiasis in Mauritius. These data given in tables IXX and XX are taken from the Medical and Health Department Annual Reports for 1958 to 1960, the latest available.

ADAMS [1934, 1935] incriminated *B. (B.) forskalii* as the intermediate host of *S. haematobium* in Mauritius, and his findings were confirmed by COWPER [1953]. During the period of ADAMS' investigations, the snail was apparently abundant but neither COWPER nor GAUD [1961] found this to be so at the time of their respective searches. COWPER was unable to locate infected snails in nature but GAUD was more successful, although the number of in-

Table XIX. Urine examinations

Laboratory	Year	Total number of examinations	Number positive for *S. haematobium*
Central Laboratory	1958	7,231	150
	1959	6,356	236
	1960	6,602	296
Civil Hospital Branch	1958	2,902	276
Laboratory	1959	2,346	391
	1960	2,596	445

Table XX. Number of patients treated for schistosomiasis

	1958	1959	1960
Hospital patients, new cases	28	32	39
Dispensary and hospital out-patients	246	391	569

fected specimens was exceedingly small. MANDAHL-BARTH [1957] showed that the host in Mauritius was a species separate from *B. (B.) forskalii* and has designated it as *B. (B.) cernicus.*

Both GAUD [1961], and McMULLEN and BUZO [1960] mention finding a species of Ancylidae in several areas in Mauritius, although no schistosome infections were encountered in this snail. McMULLEN and BUZO suggest that further studies should be conducted with this species in the light of the fact that *Ferrissia tenuis* (Family Ancylidae) transmits *S. haematobium* in a small focus in Maharashtra State in India.

References

ADAMS, A. R. D.: Ann. trop. Med. Parasit. *28:* 195 (1934).
ADAMS, A. R. D.: Ann. trop. Med. Parasit. *29:* 255 (1935).
COWPER, S. G.: Trans. roy. Soc. trop. Med. Hyg. *47:* 564 (1953).
GAUD, J.: Bull. Wld Hlth Org. *25:* 447 (1961).
MANDAHL-BARTH, G.: Bull. Wld Hlth Org. *17:* 1 (1957).
McMULLEN, D. B. and BUZO, Z. J.: Report of the preliminary survey by the Bilharziasis Advisory Team, 1959. II. Mauritius. WHO unpublished document, MHO/PA/52.60 (1960).

Table XXI

Village	Positive	Negative	Suspicious	Total examined
Estoi	23	357	4	384
Caldas de Monchique	0	102	0	102
Estômar	0	24	0	24
Faro	0	188	0	188
Portimao	0	20	0	20
Lagas	0	188	0	188
Total	23	879	4	906

Distribution of Schistosoma haematobium *in Europe*

S.haematobium was endemic in only one area in Europe – the Algarve Province of South Portugal. The 1948 survey by AZEVEDO *et al.*, covering the various localities that have reported cases at one time or another, showed that the infection was limited to Estoi village. Of 906 individuals in various age groups examined, only 23 were found to be positive, and all these came from Estoi, as shown in table XXI.

AZEVEDO [1966] reported that schistosomiasis is now apparently extinct in Portugal, as no infection could be found in 597 individuals from several former endemic areas. According to the same author the possibility still exists of new disease foci being established from imported cases in view of the occurrence of *B. (B.) truncatus* in the north and south of the country and of *Planorbarius metidjensis* in Algarve.

References

AZEVEDO, J. FRAGA DE: The distribution of *Schistosoma haematobium* in Europe. WHO un-published document BILH/INF/66.6 (1966).

AZEVEDO, J. FRAGA DE; SILVA, J.B. DA; MATOS COITO, A. DE; COELHO, J.F., and COLAÇO, E.A.: An. Inst. Med. trop., Lisboa 5: 175 (1948).

Human Schistosomes and Intermediate Hosts in South-West Asia

S.mansoni and *S.haematobium* both occur in this region, although the latter species predominates and is far more important from a public health viewpoint.

S.mansoni is extremely limited in its distribution. No autochthonous in-

Table XXII. S. mansoni in South-West Asia; estimated exposed and infected population

Country	Total population	Population exposed	Population infected
Southern Yemen	225,000	?	?
Saudi Arabia	6,600,000	200,000	20,000
Yemen	5,000,000	3,000,000	1,000,000
Israel	2,380,000	?	30,000 (mostly immigrants from Yemen)

Table XXIII. S. haematobium in South-West Asia; estimated exposed and infected population

Country	Total population	Population exposed	Population infected
Iraq	6,855,000	5,000,000	1,000,000
Iran	22,182,000	1,000,000	100,000
Syria	5,251,000	74,000	3,300
Turkey	30,256,000	1,300	100
Israel	2,380,000	100,000	50,000 (mostly immigrants)
Lebanon	2,200,000	1,000	120
Saudi Arabia	6,600,000	90,000	2,000
Yemen	5,000,000	500,000	25,000
Southern Yemen	225,000	5,000	1,000
Cyprus	589,000	–	–
Total	81,538,000	6,771,300	1,181,520

fection has been reported from Iraq, Iran, Syria, Lebanon and Turkey. The parasite is found in Saudi Arabia, Southern Yemen, and Yemen. It occurred formerly in Israel but cases have not been reported in recent years and the molluscan intermediate host is said to have disappeared from the one focus previously known.

There is a possibility of spread of infection in the countries in which *S. mansoni* already exists; host snails are not recorded from other countries of the region.

S. haematobium infection is fairly widespread in the region; it flourishes in parts of the Fertile Crescent, mainly in the lower reaches of the Euphrates and Tigris in Iraq, thus affecting the main granary in the area. The limited foci in the contiguous portion of Khuzistan in Iran present potentialities of spread. The centres along the tributaries of the Euphrates at the Syrio-Turkish border, situated as they are in the Syrian Gezir, are also of significance. In effect, the four countries that form the Tigris-Euphrates water basin (Turkey, Syria, Iraq and Iran) in which *S. haematobium* is established should be regarded as the major zone of infection in South-West Asia.

In Saudi Arabia schistosomiasis is focal in distribution, affecting widely scattered oases. The proximity of certain foci to Mecca and the possible spread of the disease along pilgrims' routes, however, make them important centres for the dissemination of infection abroad. The affected areas in Yemen, the region of the high plateau in the north, are fairly extensive, but the suspected areas in the foothills and the middle heights of Taiz and Ibb Provinces are relatively limited in extent.

Circumscribed foci also exist in Southern Yemen, contiguous with the centres in Yemen.

A new focus has been discovered at Sarafand in Lebanon in recent years (1961).

Southern Yemen

In a report on schistosomiasis HAYTHORNTWAITE [in PETRIE and SEAL, 1943] mentioned that in 1940, 12 members of the Royal Air Force who bathed in Wadi Tiban at Museimir Al Anad became infected with *S. mansoni*. The disease is still present in this area [WRIGHT, 1963a]. A focus of *S. mansoni* is also present at Wadi Hatib south of Nisab.

Autochthonous cases of *S. haematobium* were reported by GREVAL [1923]. Foci have also been reported in Subeihi at Tor al Baha and Khor Umeira, in Haushabi at Museimir and Kirsh, and in Amiri at Dhubiyat and on Jebel Jehaf [PETRIE and SEAL, 1943]. In 1959, a focus was discovered at Dirgag in Abyan in the then Western Aden Protectorate [WRIGHT, 1963a], Abyan is a district lying between Wadi Bana and Wadi Hasan, and one of lesser extent in Wadi Hasan. The rate of infection among school-children examined in Dirgag ranges up to 80%.

Urinary schistosomiasis is also known to occur in Said, a small town in Wadi Yeshbum in upper Aulaqi, not far from the border between the former Western and Eastern Protectorates of Aden, at an altitude of about 1,000 m. There are a number of similar towns in the Wadi, but Said is the only one from which urinary schistosomiasis is at present known. Cases have also been reported from Wadi Hatib, south of Nisab. It is a wide, barren and sparsely populated valley with several short, permanent streams.

'The annual report of the Aden Health Service for 1959 shows that cases of schistosomiasis have been diagnosed in school-children at Dhala, at several villages in Abyan, at Mukeiras in Audhali, Said in Upper Aulaqi and at Al Ulya and Ain in Beihan. No differentiation between intestinal and urinary schistosomiasis is made in this report, but it is probable that the majority of infections are with *S.haematobium*, because of the greater ease with which it is detected. These records, taken in conjunction with those of PETRIE and SEAL, serve to show that schistosomiasis is widespread in the Western Aden Protectorate, but at present there are no adequate indications of the intensity of infection.' [WRIGHT, 1963a].

B.pfeifferi is the intermediate host of *S.mansoni* in Southern Yemen. It has been reported from Said, Wadi Yeshbum south-east of Said near the border of the former Western and Eastern Aden Protectorates. WRIGHT [1963a] found it also in Wadi Hatib, south of Nisab and at Museimir near the Yemen border.

B.(B.)reticulatus is a potential host of *S.haematobium* in Southern Yemen, but *B.(B.)beccarii* is probably the main host. The former has been found at Marbum, near Said; in Wadi Hatib, south of Nisab; at Tafwa and Dhala; and also at Raidi al Sa'ar, in the northern regions of the Hadramaut. *B.(B.)beccarii* is reported from Wadi Hasan at Dirgag, Abyan, and in Wadi Bana and Bateis, Abyan. *B.(B.)truncatus sericinus*, a potential host, was found by WRIGHT [1963b] at Tarbak, Wadi Amhadu, a part of Wadi Hatib.

References

GREVAL, S. D. S.: Indian J. med. Res. *10:* 943 (1923).
PETRIE, P. W. R. and SEAL, K. S.: A medical survey of the Western Aden Protectorate (1939–1940). Colonial Office (Middle East No. 66); cited by WRIGHT, 1963a (1943).
WRIGHT, C. A.: Trans. roy. Soc. trop. Med. Hyg. *57:* 142 (1963a).
WRIGHT, C. A.: Bull. brit. Mus. (nat. Hist.) Zool, *10:* 259 (1963b).

Yemen

S.mansoni and *S.haematobium* are present in Yemen. From available records, *S.mansoni* appears to be the more widely distributed species and to infect more people. FAROOQ [1960] has summarized the schistosomiasis situation in Yemen and has indicated that it is one of the major public health problems of the country.

The epidemiology of the disease is related to the topography of the country, the infection being absent from the lowland coastal belt (Tihama). *S.mansoni* is the predominent species in the middle height provinces of Taiz, Ibb and Baida, while *S.haematobium* infection is related to the highlands of Sana, Hajja and Sada Provinces.

Mosques constitute a major source of infection since the molluscan intermediate hosts flourish in the ablution basins, thus accounting for the predominantly male infections. The second most important source of infection is rainwater reservoirs or magils. Agricultural practices do not appear to be related to transmission in Yemen. Females acquire infection either in streams or open conduits which are used for washing clothes. Children are exposed mainly through swimming in pools in the mosques or in the Magils.

Endemicity of *S.mansoni* is limited to the foothills and the middle height zone, elevation up to 2,000 m. Some of the most fertile agricultural lands in the Arabian peninsula are to be found in this zone, where an elaborate and intricate system of terracing permits the cultivation of steep mountain slopes and fertile valleys, which constitute the granary of the country. Over 60% of Yemen's population lives in the area and is exposed to *S.mansoni* infection.

The disease is endemic in the provinces of Taiz, Ibb, Baida and Sana. From 35 to 50% of patients examined at Taiz hospitals were found to be infected [FAROOQ, 1960]. In these areas it is estimated that nearly 3,000,000 Yemenites are exposed to the infection and a conservative estimate of 1,000,000 individuals infected with *S.mansoni* is made [FAROOQ, 1960].

KUNTZ et al. [1953] found 7% of 182 persons positive for *S.mansoni* at Hodeida, 56% of 218 positive at Taiz, 4% of 26 positive at Ma'bar and 18% of 70 positive at Sana. The Hodeida cases came from inland.

DI EGIDO [1958] reported on the examination of stools at the Royal Hospital at Taiz, to which patients come from all parts of the country. In 1955, 24.6% of 1,952 faecal specimens were positive for *S.mansoni* and, in 1957, 8.4% of 4,148 were positive.

AYAD [1956] found cases of intestinal and urinary schistosomiasis in schoolboys at Sana, Taiz and *S.mansoni* infection in people at Hodeida.

NAGATY [1963] conducted faecal examinations at various points in Yemen. At Sana and the vicinity, including Manakha, 6% of 409 persons, mostly males, were positive for *S.mansoni*. Only 2% of 185 males in Tihama, including Hodeida, were positive. Undoubtedly, these cases were imported, since intestinal schistosomiasis is apparently not endemic in the low coastal Tihama area. A total of 198 persons were examined from Taiz and the vicinity, of whom 27% were infected with *S.mansoni*. Faecal specimens from 49 males were collected from Ibb and Jibla; of these stools, only one was positive for *S. mansoni*.

Foci of *S. haematobium* are widespread in the highland plateau areas of Sada, Hajjah, Sana, Baida, Ibb and the Taiz Provinces. It has not been recorded from the northernmost province of Asir. Its distribution is rather focal and sources of infection are well delineated. Infection rates are believed to be below 10%. *S. haematobium* is absent in the lowland coastal belt (Tihama) and only a few cases are reported from the foothills and the middle heights of Yemen from the provinces of Taiz and Ibb.

It is believed that approximately 50% of the population living in the endemic areas is exposed to the infection in the highland plateau (elevation 2,000–4,000 m), which contains less than 30% of the population of Yemen, estimated between 4 and 7 million. It is reckoned that if 500,000 individuals are exposed to the infection with an over-all infection rate of 5% there would be 25,000 cases of *S. haematobium* in the country. These estimates are based on FAROOQ's reconnaissance survey of 1960.

KUNTZ *et al.* [1953] found 10% of 218 persons positive at Taiz. NAGATY [1963] conducted urine examinations at various places in Yemen and obtained infection rates for *S. haematobium* in 5% of 387 males and 5% of 97 females at Sana and Manakha, less than 1% in 67 males at Taiz and the vicinity, and slightly over 1% among 122 males at Ibb and Jibla. Since most urine and faecal examinations in Yemen have been conducted on hospitalized individuals in several of the main towns and cities, there is little available information on prevalence rates in most of the endemic areas of schistosomiasis.

Biomphalaria spp. of molluscan intermediate host have been collected from some endemic areas of *S. mansoni* and *Bulinus (B.)* spp. from those of *S. haematobium*. Specific identifications are lacking from much of the material. Presumably *B. pfeifferi* is the intermediate host of *S. mansoni* and *B. (B.) truncatus* that for *S. haematobium*. Probably *B. (B.) truncatus* is represented by a sub-species or variety, *sericinus*.

References
AYAD, N.: Bull. Wld Hlth Org. *14:* 1 (1956).
EGIDO, M. DI: Arch. ital. Sci. med. trop. *39:* 685 (1958).
FAROOQ, M.: Report on a visit to Yemen, 25 May–13 June 1960. WHO unpublished document, EM/BIL/16 (1960).
KUNTZ, R.E.; MALAKATIS, G.M.; LAWLESS, D.K., and STROME, C.P.A.: Amer. J. trop. Med. Hyg. *2:* 13 (1953).
NAGATY, H.F.: A survey of malaria, bilharziasis, onchocerciasis and other parasitic infections in the Yemen, 8 April–3 June 1962. WHO unpublished document, EM/EPID/9 (1963).

Saudi Arabia

Schistosomiasis in Saudi Arabia is characterized by its marked focal distribution. It is largely a disease of oases. Its economic importance arises from the fact that it affects the only islands of fertility in what is otherwise a sea of sandy desert and barren hills. A large proportion of the population is engaged in herding animals and leads a nomadic existence. These nomadic peoples are no doubt an important source for the spread of schistosomiasis and, because of their way of life, are not susceptible to control.

Few data are available on prevalence rates in various parts of the country. The main information on distribution of the disease was furnished through a survey by FAROOQ [1961]. Some data have been collected by personnel of the Arabian American Oil Company, largely from treatment of employees in various medical dispensaries; however, these people have originated in many different places in South-West Asia and elsewhere and it is often difficult to pinpoint the place of exposure.

KLIMOV [1963] examined 810 people for schistosomiasis in the south-west of the Arabian Peninsula and found 522 with *S. mansoni* and 288 with *S. haematobium* infections.

S. mansoni is endemic in Taif, a large oasis at 1,373 m elevation and the summer capital of Saudi Arabia. It has a population of 160,000 to 180,000. An infection rate of 13.2% has been reported in the area [FAROOQ, 1961]. Apart from this oasis no other confirmed foci of *S. mansoni* have been reported from Hejaz. In view of the growing importance of Taif, and the establishment of road and air communication between it and Mecca for the benefit of pilgrims, the dangers of the spread of infection even outside the country appear considerable.

Endemic centres in a number of oases exist in Nejd, the central Arabian province, within a short distance of each other on the outskirts of Riyadh, the capital city of the country. Of these, Diriya, Elb and Oda form a picturesque circular group of oases in a deep wadi, 20 km north-west of Riyadh. The population, an estimated 7,000 to 8,000, has an infection rate of less than 10%.

A northern group of oases, Binban and Ugla, some 50 km north of Riyadh, have been known to be endemic with epidemic outbreaks of severe forms of *S. mansoni*.

Solima oasis in Al Kharj district, 77 km south of Riyadh, is endemic. An infection rate of 25% in the school population has been obtained. The importance of this focus lies in the fact that it is very close to the extensive agricultural projects, with rich underground reservoirs of water, being developed jointly by the Government and ARAMCO at Sahaba. Water is pumped from large 'ains' 14 km away and flows in open irrigation channels. The potentialities of spread of infection in the area appear to be considerable [FAROOQ, 1961].

Endemicity of *S.haematobium* has been established in two areas in Hejjaz Province in Saudi Arabia. One in Wadi Fatima and the other in the Tabuk area.

Wadi Fatima is a valley, 70 km long and 5 to 15 km in width, which skirts Mecca on its east. It has a rich, underground source of water and in parts it is very green with luxuriant growth of date palms and fruit trees. Over 50,000 people, cultivators and nomads, inhabit scattered villages in the valley. Haematuria has been reported to be rampant in Gushashia village in the valley, about 45 km north-east of Mecca. *S.haematobium* has been reported among patients attending King's Hospital in Mecca, whose histories revealed visits to Wadi Fatima. This valley should be regarded as possessing endemic foci of *S.haematobium* with requisite potentialities for the spread of infection. Unconfirmed reports of urinary schistosomiasis have also been made from Rabigh area between Jeddah and Medina (in Barza, Khalais and Hager oases, 100 km into the interior of the Rabigh area) [FAROOQ, 1961].

Tabuk is a flourishing oasis, 500 km north of Medina on the derelict section of the old Hejjaz railway about 50 km from the border of Jordan. It has a civilian population of 5,000 and a large military camp (30,000) on its outskirts. Among the out-patients attending the military and civil hospitals in Tabuk, 7 or 8 new cases of *S.haematobium* are seen every month. Unconfirmed reports of urinary schistosomiasis have also been made from the Taima area south-east of Tabuk.

The occurrence of *S.haematobium* has been reported from parts of the southern province of Asir, bordering Yemen. Infection has been stated to be frequent among individuals coming from Qizan in the area. This important but least developed province, just north of Yemen, is also becoming a well-established centre of *S.haematobium* [FAROOQ, 1961].

In a schistosomiasis survey initiated in 1965 by the Medical Department of ARAMCO, ALIO [1967] conducted intradermal tests and observed evidence of gross haematuria in schoolboys in numerous areas. On the basis of his findings, he regarded the exposure to schistosomiasis hazard to be of moderate degree in five communities and of marked degree in seven communities.

Biomphalaria spp. of molluscan intermediate host have been collected by AZIM and GISMANN [1956] and by FAROOQ [1961]. Presumably *B.pfeifferi* is involved in transmission of *S.mansoni* but specific determination needs to be made.

B. (B.) truncatus is the intermediate host of *S. haematobium. B. (B.) forskalii* was found by FAROOQ in a masonry channel at Gushashia in Wadi Fatima and by AZIM at Ain El Khef, 25 km west of Gushashia. It is not known whether this species is involved in the transmission of urinary schistosomiasis.

According to ALIO [1967], MANDAHL-BARTH found that the genital organs of *Biomphalaria* in Saudi Arabia seemed to agree with those of *B. pfeifferi* but that the radula is reminiscent of that of *B. alexandrina*. He regarded the form as a new species which he named *B. arabica*.

References

ALIO, IVAN S.: Epidemiology of schistosomiasis in Saudi Arabia with an emphasis on geographic distribution patterns. Arabian-American Oil Co., Dhahran, Saudi Arabia. Document (1967).

AZIM, M. A. and GISMANN, A.: Bull. Wld Hlth Org. *14:* 403 (1956).

FAROOQ, M.: Report on a visit to Saudi Arabia, 24 November–26 December 1960. WHO unpublished document, EM/BIL/24 (1961).

KLIMOV, I. A.: Med. Parazit. (Mosk.) *32:* 710 (1963).

Israel

S. mansoni was long reported as rare and was considered to be of extraneous origin. FAIRLEY and FAIRLEY [1929] indicated the occurrence of both types of schistosomiasis among four persons immigrating from Palestine to Australia, who supposedly had acquired their infection in the neighbourhood of Jaffa; two of these harboured *S. mansoni*.

During a survey for hookworm conducted in the Jaffa area in 1931–1932, SCOTT *et al.* [1934] found *S. mansoni* ova in three Arabs originating from Jarisha and Yamassin Gharbiya villages. WITENBERG [1938] found eggs of both *S. haematobium* and *S. mansoni* in the urine of a large proportion of infected persons in the same villages of Jarisha and Yamassin, localities he believed to be constant dissemination foci for both forms of schistosomiasis, and he also reported the presence of both host snails in Wadi Musrara, a tributary of the Yarkon.

Indigenous cases of *S. mansoni* were also reported by FRANKL [1953], who observed early intestinal schistosomiasis in 19 youths, all born in the country. The patients were seen in 1951 and were thought to have acquired their infection in or near the River Yarkon (Auja), near Tel Aviv. FRANKL is not aware of earlier autochthonous cases and believes the parasite to have been imported by Yemenites.

WITENBERG [1951] stated: 'Over 20% of immigrants from Yemen are infected with *S. mansoni*. *S. haematobium* occurs among them also, but is rare.' HELLER [1953] wrote: 'It is conservatively estimated that 20,000–30,000 Yemenites are infected by *S. mansoni* (and in a smaller number by *S. haematobium* as well).' ELIAKIM and DAVIES [1954] examined 690 Yemenite immigrants by means of the skin test and found that 37.9% of the males and 30.4% of the females reacted positively. They reported incidence to increase with age, ranging from 21.4% in children 3 to 4 years old to 84.6% in adults over the age of 50. It may be assumed that the rates for *S. mansoni* are only slightly lower.

According to SALITERNIK and WITENBERG [1959], *Biomphalaria* had disappeared from the single known focus in the Yarkon River. There is apparently no danger of spread of infection unless the snail is again introduced.

S. haematobium: The sporadic occurrence of urinary schistosomiasis in Palestine was known to practitioners some time before the First World War, and clinical cases were reported from different parts of the country by several authors.

FELIX [1925] demonstrated the disease in various groups of Jewish school-children and students in the Jaffa area, including the Jaffa orphanage (23 of 53, or 43%) and the agricultural school of Mekveh Israel (21 of 158, or 13%). From a total of 1,256 children examined 54, or 4%, were infected.

BUXTON and KRIKORIAN [1922] proved the endemicity of the disease among Arab school-children in villages around Jaffa to be 7% (31 of 470).

Other well-authenticated cases of indigenous infection were reported from Um Khalid, near the Iskanderuna River, which the inhabitants had to wade; from Nahr Rubin; from Nahr Barideh; and from the River Auja itself.

FELIX [1925] points out that during 1921, 11 cases of urinary schistosomiasis in adults were found in his laboratory without systematic search and opposed the opinion, expressed by BUXTON and KRIKORIAN [1922], that the disease was 'apparently dying out of the area'. On the contrary, he feared that the creation of agricultural settlements would introduce new sources of infection.

In 1951, official information was obtained from the Israeli health authorities.[1] Although notifications to government health departments must be considered unreliable, it appears that a marked decrease was noted in the incidence of the disease from 1930 onwards. A total of 299 cases was reported during the 11-year span 1935 to 1945, as follows:

1   Personal communication from Health Ministry, Israel, to Dr. J. S. PETERSON, Medical, Education and Welfare Division, United Nations Relief and Works Agency for Palestine Refugees in the Near East.

Year	Number of cases	Year	Number of cases
1935	6	1941	6
1936	69	1942	1
1937	144	1943	1
1938	41	1944	3
1939	4	1945	2
1940	22		

The vast majority of these cases were of urinary schistosomiasis and had been contracted locally. From 1948 to 1950, no locally contracted cases of urinary schistosomiasis were detected in Israel. In 1952, 89 cases were detected among Arab refugees from Palestine.

Between 1948 and 1952 some 300,000 persons immigrated into Israel from schistosomiasis endemic areas; of these, 40,000 are estimated to suffer from the disease [DAVIES and ELIAKIM, 1955].

In 1955, an outbreak of urinary schistosomiasis was reported outside the endemic Jaffa area, from Tirat-Zvi, a settlement in the Beth-Shean valley, Jordan region [WITENBERG and SALITERNICK, 1955; DAVIES, 1955]. Nearly 50% of the young people were found to be infected; a systematic examination of all 451 inhabitants revealed S. haematobium infection in 97 persons (21.5%) mostly under the age of 20. It is believed that the infections were all contracted in the local swimming pools and that they were originally introduced by immigrants from Iraq and Iran living in nearby settlements. There is reason to suspect that other autochthonous foci now exist in the Beth-Shean valley.

In summary, the present state of infection in Israel should not be regarded as static. Changes in epidemiological factors may occur in the future and the possibility of spreading infection may increase [WITENBERG and SALITERNIK, 1957].

As indicated previously Biomphalaria sp. of molluscan intermediate host which transmitted S. mansoni, is no longer found in Israel.

B. (B.) truncatus is the intermediate host of S. haematobium and is widely distributed throughout the lower regions of the northern and central parts of the country. It is not generally found in hilly country, the Negev or the Arava Valley. Its absence in the hilly country may be explained by the scarcity of swamps and the absence of rivers. The Negev and the Arava Valley are poor in perennial water basins and the spring water usually has a high salt content. However, with the completion of planned irrigation projects, conditions for Bulinus breeding may be created at some places.

WITENBERG and SALITERNIK [1957] recorded *B. (B.) truncatus* from over 80 places in Israel.

References
BUXTON, P. A. and KRIKORIAN, K. S.: Trans. roy. Soc. trop. Med. Hyg. *16:* 162 (1922).
DAVIES, A. M.: Harefuah *49:* 10 (1955).
DAVIES, A. M. and ELIAKIM, M.: Ann. trop. Med. Parasit. *49:* 9 (1955).
ELIAKIM, M. and DAVIES, A. M.: Harefuah *47:* 121 (1954).
FAIRLEY, K. D. and FAIRLEY, N. H.: Med. J. Aust. *2:* 597 (1929).
FELIX, A.: Amer. J. trop. Med. *5:* 41 (1925).
FRANKL, O.: Harefuah *45:* 83 (1953).
HELLER, H.: Harefuah *44:* 243 (1953).
SALITERNIK, Z. and WITENBERG, G.: Bull. Wld Hlth Org. *21:* 161 (1959).
SCOTT, J. A.; AYOUB, G. E., and REITLER, R.: Amer. J. Hyg. *19:* 601 (1934).
WITENBERG, G.: in MAGNES anniversary book, Jerusalem, p. 319 (1938).
WITENBERG, G.: Harefuah *41:* 178 (1951).
WITENBERG, G. and SALITERNIK, Z.: Harefuah *48:* 219 (1955).
WITENBERG, G. and SALITERNIK, Z.: Bull. Res. Coun. Israel B *6:* 107 (1957).

Lebanon

The first autochthonous infection was reported from Lebanon in 1961 [AZAR *et al*.]. A boy from Sarafand was found infected with *S. haematobium* by the staff of the American University Hospital. As a consequence the American University Hospital conducted a field survey at Sarafand in 1961 and found an endemic focus in the area between Sidon and Tyre (Sur). Of 591 residents of all ages, 14.6% were found infected with *S. haematobium*. One third of the age group 10 to 19 years were infected.

The endemic focus lies in a coastal strip between Sidon and Tyre which is irrigated by a canal running northward from a dam created on the Litani River as it emerges into the coastal area [EL BITASH, 1964]. Occasionally infected persons have been found living outside this area, but it is believed that they had contracted the infection while in the endemic area. The northern limit of the area is near the terminus of the irrigation canal and the southern limit is not clearly known.

According to a report from the project [OLIVIER and BUZO, 1964], 8.5% of the 1,470 inhabitants of Old Sarafand have been found infected, and 5.3% of the inhabitants of the new coastal portion of Sarafand are infected.

S. mansoni is not present in Lebanon.

The molluscan intermediate host *B. (B.) truncatus* transmits urinary schistosomiasis in Lebanon. The snail has been found in various places

[AZIM and GIZMANN, 1956] even up the Nahr el Litani River as far as Qara'on. It has been recovered also from Saida and Sur and the intervening areas along the irrigation canal between these two towns. It was not until 1963 that the first infected snails were discovered in Sarafand [SCHACHER *et al.*, 1964]. Exposure of a gerbil *(Gerbillus gerbillus)* to cercariae shed by these snails resulted in the development of adult *S. haematobium* in the animal.

References

AZAR, J.E.; LUTTERMOSER, G.W., and SCHACHER, J.F.: Amer. J. trop. Med. Hyg. *10:* 709 (1961).

AZIM, M.A. and GISMANN, A.: Bull. Wld Hlth Org. *14:* 403 (1956).

EL BITASH, M.H.: Rapport de mission. Lutte contre la bilharziose au Liban. Report on the control of bilharziasis in the Lebanon, 28 mai–27 aout, 1964. WHO unpublished document, EM/BIL/29 (1964).

OLIVIER, L.J. and BUZO, Z.J.: Report on a visit to Lebanon by the WHO Inter-regional Bilharziasis Advisory Team, 16–21 March 1964. WHO unpublished document, MHO/PA/148.64 (1964).

SCHACHER, J.F.; DAILEY, M.D., and KHALIL, G.M.: J. Parasit. *50:* 545 (1964).

Syria

There are three distinct endemic zones of *S. haematobium* in the Syrian Jezireh (Syrian Mesopotamia) water basin which is a section of the 'Fertile Crescent' of the Middle East. Two of these zones lie at the Syrio-Turkish border in the north, and a third to the south extends from the confluence of the River Khabur with the Euphrates up to the Iraqi border:

(1) in Hazakeh governorate: the Koubour-el-Beid area, Kamishli town and adjacent villages;

(2) in Rakka governorate: the Tell Abiad area and Rakka sub-district;

(3) in Deir-ez-Zor governorate: the Saloo area and Al Hurri in Abu Kamal district.

The schistosomiasis problem was assessed in 1959 by FAROOQ (table XXIV) and in 1968 by ABDALLAH AHMED. According to the latter, the prevalence of the disease has diminished in Hazakeh governorate (12.80% in 1955 to 1.60% in 1967) due to control efforts but the discovery of new infections, particularly among the young age groups (67.4% infected) denotes that active transmission is still taking place. The situation has deteriorated in Rakka governorate where the incidence of the disease in the villages investigated ranges from 13.5 to 25.1%. In Deir-ez-Zor governorate prevalence rates of 18 to 24% have been recorded.

Table XXIV. Schistosomiasis *(S. haematobium)* endemic areas in the Syrian Jezireh, 1959[1]

Endemic zone	Foci	First found infected	Water course involved	Extent km²	Number of villages	Population exposed	Number infected	Infection rate, %
Koubour-el-Beid-Kamishli	A. Koubour-el-Beid	1937	Rivers Jarah and Sublak and their canals	350	52[2]	7,700	225	2.9
	B. Kamishli	1954	River Jagh-Jagh and canals	250	49 and 1 city	51,000	1,680	3.3
	C. Damirqapoo	1959	River Ramila	5	1	110	18	16.4
Tell Abiad-Rakka	A. Turkaman	1943	Khneiz Stream and	40	3	5,000	600	12.0
	B. Khneiz	1943	River Balekh	60	4	8,000	560	7.0
Saloo-Tobe		1956	irrigation canal from Euphrates and three lakes	3	2	2,000	170	8.5
Total				708	111 villages 1 city	73,810	3,253	4.4

1 From report by FAROOQ [1959].
2 Including four additional villages found infected in 1958 and 1959.

B. (B.) truncatus is the intermediate host of S. haematobium in Syria. The snails are well distributed along the rivers in the endemic zones, although past infection rates in the snail do not seem to be high. With prospective development of irrigation projects, distribution of the intermediate host will no doubt be extended.

References

ABDALLAH AHMED, A.: Assignment report. Schistosomiasis control in the Syrian Arab Republic. WHO unpublished document, EM/SCHIS/42 (1968).

FAROOQ, M.: Report on a visit to bilharziasis endemic areas in Syria. WHO unpublished document, EM/BIL/12 (1959).

Turkey

A focus of infection in Nusseibin involving three villages, Gundek Sadek, Grebia and Kinnik on the Sublak River, with a population of 1,300, was found in 1956, when an epidemic outbreak of S. haematobium occurred in the area [GÜRSEL, 1956]. This focus within the Turkish border is virtually a part of the Koubour-el-Beid endemic zone in Syria just across the border. FAROOQ [1959] reported 10 persons infected of the population of 1,300.

This limited focus is potentially dangerous for the Nusseibin Province in which extensive lands are being brought under perennial irrigation. The damming of the Jagh-Jagh River and the irrigation system recently completed is reported to be in danger of being infected from both the existing focus within the area and from across the border from Koubour-el-Beid and Kamishli foci in Syria [FAROOQ, 1959].

B. (B.) truncatus is the intermediate host in the endemic area. No current data are available on its distribution.

References

FAROOQ, M.: Report on a visit to bilharziasis endemic areas in the Province of Syria, UAR and Turkey. WHO unpublished document, EM/BIL/12 (1959).

GÜRSEL, A.: Türk Ij. tecr. Biyol. Derg. 16: 195 (1956).

Iraq

Iraq contains the greater part of Mesopotamia or the fertile valleys of the Tigris and the Euphrates, from the highlands of Asia Minor in the north-west to the Persian Gulf in the south-east. It also includes, on the north-eastern Iranian frontier, about one third of mountainous Kurdistan and, on the Jordan and Arabian frontiers in the south-west, a portion of the Syrian Desert (Badiet esh Sham) almost half as large as the remainder of the Iraq territory.

The valley of the twin rivers can be divided into two contrasting regions, the upper and the lower valley, the line of demarcation being formed by the prehistoric coastline of the Persian Gulf, which is still seen as a shelf running across the flood-plain at about the latitude of Baghdad. In the upper valley, the two distinct river basins cut a region of undulating steppe, pasture and ploughland. The southern alluvial plain, created by the rivers themselves within the past 7,000 years, shows the land forms associated with fluviatile deposition: braided channels, extensive marshlands, and embanked river courses (natural levees).

During and after the First World War, interest in the problem was stimulated by sporadic outbreaks of schistosomiasis among British troops stationed at Basra, Hinaidi, and Kufa. BOULENGER [1919] examined 174 male Iraqi in the central and lower valley, from Samarra to Basra, finding an average incidence of 20% and a maximum incidence of 85% in Qurna. Investigations by HALL [1925] revealed the prevalence of the disease from the latitude of Hindiya southward, particularly in the rice-fields. He found a prevalence of 80% in the rural areas of Diwaniya Province. Of 711 Basra school-children he found 47% infected.

From data contained in the Iraq Health Service reports between the years 1921 and 1928, quoted by MILLS et al. [1936] and by NEVEU-LEMAIRE [1929], it appears that schistosomiasis cases had been reported at the dispensaries, at one time or another, from all but the two northernmost provinces of Mosul and Sulaimaniya, the heaviest infection records coming from the south. From a total of 887 cases for the first quarter of 1928, 62% had been observed in Basra Province. In Nasirya, 80% of school-children were found to have schistosomiasis. Outbreaks of the disease had occurred south-east of Baghdad in 1921 and 1924.

The extent and gravity of the problem in this area today is immensely increased by the progress of plans for the construction of vast new irrigation systems which will inevitably lead to the spread of infection by S. haematobium unless exceptionally vigorous measures of prevention are undertaken. Some 50 separate new irrigation projects are under way in Iraq.

In the northern valley of the Tigris, conditions are marginal and small foci have flared up sporadically only to become spontaneously extinct, but in the middle and lower valley of the twin rivers prevalence and intensity of the disease are heavy, especially towards the south, but cease altogether south of Basra, where the tidal irrigation does not favour the establishment of *Bulinus*. The over-all prevalence of schistosomiasis in Iraq is about 20%. In certain areas, however, infection rates are much higher: in Tel Mohammed, near Baghdad, it is 80%; in the area surrounding Baghdad city the prevalence of *S.haematobium* has risen from less than 10 to over 25% owing to the great increase of lift-irrigation by pumps. It is estimated that there is at least a total of 5,000,000 exposed to the risk of infection and at least 1,000,000 individuals infected with *S.haematobium* in Iraq.

Schistosomiasis is now endemic in 10 Liwas of Central and Southern Iraq with the possibility of a few scattered foci present in the north. The endemic area extends from south of Mosul, Erbil and Kirkuk bordering the Tigris River, the Greater and Lesser Zab, the Diyala and the areas irrigated from them. The disease is also endemic in the upper reaches of the Euphrates River and throughout all Central Iraq, the Mesopotamian plain to the marsh areas of the south, the Muntifiq and Amara Provinces as far as Basra. The only species present is *S.haematobium*. The distribution of the disease in the south does not appear to be uniform. A line of demarcation exists immediately south of Basra.

Based on single urine examinations of male school-children in 10 Liwas, a prevalence rate of 29.4% was obtained in 18,647 examinations in 1955 and 17.6% in 36,753 examinations in 1956. A sample survey in 1958 in the Tarmiya area showed 34.2% positives in 483 persons examined [AZZAWI *et al.*, 1961].

In the Amara rice growing area, it has been stated that 70% of the children in one village are infected [MCMULLEN and RAINEY, 1959]. There are few published data on prevalence rates in most of the endemic areas as no general surveys have apparently been made.

The epidemiology of the disease in the Basra area in the south presents puzzling aspects. NAJARIAN *et al.* [1961] were unable to find *B. (B.) truncatus* as have others in the past. On the other hand, some investigators have had no difficulty in this respect. NAJARIAN and his associates examined 427 individuals from nine canal zones along the Shatt al Arab River in the vicinity of Basra and obtained prevalence rates varying between 86 and 2% in children in settlements along five canals. Tidal effects from the Persian Gulf had previously been held responsible for limiting the distribution of *B. (B.) truncatus*. However, it was found by NAJARIAN *et al.* [1961] that salinity in the Shatt al Arab River originated in Lake Hammar.

The endemicity of urinary schistosomiasis in Iraq is promoted by extensive systems of irrigation, which vary from privately-owned pump schemes to well-planned large government installations. Among the latter already in operation in the endemic area are Dujaila, which opened in 1945, and Latafia, which has been under cultivation since 1954. Transmission is taking place in both of these areas [WRIGHT, 1958]. The Musayeb Project south of Baghdad was opened to settlers in 1956. By 1958, 13,000 of these people had been screened for *S.haematobium* and 28% had been found positive [FAROOQ, 1958].

B. (B.) truncatus is the only demonstrated molluscan intermediate host in Iraq. It is found in all endemic areas, the possible exception is the Basra area already noted [OUGHTON and RADHAWY, 1962].

The snail occurs extensively in marshes, swamps, irrigation channels and drains in Central and Southern Iraq, principally along the courses of the Tigris and Euphrates Rivers, and in a few limited foci in the northern part of the country, where it is disappearing. As noted, it probably occurs in some of the canals in the vicinity of Basra. The species has never been recorded from the Tigris or Euphrates Rivers or from their major tributaries (the Greater and Lesser Zab and the Diyala) in Iraq [WATSON, 1958].

In irrigation canals, adult *B. (B.) truncatus* appears to be discontinuous in occurrence and tends to be localized in certain areas. However, juveniles are more generally distributed [NAJARIAN, 1961].

References

AZZAWI, J. A. H. EL; KLIMT, D. R., and BAQUIR, H.: Bull. endem. Dis. *4:* 64 (1961).

BOULENGER, C. L.: Indian J. med. Res. *7:* 8 (1919).

FAROOQ, M.: Report on a visit to the bilharziasis control project in Iraq, 22–27 June 1958. WHO unpublished document, IRAQ-15 (1958).

HALL, A. H.: J. roy. Army med. Cps *44:* 92 (1925).

McMULLEN, D. B. and RAINEY, M. B.: Report on the preliminary survey by the Bilharziasis Advisory Team. I. Iraq. WHO unpublished document, MHO/PA/18.59 (1958).

MILLS, E. A.; MACHATTIE, C., and CHADWICK, C. R.: Trans. roy. Soc. trop. Med. Hyg. *30:* 317 (1936).

NAJARIAN, H. H.: Bull. Wld Hlth Org. *25:* 435 (1961).

NAJARIAN, H. H.; ARAOZ, J. DE; KLIMT, C. R.; ANI, K. AL, and AZZAWI, J.: Bull. Wld Hlth Org. *25:* 467 (1961).

NEVEU-LEMAIRE, M.: Ann. Parasit. hum. comp. *7:* 1 (1929).

OUGHTON, J. G. and RADHAWY, I. A.: Bull. endem. Dis. *4:* 23 (1962).

WATSON, J. M.: Bull. Wld Hlth Org. *18:* 833 (1958).

WRIGHT, W. H.: Observations on bilharziasis research and control programmes in Iraq, 12–19 December, 1957. WHO unpublished document, IRAQ 15 (1958).

Iran

It is believed that urinary schistosomiasis has existed in Iran since ancient times, at least in the south-western portion (Khuzistan) where Iran and Iraq share extensive marshlands, stretching between Amara and Ahwaz. Its distribution is still confined only to Khuzistan Province which geographically constitutes the eastern prolongation of Mesopotamia. It has an area of 50,000 km² and a population of 1,500,000 [ANSARI, 1958].

There are two areas which lie near to each other and have numerous foci, with few unaffected villages between them; these are the Dasht-Mishan and the Lower Diz-Shahur areas. The first is clearly delimited on the south and east by desert or marsh; on the west its limits are less clear. The second is bordered on the west by the dry and almost uninhabited land to the west of the Karheh; its limits are much less clear to the east and north where the foci seem to be more scattered. Both areas are inhabited by Arabs.

Apart from these two areas there are small, relatively isolated foci of one to four villages which appear to be ectopic or marginal. These are the areas of Khorramshahr in the south, Zargan and Seh Boneh to the east, and Bidroubeh to the north.

It is possible to say that the areas of the Dasht-Mishan and the Diz-Shahur are probably old, or even ancient, foci of the disease. On the other hand, one gets the impression that some of the foci may be recent. It is not possible to give an opinion about the focus at Khorramshahr, but the focus at Zargan seems to be, at the most, 15 years old. Thus, it seems to date from the time water was first pumped from the Karun into this area, which previously had been in dry-farming. The focus at Seh Boneh seems to date from the time, about 30 years ago, when a small group of Arabs moved to the place amongst the Bakhtiari. Finally, the focus at Bidroubeh seems to have originated as a result of the migration of a family into the area from the Shahur about 15 years ago.

Other important foci have been discovered in recent years, including those in the Neydankhan District to the north of Dezful and the Sar-Dasht District to the east. Two additional foci lie along the Karun River between Shoushtar and Sar-Dasht.

Although it is a matter of information and opinion that is hard to verify, the impression is gained that urinary schistosomiasis may be spreading in Khuzistan and that the spread depends upon human migration and the availability of suitable snail hosts. If one considers that Khuzistan is the most eastern region in which urinary schistosomiasis transmitted by *Bulinus* spp.

is known to occur, this impression is disquieting since we have no idea as to how far east it might go eventually.

Prevalence of *S. haematobium* in the endemic areas described, varies from village to village and ranges up to 88%. Prevalence is often greater in Arab villages than in those inhabited by Luror Bakhtiari. An over-all rate of 10% in the endemic areas of Khuzistan may not be an unreasonable estimate. GAUD *et al.* [1963] estimated the total number of persons infected at 100,000 in Khuzistan.

B. (B.) truncatus is the only known intermediate host of *S. haematobium* in Iran. The snail is not uniformly distributed throughout the endemic areas and in some locations it has not been possible to locate snails even though there is evidence of transmission.

The species is found in natural water sites but more frequently in manmade habitats. Among the former are swamps, ponds, rainwater accumulations and stagnant river pools. Man-made habitats comprise irrigation canals and drains, borrow pits, water reservoirs and drains, and artificial ponds.

References

ANSARI, N.: Report on a visit to Iran. WHO unpublished document (1958).
GAUD, J.; ARFAA, F., and ZEINI, A.: Ann. Parasit. *37:* 232 (1962).
WHO: Assisted Bilharziasis Pilot Project – IRAN 0038, Dezful, Khuzistan, Iran, Quarterly Reports. Unpublished documents.

Cyprus

WILLIAMSON first reported *S. haematobium* infection from Cyprus in 1902. In 1907, out of seven boys examined from Syrianokhori ('Syrian Village') he found five had eggs of *S. haematobium* present in the urine. RONALD ROSS recorded the occurrence of 'Bilharzia disease' from the same village in 1913. LEIPER [1928], examining seven boys in the village, found four infected. This focus, a small village on Morphon Bay, is on the west coast of the island. As the name of the village indicates, the inhabitants are the descendants of Syrian immigrants, which may explain the origin of the infection, but it is also possible that it may have entered the island with the Egyptian invasions, of which there are archaeological traces in the neighbourhood of Syrianokhori [LEIPER, 1928].

The district in which the village is situated is irrigated by a series of deep artifical channels bringing water from the river at some distance upstream and there are drains below the village.

A few cases known in Morphon about 1.6 km inland from Syrianokhori, were also believed to have been acquired in the village.

The area is now considered to be free from infection as a result of the drainage work undertaken during 1928 to 1932, and may, therefore, be regarded as a rare instance of an extinct schistosomiasis focus.

References

LEIPER, R. T.: J. Helminth *6:* 117 (1928).
ROSS, R.: Report to the Colonial Office on the Prevention of Malaria in Cyprus (1913).
WILLIAMSON, G. A.: Brit. med. J. *ii:* 956 (1902).
WILLIAMSON, G. A.: Brit. med. J. *ii:* 1333 (1907).

Distribution of Schistosoma haematobium *in South Central Asia*

There is at present only one established focus of *S. haematobium* in South Central Asia, i.e. in India. In addition to the single known endemic focus in Maharashtra State there is evidence, from a few widely scattered reports, that other foci of infection are present in the country.

The history of the disease in India dates back to the time when POWELL [1903] observed urinary schistosomiasis in a man from Bombay who had never been out of the State. Subsequently there have been other reports of autochthonous cases of human urinary schistosomiasis from the Indian sub-continent. Several are reports of infection found in British soldiers who apparently were exposed while on duty in India; there is a slight possibility that they may have acquired the infection while en route either to or from India. The other four reports deserve special mention. HOOTON [1914] encountered urinary schistosomiasis in a Parsee girl aged 5, who lived in Rajkot. In 1936, DE MELLO reported a similar case in a 9-year old boy from Valpoy, Goa. ANDREASEN and SURI [1945] reported urinary schistosomiasis in an 18-year-old Sepoy who grew up in Ambala, Punjab, but had had a short tour of duty in Poona before reporting with haematuria. Finally, DE SA and MONTEIRO [1949] found a case of urinary schistosomiasis in Ratnagiri District, and it was later shown that this case originated in Gimvi.

GADGIL and SHAH [1952] confirmed the existence of an endemic focus in Gimvi village in Ratnagiri District. Gimvi, a village of about 800 people, lies in rolling country near the estuary of the Vashishti River, which enters the sea at Anjavel above Ratnagiri in Ratnagiri District, 250 km south of Bombay. It lies near the Chiplun-Guhagar road and is about 16 km from Guhagar, which is on the sea coast. The village consists of scattered groups of houses lying on sloping ground near a small stream tributary to the Vashishti River, and flowing north. The stream rises in a spring at one end of the village. No case of schistosomiasis has been found in Ratnagiri District except among inhabitants of Gimvi. In 1955, there were 71 villages in a radius of 16 km of Gimvi which were visited by public health workers who questioned the villagers about haematuria. Urine was examined only from those that had haematuria. In this way, two cases of schistosome infection were encountered in a village at some distance from Gimvi, but the two boys involved had spent some time in Gimvi and had apparently contracted their infection there. No systematic urine examinations have been made outside Gimvi.

In 1955, one urine sample was examined from each of the 528 villagers of all age groups. This constituted a large proportion of all the villagers present at the time. No adult had schistosome eggs in the urine, but 38 of 229 children were found to be infected. The oldest child was 15 and the youngest 5 years old. The infection was twice as prevalent in boys as among girls. In another study, made in 1958, a large proportion of all the villagers was again checked for schistosomiasis, but urine samples were obtained only from children from 5 to 15 years of age. Of these, 29 of 101 boys (29%), and 11 of 90 girls (1%) were infected. No adult admitted to having haematuria.

Examination of urine of 94 school-children by OLIVIER in 1961 gave an over-all infection rate of 57%; 71% of the boys and 28% of the girls were infected.

Another reported focus, in Lahager village, Rajpur District, Madhya Pradesh, is under investigation [SHRIVASTAVA and ARORA, 1969].

SHOUDA [1955] has reported recovering schistosome eggs from the faeces of Punjabis. These eggs probably came from ingestion of liver infested with S. indicum eggs.

The molluscan intermediate host of S. haematobium in India is Ferrissia tenuis.

References

ANDREASEN, A. T. and SURI, H. L.: Indian med. Gaz. 80: 93 (1945).
GADGIL, R. K. and SHAH, S. N.: Indian J. med. Sci. 6: 760 (1952).
HOOTON, A.: Indian med. Gaz. 49: 188 (1914).
MELLO, I. F. DE: An explanation to the occurrence of sporadic cases of urinary schistosomiasis in India. Proc. Indian Acad. Sci. 3: 107 (1936).
OLIVIER, L. J.: Assignment report on bilharzia control, India, January–March 1961. WHO unpublished document, SEA/BILHARZ/4 (1961).
POWELL, A.: Brit. med. J. i: 490 (1903).
SA, A. E. DE and MONTEIRO, L.: Indian J. med. Sci. 3: 376 (1949).
SHOUDA: cited by OLIVIER, 1961 (1955).
SHRIVASTAVA, K. K. and ANORA, M. M.: Personal communication to the WHO Regional Office, New Delhi (1969).

Distribution of Schistosoma japonicum *and Molluscan Intermediate Hosts in the Orient*

S. japonicum is confined to the Orient. Its endemicity is established in:
(1) China (Mainland),
(2) China (Taiwan),
(3) Japan,
(4) Philippines,
(5) Celebes,
(6) Thailand,
(7) Laos,
(8) Cambodia.

The northernmost centre in Honshu, north of Tokyo, and the southernmost focus in Celebes range between 36°, latitude north, to 3° latitude south. The northernmost centre in Japan also constitutes the easternmost limits of the infection on 140°, longitude east. The focus in Southern Thailand along 100°, longitude east, marks the most westernly limits of the infection so far known.

Over the past 50 years the infection in Japan has steadily receded to delimited areas of low prevalence with small foci of moderate endemicity. The reverse is the case with China (Mainland) and the Philippines, where the extent of the infection is not yet well defined and new areas of endemicity are still being found. In a majority of the affected areas in these two countries, endemicity ranges from moderate to high levels with foci of very high infection rates.

The foci in Celebes are confined to three villages in the northern part of central Celebes. The parasite in China (Taiwan) is a zoophilic strain and no autochthonous case of human infection has so far been found on the island.

Table XXV. Estimated number of persons exposed and infected with *S. japonicum* in the Orient

Country	Total population	Population exposed	Population infected
China	700,000,000	100,000,000	32,777,630
Japan	97,000,000	400,000	20,000
Philippines	32,000,000	1,500,000	421,500
Celebes	5,000,000	10,000	1,000
Thailand	29,000,000	?	?
Laos	2,000,000	?	?
Cambodia	6,000,000	?	?
Total	871,000,000	101,910,000	33,220,130

Limited foci of human infection have recently been discovered in Laos (1957), Thailand (1959) and Cambodia (1968). It is a well-considered view that the situation in the Mekong Valley should be kept under constant review. In view of the fact that the upper reaches of the river in China (Mainland) do have *Oncomelania* and *S. japonicum*, and that rivers in the past have made excellent pathways for the transfer of snails, it is very likely that the developments along the Mekong would produce suitable habitats for *Oncomelania* and set the stage for extensive transmission of *S. japonicum* in the area. Recently (1966) authenticated cases have been reported from the Ile de Khong in the Mekong River, in south Laos and in the Mekong Valley of Cambodia at Kratié.

China (Mainland)

The infection in China was believed, until 1911, to be confined to the central and lower Yangtze Valley between parallels 28 and 32 latitude north and from meridian 110, longitude east, to the sea and, in addition, to a portion of Siang Valley in Hunan Province, a tributary to the mid-Yangtze Valley. FAUST and MELENY [1924] recorded that, in the 12 years following, an apparently separate endemic centre was located near Shuichow, on the North River, above Canton.

MAO [1948] reported the situation as follows:

'Infection was diagnosed chiefly with the intradermal reaction, seconded, when necessary, by stool examination consisting of both the hatching technique and sedimentation method. Altogether 58,000,000 intradermal tests were undertaken last year. As a result, more accurate data concerning the distribution and the incidence of the disease were gathered: one hundred million people were estimated to be under its constant threat. The endemic area covers eleven provinces and the Municipality of Shanghai. This is an area four times the size of France or nine times that of the United Kingdom. The eleven provinces, mostly south of the Yangtze River, are Kiangsu, Chekiang, Anhwei, Fukien, Kiangsi, Kwangtung, Kwangsi, Hunan, Hupeh, Yunnan and Szechwan.'

With regard to the general distribution of the infection, FAUST and MELENEY's description [1924] still remains the best and is reproduced below:

'The greatest area of endemicity is the Yangtze Valley, including not only the territory immediately watered by the main current, but also the adjacent lakes, particularly the Great Lake (Tai Hu) of Kiangsu-Chekiang Provinces, Poyang Lake in Kiangsi Province, and Tung Ting Lake in the Hunan area, as well as the important central Yangtze tributaries, the Siang and Han Rivers. Throughout the central and lower Yangtze Valley the distribution constitutes practically one single extensive area. Above Hankow, in the main valley, reports indicate its presence as far inland as Ichang, but above that region there is a stretch of about twelve hundred miles of river length for which no positive records have been made. Only in the upper portion of the river, in the central plains of Szechuan, where the south fork flows south from Chengtu, are positive reports of the infection made. The amount of territory in which the disease is prevalent in the lower Yantze Valley is, no doubt, increased by the presence of the Grand Canal, intersecting the Yangtze River at right angles, in the vicinity of Chinkiang, allowing a direct connection, both of distribution of the mollusc host and of the spread of the disease, by human intercourse.

Coastwise, schistosomiasis japonica is not known to be present in China, north of the mouth of the Yangtze River. South of the river it is now known to exist in several localities along the coast or in the coastal river basins. Thus Taching, in southern Chekiang, Foochow, Swatow and the country above Swatow on the Mei River, Hongkong and Shuichow on the North River all report positive cases, based on laboratory examination of the stools of suspected cases. On the other hand, the West River, above Canton, reports no authentic cases.

The mountainous areas, embraced in the provinces of Kiangsi, Kweichow, and Yünnan, as well as those portions of the south-eastern coastal provinces, lying above the coastal plain, report no cases.'

Areas of major infection were reported to be: (1) the Soochow-Kashing area, (2) the Wuhu area, (3) the Kiukiang area, (4) the Wuhan area, (5) the Siaokan-Tsaoshih area, (6) the Changteh-Yochow area.

In areas of minor infection, outside the six areas named above, the following centres have been discovered: (1) the Szechuan area, (2) the Fukien area, (3) the Swatow area and the North River area.

FAUST and MELENEY [1924] summarized the situation in China as follows:

'A careful study of the information in hand indicates that by far the greatest part of the territory infected with schistosomiasis in China is the Yangtze Valley flood area. The main course of the stream is not known to be responsible for a single case of infection of schistosomiasis japonica, and the biological evidence on the habits of the molluscan host argues in favour of this view. However, all of that area which lies in the bottom land of the Yangtze basin, intermediate between the source streams and the mighty River, constitutes a reservoir of water, which in time of flood not only receives the flow from the Yangtze tributaries but also the backwater of the Yangtze itself. Thus, in the wet season, this whole area is frequently inundated, while in the dry season it is resolved into lakes, swamps, marshes and alluvial bottom land. The rich silt land is easily watered during the rice-growing season by natural or artificial canals, which usually have their source of supply in the backwaters rather than in the Yangtze River.

The other areas outside the Yangtze Valley where the infection exists are in narrow valleys, where the rice fields are usually terraced and supplied with water from mountain streams.

Beginning at the Yangtze River mouth it is confined to the south bank of the River, until the River is intersected by the Grand Canal. Here the endemic territory extends north to Yangchow and Taichow, thence across the Province line to Anhwei Province, where the northern limit of the infection is bounded by a line drawn from Chuchow to Lüchowfu. At this point the endemic region bends south to the Susong sector, following the course of the Yangtze; thence to Peichien, Siaokan, Tsaoshih and to the limit of overflow of the Han River, one hundred and fifty miles above Hankow.

The region south of the Yangtze River is less easily bounded. A heavy infection lies south of the River, but becomes less and less important as one leaves the overflow areas immediately adjacent to the Yangtze. The southern limit of the infection is extended considerably by the three large lakes, Tung Ting, Poyang, and Great Lake, centres around which heavy infections exist. In the case of each of these lakes the main water supply comes from one or more extensive river systems leading down from mountain streams. The infection exists far up near the source of Tung Ting Lake. The same may be true for Poyang Lake, although this point has not been verified. In the Great Lake area the infection has not been traced above Ishing, on the west, or Kinhwafu, on the south. Changteh, on the west, and Shanghai, on the east, mark the west and east boundaries of the infection on the south bank of the Yangtze River.

The long stretch of the Yangtze River gorges, above Ichang, is not a place for backwater of the River to accumulate. This may explain why no cases have heretofore been reported from the Yangtze basin above Ichang. On the other hand, one must keep in mind the possibility that the district of sandstone through which the Yangtze River cuts in eastern Szechuan Province may make it impossible for the molluscan host to develop in this territory.

The endemic infections in Fukien and Kwangtung Provinces are as yet little known, making it impossible to delimit them until more specific information is available.'

Komiya [1957] observes that the 'endemic foci of schistosomiasis in China are so numerous and their dimension is so vast', and reported that the foci are distributed over 12 provinces with a population of 10,000,000. The Szechuan Province, one of the endemic areas 'recently found, is as wide as Japanese Islands and believed to contain more than 60 endemic foci'.

Assuming that at least one third of the exposed population of 100,000,000 reported by Mao, is infected, Wright's estimate [1950] of 32,777,000 cases of *S. japonicum* should be regarded as appropriate.

In respect of the actual number of cases, Wright recorded the following observations in 1950:

'Calculation of the number of cases in China is difficult. Little detailed information is available concerning the local distribution of the disease and local infection-rates because reported endemic areas have not been accurately delineated and incidence figures are but little known. The most recent summary is contained in the paper by Mao, who stated that the disease is endemic in 138 of 983 hsiens in 11 provinces. The rural population of the 138 hsiens is 25,290,286. Applying the available incidence data to this population, Mao estimated that a total of 5,310,960 individuals are infected. As Mao himself indicates, this estimate does not present a true picture for the reason that relatively inefficient methods of stool examinations were used in many of the surveys upon which incidence figures are based, and because the disease is probably endemic in many hsiens other than those in which it is known at present. Evidence of the inadequacy of the above-mentioned data is furnished by

Lı who estimated on the basis of extensive investigations by himself and Chen that 38% of the population of 12,890,938 of 37 districts in Kiangsu and Chekiang Provinces are sufferers from the disease. This amounts to 4,898,556 infected persons in parts of only two provinces, a figure not materially below Mao's estimate for the entire country.'

'Stoll's calculations for China were based on an infection-rate of 20% of the population of the provinces comprising the chief centres of infection and 10% of the population of other provinces in which the disease is known to be endemic. It seems probable that the rate of 10% is too low for certain provinces and the rate of 20% too high for other provinces. I have discussed this point with many Chinese workers. As a result of their advice and on the basis of incidence data in the literature, I have accepted for the purposes of this summary the following percentages of infection for the several provinces: Anhwei, 20; Chekiang, 30; Fukien, 20; Hunan, 10; Hupeh, 10; Kiangsi, 20; Kiangsu, 10; Kwangsi, 25; Kwangtung, 10; Szechwan, 5; and Yunnan, 5. I have applied these rates to the population figures published in July 1947 by the Directorate General of Budgets, Accounts and Statistics, National Government of China, and furnished to me through the courtesy of the Chinese Embassy, Washington, D.C. According to this estimation, the number of infected persons in China would be 32,777,630.'

Conditions in China (Mainland) have changed since the work of Faust and Meleney in the early 1920's; but there is little published information on the current status of the disease. Regardless of this, it seems advisable to review the available data, meagre as they are.

Schistosomiasis japonica is now endemic in 10 provinces, one municipality (Shanghai) and one autonomous region (Kwangsi). Altogether, 324 hsiens are infected [Anon, 1959]. Considerable progress has been achieved in control of the disease through the vigorous campaign sponsored by the Ministry of Health. It is said officially that the total number of infected individuals is now 10,000,000 but, in the absence of detailed data, it is difficult to appraise this statement. Hertwig and Oberdoerster [1960] voiced the opinion that probably 100,000,000 were exposed to the disease.

In order to reduce the tremendous amount of labour entailed by faecal examinations, prevalence has been determined largely by use of the intradermal test. It is reported that in 1956 the Shanghai Institute of Parasitic Diseases produced an amount of antigen sufficient for 60 million tests. At present, no firm figures are available on prevalence rates in the various provinces. In general, prevalence is low in children under 5 years of age and reaches a peak between 15 and 30 years.

On the basis of data collected from various sources, the following represents the best evaluation possible of the current status of the disease.

Kiangsu Province, bordering the Yellow Sea, north of the mouth of the Yangtze River, is 'water country' containing many lakes and criss-crossed by rivers. The disease has a fairly high prevalence. Hertwig and Oberdoerster

[1960] estimated that there were 2,000,000 infected persons in Kiangsu Province. *S. japonicum* is found in many lower animals in the province and 2 % of the water buffaloes are said to carry the parasite.

Anhwei Province, north of the Yangtze, produces bamboo, tea and rice and is heavily infected.

Hupeh Province, north of Tung Ting Lake, offers the lake type of transmission and the disease is heavily endemic.

Hunan Province, south of Tung Ting Lake, is an important grain- and rice-growing area. Here the disease is very prevalent.

Kiangsi, south-west of Lake Payang, is also an important rice-producing region and is noted for its fisheries. The disease is reported to be under control in more than half of the province, which contains Yu Kiang County, the first to be freed of infection under the national control campaign.

Chekiang Province, in the Taihu Lake Basin, is a rice-growing area. Fishing is an important occupation. Parts of this province have been heavily infected in the past, particularly the low plains of North Chekiang [Li, 1948].

Fukien Province, situated in the Taiwan Hai Hsia (formerly Formosa Strait), is mainly hilly country and offers a type of terrain not conducive to *Oncomelania hupensis*. Latest available reports indicate that there is little schistosomiasis at present.

Kwangtung Province, situated in the Pearl River Basin, has not been a major endemic area in the past and there is apparently very little infection now.

Szechuan Province has not been a seriously endemic area. The disease is mainly confined to the southern and eastern portions with a higher infection rate in the east. Around Penhsien, YAO [1945] found 11% of 160 children infected. At Chengtu in the central part of the province, the rate in 1,578 hospital patients in 1943 was 0.13% [CHANG and LIN], and in 2,551 peasants in western Szechuan in 1944, it was 0.08% (YAO, cited by MAO, 1948). *S. japonicum* occurs frequently in cattle in Szechuan; HSIUNG [1943] reported infection in 26% of 50 such animals and KUO et al. [1945] in 17% of 41 animals.

Yunnan Province has never been an important endemic area and prevalence is still very low.

The autonomous region of Kwangsi lying east of Yunnan Province is also marked by a low endemicity. However, a former important focus was situated at Pinyang where YAO [1938] found 53.5% of 191 children infected.

Kweichow Province is entirely surrounded by provinces in which the disease is endemic but is reported to be free from the infection. The country is hilly and rugged and apparently not suited to the molluscan intermediate host.

Various lower animals may be involved to some extent in the transmission of schistosomiasis in China (Mainland). At least 29 species of mammals have been found to be naturally infected with *S. japonicum*.

Oncomelania hupensis is the sole molluscan intermediate host of *S. japonicum* in China (mainland). Its northern limit has been found at Paoying in Kiangsu Province (33°15′ latitude north). The eastern limit is the coastal regions of Kiangsu Province and its western limit is Chiench'uan in Yunnan Province (100° longitude east). The distribution of the disease corresponds closely with the above-mentioned boundary lines of the snail distribution.

Chinese workers classify endemic areas into the plain, hill and swamp regions. In the plains, *O. hupensis* abounds along the banks of small rivers and lateral irrigation canals, and along the margins of lakes. In certain areas the snails are found in furrows of the rice paddies but not usually in the paddies themselves.

In the hill regions, *O. hupensis* occurs in the terraced paddy fields irrigated with water from the valleys below. Here, exposure is mainly connected with rice planting and cultivation.

In the marsh and lake country, the snails are found in swampy ground and around the margins of the lakes. Exposure is said to be connected usually with gathering rushes or other work in the spring and autumn.

Fishermen and boatmen in the plain areas are frequently exposed and have high prevalence rates.

References

ANONYMOUS: Studies on schistosomiasis japonica in New China, compiled by the National Schistosomiasis Committee. Chin. med. J. *78:* 368, 461 (1959).

CHANG, K. and LIN, C. C.: Cited by MAO, 1948 (1943).

FAUST, E. C. and MELENEY, H. E.: Amer. J. Hyg., Monogr. Ser., vol. 3, pp. 1–268 (1924).

HERTWIG, F. and OBERDOERSTER, F.: Z. Tropenmed. Parasit. *11:* 324 (1960).

HSIUNG, T. H.: Vet. mthl. *3:* (1943).

KOMIYA, Y.: Jap. J. med. Sci. Biol. *10:* 461 (1957).

KUO, S. C.; YUI, H. W., and CHANG, C. E.: Chin. med. J. *63A:* 144 (1945).

LI, F. C.: Chin. Rev. trop. Med. *1:* 15 (1948).

MAO, C. P.: Amer. J. trop. Med. *28:* 659 (1948).

WRIGHT, W. H.: Bull. Wld Hlth Org. *2:* 581 (1950).

YAO, Y. T.: Chin. med. J. *54:* 162 (1938).

YAO, Y. T.: Cited by MAO, 1948 (1943).

YAO, Y. T.: in Personal communication to W. H. WRIGHT from S. C. KUO (1945).

Japan

The endemic areas of schistosomiasis are fairly well defined and are limited to eight of the 46 prefectures in Japan, 6 in the main island of Honshu and two in the southern island of Kyushu.

Chiba, Ibaraki and Saitama Prefectures, comprising partly the Kato Plain region of central Honshu largely to the north of Tokyo, contain foci of low endemicity. Through the northern part of this area flows the Tone River whose valley contains dispersed foci of mild infection. Similar foci are also found along the Edo River, 32 km north of Tokyo, in Saitama Prefecture. According to RITCHIE *et al.* [1953] scarcely more than 5% of the population were passing eggs of *S. japonicum*. More recent surveys have not been reported [OKABE, 1970].

Shizuoka Prefecture. The Numazu area extending westward from Numazo along the coast and up towards the mountains is a lightly endemic focus. WRIGHT *et al.* [1947] found 9% of 155 school-children infected at Sudo. Examinations conducted by the 406th General Medical Laboratory [1951] in 14 villages in the area disclosed a prevalence rate of 5% at Sudo and 26% at Kanaoka. ITO *et al.* [1963] skin tested 2,000 inhabitants of the area and obtained 6.6% positives. However, none of the positive reactors had *S. japonicum* eggs in the stools. A recent survey failed to find *Oncomelania* snails in this area, except at Kanaoka, Numazu City [OKABE, 1970].

ITO *et al.* [1962] discovered a new focus at Fujikawa-Cho in the delta of the Fuji River; 47.3% of 464 persons were positive on skin tests. Stool examinations were positive in 57, or 13.2% of the individuals. However, as a result of control efforts, snails can now rarely be found in the area [KOMIYA, 1966].

The Yamanashi region. About one third (approximately 18,000 hectares with a population of 370,000 inhabitants) of the Yamanashi Prefecture is reported to be endemic for schistosomiasis. It was one of the three relatively heavily infected areas in Japan. An over-all prevalence rate of 12% was obtained by Suguira [FAROOQ, 1956] but in 1968, 1.81% of 9,570 persons examined were found to be positive [OKABE, 1970]. Scattered communities with comparatively higher rates of infection are still encountered in this region [IIJIMA, 1966]. One such focus is Kofu in Yamanashi-Ken, which is considered the most important [YOKOGAWA, 1970].

The Hiroshima region. It is in the historic Katayama area that schistosomiasis was first encountered in Japan where it is still known as 'Katayama disease'. The infection rate in the area was found to be 6.3% in 1954 [OKINAMI, 1956]. YOKOGAWA *et al.* [1969] conducted immunological tests and stool exam-

Table XXVIa. Record of cases and deaths due to schistosomiasis; Katayama District (Hiroshima Prefecture), 1918–1955[1]

Year	Cases	Deaths	Year	Cases	Deaths
1918	–	23	1937	34	2
1919	–	18	1938	20	4
1920	2,150	11	1939	16	3
1921	1,861	11	1940	33	12
1922	1,606	19	1941	29	9
1923	1,277	15	1942	12	4
1924	1,077	17	1943	86	9
1925	810	23	1944	98	10
1926	498	7	1945	103	9
1927	348	15	1946	146	15
1928	163	15	1947	151	10
1929	126	14	1948	57	4
1930	112	21	1949	122	4
1931	102	16	1950	87	3
1932	93	12	1951	48	3
1933	88	10	1952	78	0
1934	83	14	1953	24	0
1935	81	8	1954	39	0
1936	–	–	1955	45	0

1 Source: OKINAMI, 1956.

inations on 1,027 inhabitants of the Katayama District. A total of 237, or 23%, gave positive intradermal reactions. However, none of these had S. japonicum eggs in the stools, although nine cases were positive on the complement fixation test and 20 were positive on the circumoval precipitation test. In a recent survey, only one patient was detected [OKABE, 1970].

Records maintained since 1918 show the downward trend in the area (table XXVI). It is believed that schistosomiasis has practically been eliminated from this focus.

The Fukuoka and Saga region. The endemic area in Kyushu Island covers about 8,300 hectares and has a population of approximately 74,000 persons. The centres of infection lie in the contiguous portions of Fukuoka and Saga Prefectures in the Chikugo River Valley. In Fukuoka, the range of infection recorded in 1955 was 1.8 to 4.8% while in 1967 it was 1.10% of 4,059 examined [OKABE, 1970]. In 1969, a mass stool examination conducted in Saga Prefecture indicated that 7.6% of 566 cases out of 2,272 reported from 1952 to 1967 were

Table XXVIb. Prevalence in Katayama District[1]

Year	Number examined	Positive on stool examination, %
1957	1,562	1.3
1958	4,246	0.1
1959	1,455	0.41
1964	3,070	0.03
1965	9,853	0.02
1966	9,821	0.01
1967	9,640	0.01

1 Source: OKABE, 1970.

still positive [OKABE, 1970]. In the same prefecture, however, 0.03% of 14,379 persons examined in 1967 were found to be passing eggs.

WRIGHT recorded the following in respect of the total number of cases in Japan in 1950:

'Estimates for Japan have been arrived at through the application of infection rates in the various townships and counties of the infected prefectures, as obtained by the Commission on Schistosomiasis, Office of the Surgeon General, US Army, and by Colonel G.W. HUNTER, III, 406th Medical General Laboratory, Tokyo, Japan. These have been applied to the 1946 population figures for these areas as published in the Official Gazette. Since the endemic areas have been outlined with a considerable degree of accuracy, it is believed that the estimates are valid within narrow limits. The total of 174,436 infected individuals for Japan is far under the estimated number of 1,420,982 arrived at if we were to apply STOLL's formula of 10% of the population of the infected prefectures to the 1946 census figures.'

According to KOMIYA [1966], OKABE [1970] and YOKOGAWA [1970] who has recently reviewed the schistosomiasis situation in Japan, prevalence rates in all endemic areas are now extremely low. As a result of well-planned, persistent control measures and over-all rise in economic and social standards, the infection in Japan is definitely on the wane and it is perhaps the only country where the stage seems set for the ultimate eradication of the disease.

References

FAROOQ, M.: Report of a visit to the schistosomiasis endemic areas in Japan, Sept. 12–29. WHO unpublished document (1956).

HUNTER, G.W., III: in Annual Historical Report of the 406th Medical General Laboratory, Tokyo (1948).

IIJIMA, T.: Personal commun. (1966).

ITO, J.; NOGUCHI, M.; ASAKAWA, Y.; MOCHIZUKI, H.; WATANABE, T., and SUNOUCHI, S.: Kiseichugaku Zasshi (Jap. J. Parasit.) *11:* 393 (1962).

ITO, J.; NOGUCHI, M., and MOCHIZUKI, H.: Kiseichugaku Zasshi (Jap. J. Parasit.) *12:* 437 (1963).

KOMIYA, Y.: Personal commun. (1966).

OKABE, K.: in HARINASUTA Proceedings of the Fourth South-East Asian Seminar on Parasitology and Tropical Medicine, Manila 1969, p. 9 (Bangkok 1970).

OKINAMI, M.: General outline of Katayama disease in Hiroshima Prefecture. Prefectural Health Laboratories, Hiroshima. Unpublished document (1956).

RITCHIE, L. S.; HUNTER, G. W., III; NAGANO, K., and PAN, C.: Amer. J. trop. Med. Hyg. *2:* 915 (1953).

STOLL, N. R.: J. Parasit. *33:* 1 (1947).

US Army 406th Medical General Laboratory, Tokyo: Bulletin No. 4, p. 18 (1951).

WRIGHT, W. H.; McMULLEN, D. B.; BENNETT, H. J.; BAUMANN, P. M., and INGALLS, J. W., jr.: Amer. J. trop. Med. *27:* 417 (1947).

YOKOGAWA, M.: in SASA Recent advances in researches on filariasis and schistosomiasis in Japan, p. 231 (University of Tokyo Press, Tokyo, and University Park Press, Baltimore/ Manchester 1970).

YOKOGAWA, M.; SANO, M.; ARAKI, K.; JOJIMA, S.; TSUJI, M.; SAITO, S.; INATOMI, S., and SAKUMOTO, D.: Epidemiological studies on schistosomiasis japonica in an old endemic area. Conference of Parasitic Diseases, US-Japan Cooperative Medical Science Program, Washington, D. C., August 4–6, 1969 (1969).

Philippines

Endemicity has been established so far in 6 of the 13 main islands of the archipelago: namely, Luzon, Mindoro, Samar, Leyte, Mindanao and Bohol. The endemic and potentially endemic zone covers 10% of the land mass [TEMPLEMAN-KLUIT, 1962], and is characterized by the absence of a dry season [SANTOS, 1969].

Luzon

The endemic area in the largest island of the Philippines is one of the smallest and well-circumscribed, with moderate endemicity. It lies in Irosin-Juban Valley in Sorsogon, the southernmost province of Luzon, and covers an area of about 4,200 hectares. It has a population of 27,000, with an over-all prevalence rate of 20 to 25%, and it is estimated that between 5,400 and 6,750 people are infected in the area.

Mindoro

The endemic focus in the island is confined to 3 of the 12 municipalities of its eastern province; namely, Naujan, Victoria and Pola, surrounding Lake Naujan in the north-eastern part of the province.

The endemic area covers approximately 200 km². An over-all rate of 27% is considered as approximately correct. Taking the population of 40,000 living in the three named municipalities (constituting nearly a quarter of the population of the province) as exposed to the infection, an estimate of 10,000 infected individuals in the endemic area in Mindoro may not be considered too liberal.

Samar

Mainland Samar covers an area of approximately 12,950 km², and together with its 146 small islands constitutes the Province of Samar. It has a population of about 800,000, distributed mostly in coastal settlements and partly in the 'barios and sitios' in the interior riverine valley.

Endemic foci of schistosomiasis are widely distributed in the periphery of Samar. Infection has been shown to be present in 24 of the 56 municipalities into which the province is divided, although other areas also exist where the infection is endemic.

The estimated over-all rate of infection of 22% is probably nearer the truth than the 7 to 8% previously recorded. On this basis it is estimated that there are 96,800 infected individuals in a population of 440,000 in the 24 municipalities of Samar where infection has so far been established. If it is assumed, as would certainly be the case, that the disease occurs over most of the island, one can estimate that the number of infected persons over the whole island would be close to 200,000.

Leyte

The endemic area of Leyte is one large low plain in the north-eastern part of the island. This area is roughly 11–20 km wide and 90 km long and covers about 1,200 km². The population of the endemic area is relatively dense (125 per km²) and it is estimated that about 400,000 persons live there. With an over-all infection rate of 33%, it is estimated that this single endemic area contains over one quarter of the country's exposed population and nearly one third, i.e. 132,000, of the infected population in the Philippines.

Mindanao

This island with an area of about 93,240 km² approximates Luzon in size, but has no more than 3,000,000 inhabitants, which is roughly a quarter of the population of Luzon. The island is divided into 10 provinces of which nine have been found to contain endemic foci, the exception being the Province of Oriental Misamis.

The estimated extent of the known and possible endemic areas and exposed population in the island are given in table XXVII.

With an over-all infection rate of about 43.5%, it is estimated that there are approximately 73,000 individuals infected in a total population of 167,610 in the known endemic areas of nearly 3,104 km². This figure closely approaches WRIGHT's estimate of nearly 75,000, made in 1950.

It should, however, be noted that the endemic areas in Mindanao have not been properly delineated. Until the turn of the century migration into this island from other provinces of the Philippines was very limited, but of late a great influx into this potentially rich island, with extensive fertile plains, large forests, numerous rivers, fresh water swamps and marshes, has begun from the islands of the north. There is, therefore, much exploitation of virgin land and clearing of forests, all tending to make the distribution pattern an uncertain and constantly changing one.

It is interesting to note here that in Compostela in Davao Province the major focus lies in the basin of Manat River draining northward into the Agusan River, and a subsidiary focus at Mawab draining south through Hijo River. These valleys are surrounded by primary forest-clad mountain ranges. The virgin forest floor in the northern zone has been shown to be a habitat of *Oncomelania quadrasi* and comparative studies made in other virgin forest areas in Mindanao indicate that the original habitat of the snail may have been in such virgin forests. The fact that infection has also been demonstrated among wild pigs, monkeys and rats, coupled with histories of the presence of the disease among the aboriginal people in these areas before the settlers moved in, throws some light on the probable origin of *S. japonicum*.

Bohol

A focus of schistosomiasis has recently been discovered on the island of Bohol located just east of Cebu. Several infected persons were detected in the northern part of the island in 1958. A prevalence of 30% infection has been found among the people of Trinidad and Talibon.

O. quadrasi is the intermediate host of *S. japonicum* in the Philippines; it occurs in all endemic areas. The snail is located in a variety of habitats, although its original home was apparently flood plains and swamps, in which it is still found. The largest snail habitat yet discovered lies in the Manat River swamp in Davao Province, an area approximately 20 km long by 2 to 3 km wide. The snail also occurs in abandoned rice-fields, marshy areas, meandering sluggish and vegetation-clogged streams, road-side ditches and seepage areas from spring outlets.

Table XXVII. Estimated extent of the known endemic and possibly endemic areas, with the estimated population exposed to schistosomiasis in these areas in Mindanao

Province	Endemic area, km²			Population exposed[1]		
	known	possible	total of 2 and 3	in known endemic areas	in possible endemic areas	total of 5 and 6
1	2	3	4	5	6	7
1. Davao (Upper zone Compostela)	594	554	1,148	12,000	5,235	17,235
Lower zone (Davao Penal Colony and surrounding areas)	173	287	460	5,633	11,349	16,982
2. Lanao, Zamboanga and Occ. Misamis						
Panguil Bay area	534	654	1,188	46,067	68,730	114,797
Lanao Lake area	333	133	466	20,867	7,000	27,867
3. Bukidnon	394	494	888	6,340	14,182	20,522
4. Cotabato	354	6,710	7,064	34,611	158,424	193,035
5. Agusan	455	494	949	20,435	48,461	68,896
6. Surigao	267	67	334	21,657	3,724	25,381
Total	3,104	9,393	12,497	167,610	317,105	484,715

1 Population estimates based on 1948 census of the Philippines and the Provincial Health Officers reports.

References

OLIVIER, L. J.; BUZO, Z. J., and PINTO, N.: Report on bilharziasis control in the Philippines. WHO unpublished document MHO/PA/20.64 (1963).

PESIGAN, T. P.: J. Philipp. med. Ass. *23:* 23 (1947).

PESIGAN, T. P.: J. Philipp. med. Ass. *24:* 19, 495 (1948).

PESIGAN, T. P.: J. Philipp. med. Ass. *27:* 203 (1951).

PESIGAN, T. P.; PANGILINAN, M. V., and SARMIENTO, A. P.: J. Philipp. med. Ass. *25:* 417 (1949).

PESIGAN, T. P.; FAROOQ, M.; HAIRSTON, N. G.; JAUREGUI, J. J.; GARCIA, E. G.; SANTOS, A.T ; SANTOS, B. C., and BESA, A. A.: Bull. Wld Hlth Org. *18:* 345 (1958).

SANTOS, A. T.: in HARINASUTA Proceedings of the Fourth South-East Asian Seminar on Parasitology and Tropical Medicine, Manila 1969, p. 1 (Bangkok 1970).

TEMPLEMAN-KLUIT: FAO Report No. 1468 (1962).

WRIGHT, W. H.: Bull. Wld Hlth Org. *2:* 581 (1950).

Celebes (Indonesia)

Only one small isolated focus of *S. japonicum* is known in Central Celebes. Endemicity has been established in three villages, Langko, Tomoda and Antja, situated near one another on the west shore of Lake Lindoë. This is a small inter-mountain body of water, measuring about 10 km in length by 5 to 6 km in breadth. There are several small streams flowing into the lake on its southern and eastern shores, while its outlet is to the north into a branch of the Paloe River which flows north-north-east, emptying into Makassar Strait. Endemicity was recorded as approximately 50% by BONNE and SANDGROUND [1940]. *S. japonicum* was obtained from dogs and wild deer in the area. Investigations in the regions of other lakes gave negative results [OEMIJATI, 1969].

WRIGHT [1950] made the following estimates of the number of cases of *S. japonicum* in Celebes:

'The small focus of bilharziasis in the Lake Lindoë region of Celebes was estimated by STOLL to contain a few thousand cases. So little is known about this area, however, that any figure would be merely a guess. FAUST and BONNE, in summarising information concerning the area, noted that approximately half of the 176 inhabitants of three villages were passing eggs in the stools. It is difficult to conceive that this small focus represents the only endemic area on an island with a population (according to estimates for 1944) of 4,600,000, and it is probable that other foci remain to be discovered. To err on the side of conservatism, we have taken an arbitrary figure of 1,000 cases for this island.'

According to BUCK and UHRMANN [1956] who surveyed the area, the endemic focus consists of three villages with a population of 600 to 700 people. Faecal examinations were conducted on 158 of the inhabitants of these villages and 22 to 32% contained eggs of *S. japonicum*.

A recent survey party from U.S. Naval Medical Research Unit No. 2,

Taipei, Taiwan, has found a species of *Oncomelania* in the endemic area in the Celebes. Cercariae from snails collected in the endemic area were used to infect laboratory mice.

References
BONNE, C. and SANDGROUND, J. H.: Geneesk. T. Ned.-Ind. *80:* 477 (1940).
BUCK, A. A. and UHRMANN, G.: Z. Tropenmed. Parasit. *7:* 110 (1956).
OEMIJATI, S.: in HARINASUTA Proceedings of the Fourth South-East Asian Seminar on Parasitology and Tropical Medicine, Manila 1969, p. 59 (Bangkok 1970).
U.S. Naval Medical Research Unit No. 2: Namrugram, Sept. Oct. *4:* 9.
WRIGHT, W. H.: Bull. Wld Hlth Org. *2:* 581 (1950).

Thailand

A case of *S. japonicum* was observed in 1958 in a patient treated at Siriraj Hospital in Bangkok, who came from Chawang District in Nakornsrithamaraj Province in the southern part of Thailand [CHAIYAPORN *et al.*, 1959]. The area was surveyed in 1959 and 1960 and recognized as the first endemic area in the country [HARINASUTA and KRUATRACHUE, 1960, 1962]. Eggs obtained by rectal biopsy resembled those of *S. japonicum* but differed from them by their smaller size and rounder shape [KOMIYA, 1963]. KRUATRACHUE *et al.* [1964] conducted skin tests on 2,667 persons in this area; 289 gave positive or doubtfully positive reactions. Rectal biopsy was performed on 193 of these individuals, including 64 with positive skin tests and 129 with doubtful reactions. Of these, 50 were positive on biopsy but concentration methods disclosed only three with positive stools.

LEE *et al.* [1966] reported *S. japonicum*-like eggs from a subcutaneous cyst from a woman from Phitsanuloke, 480 km north of Bangkok, and *S. japonicum* eggs from the small intestine of a male who died at Ubol, 443 km north-east of Bangkok. In the latter area which is situated west of the endemic area in Khong island in Laos new cases have been found [DESOWITZ *et al.*, 1967].

The molluscan intermediate host has not yet been demonstrated [HARINASUTA, 1969]. HARINASUTA and KRUATRACHUE [1964] were unable to infect *Oncomelania* spp. from Japan, Taiwan (Formosa) and the Philippines with the local strain of *S. japonicum*. Because the miracidia differ slightly in their structure from those of *S. japonicum* strains found in Japan, China (mainland), and the Philippines [KRUATRACHUE *et al.*, 1968], it is believed that schistosomiasis in Thailand may be caused by either a new geographical strain of *S. japonicum* or a new species of schistosome [SORNMANI, 1969].

References

CHAIYAPORN, V.; KOONVISAL, L., and DHARAMADHACH, A.: J. med. Ass. Thailand *42:* 438 (1959).

DESOWITZ, R.; HARINASUTA, C.; KRUATRACHUE, M.; CHESDAPHAN, C., and JETANASEN, S.: Trans. roy. Soc. trop. Med. Hyg. *61:* 153 (1967).

HARINASUTA, CH.: in HARINASUTA Proceedings of the Fourth South-East Asian Seminar on Parasitology and Tropical Medicine, Manila 1969, p.69 (Bangkok 1970).

HARINASUTA, CH. and KRUATRACHUE, M.: Trans. roy. Soc. trop. Med. Hyg. *54:* 280 (1960).

HARINASUTA, CH. and KRUATRACHUE, M.: Ann. trop. Med. Parasit. *56:* 314 (1962).

HARINASUTA, CH. and KRUATRACHUE, M.: Trans. roy. Soc. trop. Med. Hyg. *58:* 195 (1964).

KOMIYA, Y.: Assignment report on bilharziasis survey in Thailand, 12–25 June 1963. WHO unpublished document SEA/Bilharz/6 (1963).

KRUATRACHUE, M.; BHAIBULAYA, M.; CHESDAPAN, C., and HARINASUTA, CH.: Ann. trop. Med. Parasit. *62:* 67 (1968).

KRUATRACHUE, M.; BHAIBULAYA, M., and HARINASUTA, CH.: Ann. trop. Med. Parasit. *58:* 276 (1964).

LEE, H. F.; WYKOFF, D. E., and BEAVER, P. C.: Amer. J. trop. Med. Hyg. *15:* 303 (1966).

SORNMANI, S.: in HARINASUTA Proceedings of the Fourth South-East Asian Seminar on Parasitology and Tropical Medicine, Manila 1969, p.71 (Bangkok 1970).

Laos

Reports of clinical cases of *S. japonicum* in Laotian subjects [VIC DUPONT *et al.*, 1957; GALLIARD, 1957; BARBIER, 1966; MOST, 1966] drew attention to the island of Khong which is a large island situated in the Mekong River in the southern part of the country (Province of Sithadone) near the Cambodian border. In a WHO survey [IIJIMA and GARCIA, 1967] 1,012 inhabitants of five villages were skin-tested: 18% were positive, 32% were doubtful and 50% negative. A total of 547 inhabitants whose skin test had been positive, doubtful or negative were examined by the direct faecal smear method and 47 cases (8.6%) were found to be positive for eggs of *S. japonicum*. Eighteen more cases were found to be positive using the formalin-ether concentration method. The last survey in 1968–1969 showed 20 to 35% of school-children examined positive for eggs of *S. japonicum* [IIJIMA, 1970]. The search for possible reservoir hosts proved negative in buffaloes, cats, rodents and pigs. However, adult worms of *S. japonicum* were recovered in seven of 26 dogs autopsied [IIJIMA, 1970].

Absence of *Oncomelania* [ITO and JATANASEN, 1961; IIJIMA and GARCIA, 1967] in rice-fields and mountain streams was confirmed by VOGEL [1969] in an investigation carried out during the rainy, rice-planting season. A malacological survey conducted for one year failed to reveal human schistosome cercariae in more than 13,000 operculate snails representing 11 species, although 26 types of larvae were found, including six furocercous cercariae. Suspicion is focused so far on *Pachydrobia pellucida* [Lo, 1969] and *Hydrorissoia hospitalis*, the latter having been found to harbour sporocysts of the same morphology as those obtained from snails experimentally infected [BRANDT, 1968].

References

BARBIER, M.: Bull. Soc. Path. exot. *59:* 974 (1966).

BRANDT, R. A. M.: Arch. Moll. *98:* 213 (1968).

GALLIARD, H.: Personal commun. to Dr. N. ANSARI, WHO (1957).

IIJIMA, T.: Mekong river schistosomiasis survey. Assignment report. 13 November 1968–8 May 1969. WHO unpublished document WPR/058/70 (1970).

IIJIMA, T. and GARCIA, R. G.: Preliminary survey for schistosomiasis in South Laos. Unpublished document WHO/Bilh/67.64 (1967).

ITO, J. and JATANASEN, S.: Jap. J. med. Sci. Biol. *14:* 257 (1961).

LO, CHIN-TSONG: Mekong river schistosomiasis survey. Assignment report, 13 November 1968–8 February 1969. WHO unpublished document WPR/230/69 (1969).

MOST, H.: Personal commun. to Dr. N. ANSARI, WHO (1966).

VIC DUPONT; BERNARD, E.; SOUBRANE, J.; HALLÉ, B., and RICHIR, C.: Bull. Soc. méd. Hôp., Paris *73:* 933 (1957).

VOGEL, H.: Observations and recommendations related to bilharziasis on Khong Island. Assignment report (1969).

Cambodia

The first autochthonous case discovered in 1968 [AUDEBAUD *et al.*, 1968] led to several investigations in the area of Kratié, provincial capital on the left bank of the Mekong River. There, as well as in two villages upstream and at Stung Treng, more than 130 cases were found harbouring *S. japonicum* eggs [BARBIER and BRUMPT, 1969; BAZILLIO, 1969; KRIOUTCHOV, 1968; JOLLY *et al.*, 1970]. Another survey carried out in 1969 in four districts bordering the Mekong River confirmed the high rate of infection in the district of Kratié, in particular in the floating villages (32.8% positive on stool examination), and the existence of scattered cases between the south of Laos and the estuary of the Mekong River. A great number of cases were discovered in persons who do not work in the rice paddies and many patients suffer from an itching skin and dermatitis after having been in the river. The symptoms seem mild in comparison with those in Japan and the Philippines but many patients with enlarged liver and spleen have been seen in all endemic areas [IIJIMA, 1970].

As in Thailand and Laos, all attempts to find *Oncomelania* species and to infect such species with local human schistosomes have failed [JOLLY *et al.*, 1970]. Further investigations on the epidemiology of schistosomiasis in the Mekong River basin (Thailand, Laos and Cambodia) are in progress.

References

AUDEBAUD, G.; TOURNIER-LASSERVE, C.; BRUMPT, V.; JOLLY, M.; MAZAUD, R.; IMBERT, X., and BAZILLIO, R.: Bull. Soc. Path. exot. *61:* 778 (1968).

BARBIER, M. and BRUMPT, V.: Trans. roy. Soc. trop. Med. Hyg. *63:* 66 (1969).

BAZILLIO, R.: La bilharziose à *S.japonicum* au Cambodge. Premières observations et pre-mières études épidémiologiques; thèse. Faculté royale de Médecine de Phnom Penh (1969).

IIJIMA, T.: Assignment report 1968–1969 to Cambodia. WHO unpublished document WPR/059/70 (1970).

JOLLY, M.; BAZILLIO, R.; AUDEBAUD, G.; BRUMPT, V., and SOPHINN, BOU: Méd. trop. *30:* 462 (1970).

KRIOUTCHOV, V.S.: Rapport de fin de mission, Cambodge 0505. WHO unpublished docu-ment (1968).

TOURNIER-LASSERVE, C.; AUDEBAUD, G.; BRUMPT, V.; JOLLY, M.; CALVEZ, F.; MAZAUD, R.; IMBERT, X.; GOUBE, P., and BAZILLIO, R.: Méd. trop. *30:* 451 (1970).

Distribution of Schistosoma mansoni *and Molluscan Intermediate Hosts in the Americas*

S. mansoni is endemic in Brazil, Surinam and Venezuela in South America. Of the chain of several islands skirting the northern and eastern boundaries of the Caribbean Sea, endemic foci are known to be present in eight. They are: The Dominican Republic; Puerto Rico; Vieques; St. Martin; Antigua; Guadeloupe; Martinique; and St. Lucia.

Natural abatement has taken place in St. Kitts (St. Christopher). There were 5,600 cases reported from the island in 1932. However, infection appar-ently disappeared about 1946, even though the African green monkey, a reservoir host, was on the increase. Changes in water utilization and piping apparently led to decreased numbers of *B. glabrata*, the intermediate host. Surveys in 1958 and 1959 included examination of 188 persons of all ages, none of whom was infected. Snail collections were made of *B. glabrata* but no infected ones were found [FERGUSON *et al.*, 1960].

The snail host of *S. mansoni* is found in certain other islands and it is feared that the introduction of the parasite could establish further foci of transmission in the area. The development of the oil refining industry in certain south-central Caribbean Sea islands and the movement of labour from endemic areas point to such potentialities.

Table XXVIII. S.mansoni in the Americas; estimated exposed and infected population

Name of the country	Population	Population exposed	Numbers infected
Brazil	76,409,000	45,000,000	6,000,000
Surinam	209,681	100,000	9,300
Venezuela	7,555,799	750,000	20,000
Puerto Rico and Vieques	2,520,000	2,250,000	225,000
Dominican Republic	3,372,000	6,000	1,000
St. Martin	4,494	2,000	?
Antigua	61,000	3,000	500
Guadeloupe	297,000	150,000	15,000
Martinique	35,000	10,000	500
St. Lucia	94,000	75,000	25,000
Total	90,557,974	48,346,000	6,296,300

In continental United States of America there are no autochthonous foci. There are tens of thousands of Puerto Ricans living in the United States and the infection rate among those living in New York City is estimated at about 10%.

A summary statement of the estimated number of *S.mansoni* cases in the Americas is given in table XXVIII. Total indigenous cases (disregarding immigrants in continental United States) amount to over six million, the main bulk of cases coming from Brazil and Puerto Rico.

Reference

FERGUSON, F. F.; RICHARDS, C. S.; SEBASTIAN, S. T., and BUCHANAN, J. C.: Publ. Hlth, Lond. *74:* 261 (1960).

Brazil

The only human schistosome reported from Brazil is *S.mansoni*.

Schistosomiasis is spread over extensive territories in Brazil occupying a continuous area from the north-eastern State of Rio Grande do Norte to the central State of Minas Gerais.

Isolated foci were identified in the Amazon region (Fordlandia and Bragança in the State of Pará) and in the State of Ceará. In the southern states, isolated foci are found in the States of Espírito Santo, Rio de Janeiro, Guanabara, São Paulo, and Paraná. Isolated foci were found recently in Goiania (State of Goiás) and Brasilia.

Infection Rates

Active transmission of schistosomiasis is known to occur in 15 out of the 22 Brazilian States. However the infection rates vary a great deal.

The well-known old endemic area in Brazil is represented by a continuous territory from the State of Rio Grande do Norte to Minas Gerais. Within that area one can recognize two sub-areas according to the prevalence rates, high and low endemic areas.

The infection rates vary a great deal and are those rates given in table XXIX which was prepared from data by PELLON and TEIXEIRA [1950], who made an initial survey in Brazil covering the States of Maranhão, Piauí, Ceará, Rio Grande do Norte, Paraíba, Pernambuco, Alagoas, Sergipe, Bahia, Espírito Santo and Minas Gerais. These States were those in which schistosomiasis was supposed to be endemic. In this survey 440,786 faecal specimens were examined by the HOFFMAN, PONS and JANNER technique and the age group examined was school-children from 7 to 14 years. The survey was limited to towns or villages having more than 1,500 inhabitants. Of the samples examined 10.09% showed eggs of *S.mansoni*.

Following this [PELLON and TEIXEIRA, 1953], a new survey was made in States where schistosomiasis was not supposed to be endemic (central and southern States: Rio de Janeiro, Paraná, Santa Catarina, Goiás and Mato Grosso). The survey revealed only 0.08% positives. At that time it was estimated that 5,200,000 persons were infected with *S.mansoni*.

New evidence shows that schistosomiasis is spreading to territories where negative results had been previously obtained by PELLON and TEIXEIRA. Several recent surveys made locally by the 'Departamento Nacional de Endemias Rurais' have shown higher infection rates than those presented by PELLON and TEIXEIRA. This is particularly true in the northern States of Maranhão and Rio Grande do Norte. In addition, new isolated foci were found in northern as well as in southern States. The best example of the reason for this is in the northern region of the southern State of Paraná. Migration of a large group of people to Paraná, from infected areas of northeastern Brazil, seeking better working conditions, and a greater demand for labour, resulted in the establishment of several new foci of the disease.

The figures in table XXIX give some idea of the prevalence of schistosomiasis in the country, but the examination of data from certain physio-

Table XXIX. Number of localities in several states of Brazil with infection rates 10.1–30, 30.1–50, 50.1–70 and 70.1% and over [organized from PELLON and TEIXEIRA, 1950]

State	Number of school-children examined	Total infection rate per State, %	Total number of localities surveyed	Number of localities with infection rates			
				10.1–30%	30.1–50%	50.1–70%	70.1% and over
Maranhão	12,716	0.46	31	1	0	0	0
Piauí	10,420	0.04	16	0	0	0	0
Ceará	40,314	0.94	79	0	1	1	0
R. G. do Norte	18,662	2.32	45	0	0	0	1
Paraíba	21,488	7.53	47	13	1	0	1
Pernambuco	50,363	25.17	79	26	9	20	5
Alagoãs	14,965	20.48	23	8	4	5	1
Sergipe	14,676	30.13	31	12	4	5	5
Bahia	74,590	16.55	230	64	44	9	2
Espírito Santo	12,822	1.63	23	2	0	0	0
Minas Gerais	158,039	4.41	264	12	3	7	0

Table XXX

Year	Authors	Animals infected
1953	AMORIM	Several wild rodents
1953	BARBOSA *et al.*	*Rattus rattus frugivorus*
1954	BARBOSA *et al.*	*Didelphis p. paraguayensis*
1954	BARBOSA *et al.*	*Cavia aperea aperea*
1955	MARTINS *et al.*	Wild rodents
1955	MARTINS *et al.*	*Didelphis p. paraguayensis*
1959	BARRETO	*Rattus norwegicus*
1962	BARBOSA *et al.*	*Bos tauros*

graphical areas indicates that the prevalence is much higher, as in the humid forest area of Pernambuco (25.16%) and of Alagoas (56.44%). In the central area of the State of Sergipe the infection rate attained the figure of 86.57% and in the littoral area of the same State, 28.49%.

In the State of Bahia the following figures are found: 34.52% for Jacobina area, 'matas do Orobó' 22.97% and the littoral north 26.42%.

Other important endemic areas are located in the State of Minas Gerais: 30.02% for Murici area and 16.62% for 'Médio São Francisco'.

Reservoir Hosts

Several animals have been found naturally infected in Brazil: wild and domestic rodents, the opossum and cattle (table XXX).

The following resumé of the current situation in Brazil is based on the latest available records:

In Pará, the limited focus of Belterra seems to have disappeared spontaneously. Little is known of the focus located in the north-eastern part of the State (near Bragança).

In Maranhão, the few known foci are now so numerous that the north-western part of the State can be considered as a limited endemic area. Prevalence is low in general but rates between 50.1 and 70% were found in two places.

In Ceará, the disease occurs in isolated foci and prevalence is low, with a few exceptions where the rate reaches 70%.

From Rio Grande do Norte down to the State of Alagôas, schistosomiasis is distributed over the entire eastern part of these States and infection rates are usually high.

In Sergipe, the disease is found in most of the State, except in the north-west, and high infection rates are found.

In Bahia the disease distribution is extensive and includes the main part of the State except the west and north-west. In the interior, prevalence rates are low but the rate is as high as 70% in a few places. Along the coast, infection rates are generally heavy.

Minas Gerais is heavily infected. Prevalence is high along the coast and westward from Espírito Santo beyond Belo Horizonte, following the Rio Doce valley.

Espírito Santo has scattered foci but prevalence is generally relatively low.

In the State of Rio de Janeiro, of a total of 1,145,952 persons examined between 1955 and 1961, 0.2% were positive for *S. mansoni*. However, of 2,778 cases disclosed by the surveys, only 281 were autochthonous. Five municipalities in the State were found to be transmission foci.

The State of Guanabara has a few foci [VINHA and MARTINS, 1962].

In São Paulo, the influx of people from north-eastern Brazil has led to the establishment of new foci. Formerly, the only known focus in the State was a long existing one at Santos on the coast. PIZA [1965] reported a total of 1,890 new autochthonous cases from 23 municipalities between the years 1951 and 1963. The disease is now rather widely spread in the northern part of the State.

Paraná has become infected through migrations from north-eastern Brazil, although prevalence is apparently at a low level. LIMA and LUZ [1962] reported that surveys since 1956 had revealed foci in 22 localities in the State with infection rates up to 6.25% for *B. glabrata*. However, snail infections were as low as 0.3% or even less in many areas. LUZ [1963] conducted surveys in the Joachim Tavora Administrative area; intradermal tests were conducted on the total population (about 15,000) and 69 positives were obtained. Eggs of *S. mansoni* were recovered from the stools of 31 persons, and 22 of these represented autochthonous infections. A total of 52 of 2,274 *B. glabrata* were infected.

The southernmost States of Santa Catarina and Rio Grande do Sul have not been reported to be infected.

Autochthonous cases have been reported from the State of Goaias and in Brasilia, and it is questionable whether or not infection is locally propagated in the State of Mato Grosso.

The total cases of *S. mansoni* infection in Brazil amount to an estimated four to six million.

The Molluscan Intermediate Hosts of Schistosoma mansoni *in Brazil*
Eight species of *Biomphalaria* have been recognized so far in Brazil:

B. glabrata [SAY, 1818], *B. straminea* [DUNKER, 1848], *B. tenagophila* [ORBIGNY, 1835], *B. peregrina* [ORBIGNY, 1835], *B. philippiana* [DUNKER, 1848], *B. schrammi* [CROSSE, 1864], *B. intermedia* [PARAENSE and DESLANDES, 1962] and *B. amazonica* [PARAENSE, 1966]. The first three are actual hosts of schistosomiasis mansoni, *B. peregrina* is a potential host, and the last four have proved insusceptible to the infection.

The geographical distribution of the above-mentioned species is being steadily investigated but, owing to the vastness of the country and to the small number of interested workers, wide areas still remain to be surveyed, chiefly in the central, western and Amazonian regions.

Relative to the other two transmitting hosts, *B. glabrata* shows its highest degree of dominance and frequency in a quadrantal area, between parallels 13° and 21° S, and meridians 39° and 45° W, corresponding to south-eastern Bahia, northern Espírito Santo and to the part of Minas Gerais east of the São Francisco River. From that area it spreads continuously in all directions, chiefly to the north and to the south-west. It extends northward along the coastal belt and adjoining inland areas of the States of Sergipe, Alagoas, Pernambuco, Paraíba and Rio Grande do Norte. A number of peripherally isolated populations, more or less distant from the main body of the species range, are found in the States of Maranhão, Pará, Goías, Minas Gerais, São Paulo and Paraná. In the last-mentioned State *B. glabrata* reaches, at Curitiba, the southernmost point of its range (25° 25′ S). In the State of Guanabara there is a population, still restricted to the district of Manguinhos, descended from specimens introduced there in 1917 [JANSEN, 1944].

Most populations of *B. glabrata* inhabit permanent bodies of water in zones of moderate rainfall, but it may also be found in zones of drier climate. In either situation it may colonize habitats subject to seasonal drought, developing more or less marked resistance to desiccation [COUTINHO et al., 1940; BARBOSA and DOBBIN, jr., 1952]. This happens typically in north-eastern Brazil, especially in the transitional zone between the humid coast and the semi-arid hinterland. The single record of *B. glabrata* in the last-mentioned zone, at Cajazeiras, State of Paraíba [LUCENA, 1956], shows how well endowed it is with potentialities for settling in such highly adverse environment. However, the fact that under conditions of drier climate it gives way to *B. straminea* shows that the latter is better adapted to those conditions.

With few exceptions, the studied populations of *B. glabrata* are associated with schistosomiasis. Although usually highly susceptible to infection with *S. mansoni*, they show local variations in susceptibility [PARAENSE and CORRÊA, 1963a], but even the less susceptible ones, as those of Salvador,

Bahia, are responsible for a high prevalence of schistosomiasis in human populations.

B. straminea is dominant and most frequent in the area bounded by meridian 41° W, parallel 11° S and the seashore. Its range is much wider than those of the other two species. It is present in all drainage systems of the Brazilian territory, with the few exceptions of the eastern side of the Paraná basin, of the Uruguay basin and of the area that drains into the Atlantic from 21° southward. It overlaps all the range of *B. glabrata*, except for the periphery of the latter south of parallel 20°. It also overlaps *B. tenagophila*, in the little-studied central and south-western regions.

B. straminea is a most successful species, inhabiting both permanent and temporary bodies of water and being well adapted to all climatic varieties in Brazil. Its absence from the southern temperate zone is not a result of mere climatic influence, as it also occurs in the region of Buenos Aires, Argentina, which belongs to the same zone of rainy temperate climate.

A special reference should be made to the occurrence of *B. straminea* in the state of Paraná. It was recorded by LUCENA [1956], on a conchological basis, at the Paraguayan border (Guaira and Foz do Iguaçu) and in the east, about 80 km from the coast (Timbu). LÔBO and LUZ [1954], also based on shell characteristics, recorded it in 9 municipalities. Subsequently, LIMA and LUZ [1960], adopting the anatomical criteria, showed that *B. peregrina* occurs in 7 of those municipalities, but failed to find either species in the remaining two and were unable to recognize *B. straminea* in the State.

B. straminea is much more important than *B. glabrata* as a host of schistosomiasis in north-eastern Brazil [LUCENA, 1950b], due to its much wider distribution and to its association with high human infection rates [BARBOSA and COELHO, 1956; LUCENA, 1963], in spite of being much less susceptible to *S. mansoni* infection [BARBOSA and COELHO, 1954a, b]. Outside this area, it has been recognized as a host in only two isolated foci. One of them is situated in the Amazonian region, at Fordlândia, on the lower Tapajós River (State of Pará), where the disease was introduced by immigrants from the north-eastern states [MACHADO and MARTINS, 1951]. The other focus was recently detected at Goiânia, State of Goiás [SOUZA *et al.*, 1965]. In other parts of its range there have been no indications of *B. straminea* acting as an intermediate host.

B. tenagophila is a rather southern species which concentrates in a narrow zone (21° to 24° S and 42° to 52° W), covering Rio de Janeiro and Guanabara States and a considerable part of São Paulo. From here it spreads to all areas (except through the São Francisco Basin), northward to latitude 16° S and west and south to the neighbouring countries (Bolivia, Paraguay, Argentina and Uruguay). This species seems to be unable to withstand environmental drought, and so it only thrives in permanent water bodies.

Transmission of schistosomiasis by *B. tenagophila* has only been verified in small parts of its range, in the States of Guanabara (Jacarepaguá), Rio de Janeiro (Niterói) and São Paulo (region of Santos, Itariri, Campinas and an important section of the River Paraíba valley). Investigations by PARAENSE and CORRÊA [1963b] have pointed to an adaptation of *S. mansoni* to *B. tenagophila*, through the evolution of strains or biological races capable of infecting, more or less easily, the populations of this snail in the areas of its range still free from schistosomiasis.

Despite the extensively overlapping ranges of the three planorbid species concerned, only rarely have they been found together in the same biotope. A single instance of co-existence of *B. glabrata* and *B. straminea*, reproductively isolated, has been observed in the Córrego do Bambu, a creek at Governador Valadares, Minas Gerais [PARAENSE and DESLANDES, 1955]. In Guanabara State a sample of *B. glabrata* from Aracaju, introduced in 1917 into a breeding place of *B. tenagophila* at the district of Manguinhos, gave rise to a population that excluded the autochthonous species from that biotope. The reverse occurred at Belo Horizonte, where the offspring of a sample of albino *B. tenagophila* from São Paulo, introduced with ornamental plants into a pond at the district of Baleia, replaced in about five years a population of the autochthonous *B. glabrata*. No instance of co-existence of *B. straminea* and *B. tenagophila* has been recorded yet. These facts suggest that competitive exclusion should be considered one of the factors that influence the distribution of the populations of the three species studied.

Localities

The following list comprises the localities where the three species of *Biomphalaria* concerned have been found, references being made only to the first author for each locality.

(a) Biomphalaria glabrata

State of Pará. Quatipuru, formerly a district of Capanema [PARAENSE and DESLANDES, 1959].

State of Maranhão. Cururupu, São Luiz [LUCENA, 1956]; Alegre, Paço do Lumiar, São Bento [PARAENSE, unpublished].

State of Rio Grande do Norte. Estremoz Lake, Nísia Floresta, formerly Paparí [BAKER, 1913]; Arês, Touros [LUCENA, 1956, as *Australorbis bahiensis*]; Ceará Mirim [PARAENSE, unpublished], Pureza [BARBOSA and FIGUEIREDO, 1969].

State of Paraíba. João Pessôa [LUCENA, 1946, as *Planorbis olivaceus*]; Gramame [LUCENA, 1948]; Alhandra, Cajazeiras, Ponta de Lucena, Santa Rita [LUCENA, 1956].

State of Pernambuco. Recife [CHAGAS, 1938, as *Planorbis olivaceus*]; Pontezinha [COUTINHO, 1938, as *Planorbis olivaceus*]; Peixinhos [SILVA, quoted by MEIRA, 1947, as *Planorbis olivaceus*]; Canhotinho, Olinda, Pau Amarelo, Paulista, Quipapá [LUCENA, 1948]; Bom Conselho [LUCENA, 1949]; Goiana, Poço Comprido, São João de Garanhuns [LUCENA, 1950a]; Correntes, Garanhuns [LUCENA, 1951]; Lagoa dos Gatos [LUCENA, 1951, as *Australorbis bahiensis*]; Jaboatão [BARBOSA *et al.*, 1952].

State of Alagoas. Penedo [LUCENA, 1947]; Marechal Deodoro [LUCENA, 1949]; Coruripe, Junqueiro, Maceió, Viçosa [LUCENA, 1950a]; Utinga [LUCENA, 1956]; Pilar [PESSÔA and AMORIM, 1957]; Atalaia, Murici, Palmeira dos Indios, Piassabuçu [LUCENA, 1963]; Anadia, Capela, Girau do Ponciano, Limoeiro de Anadia, Maragogi, Quebrangulo, São José da Lage, São Miguel dos Campos, Traipu, União dos Palmares [BARBOSA and FIGUEIREDO, 1969].

State of Sergipe. Aracaju [LUTZ, 1918, as *Planorbis olivaceus*]; Murta, on an affluent of the Japaratuba River, Timbó [LUTZ and PENNA, 1918, as *Planorbis olivaceus*]; Ipiranga, Riachuelo [PESSÔA and COUTINHO, 1950, as *Australorbis glabratus* and *A. olivaceus*]; Itaporanga d'Ajuda, Salgado [REY and PESSÔA, 1953]; Buquim, Cristianápolis, Estancia, Lagarto, Laranjeiras, Nossa Senhora do Socorro, Riachão do Dantas, Rosário do Catete, São Cristovão, Siriri, Umbaúba [MELLO and BARBOSA, 1969].

State of Bahia. Almada, Ilhéus [SPIX and WAGNER, 1827, as *Planorbis olivaceus, P. ferrugineus, P. nigricans, P. albescens, P. viridis* and *P. lugubris*]; Salvador [MORICAND, 1853, as *Planorbis dentifer*]; Alagoinhas, Cachoeira, Feira de Santana [LUTZ and PENNA, 1918, as *Planorbis olivaceus*]; Djalma Dutra, formerly Pocões [CONI, 1933, as *Planorbis bahiensis*]; Itabuna [COUTINHO, 1951, wrongly referred to Ilhéus: see PARAENSE, 1961, p. 290]; São Desidério [PINTO and DESLANDES, 1953]; Vila Nova [GARBE, quoted by

MORRETES, 1953, as *Australorbis olivaceus*]; Jequié, Muritiba, Santa Terezinha [LUCENA, 1956]; Baixão, Itambé, Itaparica, Irará, Santo Amaro [PARAENSE, unpublished].

State of Espírito Santo. Baixo Guandu, Colatina, Mascarenhas [BASSÈRES and PANTOJA, 1947, as *Australorbis olivaceus*]; Itapina, Santa Joana [PINTO and DESLANDES, 1953]; Afonso Cláudio, Itaguaçu, Itaimbé, Itarana [PARAENSE and DESLANDES, 1959]; Alto Mutum, Mutum Prêto, Santa Tereza, Serra Pelada [PARAENSE, unpublished].

State of Rio de Janeiro. Duas Barras [PARAENSE and DESLANDES, 1959]; Barra do Piraí [PARAENSE, unpublished].

State of Guanabara. Manguinhos [JANSEN, 1944, as *Australorbis olivaceus*].

State of Minas Gerais. Belo Horizonte, Formiga, Pedra Azul, formerly Fortaleza [MARTINS, 1938]; Francisco Sá, formerly Brejo das Almas, Montes Claros, Salinas [MARTINS and VERSIANI, 1938]; Itambacuri [PINTO, 1944]; Governador Valadares [PINTO and ALMEIDA, 1944]; Caratinga, Malacacheta, Teófilo Otoni [PINTO and ALMEIDA, 1945a, as *Australorbis olivaceus*]; Bom Jesus do Galho [PINTO and ALMEIDA, 1945b]; Januária [BAKER, 1945]; Aimorés, Conselheiro Pena, Crenaque, Cuietê, Derribadinha, Itueta, Resplendor, Tumiritinga [BASSÈRES and PANTOJA, 1947, as *Australorbis olivaceus*]; Medina [BARBOSA and DOBBIN, jr., 1951]; Jaboticatubas [RUIZ, 1951]; Mariana, Neves [RUIZ, 1952]; Bambuí [DIAS, 1953]; Lagoa Santa [PARAENSE and SANTOS, 1953, as *Australorbis olivaceus*]; Alvinopolis, Baldim, Barão de Cocais, Caeté, Monlevade, Nova Era, Ouro Prêto, Sabará, Santa Bárbara [PINTO and DESLANDES, 1953]; Tarumirim [PARAENSE *et al.*, 1954]; Santa Luzia [PARAENSE, 1955]; Divino, Pedro Leopoldo [LUCENA, 1956]; Acesita, Dom Joaquim, Ferros, Iapu, Inhapim, Itanhomi, Mesquita, Mutum, Nossa Senhora das Graças, Peçanha, Santa Maria de Itabira, Santa Rita, Sao Joao Evangelista [ANDRADE, 1956]; Jequitinhonha [PARAENSE and DESLANDES, 1959]; Agua Boa, Almenara, Alterosa, Araxá, Assaraí, Barreiro de Cima, Betim, Bocaiuva, Brasília, Braúnas, Calciolândia, Capoeirão, Carlos Bernardes, Centenário de Ipanema, Cinco Ilhas, Comercinho, Conceição da Aparecida, Conceição do Capim, Conceição do Mato Dentro, Conselheiro Lafaiete, Coração de Jesús, Coronel Fabriciano, Curvelo, Desembargador Trindade, Diamantina, Dores do Indaía, Entre Fôlhas, Florestal, Galiléia, Guanhães, Jampruca, João Pessoa, Juiz de Fora, Manhuaçu, Nova Lima, Novo Cruzeiro, Pains, Penha do Capim, Piau,

Ponto Nova, Rio Pardo de Minas, Rio Piraciacaba, Sabinópolis, Santa Maria do Suaçuí, Santo Antônio do Grama, São João do Paraíso, São Pedro do Suaçuí, São Raimundo, São Sebastião do Rio Prêto, Sapucaia, Sete Laboas, Taboleiro, Ubá, Vespasiano, Viçosa [PARAENSE, unpublished].

State of Goías. Formosa [PARAENSE and DESLANDES, 1959]; Brasília, D. F. [CRESPO *et al.*, 1965].

State of São Paulo. Ourinhos [REY, 1952]; Ipauçu, Palmital, Salto Grande [REY, 1956]; Cândido Mota, Santa Cruz do Rio Pardo [PIZA and RAMOS, 1960]; Assis, Xavantes [CORRÊA *et al.*, 1962].

State of Paraná. Jacarèzinho [COUTINHO and PESSÔA, 1949, as *Australorbis* spp.]; Uraí [REY *et al.*, 1953]; Abatiá, Assaí, Cambará, Cinzas, Jataizinho, Santo Antônio da Platina, Tomazina [LÔBO and LUZ, 1954]; Curitiba [LIMA *et al.*, 1959]; Amoreira, Bandeirantes, Cornélio Procópio, Ibiporã, Leópolis, Londrina, Pinhalão, Porecatu, Primeiro de Maio, Ribeirão Claro, Sertaneja, Sertanópolis [LIMA and LUZ, 1960]; Conselheiro Mayrink, Joaquim Távora, Rancho Alegre [LIMA and LUZ, 1962]; Andirá, Apucarana, Itambaracá, Nova Fátimá, Santa Amélia, Santa Mariana [LIMA, 1965].

(b) Biomphalaria straminea
State of Acre. Cruzeiro do Sul, Rio Branco [PARAENSE, unpublished].

State of Amazonas. Calado Lake near Manacapuru, on Solimões River; Comprido and Matafome Lakes near Três Casas, on Madeira River [HAAS, 1949a, as *Tropicorbis paparyensis*].

State of Pará. Aniperi River, right tributary of São Manoel River, close to its mouth; Cupari River, near its mouth; Fordlândia; Grande Curuaí Lake, west of Santarém; Santarém; Tostao Lake, between Alenquer and Obidos [HAAS, 1949a, as *Tropicorbis paparyensis*]; Belterra, Timbó Lake near Curí, on lower Tapajós River; Caxias Lake, Curuçá Lake and Flechal, on Cupari River; Salgado and Tracoá Lakes, on Cuminá River near Oriximiná; Cuminá River near Obidos [HAAS, 1949b, as *Tropicorbis paparyensis*]; Jacaré, on Tapajós River [HAAS, 1952, as *Tropicorbis paparyensis*]; Belém [PINTO and DESLANDES, 1953, as *Australorbis centimetralis*]; Igarapé-Açu, João Coelho, Nova Timboteua (COSTA *et al.*, quoted by Maroja, 1953, as *Australorbis centimetralis*]; Livramento, Monto Alegre, Quatipuru [PARAENSE, unpublished].

State of Maranhão. São Luiz [LUCENA, 1956]; Paço do Lumiar, São Bento [PARAENSE, unpublished].

State of Ceará. Redenção [ALENCAR, 1940, as *Australorbis centimetralis*]; Aquiraz [BAKER, 1945]; Campos Sales, Caucaia, Coreaú, Crateús, Fortaleza, Independência, Ipu, Itapipoca, Jaguaruana, Licânia, Nova Russas, Pacatuba, Pacoti, Reriutaba, Sobral, Tamboril, Tauá [LUCENA, 1950a, as *Tropicorbis centimetralis*]; Acarape, Aracati, Ipueiras, Russas [LUCENA, 1951]; Aracoiaba, Baturité, Granja, Maranguape, Pacajus [BEZERRA, 1955]; Saboeiro [LUCENA, 1956]; Amontada, Crato, Croatá, Itaiçaba, Juazeiro do Norte, Limoeiro do Norte, Massapê, Sapupara, Senador Pompeu [PARAENSE, unpublished]. Acaraú, Acopiara, Aiuaba, Antonina do Norte, Araripe, Arneiroz, Assaré, Aurora, Baixio, Barbalha, Boa Viagem, Brejo Santo, Camocim, Canindé, Cariré, Carnaubal, Cascavel, Cedro, Farias Brito, Frecheirinha, General Sampaio, Icó, Iguaretama, Iguatu, Ipaumirin, Itapagé, Itapiuna, Jaguaribe, Jardim, Jati, Jucás, Lavras da Mangabeira, Mauriti, Milagres, Missão Velha, Mombaça, Morada Nova, Morrinhos, Nova Olinda, Orós, Panaforte, Parambu, Pedra Branca, Pentecoste, Pereiro, Piquet Carneiro, Porteiras, Queixeré, Quixadá, Quixeramobim, Santa Quitéria, Santana do Acaraú, Santana do Cariri, São Benedito, São Gonçalo do Amarante, Solonópole, Tabuleiro do Norte, Umari, Uruburetama, Uruoca, Várzea Alegre [BARBOSA and FIGUEIREDO, 1969].

State of Rio Grande do Norte. Ceará Mirim, Papari Lake [BAKER, 1913]; Estremoz Lake [LUTZ, 1918, as *Planorbis centimetralis*]; Natal [LUTZ and PENNA, 1918, as *Planorbis centimetralis*]; Cerro Corá, Currais Novos, Mossoró, Santa Cruz [CHAGAS, 1938, as *Planorbis centimetralis*]; Angicos, Baixa Verde, Felipe Camarão, Goianinha, Massangana, Nisía Floresta, formerly Papari, Nova Cruz, Padre Miguelinho, São José de Mipibu, São Paulo de Potengi, São Tomé, Touros [LUCENA, 1950a, as *Tropicorbis centimetralis*]; Acari, Açu, Agua Nova, Alexandria, Apodi, Augusto Severo, Caiçara do Rio do Vento, Caiçó, Caraúbas, João Câmara, Jardim de Piranhas, Jardim do Seridó, Jucurutu, Lagoa d'Anta, Macaíba, Macau, Martins, Maxaranguape, Parazinho, Parelhas, Patu, Pau dos Ferros, Pedro Avelino, Portalegre, Pureza, Santana do Matos, Santo Antonio, São Bento do Norte, São José do Campestre, São Miguel, Serra Negra do Norte, Sítio Nôvo, Taipu, Tangará [BARBOSA and FIGUEIREDO, 1969].

State of Paraíba. João Pessoa, formerly Paraíba [LUTZ, 1918, as *Planorbis centimetralis*]; Alagoa Grande, Alagoa Nova, Alagoinha, Campina Grande, Mulungu, Sapé [CHAGAS, 1938, as *Planorbis centimetralis*]; Areia, Bodocongó, Cabaceiras, Cabedelo, Cuitegi, Marinho, Remígio, Santa Rita [LUCENA, 1949, as *Tropicorbis centimetralis*]; Bananeiras, Caiçara, Mamanguape, Umbuzeiro [LUCENA, 1950a, as *Tropicorbis centimetralis*]; Alagoa do Monteiro [LUCENA, 1951]; Araruna, Bonito de Santa Fé, Brejo das Freiras, Cajazeiras, Catolé do Rocha, Ingá, Itabaiana, Itaporanga, Jatobá, Monteiro, Patos, Pilar, Pombal, Princesa, Santa Luzia, São João do Cariri, Serraria, Souza [LUCENA, 1956]; Arara, Borborema, Cruz do Espírito Santo, Guarabira, Maia, Pirpiribuba, Rio Tinto [LUCENA, 1963]; Antenor Navarro, Araçagi, Barra de Santa Rosa, Boqueirão, Brejo do Cruz, Cacimba de Dentro, Conceição, Coremas, Esperança, Juàzeirinho, Mogeiro, Pedra Lavrada, Piancó, Picuí, Pilões, São José de Piranhas, São Sebastião do Umbuzeiro, Solânea, Soledade, Taperoá, Teixeira [BARBOSA and FIGUEIREDO, 1969].

State of Pernambuco. Jaboatão, Socorro [LUTZ, 1918, as *Planorbis centimetralis*]; Belo Jardim, Bezerros, Campo Grande, Caruaru, Gonçalves Ferreira, Lagoa do Carro, Limoeiro, Palmares, Paudalho, Vitória [LUTZ and PENNA, 1918, as *Planorbis centimetralis*]; Catende [JANSEN, 1943, as *Australorbis centimetralis*]; Aldeia Velha, Altinho, Angelim, Bebedouro, Belém de Maria, Calçado, Canhotinho, Garanhuns, Gravata, Igaraçu, Olho Dágua dos Pombos, Panelas, Quipapa, Recife, Salgadinho, São Bento do Una, São Caetano, São João, São Joaquim, Timbaúba [LUCENA, 1948, as *Tropicorbis centimetralis*]; Bom Jardim, João Alfredo, Orobo, Russinha, Surubim, Vertentes [LUCENA, 1949, as *Tropicorbis centimetralis*]; Agua Preta, Bom Conselho, Bonito, Brejo da Madre de Deus, Correntes, Escada, Fazenda Nova, Frei Miguelinho, Gameleira, Glória do Goitá, Maraial, Poço Comprido, Ribeirão, São Pedro de Garanhuns [LUCENA, 1950a, as *Tropicorbis centimetralis*]; Afogados de Ingazeira, Araripina, Bodocó, Custódia, Exú, Flôres, Jupi, Maniçobal, Nazaré da Mata, Ouricuri, Parnamirim, Paulista, Pesqueira, Salgueiró, Sanharo, São José do Egito, Serra Talhada, Serrita, Sertânia, Triunfo [LUCENA, 1951]; Olinda, São Lourenço da Mata [BARBOSA *et al.*, 1952, as *Tropicorbis centimetralis*]; Cabo, Goiana, Moreno, Vicência [BARBASO and COELHO, 1954a, b as *Tropicorbis centimetralis*]; Aguas Belas [LUCENA, 1956]; Carpina, Chã da Alegria, Macaparana [BARBOSA and COELHO, 1956, as *Tropicorbis centimetralis*]; Abreu e Lima, Agrestina, Aliança, Barreiros, Cachoeirinha, Camocituba, Capibaribe, Condado, Cupira, Ipojuca, Itapissuma, Jurema, Lagoa dos Gatos, Lajedo, Manoel Borba, Pombos, Pontas de Pedras, Pontezinha, Rio Formoso, São Joaquim do Monte, Siriji, Sirinhaém, Tacaimbó, També, Taquaritinga, Toritama [Lucena, 1963]; Afrânio, Amaraji, Arco-verde, Belém de São Francisco, Betânia, Bodocó, Buique, Cabrobó, Carnaiba, Floresta, Ibimirim, Inajá, Itapetim, Itaquitinga, Logoa do Ouro, Mirandiba, Passira, Pedra, Petrolândia, Petrolina, Santa Cruz do Capibaribe, Santa Maria da Boa Vista, Tabira, Tacaratu, Taquaritinga do Norte, Tracunhaém, Trindade, Venturosa, Verdejante, Vitória de Santo Antão [Barbosa and Figueiredo, 1969].

State of Alagoas. Penedo [Lucena, 1947, as *Tropicorbis centimetralis*]; Delmiro, Igreja Nova, Pôrto Real do Colégio [Lucena, 1949, as *Tropicorbis centimetralis*]; Arapiraca, Assembléia, Atalaia, Barra do Canhoto, Cana-fístula, Colônia de Leopoldina, Conceiçao do Paraíba, Limoeiro de Anadia, Murici, Palmeira dos Indios, Quebrangulo, Salomé, São José da Laje, São Miguel dos Campos [Lucena, 1950a, as *Tropicorbis centimetralis*]; Rio Largo, Viçosa [Lucena, 1951]; Maceió, Utinga [Lucena, 1956]; Flexeiras [Pessôa and Amorim, 1957, as *Tropicorbis centimetralis*]; Anadia, Capela, Coruripe, Passo de Camaragibe, Piassabuçu, Pilar, Pôrto Calvo, São Luis do Quitunde [Lucena, 1963]; Agua Branca, Cacimbinhas, Delmiro Gouveia, Girau do Ponciano, Igaci, Junqueiro, Major Isidoro, Marimbondo, Mata Grande, Olho d'Agua das Flôres, Olho d'Agua do Casado, Pão de Açúcar, Piranhas, Pôrto de Pedras, Santana do Ipanema, São Brás, São José da Tapera, União dos Palmares [Barbosa and Figueiredo, 1969].

State of Sergipe. Propriá [Lutz and Penna, 1918, as *Planorbis centimetra-lis*]; Neópolis [Lucena, 1949, as *Tropicorbis centimetralis*]. Aguidabã, Capela, Graccho Cardoso, Itabaiana, Japoatã, Lagarto, Maruim, Muribeca, Nossa Senhora da Glória, Ribeirópolis, Sirirí, Tobias Barreto [Mello and Barbosa, 1969].

State of Bahia. Itabuna [Pessôa and Coutinho, 1950, as *Tropicorbis cen-timetralis*]; Juazeiro, Paulo Afonso [Pinto and Deslandes, 1953, as *Australor-bis centimetralis*]; Muritiba [Lucena, 1956]; Ilhéus [Paraense, 1961].

State of Espirito Santo. Mascarenhas [Paraense, unpublished].

State of Minas Gerais. Belo Horizonte [Teixeira, 1919, as *Planorbis centi-metralis*]; Rio Casca [Barros, 1934, as *Planorbis centimetralis*]; Governador Valadares [Penido *et al.*, 1951, as *Australorbis centimetralis*]; Cordis-burgo, Vespasiano [Pinto and Deslandes, 1953, as *Australorbis centi-

metralis]; Matosinhos [LUCENA, 1956]; Arcos, Bocaiuva, Buenópolis, Calciolândia, Corinto, Coronel Fabriciano, Curvelo, Derribadinha, Francisco Sá, Itinga, Jacinto, Jequitaí, Lagoa Santa, Lontra, Montes Claros, Paracatu, Pedro Leopoldo, Pirapora, Porteirinha, Salinas, Salto da Divisa, São Pedro do Suaçuí, São Romão, Sete Lagoas, Teófilo Otoni [PARAENSE, unpublished].

State of Goiás. Anápolis, Goiania, Trindade [SOUZA *et al.*, 1965]; Arraias [CUNHA NETO, personal cummunication].

State of Mato Grosso. Ponta Porã [LUCENA, 1956].

State of Paraná. Foz do Iguaçu, Guaíra, Timbu [LUCENA, 1956].

(c) Biomphalaria tenagophila
State of Bahia. Caravelas [LUTZ, 1918, as *Planorbis nigricans*].

State of Espírito Santo. Vitória [BAKER, 1945, as *Australorbis bahiensis*]; Linhares [PINTO and DESLANDES, 1953, as *Australorbis nigricans*].

State of Rio de Janeiro. Campos [BAKER, 1945, as *Australorbis bahiensis*]; Petrópolis [PILSBRY, 1951, as *Australorbis bahiensis megas*]; Itaipava [PINTO and DESLANDES, 1953, as *Australorbis nigricans*]; Niteroi [MARTINS, 1957, as *Australorbis nigricans*]; Macaé, Magé, São Gonçalo, Terezópolis [BARBOSA and CARNEIRO, 1958, as *Australorbis nigricans*]; Cabo Frio, Cantagalo, Três Rios [PARAENSE and DESLANDES, 1959]; Bocaininha, Cordeiro, Duque de Caxias, São Joaquim [PARAENSE, unpublished].

State of Guanabara. Rio de Janeiro [ORBIGNY, 1835, as *Planorbis ferrugineus*].

State of Minas Gerais. Juiz de Fora, Nova Era [PINTO and DESLANDES, 1953, as *Australorbis nigricans*]; Itajubá [PARAENSE and DESLANDES, 1955, as *Australorbis nigricans*]; Belo Horizonte (albino population introduced from São Paulo) [BARBOSA and CARNEIRO, 1958, as *Australorbis nigricans*]; Betim, Retiro, Rio Novo, Ubá [PARAENSE, unpublished]. Brasília, D. F. [CRESPO *et al.*, 1965].

State of Mato Grosso. Pôrto Esperança [LUCENA, 1951, as *Australorbis bahiensis*]; Várzea Grande [PARAENSE and DESLANDES, 1959]; Campo Grande [PARAENSE, unpublished].

State of São Paulo. São Paulo [MACIEL, 1920, as *Planorbis nigricans*]; Santos [ARANTES, 1923, as *Planorbis centimetralis*]; Santo Amaro [LUCENA, 1951, as *Australorbis bahiensis*]; Bauru [RUGAI, 1954]; Campinas [MACHADO and ABREU, 1955]; Pindamonhangaba [CORRÊA *et al.*, 1956, as *Australorbis nigricans*]; Ana Dias, in Itariri [REY, 1956, as *Australorbis nigricans*]; Aparecida, Caçapava, Cachoeira, Cruzeiro, Cunha, Guaratinguetá, Jacareí, Lagoinha, Lorena, Piquete, Roseira, Taubaté, Tremembé [PIZA *et al.*, 1959, as *Taphius nigricans*]; São José dos Campos [TOLEDO, quoted by PIZA *et al.*, 1959, as *Taphius nigricans*]; Cubatao, Santo André, São Bernardo do Camp, São Vicente [PARAENSE and DESLANDES, 1959]; Araraquara, Guarujá, Iguape, Miracatu, Piraçununga, Rincão, [CODA *et al.*, 1959, as *Taphius nigricans*]; Alfredo Marcondes, Jambeiro, Pedro de Toledo, São Caetano do Sul [PIZA and RAMOS, 1960]; Alto Alegre, Alvares Machado, Anhumas, Araçatuba, Avanhandava, Bananal, Barbosa, Birigui, Boituva, Braúna, Cordeirópolis, Coroados, Fartura, Florínea, Garça, Glicério, Guararapes, Iacanga, Indiana, Itanhaém, Itapecerica da Serra, Itaquaquecetuba, Lagoinha, Laranjal Paulista, Leme, Lençois Paulista, Limeira, Lins, Lutécia, Macatuba, Marabá Paulista, Marília, Martinopólis, Maua, Mirante do Paranapanema, Mogi das Cruzes, Oriente, Oscar Bressane, Penápolis, Peruibe, Piacatu, Piracicaba, Pirapòzinho, Pompéia, Pôrto Feliz, Presidente Bernardes, Presidente Prudente, Presidente Wenceslau, Promissão, Rinópolis, Rio Claro, Rubiácea, Santana do Parnaíba, Santopólis do Aguapeí, Sao Miguel Arcanjo, São Roque, Sorocaba, Suzano, Taciba, Tietê, Tupã, Valinhos, Valparaíso, Vera Cruz, Xavantes [CORRÊA *et al.*, 1962]; Ribeirão Prêto, São Carlos, São Luís do Paraitinga [PARAENSE, unpublished].

State of Paraná. Curitiba [MORRETES, 1949, as *Australorbis lugubris*]; Guaíra [LUCENA, 1951, as *Australorbis bahiensis*]; Paranaguá [PINTO and DESLANDES, 1953, as *Australorbis nigricans*]; Assaí [LÔBO and LUZ, 1954]; Morretes, Porecatu [LUCENA, 1956]; Jacarèzinho [PARAENSE and DESLANDES, 1959]; Antonina, Itaguajé [LIMA and LUZ, 1960]; Itambaracá, Londrina, Sertanópolis [LIMA, 1965].

State of Rio Grande do Sul. Pôrto Alegre [MARTENS, 1868]; Riacho Partenon [LUCENA, 1951]; Guaíba, Tramandaí [PARAENSE and DESLANDES, 1959]; Capão Sêco, Chuí, Curral Alto, Pelotas [PARAENSE, unpublished].

References

ALENCAR, J. E.: Ceará méd. *20:* 16 (1940).

AMORIM, J. P. DE: Rev. bras. Malar. *5:* 219 (1953).

AMORIM, J. P. DE: Rev. Inst. Med. trop., S. Paulo *4:* 397 (1962).

AMORIM, J. P. DE: Arch. Hig., S. Paulo *27:* 335 (1962a).

AMORIM, J. P. DE; ROSA, D. DA, and LUCENA, D. T. DE: Rev. bras. Malar. *6:* 13 (1954).

ANDRADE, R. M. DE: Rev. bras. Malar. *8:* 387 (1956).

ARANTES, A.: An. paul. Med. Cirurg. *4:* 95 (1923).

BAKER, F. C.: Proc. Acad. nat. Sci., Philad. *65:* 618 (1913).

BAKER, F. C.: The molluscan family Planorbidae (University of Illinois Press, Urbana 1945).

BARBOSA, F. S. and CARNEIRO, E.: Cienc. e Cult. *10:* 144 (1958).

BARBOSA, F. S. and COELHO, M. V.: Publ. avuls. Inst. Aggeu Magalhães *3:* 1 (1954a).

BARBOSA, F. S. and COELHO, M. V.: Publ. avuls. Inst. Aggeu Magalhães *3:* 55 (1954b).

BARBOSA, F. S. and COELHO, M. V.: Publ. avuls. Centro Pesq. Aggeu Magalhães *5:* 31 (1956).

BARBOSA, F. S. and DOBBIN, J. E., jr.: Publ. avuls. Inst. Aggeu Magalhães *1:* 1 (1951).

BARBOSA, F. S. and DOBBIN, J. E., jr.: Publ. avuls. Inst. Aggeu Magalhães *1:* 145 (1952).

BARBOSA, F. S. and FIGUEIREDO, T.: Rev. Inst. Med. trop. S. Paulo *11:* 285 (1969).

BARBOSA, F. S.; BARBOSA, I., and ARRUDA, F.. Science *138:* 831 (1962).

BARBOSA, F. S.; DOBBIN, J. E., jr., and COELHO, M. V.: Publ. avuls. Inst. Aggeu Magalhães *2:* 43 (1953).

BARBOSA, F. S.; DOBBIN, J. E., jr., and VIEIRA, A. E.: Publ. avuls Inst. Aggeu Magalhães *1:* 99 (1952).

BARRETTO, A. C.: Bol. Fund. Gonçalo Moniz *14:* 1 (1959).

BARROS, J. R. DE: Rev. méd. Minas *1:* 25 (1934).

BASSÈRES, M. S. and PANTOJA, W. P.: Rev. Serv. Saúde públ., Rio de J. *1:* 149 (1947).

BEZERRA, O. F.: Rev. bras. Malar. *7:* 351 (1955).

CHAGAS, E.: Hospital, Rio de J. *14:* 1323 (1938).

CODA, D.; FALCI, N., and MENDES, F. A. T.: Rev. Inst. A. Lutz, S. Paolo *19:* 25 (1959).

CONI, A. C: Rev. méd. Bahia *1:* 193 (1933).

CORRÊA, R. R.; CODA, D., and OLIVEIRA, U. A.: Fol. clin. biol., S. Paulo *26:* 85 (1956).

CORRÊA, R. R.; PIZA, J. DE T.; RAMOS, A. DA S., and CAMARGO, L. V. DE: Arch. Hig., S. Paulo *27:* 139 (1962).

COUTINHO, B.: Neurobiologia *1:* 212 (1938).

COUTINHO, B.; GOUVÊA, L., and LUCENA, D.: Mem. Inst. Osw. Cruz *35:* 207 (1940).

COUTINHO, J. O.: Arch. Hig., S. Paulo *16:* 3 (1951).

COUTINHO, J. O. and PESSÔA, S. B.: Hospital, Rio de J. *35:* 531 (1949).

CRESPO, V. M.; VERANO, O. T., and BARBOSA, J. A.: Rev. goiana Med. *11:* 59 (1965).

CRESPO, V. M.; VERANO, O. T., and BARBOSA, J. A.: Rev. bras. Malar. *17:* 367 (1966).

CROSSE, H.: J. Conchyl. *12:* 152 (1864).

CUNHA, A. S. DA: Esquistossomose mansoni; Universidade de S. Paulo, S. Paulo (1970).

DIAS, E.: Rev. bras. Malar. *5:* 211 (1953).

DUNKER, W.: Proc. Zool. Soc. Lond. *16:* 40 (1848).

HAAS, F.: An. Inst. Biol., Mex. *20:* 301 (1949a).

HAAS, F.: Arch. Molluskenk *78:* 149 (1949b).

HAAS, F.: Fieldiana, Zool. *34:* 107 (1952).

JANSEN, G.: Mem. Inst. Osw. Cruz *39:* 335 (1943).

JANSEN, G.: Mem. Inst. Osw. Cruz *40:* 201 (1944).

LIMA, E. C.: Esquistossomose mansoni no Estado do Parana; Thesis, Faculty of Medicine, University of Paraná, Curitiba (1965).

LIMA, E. C. and LUZ, E.: An. Fac. Med. Paraná *3:* 17 (1960).

LIMA, E. C. and LUZ, E.: An. Fac. Med. Paraná *5:* 105 (1962).

LIMA, E. C.; LUZ, E., and DESLANDES, N.: An. Fac. Med. Paraná *2:* 6 (1959).

LÔBO, A. G. S. and LUZ, E.: Rev. bras. Malar. *6:* 545 (1954).

LUCENA, D. T. DE: An. Soc. biol., Pernambuco *6:* 50 (1946).

LUCENA, D. T. DE: An. Soc. biol., Pernambuco *7:* 37 (1947).

LUCENA, D. T. DE: Bol. Secret. Agric. Ind. Com., Pernambuco *15:* 134 (1948).

LUCENA, D. T. DE: Bol. Secret. Agric. Ind. Com., Pernambuco *16:* 126 (1949).

LUCENA, D. T. DE: Bol. Secret. Agric. Ind. Com., Pernambuco *17:* 32 (1950a).

LUCENA, D. T. DE: An. Soc. Med., Pernambuco *2:* 12 (1950b).

LUCENA, D. T. DE: Pap. avuls. Dep. Zool., S. Paulo *10:* 93 (1951).

LUCENA, D. T. DE: Resenha sistematica dos planorbideos brasileiros; Thesis, Recife (1956).

LUCENA, D. T. DE: Rev. bras. Malar. *15:* 13 (1963).

LUTZ, A.: Mem. Inst. Osw. Cruz *10:* 65 (1918).

LUTZ, A. and PENNA, O.: Mem. Inst. Osw. Cruz *10:* 83 (1918).

LUZ, E.: An. Fac. Med., Paraná *6:* 79 (1963).

MACHADO, P. A. DE and ABREU, L. G. S.: Rev. Inst. A. Lutz, S. Paulo *15:* 235 (1955).

MACHADO, W. G. and MARTINS, C.: Hospital, Rio de J. *39:* 289 (1951).

MACIEL, J.: Bol. Soc. Med. Cirurg., S. Paulo *2:* 262 (1920).

MAROJA, R. C.: Rev. Serv. Saúde públ., Rio de J. *6:* 211 (1953).

MARTENS, E.: Malakozool. Blät. *15:* 169 (1868).

MARTINS, A. V.: Mem. Inst. biol. E. Dias *2:* 5 (1938).

MARTINS, A. V.: Bull. Wld Hlth Org. *18:* 931 (1958).

MARTINS, A. V. and VERSIANI, A. W.: Brasil-méd. *52:* 812 (1938).

MARTINS, A. V.; MARTINS, G., and BRITO, J. S. DE: Rev. bras. Med. *11:* 165 (1954).

MARTINS, A. V.; MARTINS, G., and BRITO, J. S. DE: Rev. bras. Malar. *7:* 259 (1955).

MARTINS, R. S. DE: Rev. bras. Malar. *9:* 361 (1957).

MEIRA, J. A.: Arch. Fac. Hig., S. Paulo *1:* 5 (1947).

MELLO, D. A. and BARBOSA, F. S.: Gaz. méd. Bahia *69:* 123 (1969).

MORICAND, S.: J. Conchyl. *4:* 37 (1853).

MORRETES, F. L.: Arq. Mus. Paranaense *7:* 1 (1949).

MORRETES, F. L.: Arq. Mus. Paranaense *10:* 37 (1953).

ORBIGNY, A. D': Mag. Zool. *5:* 26 (1835).

PARAENSE, W. L.: Mem. Inst. Osw. Cruz *53:* 285 (1955).

PARAENSE, W. L.: Rev. bras. Biol. *21:* 287 (1961).

PARAENSE, W. L.: Rev. bras. Biol. *26:* 115 (1966).

PARAENSE, W. L. and CORRÊA, L. R.: Rev. Inst. Med. trop., S. Paulo *5:* 15 (1963a).

PARAENSE, W. L. and CORRÊA, L. R.: Rev. Inst. Med. trop., S. Paulo *5:* 23 (1963b).

PARAENSE, W. L. and DESLANDES, N.: Rev. bras. Biol. *15:* 341 (1955).

PARAENSE, W. L. and DESLANDES, N.: Amer. J. trop. Med. Hyg. *8:* 456 (1959).

PARAENSE, W. L. and DESLANDES, N.: Rev. bras. Biol. *22:* 343 (1962).

PARAENSE, W. L. and SANTOS, J. M.: Rev. bras. Malar. *5:* 253 (1953).

PARAENSE, W. L.; PEREIRA, O., and PINTO, D. B.: Trans. roy. Soc. trop. Med. Hyg. 48: 540 (1954).

PELLON, A. B. and TEIXEIRA, I.: Distribuição geográfica da esquistossomose mansônica no Brasil. Publication of the 'Divisão de Organisação Sanitaria', Ministry of Health, Brazil, Rio de Janeiro (1950).

PELLON, A. B. and TEIXEIRA, I.: O inquérito helmintologico escolar em cinco Estados das regiões Leste, Sul e Centro-Oeste. Publication of the 'Divisao de Organisação Sanitaria', Ministry of Health, Brazil, Rio de Janeiro (1953).

PENIDO, H. M.; PINTO, D. B., and DESLANDES, N.: Rev. Serv. Saúde públ., Rio de J. 4: 383 (1951).

PESSÔA, S. B. and AMORIM, J. P.: Rev. bras. Malar. 9: 5 (1957).

PESSÔA, S. B. and COUTINHO, J. O.: Fol. clin. biol., S. Paulo 16: 123 (1950).

PILSBRY, H. A.: Nautilus 65: 3 (1951).

PINTO, C.: Mem. Inst. Osw. Cruz 40: 209 (1944).

PINTO, C. and ALMEIDA, A. F.: in PINTO, C., 1944, p. 291 (1944).

PINTO, C. and ALMEIDA, A. F.: Rev. bras. Med. 2: 912 (1945a).

PINTO, C. and ALMEIDA, A. F.: Rev. bras. Med. 2: 1000 (1945b).

PINTO, D. B. and DESLANDES, N.: Rev. Serv. Saúde públ., Rio de J. 6: 135 (1953).

PIZA, J. T. DE: Contribuicao para o Simposio sobre esquistossomose; Associação Médica Brasileira, São Paulo (1965).

PIZA, J. T. DE and RAMOS, A. S.: Arch. Hig., S. Paulo 25: 261 (1960).

PIZA, J. T. DE; RAMOS, A. S.; BRANDÂO, C. S. H., and FIGUEIREDO, C. G.: Rev. Inst. A. Lutz, S. Paulo 19: 97 (1959).

REY, L.: Rev. clin., S. Paulo 28: 57 (1952).

REY, L.: Contribuição para o conhecimento da morfologia, biologia e ecologia dos planor-bídeos brasileiros transmissores da esquistossomose. Serviço Nacional de Educação Sanitaria, Rio de Janeiro (1956).

REY, L. and PESSÔA, S. B.: Rev. clin., S. Paulo 29: 85 (1953).

REY, L.; AMATO NETO, V.; CAMPOS, R., and SILVA, L. H. P.: Fol. clin. biol., S. Paulo 20: 215 (1953).

RUGAI, E.: Rev. Inst. A. Lutz, S. Paulo 14: 9 (1954).

RUIZ, J. M.: An. Fac. Farm. Odont., S. Paulo 9: 51 (1951).

RUIZ, J. M.: Mem. Inst. Butantan 24: 63 (1952).

SOUZA, A. H. S.; CUNHA NETO, A. G., and LIMA, M. I.: Rev. bras. Malar. (1965).

SPIX, J. B. and WAGNER, J. A.: Testacea fluviatilia brasiliensia (Munich 1827).

TEIXEIRA, J. M.: A schistosomose mansônica na infância, em Belo Horizonte; Thesis, Faculty Medicine of Minas Gerais, Belo Horizonte (1919).

VINHA, C. and MARTINS, M. R. S. DE: Rev. bras. Malar. 14: 423 (1962).

Surinam

Surinam has a coastline of about 345 km and a width of about 500 km. Almost 80% of the population lives in a portion of the coastal strip having an area of about 4,400 km². About half of the people in the area live in the capital,

Paramaribo, and the remainder live in small villages or scattered in the farming area. Schistosomiasis is endemic only in the central part of the coastal region where the sandy ridges occur; this area contains about 600 km² and lies both east and west of the capital [OLIVIER and BUZO, 1962].

Surveys carried out in the Saramacca District by the Bureau of Public Health showed a prevalence of 23% in a population of about 10,000 persons. Spread of the disease is indicated by several reports [PAULINI, 1969].

About 100,000 people live in the known endemic area. The prevalence in 19 localities studied in 1956–1957 ranged from 1.5 to 30.5% with on over-all rate of 12.7%. It has been estimated that 9,300 are infected.

The only known molluscan intermediate host for *S. mansoni* in Surinam is *B. glabrata*. At certain seasons of the year this species occurs in enormous numbers in ditches, canals and rice-fields throughout the endemic area. Distribution is incompletely known. However, the snail is not confined to the endemic areas, since it is found in Coronie and Nickexie, although in these districts human infection is uncommon or absent.

References

OLIVIER, L.J. and BUZO, Z.J.: Report of the WHO Bilharziasis Advisory Team Visit to Surinam, 20–25 January 1962. WHO unpublished document, MHO/PA/117.64 (1962).
PAULINI, E.: A report on schistosomiasis in Surinam. Unpublished PAHO/WHO document, CD-AMRO-0901/A (1969).
VAN DER KUYP, E.: Bureau voor Openbare Gezondheidszorg Suriname, Publ. No. 2 (1964).
VAN DER KUYP, E.: Bureau voor Openbare Gezondheidszorg Suriname, Publ. No. 3 (1964).

Venezuela

S. mansoni endemic areas are confined to the north central part of Venezuela. They affect the Federal District and the States of Miranda, Aragua, Carabobo, Guárico and Maracay, covering an area of roughly 35,000 km². It is estimated that about 12% (750,000) of the country's population live in the endemic zone and that about 20,000 persons are now infected. Over-all prevalence in the endemic zone is, therefore, estimated to be about 4%.

An effective control campaign has been in progress since about 1940, and has resulted in material reductions in the prevalence rates in various parts of the endemic areas. The following data present the level of infection prior to 1950:

26.6% in the total population in the coastal valley;

31.6% in the rural areas of the 900-m altitude Caracas valley;

1–50% in other smaller valleys of the northern range, the highest rates being found below 900 m;

7% at altitudes of 1,200 m above sea-level.

In 1964, 9.4% of 13,139 persons examined in the Aragua State were positive. The rate in children of less than 10 years of age was 6.2% and that in individuals above 10 years of age was 13.6%.

In the same year, examinations in the State of Carabobo revealed an infection rate in 6% of 7,991 individuals, with a rate of 1.8% in those of less than 10 years of age and a rate of 8.9% in those above 10 years of age.

In Guárico State, 5.6% of 1,833 persons were infected. The prevalence rate in persons under 10 years of age was 2.6% and in those over that age, 11.2%.

B. glabrata is apparently the sole intermediate host of S. mansoni in Venezuela. The species occurs in irrigation canals, drainage ditches, small reservoirs and concrete lakes for irrigation or other purposes, swamps, ponds and sluggish streams. The snail is distributed generally throughout the endemic areas. It has been reported also from the States of Falcon, Cojedes and Monagas, where S. mansoni does not occur. HUBENDICK [1961] reported B. prona and B. schrammi from Venezuela. These species are apparently not susceptible to S. mansoni infection. He also found B. straminea, an efficient intermediate host of the parasite in Brazil, and B. obstructa, which has been infected experimentally. However, these two species are not known to be involved in the epidemiology of the parasite in Venezuela.

References

GABALDON, A.: Recent developments in the control of bilharziasis in Venezuela. WHO unpublished document, BILH/Exp. Com. 3/WP/31 (1964).

HUBENDICK, B.: Meddn. Göteborgs Musei Zool. Avdelning, Ser. B. 8: 3 (1961).

VENEZUELA, MINISTERIO DE SANIDAD Y ASISTENCIA SOCIAL: Memoria y Cuenta 1964, p. 368 (1965).

St. Lucia

St. Lucia is a small island, with an area of 593 km², situated in the Windward Group of the West Indies. Rugged hills and mountains ranging up to 915 m cover most of the island.

S. mansoni is the only schistosome infecting man in St. Lucia. Infection was first recognized on the island in 1925 at Soufriere, and for a time cases were not recognized in other parts of the island. In 1951, a rough survey in

Soufriere disclosed a prevalence rate of 50% [PANIKKAR, 1961]. The same author reported prevalence rates ranging from 2 to 69% in school-children in 14 locations in the island. MALEK [1962] conducted faecal examinations in 11 localities among persons ranging in age from 2 to 60 years and obtained positive results in 10 places. Prevalence rates varied between 17.9 and 74.2%. LEES [1965] examined 640 children varying in age from 4 to 14 years in five villages along the Cul de Sac River south of Castries and found 45.9% infected.

MALEK [1962] was unable to find *S. mansoni* in some domestic and feral animals on the island.

B. glabrata is apparently the only snail involved in the transmission of *S. mansoni* in St. Lucia. It is limited in distribution and flourishes only in certain scattered habitats. It is absent from fast-flowing streams but prevalent in quiet, sheltered areas. The snail occurs on flooded embankments, in swampy areas close to rivers, and in the headwaters of the streams where there is ample vegetation and the water movement is slow. Additional sites of infestation include ponds, drainage ditches and rice fields. MALEK [1962] noted infection rates in the intermediate hosts varying from 5.8% at the Ravine Poisson to 17.8% near Sulphur Spring, Soufriere. Opportunities for transmission would, therefore, seem to be intense in certain localities.

References

LEES, R. E. M.: W. Indian med. J. *14:* 82 (1965).
MALEK, E. A.: Report on precontrol studies of bilharziasis in St. Lucia. PAHO/WHO unpublished document (1962).
OLIVIER, L. J. and BUZO, Z. J.: Report of the WHO Bilharziasis Advisory Team visit to Saint Lucia. WHO unpublished document, MHO/PA/118.64 (1962).
PANIKKAR, M. K.: J. trop. Med. Hyg. *64:* 251 (1961).

Martinique

S. mansoni is endemic on the island. According to DESCHIENS *et al.* [1953] the average prevalence rate is 6.4% and the average morbidity is 43%.

Schistosomiasis is present in the Cantons of Fort-de-France, Basse-Pointe, Trinité, Carbet, Lamentin, Saint-Esprit and Marin. Endemicity is widespread and is governed to some extent by the nature of the terrain and climatic factors. In the north where forest predominates and the flow of the coastal rivers is favourable, the molluscan intermediate host finds suitable breeding places. In the more arid southern part of the island, the river flow is irregular and conditions are not conducive to snail infestation.

B. glabrata is the sole molluscan intermediate host. The snails abound in slow-flowing streams, ponds and marshy areas. DESCHIENS [1952] stated that they even occur in the lakes and ponds and drainage ditches in the public gardens in Fort-de-France.

References

DESCHIENS, R.: Le problème sanitaire des bilharzioses dans les territoires de l'Union française. Soc. Path. exot., Monogr. V, p. 25 (Masson, Paris 1952).
DESCHIENS, R.; LAMY, L., and MAUZÉ, J.: Bull. Soc. Path. exot. *46:* 810 (1953).

Guadeloupe

The island has a total population of 283,000 distributed over an area of 1,509 km². *S. mansoni* was first found to be present in 1909. DESCHIENS *et al.* [1953] stated that the prevalence rate, based on statistics for the years 1948 to 1951, was 7.8%. The morbidity rate was said to average 28%. Chronic colitis and dysentery are common complaints. The disease is widely distributed throughout Guadeloupe and Grande-Terre and apparently occurs also on Marie-Galante and La Desirade, since collections of *B. glabrata*, the molluscan intermediate host, have been made from the latter islands.

B. glabrata is found in slow-moving streams, ponds, covered reservoirs, drainage and irrigation canals, and in stagnant water collections. Snails are distributed in the above-mentioned islands but apparently have not been found in the Iles des Saintes.

DESCHIENS *et al.* [1953] studied the distribution of the snail and infection rates. The malacological index of the various endemic areas was as follows: Pointe-à-Pitre 30 to 90%; Basse-Terre 12 to 56%; Baie-Mahault 40%; Lamentin 20%; Sainte-Rose 40%; Abymes 80%; and Sainte-Anne 4 to 5%.

COURMES *et al.* [1964] added a considerable number of snail-infested localities in their survey. In Guadeloupe, 47 locations were searched, of which 32 were infested with *B. glabrata*. Of 1,992 specimens collected, 10% were infected with *S. mansoni*. In Grande-Terre 58 of 68 localities were found to have *B. glabrata;* the infection rate in 2,474 snails was 0.60%. In one locality on Marie-Galante, none of 17 specimens was infected.

The above-mentioned workers examined 184 school-children at Baie-Mahault and found 43, or 23.3%, infected with *S. mansoni*. At Morne-à-l'Eau on Grande-Terre, none of 42 school-children was infected.

References
DESCHIENS, R.; LAMY, L., and MAUZÉ, J.: Bull. Soc. Path. exot. *46:* 810 (1953).
COURMES, E.; AUDEBAUD, G., and FAURAN, P.: Bull. Soc. Path. exot. *57:* 1071 (1964).

Antigua

Infection was detected in 1929. Sluggish streams and ponds are found all over the island, in many cases covered with beautiful water hyacinths sheltering snail hosts. According to JONES [1932] the inhabitants of the country districts endeavour to escape from the rather brackish water which is piped to the villages, preferring to drink the fresh water of the ponds. One of the villages adjoining the main collecting stream which is the source of water to the reservoir supplying the city of St. John, the capital of the island of Antigua, was reported to have an *S. mansoni* infection rate of 60% of the inhabitants.

Dr. UTTLEY [1965], Senior Medical Officer of Antigua, advised that medical records prior to 1950 had been destroyed by fire. One case of schistosomiasis was diagnosed by laboratory examination in the general hospital in 1962 but none in 1963 and 1964. Between 1949 and 1964, 14 cases were diagnosed at public dispensaries; these diagnoses were based on clinical evidence and may have been unreliable.

According to Dr. UTTLEY, *B. glabrata* is commonly found in ponds. In the island area of 280 km², there are 180 ponds, many of which dry up in the dry season. Many others, falling into disuse are not being maintained and are now permanently dry. There are no permanent streams on the island.

References
JONES, S. B.: J. trop. med. Hyg. *35:* 129 (1932).
UTTLEY, K. H.: Personal commun. to W. H. WRIGHT (1965).

St. Martin

HOFFMAN [1930] reported *S. mansoni* at Colombier in the French (northern) part of the island. EMANUEL [1933] reported several cases of *S. mansoni* from the same region. However, no indigenous case has ever been reported from Dutch St. Martin. *B. glabrata* has been reported from French St. Martin.

References
EMANUEL, J.: Geneesk. T. Ned.-Ind. *73:* 286 (1933).
HOFFMAN, W. A.: Puerto Rico J. publ. Hlth *5:* 357 (1930).

Puerto Rico and Vieques

The island of Puerto Rico has an area of 8,897 km². The population is fairly dense, averaging 686 individuals per 2.59 km². Schistosomiasis was first discovered at Mayaguez in 1904 by GONZALEZ-MARTINEZ and has been studied by numerous workers since that time.

There is some evidence to indicate that the over-all prevalence of schistosomiasis in Puerto Rico has not declined materially in spite of the marked improvement of economic conditions on the island. It is difficult to pass final judgement on the question because of the lack of extensive surveys during the early years, and because of varying techniques.

WHITE et al. [1957], in 1953 to 1955, examined over 10,000 schoolchildren in the first 12 grades (ages 5 to 18 years), with one exception where the age group was 1 to 16 years; the schools selected for study were in various parts of the island. As the result of the single stool examination, the prevalence rate was found to be 10%, with a rate of 12.5% in males and 8.1% in females.

MALDONADO and OLIVER-GONZALEZ [1958] examined a total of 23,262 individuals in six endemic foci of schistosomiasis, including Comerio, Barranquitas, Utuado, Jayuya, Guayama and Ceiba; a large majority was under 15 years of age. The average prevalence fell from about 22% in 1953 to 11% in 1955. No definite control measures had been instituted except for limited molluscicidal activity in Guayama, and chemotherapy among infected individuals in a small focus in another area. The data indicated that the majority of cases arise between 10 and 20 years of age.

MALDONADO and OLIVER GONZALEZ [1962] conducted another survey in 1960 in the same six localities investigated in the above-mentioned study. A single stool examination was made from 6,780 individuals, 85% of whom were school-children in the 6- to 15-year age group. The average prevalence rate was 4.8%. Again infection rates were usually higher in males than in females. The authors stated that the disease has shown no tendency to decrease; a sharp drop in positive stools occurred in one area, and a sharp increase in another.

FERGUSON [1965] summarized the status of schistosomiasis in Puerto Rico. According to FERGUSON, a total of 139 surveys for S. mansoni had been made up to 1963. At that time 9,047, or 7%, of 126,244 faecal specimens were positive. He also cited surveys among school-children in control projects, based on examination of single stools from selective years. The surveys were apparently conducted between 1954 and 1958. Infection rates varied between 32% at Mariana and Daguao to less than 1% in the Lajas Valley. The above-mentioned author thought that a 15-percent rate might be estimated for the island as a whole plus those Puerto Ricans who had immigrated to the United States. However, in the endemic sectors of the island homeland, he considered that a rate of 20% reflected the current status of infection.

KAGAN *et al.* [1966] conducted a careful, statistically planned survey by means of the intradermal test to determine prevalence of infection in Puerto Rico. The subjects consisted of a randomly selected population of school-children in the fifth grade, ranging from 10 to 13 years of age. The project involved 10,824 children in 396 schools, who were tested between December 1962 and June 1963. Data were compiled on the basis of 30 major watersheds which were sub-divided for detailed analysis. The percentage of positive reactors varied considerably in various areas (urban and rural) and ranged from 36.3 to 3.4. The general over-all prevalence was 12%. Surprisingly, children in urban schools showed a higher average rate than did children in rural schools. This was attributed to the influx of rural students into urban schools. The eastern third of the island on a line from Loiza to Santa Isabel had the highest endemicity with a rate of 20%. This part of the island has more rainfall and contains the greatest number of streams. It is also the most populous side of the island. Except for the area with the towns Utuado and Jayuya, and the area with Mayaguez, the prevalence of schistosomiasis in the western third of the island is uniformly low compared with the eastern third. In the Ponce area, the endemicity was very low.

Vieques

This is a small island off the east coast of Puerto Rico. FERGUSON [1965] reported that a survey among 222 school-children in 1955 revealed that 21, or 10%, were positive for *S. mansoni*. KAGAN *et al.* [1966] skin-tested school-children in certain parts of the island and found 11.2% to be positive.

B. glabrata is the sole intermediate host of *S. mansoni* in Puerto Rico and Vieques. The snail is widely distributed, occurring in some rivers and in many low-gradient small streams which in many places are partially clogged with vegetation. It is also found in disjunct marginal pools, artificial lakes, irrigation canals, ponds, rainwater accumulations, roadside ditches, marshes, swamps and borrow pits. In some parts of the island, snail infestation is seasonal but in protected upland alluvial plains and in limited paralotic sites such as pasture land and small creek tributaries, *B. glabrata* is permanently established. In the high-gradient streams, pockets of infestation may occur but are usually flushed out during the rainy season [HARRY and CUMBIE, 1956].

RICHARDS [1963] obtained shedding of cercariae of *S. mansoni* following experimental infection of *B. peregrina* and *B. heliophila* but these species are not thought to be involved in the transmission of *S. mansoni* in Puerto Rico.

References

FERGUSON, F. F.: Publ. Hlth Rep., Wash. *80:* 339 (1965).

GONZALEZ-MARTINEZ, I.: Memoria leída en la Asamblea General de la Associación Médica de Puerto Rico, 3 de Abril 1904. Tip Boletin, p. 32 (1904).

HARRY, H. W. and CUMBIE, B. G.: Amer. J. trop. Med. Hyg. *5:* 742 (1956).

KAGAN, I. G.; NEGRON, H.; ARNOLD, J. C., and FERGUSON, F. F.: A skin test survey for the prevalence of schistosomiasis in Puerto Rico. Washington Public Health Service Publication No. 1525 (1966).

MALDONADO, J. F. and OLIVER-GONZALEZ, J.: Amer. J. trop. Med. Hyg. *7:* 386 (1958).

MALDONADO, J. F. and OLIVER-GONZALEZ, J.: Bol. Asoc. Méd., Puerto Rico *54:* 133 (1962).

RICHARDS, C. S.: Amer. J. trop. Med. Hyg. *12:* 26 (1963).

WHITE, P. C., jr.; PIMENTEL, D., and GARCIA, F. C.: Amer. J. trop. Med. Hyg. *6:* 715 (1957).

Dominican Republic

The first autochthonous cases of schistosomiasis in the Dominican Republic were discovered in the laboratory of the San Antonio Hospital in San Pedro de Macoris by Dr. PONCE PINEDO. Additional cases were observed during the next few months and in 1943–1944 PONCE PINEDO summarized the findings in his doctoral thesis before the Faculty of Medicine of the University of Santo Domingo. All of the observed cases came from the vicinity of Hato Mayor, a town some 35 km from San Pedro de Macoris. In 1945, READ summarized the situation and noted that a total of 11 cases had been recognized. PONCE PINEDO published his findings in 1945 and 1947.

OLIVIER *et al.* [1952] investigated the focus at Hato Mayor. Faecal examinations of 243 children between the ages of 5 and 15 years living in Hato Mayor revealed 52 infections with *S. mansoni*. The population of the town at that time was 3,911 and it was estimated that 28%, or about 1,100, of these were children within the age group surveyed. It was believed that about 220 children in this age group were infected.

MARTINEZ LARRÉ and RAVELO DE LA FUENTE reported a new focus of infection at Las Palmillas, 4 km from Hato Mayor, which they regarded as an extension of the focus at Hato Mayor.

B. glabrata was collected by OLIVIER *et al.* in various locations around Hato Mayor, in the arroyo Las Guamas, the arroyo Pana Pana, the Rio Magua and the arroyo Jagua. Many of the snails harboured cercariae which developed into *S. mansoni* in exposed mice.

ETGES [1969] has reported other foci of *B. glabrata* at Miches, Nisibón, Cotui and Nagua.

References

ETGES, F.J.: The present status of bilharziasis in the Dominican Republic. Conference of Parasitic Diseases, US-Japan Cooperative Medical Science Program, Washington, D.C., August 4–6 (1969).

MARTINEZ LARRÉ, M. and RAVELO DE LA FUENTE, J.J.: Rev. méd. domin. *8:* 44 (1953).

OLIVIER, L.; VAUGHN, C. M., and HENDRICKS, J.R.: Amer. J. trop. Med. Hyg. *1:* 680 (1952).

PONCE PINEDO, A. M.: in Congress Medico Dominicano del Centenario, 1944, p. 382 (1945).

PONCE PINEDO, A. M.: Puerto Rico J. publ. Hlth trop. Med. *22:* 308 (1947).

READ, H.: Bol. Asoc. méd. P. Rico *37:* 105 (1945).

The Schistosome-Intermediate Host Complex

Africa

Many valuable records now exist of species and sub-species of African Planorbidae which are susceptible and refractory to *S. mansoni* and *S. haematobium*. Many of these data have been derived from experimental infections of snails in the laboratory, but information on the relative susceptibilities of the molluscan intermediate hosts to these schistosomes and their significance in the transmission picture is inconclusive, since much of the above-mentioned work was not carried out under standardized conditions, and successful infection in the laboratory does not necessarily correspond to epidemiological fact. Various factors exert an influence upon the infection of snails by miracidia including: the age and susceptibility of the snails and virulence of miracidia; the dispersion of snails and miracidia; the length of contact time; the number of miracidia per snail; the temperature of exposure and the temperature at which snails are maintained during the pre-patent period. Each or all of these factors may be responsible for unsuccessful exposure and greater care should be exercised in experimental work of this kind, and in the critical appraisal of results made, prior to reporting them in the literature.

S. mansoni

The present distribution of *S. mansoni* covers Egypt, Sudan and most of Africa south of the Sahara (including Madagascar), and all of the intermediate hosts of this parasite in Africa belong to the planorbid genus *Biomphalaria*. There seems little reason to doubt the extensive intermediate-host capacity of

Biomphalaria and while differences in the degree of susceptibility have been noted, there appears to be a general compatibility of various strains of *S. mansoni* and *Biomphalaria*.

Though many problems continue to be presented by the taxonomic relationships of medically important snails, a framework for the basic identification of material has been provided by the introduction of the species-group concept into the taxonomy of the African forms, by MANDAHL-BARTH [1957a, b]. Four main groups are recognized in this classification of *Biomphalaria*:

(1) *pfeifferi* group, which comprises several forms and is represented in nearly all parts of Africa south of the Sahara;

(2) *choanomphala* group, which comprises a few forms which are restricted to certain of the Great Lakes;

(3) *alexandrina* group, which comprises a few forms which have a curiously isolated and restricted distribution in North Africa, but includes *B. angulosa* (Mandahl-Barth), which is widespread in distribution in South-East Africa and is closely related in its soft parts to *B. alexandrina alexandrina* (Ehrenberg);

(4) *sudanica* group, which comprises a West African and an East African species, each with two sub-species.

As the result of examining many new collections of material MANDAHL-BARTH [1960] concluded that it seems wiser not to divide *B. pfeifferi pfeifferi* (Krauss) into sub-species, a solution which is acceptable from the medical point of view, especially as all forms act as intermediate hosts of *S. mansoni*. It seems most likely that the areas around Lakes Kivu and Tanganyika are the centres from which forms of *B. pfeifferi* have spread.

The local role of *Biomphalaria* as an intermediate host of *S. mansoni* is usually accepted on general epidemiological evidence or after observing the shedding of schistosome cercariae and proving their identity by infection of laboratory animals, and this capacity has been demonstrated in some areas by completion of the life cycle in the laboratory.

Laboratory demonstration of the intermediate-host capacity of *B. alexandrina alexandrina* (Ehrenberg) in Egypt, and of *B. alexandrina* and *B. pfeifferi* in Khartoum in the Sudan was made by ARCHIBALD [1933], while MALEK [1950] described the susceptibility of *B. boissyi* (now designated *alexandrina*, MANDAHL-BARTH, 1957a), to infection with certain strains of *S. mansoni*. GAUD [1955] tabulated the localities of the infected *Biomphalaria* for former French administrative areas in Africa and detailed records for the former Belgian Congo and Ruanda Urundi were given by GILLET and WOLFS [1954].

These authors listed various sub-species of *B.pfeifferi*, the differentiation of which, as stated above, has now been discontinued. MALEK [1958] described the distribution of intermediate hosts of schistosomiasis in relation to hydrography with special reference to the Nile Basin and Sudan and including the former Belgian Congo, Kenya, Uganda, Ethiopia and former French Equatorial Africa.

B.pfeifferi has been successfully infected in the laboratory in the Republic of South Africa, Mozambique, Rhodesia, Liberia, Sierra Leone, Ghana, Zaire, Uganda, Kenya, Tanzania and Sudan.

In East Africa, CRIDLAND [1955] found that all the species of *Biomphalaria* from Uganda and the adjacent territories were susceptible in varying degrees to *S.mansoni* of local origin. PITCHFORD [1958] in a survey of Swaziland, recorded *B. pfeifferi* as widespread in the lowveld, but diminishing or disappearing towards the middleveld. PITCHFORD and VISSER [1962] found naturally infected *B. pfeifferi* in irrigation canals in the Transvaal and demonstrated that well-defined seasonal transmission patterns of *S.mansoni* occur there.

McCLELLAND [1956] isolated *S.mansoni* in mice from naturally infected *B.sudanica* (Martens), collected at Kisumu, Kenya, and TEESDALE [1962] found *B.pfeifferi* naturally infected with *S.mansoni* at Nairobi and Kitui in Kenya. WEBBE [1962a, 1965] found *B.sudanica tanganyicensis* (Smith), and *B.pfeifferi* naturally infected with *S.mansoni*, in water courses in the western and lake regions of Tanzania, and has demonstrated well-defined seasonal transmission patterns there. *B.pfeifferi* is also widespread in distribution in the northern region of Tanzania and spreading eastward, but disappearing in the coastal plains of Tanzania and Kenya, and STURROCK [1965a] has discussed the apparent absence of *Biomphalaria* and *S.mansoni* at certain latitudes in both East and West Africa in relation to temperature. *B.camerunensis camerunensis* (Boettger) and *B.camerunensis manzadica* (Mandahl-Barth) are the West African representatives of the *sudanica* group, where they are known only from the type localities in Cameroon and lower Zaire, respectively. STURROCK [1965b] infected *B.angulosa* with a Mwanza strain of *S.mansoni*, and found that the course of infection was similar to that found in other *Biomphalaria* spp. which transmit *S.mansoni*. According to LE ROUX these species, together with *B.pfeifferi*, are also intermediate hosts of *S.mansoni* in Rhodesia, while *B.angulosa* has also been seen infected with schistosome cercariae in Malawi.

COURTOIS and WANSON [1949] and SCHWETZ [1949] reported *B. choanomphala* (Martens) to be naturally infected with *S.mansoni* on the Congo shore of Lake Albert, but NELSON [1958] quoted MANDAHL-BARTH as believing the snails in question to be *B. stanleyi* (Smith), and this view was also held by BEQUAERT [quoted by FAIN, 1953, who also found naturally infected snails in Lake Albert]. WEBBE [1962a] and McCLELLAND and JORDAN [1962] found *B. choanomphala*, naturally infected with *S. mansoni*, at Mwanza and Bukoba, respectively, in Lake Victoria.

LE ROUX [1961] stated that all African *Biomphalaria* are susceptible to *S. mansoni*, and supports this by reporting the successful infection of *Biomphalaria* spp. from Addis Ababa with a Tanzania strain of the parasite. However, WRIGHT [1962] reported having failed to infect *B. sudanica* from Sudan with a strain of *S. mansoni* from Komatipoort in the Transvaal, but successfully infected *B. pfeifferi* from Gambia and *B. glabrata* (Say) from Brazil, with the same strain of parasite. COWPER [1947] found that *B. alexandrina* from Egypt was susceptible to a Uganda strain of *S. mansoni* and FILES and CRAM [1949], found that *B. pfeifferi* from Liberia was susceptible to an Egyptian strain, while DE MEILLON [1956], reported that *Biomphalaria* from Botswana (Bechuanaland) was susceptible to the Transvaal strain of *S. mansoni*.

There is no doubt that strains of *S. mansoni* exist, but supporting evidence other than snail infection experiments has been lacking. SAOUD [1965a], however, carried out comparative studies on the characteristics of some geographical strains of *S. mansoni* from Egypt, Tanzania and Puerto Rico in mice and hamsters. He showed from the collective evidence of variation in the morphological and biological characters of different strains that *S. mansoni* is not a uniform species, but that distinct infra-specific and inter-strain variations do occur. SAOUD [1965b] reported the susceptibility of various snail intermediate hosts of *S. mansoni* to different strains of the parasite. From the epidemiological point of view it is of great interest to note that the Neotropical *B. glabrata* from Puerto Rico was more highly susceptible to its local strain of *S. mansoni* (96%), when compared with *B. alexandrina alexandrina* and *B. sudanica tanganyicensis*, exposed to the Egyptian and Mwanza (Tanzania) strains, respectively (51.6 and 61.5%). It was also observed that those *B. glabrata* (Puerto Rico) which became positive were shedding greater numbers of cercariae than those which were shed by the African *Biomphalaria* spp., when infected with their local strains of the parasite, and it is considered that this points to the closer compatibility between the parasite and its intermediate host in the Western Hemisphere than in Africa. It was found that *B. alexandrina alexandrina*, was partially refractory to infection with all the strains of *S. mansoni* other than the Egyptian strain. COWPER [1948] failed to infect *B. alexandrina alexandrina* with *S. mansoni* from Liberia.

Biomphalaria also transmit the related schistosomes of the *mansoni* group, including *S. rhodaini* (Brumpt). There appears to be only one record of *S. rhodaini* from man [D'HAENENS and SANTELE, 1955]. SCHWETZ *et al.* [1951] exposed several species of planorbid snails to *S. rhodaini* miracidia and FAIN *et al.* [1953], BERRIE and GOODMAN [1962] and FRIPP [1964] have reported on the laboratory maintenance of *S. rhodaini*. Both *B. sudanica* [SCHWETZ, 1953; BERRIE and GOODMAN, 1962] and *B. pfeifferi* [SCHWETZ *et al.*, 1951] have been shown to be hosts of *S. rhodaini*, while FRIPP [1964] has reported infection rates obtained with *B. sudanica tanganyicensis*.

It is considered that *S. mansoni* var. *rodentorum* is nothing more than *S. mansoni* in rodents [TEESDALE and NELSON, 1958] and, more recently, PITCHFORD and VISSER [1960] have produced further evidence to support this, and have shown that the shape of the eggs depends upon the host species and its diet and that eggs identical with those described by SCHWETZ [1953] as *S. mansoni* var. *rodentorum*, are commonly seen in rodents infected with *S. mansoni*.

McCULLOUGH [1965] recorded *B. sudanica* from Ghana and found it susceptible to the West African strain of *S. mansoni*.

S. haematobium

As in *Biomphalaria*, MANDAHL-BARTH [1957b] has introduced the species group system into the genus *Bulinus* and thereby replaced the earlier sub-genera with divisions which are biologically more realistic. There are four main groups of importance because of their differing host-parasite relationships. The *africanus* group is confined to the Ethiopian zoogeographical region (south of the Sahara) and in that area its members are important hosts for schistosomes with terminal-spined eggs parasitic in man and domestic animals; the *tropicus* group has a similar distribution but is largely absent in West Africa and its species are not known to be hosts for schistosomes. The *truncatus* group is present throughout the Middle East and Mediterranean region of Africa where its species are the hosts of human and cattle schistosomiasis, and its distribution extends into West Africa as far south as Angola, also into the Great Lakes region of East Africa. The *forskalii* group has an almost pan-African distribution, and is also present in Mauritius and Madagascar, but with only two of its species confirmed hosts for urinary schistosomiasis.

Specific identifications within these groups are not always easy, and to variation in morphological characters between populations of *B. truncatus truncatus* (Audouin), can now be added differences in the chromatographical pattern of fluorescent substances in the body-surface mucous, reported by WRIGHT [1959].

Various reports have appeared in the literature concerning apparent incompatibility between local races of *Bulinus* spp. and strains of *S.haematobium* [LE ROUX, 1954a; CRIDLAND, 1955]. MCCULLOUGH [1957], working in Ghana, found that *S.haematobium* from an endemic area where *B.(Ph.) globosus globosus* (Morelet) (*africanus* group) was the intermediate host, did not develop in *B.truncatus rohlfsi* (Clessin), and that the reverse was also true. Repeated attempts in the laboratory to infect members of the *africanus* group with miracidia of parasites normally using snails of the *truncatus* group have failed and *truncatus* species have always proved refractory to parasites normally developing in the *africanus* group. LE ROUX [1958] suggested that these are separate species of parasites, the *truncatus* born from being known as *S.haematobium*, and that developing in the *africanus* group as *S.capense* [HARLEY, 1864]. NELSON *et al.* [1962] considered that there are insufficient grounds for resurrecting *S.capense* to distinguish the South African from the Egyptian strain of *S.haematobium*. WRIGHT [1962], however, points out that although proof is not yet available, it seems likely that this dichotomy is the exact parallel of that between the two common African schistosomes of cattle, *S.mattheei* developing in snails of the *africanus* complex and *S.bovis* which used the *truncatus* group. This author also commented on the difficulties of obtaining consistent results in the infection of *Bulinus* spp., with *S.haematobium*, which are well known and have been reviewed by MOORE *et al.* [1953]. This fact coupled with the recent recognition of the separate identities of *S.haematobium* and *S.capense* renders many of the early studies on intermediate host-parasite relationships unreliable as sources of information on strain differences in the parasite.

Apart from the technical difficulties involved in the routine infection of *Bulinus* spp. with *S.haematobium* and *S.capense*, it has recently become apparent that interpretation of the results must be based on more than percentages of surviving snails shedding cercariae. WRIGHT [1963a] tested the susceptibility of *B.truncatus rohlfsi* from Angola to *S.haematobium* from Khartoum and Cairo, and showed that although the percentages of Angolan snails shedding cercariae were similar to the percentages obtained with Khartoum and Cairo snails, the Angolan species shed fewer cercariae per snail and frequently lost the infection after some days.

WRIGHT [1962] recorded the results of experimental infections to show the susceptibility of different *Bulinus* snails to *S.haematobium* strains of different origins, and considers that the evidence for the existence of local strains of *S. haematobium* and *S. capense* is quite overwhelming, and that apparently many of these strains have an almost parochial distribution.

B. truncatus is the demonstrated intermediate host of *S. haematobium* in certain localities of Egypt, North Africa and the nilotic Sudan. In the steppe region of Sudan the assumed intermediate hosts fall within the *truncatus* group, and the snails implicated in Mauritania are quoted by DESCHIENS [1951] as also belonging to this group. Their intermediate host role for *S. bovis* has been demonstrated in Tunisia by ANDERSEN and GOBERT [1934], and in Morocco by BLANC and DESPORTES [1936].

LE ROUX [1954b] found experimentally that *B. coulboisi* (Bourguignat) (*truncatus* group), from Lake Tanganyika, was susceptible to an Egyptian strain of *S. haematobium*. CRIDLAND [1955], however, failed to infect *B. truncatus trigonus* (Martens) and *B. transversalis* (Martens), also *truncatus* group, with local strains of *S. haematobium*.

South of the Sahara and at corresponding latitudes in the east most of the acknowledged intermediate hosts of *S. haematobium* are contained in the *africanus* group. *B. (Ph.) globosus* is a commonly accepted transmitter of urinary schistosomiasis, has a wide distribution in all Africa south of the Sahara and is found in a variety of habitats. It shows a wide range of variability and some of the variations may probably be those of true geographical races. This species has frequently been placed in synonomy with *B. (Ph.) africanus africanus* (Krauss), or *B. (Ph.) africanus ovoideus* (Bourguignat), which are species of southern and eastern Africa. It is extremely difficult by shell characters alone to distinguish *B. (Ph.) africanus* from *B. (Ph.) globosus* but the differences in structure of the copulatory organ seems to be a fairly reliable determining character. In Somalia and southern Ethiopia, *B. (Ph.) abyssinicus* (Martens) is present and was shown to be an intermediate host. The role of *B. (Ph.) globosus* as an intermediate host of *S. haematobium* has been demonstrated in Sierra Leone by GORDON *et al.* [1934], in Portuguese Guinea by PINTO [1955], in Ghana by EDWARDS and McCULLOUGH [1954], in East and West Congo by GILLET and WOLFS [1954] and in Uganda by CRIDLAND [1955]. The closely-related form *B. (Ph.) ugandae* (Mandahl-Barth) occurs in similar habitats around Lake Victoria, but is not apparently capable of transmitting *S. haematobium* [CRIDLAND, 1955; MANDAHL-BARTH, 1962], but BERRIE [1964] confirmed this species as an intermediate host of a bovine schistosome. The intermediate host role of *B. (Ph.) africanus* was first demonstrated in South Africa by BECKER [1916], but LE ROUX considers that the parasite concerned was *S. mattheei*. STURROCK [1965a] recorded that *B. (Ph.) africanus africanus*, the form from South Africa which transmits *S. haematobium* there, is present in the Southern Highlands area of Tanzania, in rivers, swamps and temporary water courses, and he found that it is capable of transmitting East African strains of *S. haematobium*, but no naturally infected specimens have yet been found. *B. (Ph.) africanus ovoideus* occurs both in the coastal plain and inland in East Africa, usually in temporary streams, swamps and dams, and it has been shown by TEESDALE and NELSON [1958] to transmit *S. haematobium* and *S. bovis* in Kenya and both these schistosome species in the Lake Region of Tanzania, where the evidence produced by KINOTI [1964a] suggests that it is entirely responsible for the transmission of *S. bovis*. KINOTI [1964b] has also reported on the susceptibility of *B. (Ph.) globosus* and *B. (Ph.) africanus ovoideus* to a Tanzanian strain of *S. bovis* and a South African strain of *S. mattheei*. Both schistosomes were found to develop well in *B. (Ph.) africanus ovoideus*, but *B. (Ph.) globosus* was only slightly susceptible to either. *S. bovis* developed also in *B. (Ph.) africanus africanus* and in *B. (B.) forskalii* (Ehrenberg), but *S. mattheei* failed to develop in *B. (Ph.) nasutus productus* (Mandahl-Barth), as did *S. bovis* in a form intermediate between *B. (B.) tropicus tropicus* (Krauss) and *B. (B.) coulboisi* (Bourguignat) (*truncatus* group), or in *B. (B.) tropicus alluaudi* (Dautzenberg).

TEESDALE and NELSON [1958], working in Kenya, recorded that in spite of the wide distribution of cercariae of *S. bovis* in water used by local people the parasite had not been seen in man. Further south, *S. bovis* is replaced by *S. mattheei*, in both domestic and wild animals, and according to PITCHFORD [1959], in South Africa man is obviously more susceptible to this parasite than to *S. bovis*. This author has not seen any areas, however, where the whole human population is infected with *S. mattheei*, as recorded by FISHER [1934], in the *S. intercalatum* area at Yakusu in Zaire, which is transmitted by *B. (Ph.) africanus* (? *globosus*). Further, *S. mattheei* has, on almost all occasions, been found in association with either *S. mansoni* or *S. haematobium*, suggesting that *S. mattheei* is not well adapted to man whereas *S. intercalatum* exists as pure infections. CRIDLAND [1955] demonstrated the host role of the East African species *B. (Ph.) nasutus nasutus* (Martens), which is found in swampy pools and temporary water courses throughout East Africa and which is replaced around Lake Victoria by *B. (Ph.) nasutus productus*. To the south of Mwanza in the Lake Region of Tanzania, it is generally confined to small temporary pools and seepages and is the principal intermediate host of *S. haematobium*, showing a well-defined transmission pattern [WEBBE, 1962b]. It does not apparently transmit *S. bovis* in this area [WEBBE, 1962b; KINOTI, 1964a]. Snails of the *tropicus* group have a similar distribution to those of the *africanus* group, but are generally absent in West Africa, while most of the species which comprise this group are not known to be hosts of schistosomes. The claim of PORTER [1938], regarding *B. tropicus* in South Africa, could never be substantiated. An interesting position, however, exists in Gambia where SMITHERS [1956] has found multiple intermediate hosts of *S. haematobium. B. (B.) guernei* of the *tropicus* group, and *B. (Ph.) jousseaumei* (Dautzenberg), were shown to act as natural hosts while *B. (B.) senegalensis* (Muller) was found naturally infected with *S. haematobium*, and *S. bovis* and laboratory bred *B. (B.) forskalii* were found to be receptive to both *S. haematobium* and *S. bovis; B. (B.) forskalii* and *B. (Ph.) globosus* were suspected on epidemiological grounds of being natural hosts of *S. haematobium*. In Guinea a little further south, GILLET [1956a] showed that *B. (Ph.) globosus* is the intermediate host of *S. haematobium*, and *B. (Ph.) jousseaumei* is a suspected host only.

Snails of the *forskalii* group are extremely prevalent in West Africa in small water bodies, and have been described as the dominant species in certain parts of Nigeria, Liberia, Senegal and Gambia. They are also reported to be common in other regions including the Lira district of Uganda, Kenya, Tanzania and western Botswana. The members of the group which are definitely known to act as hosts for urinary schistosomiasis are *B. (B.) cernicus* (Morelet) in Mauritius and *B. (B.) senegalensis* in West Africa. The parasites carried by these two hosts have not been adequately compared with other strains for a proper assessment of their relationships to be made. COWPER [1953] attempted to infect *B. (B.) truncatus* from Egypt with the Mauritian strain, but without success. *B. (B.) senegalensis* from Gambia is readily susceptible to the Cairo strain of *S. haematobium* and this species of snail is also slightly susceptible to *S. capense* from Kenya. WRIGHT [1956] believes the snails termed *B. (B.) forskalii* and found susceptible to *S. haematobium* in Gambia, to be *B. (B.) senegalensis* or possibly *B. (B.) ludovicianus* (Mittre), although *B. (B.) forskalii* also occurs there.

Snails of the *forskalii* group have been reported as harbouring mammalian-type schistosome cercariae in various other parts of Africa: in Nigeria near Kaduna; in the former French Sudan by GILLET [1956b] and KERVRAN [1947]; in the former French Cameroons by GAUD [1955]; in Egypt by EL GINDY [1955] and AYAD [1956]; in Mozambique by AZEVEDO *et al.* [1954]; and in Kenya by MCCLELLAND [1955], where TEESDALE [1962] also considered that it may act as a host for *S. haematobium* but is of little importance.

Snails of this group were found to be susceptible to experimental infection with *S. haematobium* to a small degree in Egypt, and to a higher degree in the Transvaal, South Africa [DAWOOD and GISMANN, 1956; KUNTZ, 1955]. The number of cercariae shed is generally described as small, and this is attributed to the small size of the snails. Failure to infect snails of this group upon exposure to *S. haematobium* miracidia has been recorded for various regions including Egypt and the former Belgian Congo, for *B. (B.) scalaris* (Dunker) and *B. (B.) forskalii* in Uganda by CRIDLAND [1955], and for *B. (B.) forskalii* in Ghana by McCULLOUGH [1955] and Rhodesia by ALVES [1956].

STURROCK [1965a] records that *B. (B.) reticulatus* (Mandahl-Barth) occurs sporadically in Tanzania, as it does in Kenya and Rhodesia, and it was shown by WRIGHT [1963b] to transmit *S. haematobium* in Southern Yemen. MANDAHL-BARTH [1957b] commented, however, that this species (*forskalii* group), could just as well be referred to the *truncatus* group.

Conclusions

Difficulties appear to arise from the many intermediate forms of medically important snails which occur and from insufficient knowledge of ecophenotypical variation, indicating that more laboratory experiments must be carried out to determine which characteristics are due to genetic factors and which are caused by environmental factors of the habitat. It is essential, therefore, that snail collecting activities should be continued together with mapping of the distribution of various species, and further clarification may depend upon the use of techniques such as chromosome studies and chromatography of blood and mucous protein.

It must be emphasized that accurate information on the relative susceptibilities of molluscan intermediate hosts to the principal human schistosomes can only be obtained if such work is carried out under carefully standardized laboratory conditions, while greater efforts should be made to link such work with epidemiological fact.

It is evident that many early studies on host-parasite relationships are unreliable as sources of information of strain differences in the parasites, and it now appears that interpretation of results should be based on more than percentages of surviving snails shedding cercariae.

References

ALVES, W.: A note on 'immunity'. WHO unpublished document, WHO/Bilh. Conf./32 (1956).

ANDERSON, C. and GOBERT, E.: Bull. Soc. Path. exot. *27:* 850 (1934).

ARCHIBALD, R. G.: J. trop. med. Hyg. *36:* 345 (1933).

AYAD, N.: Bull. Wld Hlth Org. *14:* 1 (1956).

AZEVEDO, J. FRAGA DE; CAMBOURNAC, F., and PINTO, A. R.: in Ve Congrès internationaux de Médecine tropicale et du Paludisme. Communications, vol. 2, p. 311 (1954).

BECKER, J. G.: Med. J. S. Afr. *11:* 156 (1916).

BERRIE, A.D.: Ann. trop. Med. Parasit. *58:* 457 (1964).

BERRIE, A.D. and GOODMAN, J.D.: Ann. trop. Med. Parasit. *56:* 297 (1962).

BLANC, G. and DESPORTES, C.: C.R. Soc. Biol., Paris *123:* 766 (1936).

COURTOIS, G. and WANSON, M.: Ann. Soc. belge Méd. trop. *29:* 447 (1949).

COWPER, S.G.: Ann. trop. Med. Parasit. *41:* 173 (1947).

COWPER, S.G.: Trans. roy. Soc. trop. Med. Hyg. *47:* 564 (1953).

CRIDLAND, C.C.: J. trop. med. Hyg. *58:* 1 (1955).

DAWOOD, M.M. and GISMANN, A.: in World Atlas of Epidemic Diseases (Falk-Verlag, Hamburg 1956).

DESCHIENS, R.: Bull. Soc. Path. exot. *44:* 631 (1951).

D'HAENENS, G. and SANTELE, A.: Ann. Soc. belge Méd. trop. *35:* 497 (1955).

EDWARDS, E.E. and McCULLOUGH, F.S.: Ann. trop. Med. Parasit. *48:* 164 (1954).

EL GINDY, M.S.: J. Egypt. med. Ass. *38:* 166 (1955).

FAIN, A.: Mém. Inst. colon. belge Sci. nat. 22, fasc. 5 (1953).

FAIN, A.; THIENPONT, D.; HERIN, V., and DERAMÉE, O.: Ann. Soc. belge Méd. trop. *33:* 423 (1953).

FILES, V.S. and CRAM, E.B.: J. Parasit. *35:* 555 (1949).

FISHER, A.C.: Trans. roy. Soc. trop. Med. Hyg. *28:* 277 (1934).

FRIPP, P.J.: Ann. trop. Med. Parasit. *58:* 224 (1964).

GAUD, J.: Bull. Wld Hlth Org. *13:* 209 (1955).

GILLET, J.: Bilharziasis in Portuguese Guinea. WHO unpublished document, WHO/Bil. Conf./44 (1956a).

GILLET, J.: Bilharziasis in French West Africa. WHO unpublished document, WHO/Bil. Cong./41 (1956b).

GILLET, J. and WOLFS, J.: Bull. Wld Hlth Org. *10:* 315 (1954).

GORDON, R.M.; DAVEY, T.H., and PEASTON, H.: Ann. trop. Med. Parasit. *28:* 323 (1934).

HARLEY, J.: Med.-chir. Trans. *47:* 55 (1864).

KERVRAN, P.: Bull. Soc. Path. exot. *40:* 349 (1947).

KIKUTH, W. and GÖNNERT, R.: Ann. trop. Med. Parasit. *42:* 256 (1948).

KINOTI, G.: Bull. Wld Hlth Org. *31:* 815 (1964a).

KINOTI, G.: Ann. trop. Med. Parasit. *58:* 270 (1964b).

KUNTZ, R.E.: Amer. J. trop. Med.Hyg. *4:* 383 (1955).

LE ROUX, P.L.: J. Helminth. *11:* 57 (1933).

LE ROUX, P.L.: Trans. roy. Soc. trop. Med. Hyg. *48:* 5 (1954a).

LE ROUX, P.L.: Trans. roy. Soc. trop. Med. Hyg. *48:* 4 (1954b).

LE ROUX, P.L.: Trans. roy. Soc. trop. Med. Hyg. *52:* 12 (1958).

LE ROUX, P.L.: J. Helminth. (R.T. LEIPER supplement), p. 117 (1961).

MALEK, E.T.A.: Amer. J. trop. Med. *30:* 887 (1950).

MALEK, E.T.A.: Bull. Wld Hlth Org. *18:* 691 (1958).

MANDAHL-BARTH, G.: Bull. Wld Hlth Org. *16:* 1103 (1957a).

MANDAHL-BARTH, G.: Bull. Wld Hlth Org. *17:* 1 (1957b).

MANDAHL-BARTH, G.: Intermediate hosts of Schistosoma, African *Biomphalaria* and *Bulinus.* Wld Hlth Org. Monogr. Ser. No. 37 (1958).

MANDAHL-BARTH, G.: Bull. Wld Hlth Org. *22:* 565 (1960).

MANDAHL-BARTH, G.: Bull. Wld Hlth Org. *27:* 135 (1962).

McCLELLAND, W.F.J.: Trans. roy. Soc. trop. Med. Hyg. *49:* 295 (1955).

McClelland, W. F. J.: J. trop. med. Hyg. *59:* 227 (1956).
McClelland, W. F. J. and Jordan, P.: Ann. trop. Med. Parasit. *56:* 396 (1962).
McCullough, F. S.: Nature, Lond. *176:* 981 (1955).
McCullough, F. S.: W. afr. med. J. *6:* 98 (1957).
McCullough, F. S.: Ann. trop. Med. Parasit. *59:* 312 (1965).
Meillon, B. de: Med. Klin. *51:* 670 (1956).
Moore, D. V.; Thillet, C. J.; Carney, D. M., and Meleney, H. E.: J. Parasit. *39:* 215 (1953).
Nelson, G. S.: E. afr. med. J. *35:* 335 (1958).
Nelson, G. S.; Teesdale, C., and Highton, R. B.: in Bilharziasis. Ciba Foundation Symposium, p. 127 (Churchill, London 1962).
Pinto, A. R.: An. Inst. Med. trop., Lisboa *12:* 653 (1955).
Pitchford, R. J.: Bull. Wld Hlth Org. *18:* 735 (1958).
Pitchford, R. J.: Trans. roy. Soc. trop. Med. Hyg. *53:* 285 (1959).
Pitchford, R. J. and Visser, P. S.: Ann. trop. Med. Parasit. *54:* 247 (1960).
Pitchford, R. J. and Visser, P. S.: Trans. roy. Soc. trop. Med. Hyg. *56:* 294 (1962).
Porter, A.: Publ. S. afr. Inst. Med. Res. *842:* 492 (1938).
Saoud, M. F. A.: J. Helminth. *39:* 101 (1965a).
Saoud, M. F. A.: J. Helminth. *39:* 363 (1965b).
Schwetz, J.: Ann. Soc. belge Méd. trop. *29:* 491 (1949).
Schwetz, J.: Ann. trop. Med. Parasit. *47:* 183 (1953).
Schwetz, J.; Baumann, H., and Fort, M.: Ann. Parasit. hum. comp. *26:* 407 (1951).
Sturrock, R. F.: Bull. Wld Hlth Org. *32:* 225 (1965a).
Sturrock, R. F.: Ann. trop. Med. Parasit. *59:* 1 (1965b).
Teesdale, C.: Bull. Wld Hlth Org. *27:* 759 (1962).
Teesdale, C. and Nelson, G. S.: E. afr. med. J. *35:* 433 (1958).
Webbe, G.: in Bilharziasis. Ciba Foundation Symposium, p. 7 (Churchill, London 1962a).
Webbe, G.: Bull. Wld Hlth Org. *27:* 59 (1962b).
Webbe, G.: Bull. Wld Hlth Org. *33:* 155 (1965).
Wright, C. A.: Nature, Lond. (Correspondence) *177:* 33 (1956).
Wright, C. A.: J. Linn. Soc. (Zool.) *44:* 222 (1959).
Wright, C. A.: in Bilharziasis. Ciba Foundation Symposium, p. 103 (Churchill, London 1962).
Wright, C. A.: Bull. brit. Mus. (nat. Hist.) Zool. *10:* 449 (1963a).
Wright, C. A.: Trans. roy. Soc. trop. Med. Hyg. *57:* 142 (1963b).

South-West Asia

The schistosome-intermediate host complex in this region has not been extensively investigated. *B. (B.) truncatus truncatus* is the main host of *S. haematobium*. When this species from Israel was exposed to strains of the parasite from Morocco and Yemen, no infections were obtained [Witenberg and Saliternik, 1957]. The same authors found that only 4% of snails exposed to an Iraqui strain became infected. Wright [1963a] found that two Aden strains of the parasite would not experimentally infect *B. (B.) truncatus*.

WRIGHT [1963b] believed that the highland form of this snail should be regarded as a separate species, which he has named *B. (B.) sericinus*. MAN-DAHL-BARTH [1965] apparently preferred to treat it as a variety of *B. (B.) truncatus*. WAJDI [1964] reported that *S. haematobium* from Aden developed in *B. (B.) beccari* and *B. (B.) reticulatus* but not in *B. (B.) truncatus*. Partial development occurred in *B. (B.) forskalii* but no cercariae were shed. WITEN-BERG and SALITERNIK [1957] found that a strain of *S. mansoni* from Yemen developed in about 40% of *B. glabrata* but in only 17% of a local strain of *B. alexandrina*.

References

MANDAHL-BARTH, G.: Bull. Wld Hlth Org. *33:* 33 (1965).
WAJDI, N.: J. Helminth. *38:* 383 (1964).
WITENBERG, G. and SALITERNIK, Z.: Bull. Res. Counc. Israel B *6:* 107 (1957).
WRIGHT, C. A.: Bull. brit. Mus. (nat. Hist.) Zool. *10:* 257 (1963a).
WRIGHT, C. A.: Trans. roy. Soc. trop. Med. Hyg. *57:* 142 (1963b).

The Orient

S. japonicum has been reported from China (Mainland), China (Taiwan), Japan, the Philippines, Celebes, Laos, Cambodia and Thailand. Its intermediate host, the oncomelanian snail, has been known only in China (Mainland), China (Taiwan), Japan and the Philippines.

Generic Complex

The snails known to be naturally infected with *S. japonicum* belong to the sub-family Pomatiopsinae, family Hydrobiidae. In the past, different generic names have been used for the snails in the four main geographical areas. *Oncomelania, Hemibia, Prososthenia, Katayama* and *Schistosomophora* have been used for the snails in China (Mainland); *Blanfordia, Katayama, Tricula* and *Oncomelania,* for the snails in China (Taiwan); *Hypsobia, Katayama, Blanfordia* and *Oncomelania,* for the snails in Japan; and *Prososthenia, Oncomelania, Blanfordia* and *Schistosomophora,* for the snails in the Philippines. The shape of the shell, the presence or absence of vertical ribs on the shell, the rachidian-tooth formula, the whorls in the operculum, and the structure of the central nervous system were considered important generic characteristics. As these characteristics were often found to be variable, the generic definitions and synonyms were at variance among different taxonomists.

The method of classical systematics came to its full use when BARTSCH [1936] grouped all the snail hosts of *S. japonicum* under three genera, *Oncomelania*, *Katayama* and *Schistosomophora*. *Schistosomophora* differs from *Katayama* and *Oncomelania* in the number of cusps on the anterior edge of the rachidian tooth and in the number of whorls in the operculum. The main reason for separating *Katayama* from *Oncomelania*, besides the number of basal denticles of the rachidian tooth and the number of opercular whorls, is the absence of vertical ribs on the shells. The snails in Japan and China (Taiwan) belong to the genus *Katayama*; in the Philippines, to *Schistosomophora*; and in China (mainland), to both *Oncomelania* and *Katayama*. After studying the variations of snails in different geographical populations, ABBOTT [1948] found that the generic characteristics used by BARTSCH to differentiate oncomelanian genera are so inconsistent and variable that they merit no generic value. He declared that all the known intermediate hosts of *S japonicum* in the Orient belong to one genus, *Oncomelania*.

In 1962, HABE and MIYAZAKI reported a new hydrobiid snail, *Tricula chiui*, from Alilao, Taiwan. This snail was proved to be experimentally susceptible to the infection with the four main geographical strains of *S. japonicum* [CHIU, 1965, 1967; HSÜ, S.Y., and HSÜ, 1966; HSÜ, H.F., and HSÜ, 1967], although natural infection with this schistosome has not been reported. Recent studies, however, showed that *Tricula chiui* is an oncomelanian snail which is either a geographical race of *Oncomelania formosana* [HSÜ and HSÜ, 1967] or a sub-species of *Oncomelania hupensis* [DAVIS, 1967].

It is the consensus that all of the intermediate hosts of *S. japonicum* (actual or potential) known at present in the endemic areas belong to a single genus, *Oncomelania*.

Specific Complex

A number of oncomelanian species have been reported as intermediate hosts of *S. japonicum*. In China (Mainland), 20 species have been incriminated: *O. hupensis*, *O. schmackeri*, *O. carectorum*, *O. luteola*, *O. crassa*, *O. costulata*, *O. moellendorffi*, *O. sublaevis*, *O. longiscata*, *O. nosophora*, *O. elongata*, *O. multicosta*, *O. fausti*, *O. cantoni*, *O. anhuinensis*, *O. vlii*, *O. tangi*, *O. yaoi*, *O. robertsonia* and *O. slateri*; in China (Taiwan), one species, *O. formosana*; in Japan, one species with two sub-species, *O. nosophora nosophora* and *O. nosophora yoshidai*; and in the Philippines, two species, *O. quadrasi* and *O. hydrobiopsis*, were given. Old school taxonomists differentiated these species by minute and inconsistent external morphological characteristics such as the shape, size, number of whorls, and the degree of the development of ribs of the shell; and the internal characteristics such as the dental formula of the radular teeth. In his extensive study of the variability of oncomelanian species, ABBOTT [1948] reduced the above-mentioned number of species into four species and one sub-species, *O.hupensis*, *O.nosophora*, *O.nosophora slateri*, *O.formosana* and *O.quadrasi*. *O.hupensis* measures 7 to 9 mm in shell length and can be differentiated from the other species by the presence of axial ribs on the shells; it is found in China (Mainland). *O.nosophora* measures up to 10 mm in length but its shell is smooth; it can be differentiated from *O.formosana* and *O.quadrasi*, besides its greater shell length, by the fact that the length of the last whorl of its shell is equal to, or less than, that of the remaining whorls in the spire. It occurs in Japan and is also said to be found in China (Mainland). *O.nosophora slateri* is distinguished from *O.nosophora* by the last whorl of the shell, which is always greater than half the height of the entire shell; it occurs in Szechuan, in China (Mainland). *O.formosana* is characterized by its smooth shell; it can be differentiated from *O.nosophora* by its small shell size (only 4 to 6 mm in length) and by the large size of the last whorl (the length of its last whorl is always greater than that of the remaining whorls in the spire). It occurs in China (Taiwan). *O.quadrasi* has a smooth shell and its whorl is always greater in length than the remaining whorls in the spire; it is, therefore, very similar to *O.formosana* but can be differentiated by its still smaller shell length, (3–5 mm). It occurs in the Philippines.

Studying the morphological characteristics of oncomelanian snails collected from 16 localities in 11 provinces in China (Mainland), KUO and MAO [1957] assert that the gross differences in the shell of oncomelanian snails result from environmental conditions and are of no taxonomic value. They indicate that the other morphological characteristics which have been commonly used for specific differentiation of the oncomelanian species in China (Mainland) are also not well defined. They propose that all the oncomelanian snails which are involved in the transmission of *S.japonicum* in China (Mainland) should belong to one species, *O.hupensis*. Thus, the intermediate host species complex of *S.japonicum* has been reduced to four geographical species: *O.hupensis* in China (Mainland), *O.formosana* in China (Taiwan), *O.nosophora* in Japan, and *O.quadrasi* in the Philippines. According to DAVIS [1967], they do not differ greatly in their internal anatomy. Their external differences are mainly those of size, ribs on the shells of some populations of *O.hupensis*, and variance in the intensity of external pigmentation and in the yellow coloration of the granules surrounding the medial surface of the eye. In shell shape, there is a north-south cline, with *O.nosophora* from Japan having a long, slender shell; *O.quadrasi* from the Philippines having a relatively more short and broad shell; and *O. formosana* from China (Taiwan) being intermediate.

Following the modern trend of the new systematics, variations in the populations have been studied. ABBOTT [1948] reported that in his study of the shell characteristics of 500 *O. formosana* from China (Taiwan), 5% of his specimens were indistinguishable from *O. quadrasi* from the Philippines and 10% were the same shape and size as *O. nosophora* from Japan and China (Mainland). In the same paper, ABBOTT also gave a vivid description of the ecological effect on the shell morphology of *O. hupensis*. KUO and MAO [1957] proved by experiment the effect of the environmental conditions upon the characteristics of the shells. The colour of the shell of *O. hupensis* has been shown to be variable under different environmental conditions [MAO and LI, 1948]. The resistance to desiccation of *O. nosophora* varies in snails collected from dry habitats compared with those from wet habitats [KOMIYA and IIJIMA, 1958]. These facts and other relevant evidence indicate that the species problem of the intermediate hosts of *S. japonicum* cannot be solved merely by morphological studies of the external and internal characteristics.

Studies of the biological characteristics of the four geographical oncomelanian species in recent years afford information for numerical taxonomists to evaluate complicated data. WAGNER and MOORE [1956] reported that the effects of water level fluctuation on egg laying differ in *O. nosophora* and *O. quadrasi*. WAGNER and WONG [1956] also found the egg-laying habits different in these two species. CHI and WAGNER [1957] showed that certain phenomena in the reproduction and growth of the snails were different among *O. quadrasi*, *O. formosana*, and *O. nosophora*. A gradient difference in temperature and moisture response was found in the above-mentioned geographical species [VAN DER SCHALIE and GETZ, 1963]. Interesting findings were made on the differences in the susceptibility of the four geographical species of oncomelanian snails, *O. hupensis*, *O. formosana*, *O. nosophora* and *O. quadrasi* to the infection of the four geographical strains of *S. japonicum*, Chinese (Mainland), Chinese (Taiwan), Japanese, and Philippine [HUNTER et al., 1952; DEWITT, 1954; HSÜ, S. Y. and HSÜ, 1960, 1966, 1967; HSÜ, H. F. and HSÜ, 1967; MOOSE and WILLIAMS, 1963, 1964; CHIU, 1965, 1967]. It is also interesting to report that the immunological studies made on the snail antigen-antibody by the Ouchterlony double diffusion technique indicated that there are certain differences among the four geographical species [DAVIS, 1968].

While the four geographical oncomelanian species, *O. hupensis*, *O. nosophora*, *O. formosana* and *O. quadrasi* seem to be distinct biologically in many respects, they were mostly interbred successfully in different species-crossing combinations [KOMIYA and KOJIMA, 1958; WAGNER and CHI, 1959; DAVIS *et al.*, 1965; DAVIS, 1968]. In addition, BURCH [1960, 1964] found that the chromosome number of these four species is the same and that in their F_1 hybrids no apparent anomalies occurred in chromosome pairing that did not occur as prevalent in the normal parent. He further expressed that if reproductive isolation (including chromosomal homology) is used as a main criterion for determining which populations are distinct species and which are not, all the known oncomelanian snails are in reality no more than one species with several geographical races. In agreement with BURCH's opinion and with the support of the finding that among thousands of hybrids of all four species of *Oncomelania* observed, only one abnormal snail was found [DAVIS *et al.*, 1965], DAVIS [1967] declared that the so-called *Oncomelania* species of most previous authors should be considered sub-species of *O. hupensis*. In the following year, DAVIS [1968] classified the hydrobiid snails from Alilao, Taiwan (first known as *Tricula chiui*) also as a sub-species of *O. hupensis*. Thus, the genus *Oncomelania* contains only one species, *O. hupensis*, which consists of five sub-species: *O. hupensis hupensis*, *O. hupensis nosophora*, *O. hupensis quadrasi*, *O. hupensis formosana* and *O. hupensis chiui*. However, HSÜ, H. F., and HSÜ [1967] were of the opinion that the four geographical oncomelanian species, *O. hupensis*, *O. nosophora*, *O. quadrasi* and *O. formosana*, should still be maintained at their species level and the snails from Alilao, Taiwan, should be regarded as a geographical race of *O. formosana*.

Based upon the following reasons, it seems appropriate to divide the known oncomelanian snails into four species as we suggested previously [HSÜ, H. F., and HSÜ, 1967].

1. Reproductive isolation. Although successful interbreeding between different oncomelanian species has been reported experimentally, the percentage of successful homospecific mating between *formosana* and *formosana*, between *quadrasi* and *quadrasi*, and between *nosophora* and *nosophora* was 71–90, 73–88, and 53–59 respectively, whereas the percentage of successful heterospecific mating between *quadrasi* and *formosana*, between *nosophora* and *formosana*, and between *nosophora* and *quadrasi* was only 7, 45, and 56 respectively [WAGNER and CHI, 1959]. Negative interbreeding between the Alilao race of *O. formosana* and *O. quadrasi* was also recorded [DAVIS, 1968]. It should be stated that all these interbreeding experiments were performed in a compulsory situation, i.e. heterospecific interbreeding had to take place because of the absence of snails of the opposite sex of the same species. Even under such a compulsory condition, the proportion of successful breeding was much lower in heterospecific snails than in homospecific snails. Furthermore, there is no experimental evidence to indicate that under competitive conditions, i.e. the presence of both sexes of heterospecific and homospecific snails, inter-breeding between different species did occur. We have to consider also that *O.nosophora*, *O.formosana*, and *O.quadrasi* are insular species; they have been reproductively isolated from each other and from the continental species, *O.hupensis*, for about a million years. Although interbreeding is still possible under a very artificial experimental condition, the results obtained by WAGNER and CHI, and DAVIS, as mentioned above, indicate that a certain degree of reproductive isolation of these four species has been demonstrated.

    2. Characters for species determination. A species should be established from the combined weights of characters obtained from different fields of in-vestigation, i.e. morphology, physiology, biology, genetics, cytology, phy-logeny, parasitology, chemistry, serology, immunology, etc. A specific de-termination should not be based upon one or two characters, even though they have resulted from genetic or cytological studies. In considering the combined weight of the distinct characters of the four main geographical oncomelanian species, it is apparent that each of them has reached a species level, and the four specific names *O.hupensis*, *O.nosophora*, *O.formosana*, and *O.quadrasi*, should be retained.

    3. Sub-species in taxonomy. SOKAL [1964] labelled the sub-species concept a myth in relation to descriptive taxonomic work. This is especially true in the taxonomy of oncomelanian snails. According to HSÜ, S.Y., and HSÜ [1967], there are four races of *O.formosana* in Taiwan. If *O.formosana* is to be called *O.hupensis formosana*, the question will arise how to name the four races of oncomelanian snails in Taiwan. While numerical taxonomist [CAIN, 1959] attempts to abandon the binomen on account of its encumbrance and to take a monomian system, we should not go back to trinomen. WILSON and BROWN [1953] pointed out that as the analyses of geographical variations become more complete, the trinomial nomenclatorial system will be revealed as inefficient and superfluous. This system itself is top-heavy and cumbersome and we should try to avoid it as much as possible. We, therefore, prefer, for instance, *O.formosana* to *O.hupensis formosana* unless the name *O.formosana* has been definitely proved to be untenable.

Infraspecific Complex

    Results of investigation made in recent years indicate that the geographi-cal species may be a complex itself, especially *O.hupensis* in China (Mainland) and *O.formosana* in China (Taiwan). On the Chinese mainland, YUAN [1958] found that *O.hupensis* from various localities differs in susceptibility to the infection of local strains of *S. japonicum*. Snails from Tsinpu, Kiangsu; Kiukiang, Kiangsu; and Yoyang, Hunan, were susceptible to infection of *S. japonicum* from these three localities, but they could not readily be infected by the strains of *S. japonicum* from Tali, Yunnan, and from Mienchu, Szechuan. Similarly, *O. hupensis* from the latter two localities was refractory to the infection of *S. japonicum* from the former three localities.

In China (Taiwan), Hsü, H. F., and Hsü [1967] recognized four geographical races of *O. formosana* by the different degrees of infectivity with the various geographical strains of *S. japonicum*. They are: Alilao race (syn.: *Tricula chiui*, *Oncomelania hupensis chiui*), Changhua race (syn.: Pu Yen population); Ilan race, and Kaohsiung race (syn.: Yueh Mei population). The Alilao race is distinguished by its high susceptibility to all the geographical strains of *S. japonicum* (infection rate: 54–98%); and the Kaohsiung race, by its low susceptibility or non-susceptibility (infection rate: 0.0–1.8%). Both the Changhua and the Ilan races are characterized by their low susceptibility to the three human strains of *S. japonicum* which occur outside Taiwan (the Chinese mainland, the Japanese, and the Philippine strains), their comparatively high susceptibility to the non-human strain which occurs in the same areas with the snail race, and their comparatively low susceptibility to the non-human strain which occurs on the same island but in different areas [for detailed information, see table III, Hsü, H. F., and Hsü, 1967]. As previously mentioned, although the Alilao race is susceptible to all the geographical stains of *S. japonicum*, originating either on Taiwan or outside Taiwan, natural schistosome infection of this snail race was not found locally. Hsü, H. F., and Hsü [1967] also made comparative studies of the shell size and the habitat of the four geographical races of *O. formosana*. They noticed that the size of the Alilao race is definitely smaller than that of the other three races and that the mean lengths of the female specimens of the Changhua, the Ilan, and the Kaohsiung races are statistically different each from the other, although there are no significant differences in the mean lengths of the males of these three races. It is evident that morphological differences have begun to develop in these four races. As to their habitat, the results of their studies seem to indicate that the habitats of each of the four races are distinct. They asserted, however, that a close examination of the results indicates that, fundamentally, the habitats of the four races are the same, varying only according to the environmental situations and evolutional development.

Recently, DAVIS [1968] made an excellent study on the anatomy, hybridization, electrophoretic analysis and antigen-antibody reactions of the foot muscles of the Alilao race and other races of *O. formosana*. While there were a few minor anatomical dissimilarities, the results obtained from hybridization and from the antigen-antibody systems show that there are no specific differences. Special mention should be made that the antigen-antibody precipitating reaction of the foot muscles by the Ouchterlony double diffusion method showed a complete homogeneity among the four geographical races of *O. formosana*, and that there is no complete homogeneity in this reaction between *O. formosana* and the other three oncomelanian species: *O. hupensis*, *O. nosophora*, and *O. quadrasi*. The result of this finding strongly supports the supposition that the oncomelanian snail in Alilao, Taiwan, should be regarded as a geographical race of *O. formosana*, although its size is definitely smaller than that of the other geographical races of this species.

It is a well-known fact that microgeographical races are especially prominent in snails because of the sedentary habits of these organisms and their tendency to form isolated local colonies. It is expected that more than one geographical race of oncomelanian snails may be found in one main geographical area. In the future, the origin or locality of the snails must be mentioned in all parasitological and epidemiological publications in which oncomelanian snails are involved in experimental studies. Such usage as *O. hupensis* from China (Mainland) or *O. formosana* from China (Taiwan), is not sufficient for denoting the nature of the snails.

Potential Intermediate-Host Complex

Experimentally, two more hydrobiid species of snails, *Pomatiopsis lapidaria* and *P. cincinnatiensis*, were reported to be susceptible to infection by *S. japonicum*. Cercariae of *S. japonicum* were found in *P. lapidaria* by experimental infection [BERRY and RUE, 1948]; and sporocysts, in *P. cincinnatiensis* [VAN DER SCHALIE and BASCH, quoted from GETZ, 1962]. *Pomatiopsis* is found in North America. Many morphological and biological similarities were noticed between *Oncomelania* and *Pomatiopsis* [ABBOTT, 1948; VAN DER SCHALIE and DUNDEE, 1955, 1956; DUNDEE, 1957; VAN DER SCHALIE and GETZ, 1963; DAVIS, 1967]. Crossing of *P. lapidaria* and *O. quadrasi* produced an F_2 generation and crossing of *P. lapidaria* and *O. formosana* produced offspring which died before adult characters became evident [VAN DER SCHALIE et al., 1962]; VAN DER SCHALIE and DUNDEE [1956] suggested that further study may reveal that *Pomatiopsis* and *Oncomelania* could be grouped under one genus. DAVIS [1967], however, reported that *P. lapidaria* will not produce a hybrid F_1 generation when interbred with *Oncomelania*. Based upon the results of BURCH's cytological studies [BURCH, 1960], DAVIS drew a further conclusion that crosses between *P. lapidaria* and species of *Oncomelania* are improbable because of the apparent differences in the sex determinant mechanism. After making a comparative study of the anatomy, hybridization, electrophoretic properties, and ecology of *P. lapidaria* and *O. formosana*, DAVIS [1967] concluded that *Oncomelania* and *Pomatiopsis* are distinct genera within the sub-family Pomatiopsinae. Thus, *Pomatiopsis* species and *Oncomelania* species are still very closely related taxonomically, although they cannot be grouped together as one genus. Experimentally, *Pomatiopsis* species may be a potential intermediate host of *S. japonicum* in North America, but they may not eventually become a natural host of this parasite because their degree of susceptibility to the experimental infection is very low [DEWITT, 1954], even though human cases of schistosomiasis japonica may be occasionally brought into this area.

Another interesting potential intermediate host of *S. japonicum* is the Alilao race of *O. formosana* in Alilao, Taiwan. As mentioned above, a natural infection of this geographical race of oncomelanian snail has never been reported, but experimentally it is very highly susceptible to all the strains of *S. japonicum*. As the habitat of the Alilao race is confined to the bases of waterfalls at the seashore of mountainous hills, the mammalian hosts may have no opportunity to reach these places and disseminate the schistosome eggs [HsÜ, H. F., and HsÜ, 1967]. For this reason, this oncomelanian race has remained as an innocent potential intermediate host of *S. japonicum*.

Evolution of the Intermediate-Host Complex

The intermediate-host complex of *S. japonicum* presents a complicated but interesting problem. However, if it is examined from the evolutional point of view, the problem will become not only simpler but even more interesting. HsÜ, H. F., and HsÜ [1958] formulated an evolutional theory for the development and formation of the geographical strains of *S. japonicum*. The same idea was later applied to the origin of the four geographical oncomelanian species [HsÜ, S. Y., and HsÜ, 1960] and of the four geographical races of *O. formosana* in Taiwan [HsÜ, H. F., and HsÜ, 1967]. It seems appropriate to conclude the present discussion with some elaboration of this theory.

It has been assumed that the main pattern of dispersal of animals is apparently due to the evolution of successive dominant groups in the most favourable area of the Old World tropics, and consequent spread with successive replacement into smaller and/or less favourable areas. The animals found on continents are apparently always dominant over those on islands, and dispersal is almost always from continents to islands. It may be assumed that the ancestors of oncomelanian snails originated somewhere around the border

of India, Burma, and Yunnan. According to ANNANDALE [1924], fossil specimens of oncomelanian snails have been found in the Shan plateau, upper
Burma; from there they probably radiated to China and Japan. Crossing the
Bering Bridge, they extended further to North America. From South China,
they branched out into Taiwan and the Philippines (probably also into Thailand, Laos, and Celebes). The dispersion should have been completed before
the above-mentioned islands were separated from the Asiatic continent and
before the Bering Strait severed the connexion between Asia and North
America. All these events should have taken place before or during the Pleistocene period.

During the process of evolution, these snails were constantly multiplying
in certain places, spreading into other places, receding and becoming extinct
in others, and thus forming the present apparently discontinuous pattern of
geographical distribution. Mutation may occur among isolated populations.
As the survival and spread of mutations may proceed most rapidly in relatively
small, isolated populations, this type of evolution may produce a new species
or a new genus on the islands of Japan, Taiwan, and the Philippines as well
as on the North American continent that had separated from Asia. The
mutations that happen to be advantageous under special conditions are
selected. The time lapse between the Pleistocene period and the present has
been about a million years. Oncomelanian snails on these islands and in North
America should have undergone sufficient reproductive isolation, ecological
differences, and general adaptation to have characteristics distinct from their
ancestral form on the Asiatic continent. As the ecological conditions and
general adaptations were different in different isolated areas, the characteristics of various populations in different main geographical areas, i.e. Japan,
China (Taiwan), the Philippines, and North America, should have developed
differently. Physiological differentiations of isolated populations sometimes
proceed more rapidly than morphological changes. The insular populations
of oncomelanian snails have, indeed, become distinct in physiological characteristics and certain minor morphological differences have also been noted.
This explains the evolutional history of *O. hupensis*, *O. nosophora*, *O. formosana* and *O. quadrasi* as well as *P. lapidaria* and *P. cincinnatiensis*. Because
S. japonicum has never been established in North America, there has been no
host-parasite relationship between *Pomatiopsis* and *S. japonicum* under natural
conditions. By its genetic constitution, however, *Pomatiopsis* remains as a
potential host of *S. japonicum*.

Special note should be given to the evolution of the four geographical
races of *O. formosana* in China (Taiwan). As mentioned above, oncomelanian

snails were assumed to exist on Taiwan before this island was separated from the Chinese mainland. After the separation of the island from the mainland, the oncomelanian snail in Taiwan underwent reproductive isolation and ecological differentiation, resulting in forming a different species, *O. formosana*. At first, *O. formosana* may have inhabited the mountain streams in the highland on Taiwan. The Central Ridge, being the backbone ridge of this island, is the main water divider between the eastern and the western slopes. As the geophysical and ecological conditions in different valleys are dissimilar, oncomelanian snails can thrive and reproduce only in those valleys where they can adapt, i.e. the Tatun Mountain in the north, the Ilanchoshui Valley in the north-east, the Choshui Valley in the mid-west, and the Laonung and Nantzehsien Valleys in the south-west. As soon as the snails adapted themselves in these valleys, they became isolated populations. Following the development of the alluvial plains, the snails inhabiting these valleys gradually migrated into their respective plains, especially along the irrigation ditches. From the Ilanchoshui Valley, the snails migrated into the Ilan plain; from the Choshui Valley, into the Changhua plain; and from the Laonung and Nantzehsien Valley into the Kaohsiung plain. However, the situation in the Tatun mountains in the north was different; because the Tatun mountains ended abruptly at the sea, the snails in this area have remained in the waterfalls of the foothills at the Alilao area. As the ecological conditions and general adaptibility are dissimilar in different isolated valleys and plains, eventually four distinct races of *O. formosana* developed on Taiwan. Physiological differentiations of isolated populations usually proceed more rapidly than morphological changes and this is the present situation with respect to the Changhua, the Ilan, and the Kaohsiung races. Because the shell of the Alilao race is definitely smaller than those of the other three races, one must conclude that a morphological change also developed in addition to physiological changes [HSÜ, H. F., and HSÜ, 1967]. It is of great interest to note again that antigenically there is no change in the foot muscles of the four races [DAVIS, 1968].

The limnic fauna, to which oncomelanian snails belong, is relatively undiversified on the species level and upward; this indicates a comparatively slow or inefficient evolution [HUBENDICK, 1962]. This is well exemplified by the present status of the oncomelanian taxa. As mentioned above, the four geographical species of *Oncomelania* can be experimentally interbred with each other in most cases, although to a reduced degree. This shows that although geographical species have been formed, their genetic divergence is still not very complete.

As oncomelanian snails are limnic organisms, their evolution in one main geographical area very often leads to micro-geographical races. The lifetime of the isolated populations is generally too short, so that the micro-geographical races comparatively seldom evolve into distinct species [HUBENDICK, 1954]. This explains the reason why there are possibly several micro-geographical races but one oncomelanian species, *O. hupensis*, on the Chinese mainland. This holds true also for the oncomelanian taxa on Taiwan; one species, *O. formosana*, but four races.

Conclusion

For a better understanding of the intermediate-host complex of *S. japonicum*, an intensive study of the external morphology, internal anatomy, histology, cytology, physiology, biochemistry, serology, and behaviour of the snail hosts in the different geographical areas had to be made. A species cannot be established by a single character. Modern empirical or numerical taxonomists emphasize the study of as many characters as possible. As knowledge of the characters of the intermediate-host complex of *S. japonicum* is far from complete, more research along these lines is necessary.

The segregation of the four geographical species of *Oncomelania* in China (mainland), Japan, China (Taiwan), and the Philippines, and of *Pomatiopsis* in North America has been so definite that their gene flow has stopped for nearly a million years. As a good working basis and as a sound taxonomical concept, *O. hupensis* on the Chinese mainland, *O. formosana* on Taiwan, *O. nosophora* in Japan, and *O. quadrasi* in the Philippines should be regarded as separated species, and *Pomatiopsis* species in North America as a separated genus. In each main geographical area, the oncomelanian species may have more than one geographical race as exemplified by four races of *O. formosana* on Taiwan. It will be of great additional interest to study the characters of the snail hosts of *S. japonicum* in Thailand, Laos, Cambodia and Celebes when they become known.

References
ABBOTT, R. T.: Bull. Mus. comp. Zool. Harv. *100:* 245 (1948).
ANNANDALE, N.: Amer. J. Hyg. Monogr. Ser. *3:* 269 (1924).
BARTSCH, P.: Smithson misc. Collns *95:* 1 (1936).
BERRY, E. G. and RUE, R. E.: J. Parasit. *34:* suppl., p. 15 (1948).
BURCH, J. B.: Amer. Malacol. Union Ann. Reps. *26:* 15 (1960).
BURCH, J. B.: Amer. Malacol. Union Ann. Reps. *31:* 28 (1964).
CAIN, A. J.: Proc. Linn. Soc., Lond., Session 170, 1957–1958, p. 234 (1959).
CHI, L. W. and WAGNER, E. D.: Amer. J. Trop. med. Hyg. *6:* 949 (1957).
CHIU, J. K.: J. Parasit. *51:* 206 (1965).

CHIU, J. K.: Malacologia *6:* 145 (1967).

DAVIS, G. M.: Malacologia *6:* 1 (1967).

DAVIS, G. M.: Malacologia *7:* 17 (1968).

DAVIS, G. M.: in HARINASUTA Proceedings of the Fourth South-East Asian Seminar on Parasitology and Tropical Medicine, Manila 1969, p. 93 (Bangkok 1970).

DAVIS, G. M.; MOOSE, J. W., and WILLIAMS, J. E.: Malacologia *2:* 209 (1965).

DEWITT, W. B.: J. Parasit. *40:* 453 (1954).

DUNDEE, D. S.: Mus. Zool. Univ. Mich., Misc. Publ. *100:* 1 (1957).

GETZ, L. L.: J. Parasit. *48:* 498 (1962).

HABE, T. and MIYAZAKI, I.: Kyushu J. med. Sci. *13:* 47 (1962).

HSÜ, H. F. and HSÜ, S. Y.: in Proceedings of the Sixth International Congresses on Tropical Medicine and Malaria, vol. 2, p. 58 (1958).

HSÜ, H. F. and HSÜ, S. Y.: Z. Tropenmed. Parasit. *18:* 417 (1967).

HSÜ, S. Y. and HSÜ, H. F.: J. Parasit. *46:* 793 (1960).

HSÜ, S. Y. and HSÜ, H. F.: J. Parasit. *52:* 800 (1966).

HSÜ, S. Y. and HSÜ, H. F.: J. Parasit. *53:* 654 (1967).

HUBENDICK, B.: Proc. malac. Soc., Lond. *31:* 6 (1954).

HUBENDICK, B.: Oikos *13:* 249 (1962).

HUNTER, G. W.; RITCHIE, L. S., and OTORI, Y.: J. Parasit. *38:* 492 (1952).

KOMIYA, Y. and IIJIMA, T.: Jap. J. med. Sci. Biol. *11:* 455 (1958).

KOMIYA, Y. and KOJIMA, K.: Jap. J. med. Sci. Biol. *11:* 185 (1958).

KUO, Y. H. and MAO, S. P.: Chin. med. J. *75:* 824 (1957).

MAO, S. P. and LI, L.: J. Parasit. *34:* 380 (1948).

MOOSE, J. W. and WILLIAMS, J. E.: J. Parasit. *49:* 702 (1963).

MOOSE, J. W. and WILLIAMS, J. E.: in [US] 406th Medical Laboratory Research Report 1964, vol. 1 (1964).

SCHALIE, H. VAN DER and DUNDEE, D. S.: Trans. amer. microscop. Soc. *74:* 119 (1955).

SCHALIE, H. VAN DER and DUNDEE, D. S.: Occ. Pap. Mus. Zool. Univ. Mich. *579:* 1 (1956).

SCHALIE, H. VAN DER and GETZ, L. L.: Ecology *44:* 73–83 (1963).

SCHALIE, H. VAN DER; GETZ, L. L., and DAZO, B. C.: Amer. J. trop. Med. Hyg. *11:* 418 (1962).

SOKAL, R. R.: in LEONE Taxonomic Biochemistry and Serology, pp. 33–48 (Ronalds Press, New York 1964).

WAGNER, E. D. and CHI, L. W.: Amer. J. trop. Med. Hyg. *8:* 195 (1959).

WAGNER, E. D. and MOORE, B.: Amer. J. trop. Med. Hyg. *5:* 553 (1956).

WAGNER, E. D. and WONG, L. W.: Amer. J. trop. Med. Hyg. *5:* 544 (1956).

WILSON, E. O. and BROWN, W. L., jr.: System. Zool. *2:* 97 (1953).

YUAN, H. C.: Chin. med. J. *77:* 575 (1958).

The Americas

Many variations have been noted in the susceptibility of geographical races or strains of molluscan intermediate hosts in the Americas to infection with *S. mansoni*. *B. glabrata* is usually highly prone to infection and the parasite is seldom inhibited in its development in this species. However, exceptions do occur.

FILES and CRAM [1949] reported that *B. glabrata* from Puerto Rico could be infected with Puerto Rican, Venezuelan and Brazilian-Puerto Rican cross-strains of *S. mansoni*. Venezuelan *B. glabrata* likewise became infected with all strains of the parasite employed but showed a higher rate of infection with the Brazilian-Puerto Rican cross-strain than with a Venezuelan strain. However, *B. glabrata* from Brazil could not be infected with all of the *S. mansoni* strains; only 7% took a Puerto Rican human strain, and none was infected with a Puerto Rican animal strain or with the Venezuelan strain. Later, FILES [1951] demonstrated resistance of a strain of *B. glabrata* from Salvador, Bahia, Brazil to infection with exotic strains of *S. mansoni*. NEWTON [1952] exposed this same strain of snail to a strain of *B. glabrata* from Puerto Rico. The parasite was destroyed and removed, usually within 24 to 48 h after penetration, although *B. glabrata* from Puerto Rico was highly susceptible to infection. Later, NEWTON [1953] demonstrated that susceptibility of *S. mansoni* infection in *B. glabrata* is a heritable character, and that several genetic factors are probably involved. BARBOSA [1959] showed that the Bahia snail was a very poor host even for a Brazilian strain of the parasite.

B. tenagophila has been considered a poor host for *S. mansoni* but studies by RAMOS *et al.* [1961] would indicate that it can be an important factor in transmission when pollution of streams is at a high level. *B. straminea* is a less favourable host than is *B. glabrata* [BARBOSA and COELHO, 1954].

In more recent studies, PARAENSE and CORRÊA [1963a] sampled 23 populations of *B. glabrata* scattered over the range of the species. These were exposed to 10 miracidia per snail of a strain of *S. mansoni* from Belo Horizonte, Brazil. A great majority of populations were highly susceptible, showing infection rates above 50%. Six populations, however, were less susceptible or even highly resistant to infection with rates of 48, 24.1 and 0%. Strains from Salvador, Bahia, Brazil were entirely resistant when exposed to as many as 1,000 miracidia.

PARAENSE and CORRÊA [1963b] found that *B. tenagophila* from Pindamonhangaba, São Paulo, Brazil, was insusceptible to infection with *S. mansoni* from Belo Horizonte, Brazil, when exposed to 50 miracidia. Exposure to 1,000 miracidia resulted in infection in only one of 54 specimens. On the other hand, *B. tenagophila* from São Jose dos Campos, São Paulo, Brazil, which was insusceptible to infection, was easily infected with a local strain of *S. mansoni*. The latter strain, however, failed to infect *B. glabrata* from Belo Horizonte, Brazil, which was highly susceptible to local *S. mansoni*.

KAGAN and GEIGER [1965] exposed pigmented *B. glabrata* from Puerto Rico and Brazil and an albino strain from Brazil to three strains of *S. mansoni*, including one from Puerto Rico, one from Brazil, and the third an adaptation of the Brazilian schistosome to the Brazilian albino snail. Variations in infection rates indicated snail susceptibility. The pigmented and albino snails from Brazil were both less susceptible to infection with the Puerto Rican schistosome, whereas the Puerto Rican snail did not give evidence of loss of susceptibility against the Brazilian strains. Initially, the Brazilian albino snail could not be readily infected with the Brazilian parasite; however, exposure to miracidia of the adapted Brazilian strain resulted in an increase in infectivity.

COELHO [1962] studied the resistance of *B. tenagophila* in Brazil to schistosome infection. He exposed 1,433 specimens of this species from 14 districts of the States of São Paulo, Guanabara, Rio de Janeiro, Minas Gerais and Rio Grande do Sul to *S. mansoni* miracidia. After 35 days, cercariae and secondary sporocysts could be found in only 0.5% of the 1,019 surviving specimens. The percentage of infection among 195 *B. glabrata* and 50 *B. straminea* used as controls was 80 and 5.5% respectively. Histological preparations from the cephalopodal region of 49 *B. tenagophila* from seven districts of São Paulo, killed 36 and 74 h after exposure, revealed granuloma formation between 88.7 and 93% of the primary sporocysts which were undergoing resorption.

RICHARDS [1963] exposed 1,521 Puerto Rican freshwater molluscs of 22 species to miracidia of *S. mansoni*. Frequency of observed penetration in descending order was as follows: *B. obstructa, B. glabrata, B. peregrina, B. heliophila, Aplexa marmorata, Pleisophysa hubendicki,* and *Drepanotrema simmonsi.* Successful infection with shedding of cercariae was observed in *B. glabrata, B. peregrina* (under the name of *Tropicorbis riisei*) and *B. heliophila* (under the name of *Tropicorbis albicans*).

BARBOSA *et al.* [1958] had previously found *B. peregrina* (under the name of *Tropicorbis philippianus*) from Ecuador susceptible to *S. mansoni.*

RICHARDS and FERGUSON [1965] conducted studies on the variability of *B. glabrata.* Detailed morphological analyses were made on fresh and preserved specimens, together with comparative measurements of 204 shells collected from a wide range of freshwater habitats at 40 sites in Puerto Rico, Surinam, St. Kitts and Antigua. Shell characteristics were compared with certain internal features in the 21 strains from 17 geographically isolated areas. Characteristics in the shell and internal morphology which show consistent differences in geographically or ecologically isolated populations were ratio of shell height to diameter, ratio of width of body whorl at aperture to diameter, average shell diameter at puberty, egg capsule diameter, type of spermatheca, and whether crossed with albino *B. glabrata.* Studies of internal morphology, laboratory culture, and crossing with an albino strain demonstrated that such characters represented striking intraspecific variation. However, the data did not support establishment of any new species.

Other species of *Biomphalaria* in the Americas have been found susceptible to *S. mansoni* infection. These include *B. chilensis* from Chile tested by BARBOSA and BARBOSA [1958] and *B. sericea* from Los Rios, Ecuador by BARBOSA *et al.* [1958]. CRAM *et al.* [1945] and McQUAY [1952] demonstrated susceptibility of *B. obstructa* (under the name of *Tropicorbis havanensis*) from a lake at Baton Rouge, La., USA, to *S. mansoni*. However, a strain of the same snail from lagoons in a park in New Orleans, La., was reported by BROOKS [1953] to be completely refractory.

A number of other species of *Biomphalaria* which occur in the Americas are either resistant to *S. mansoni* infection or are not known to be involved in the epidemiology of schistosomiasis. These include the following:

Species	Type locality
B. andecola	Lake Titicaca, Bolivia
B. philippiana	Cochabamba, Bolivia
B. prona	Lago de Valencia, Venezuela
B. schrammi	Guadeloupe
B. intermedia	Valparaiso, São Paulo, Brazil

A PAHO/WHO publication entitled. 'A guide for the identification of the snail intermediate hosts of schistosomiasis in the Americas' contains detailed information on the subject.

References

BARBOSA, F.S.: in Proceedings of the 15th International Congresses of Zoology, London 1958, p. 691 (1959).

BARBOSA, F.S. and BARBOSA, I.: Bol. Chileno Parasitol. *13:* 7 (1958).

BARBOSA, F.S. and COELHO, M.V.: Publ. avuls. Inst. Aggeu Magalhaes *3:* 55 (1954).

BARBOSA, F.S.; BARBOSA, I., and CARNEIRO, E.: An. Inst. Med. Trop. *15:* 397 (1958).

BARBOSA, F.S.; BARBOSA, I., and RODRIGUEZ, J.D.: J. Parasitol. *44:* 622 (1958).

BROOKS, C.P.: J. Parasitol. *39:* 159 (1953).

COELHO, M.V.: Rev. Inst. Med. trop., S. Paulo *4:* 289 (1962).

CRAM, E.B.; JONES, M.F., and WRIGHT, W.H.: Science *101:* 302 (1945).

FILES, V.S.: Parasitology *41:* 264 (1951).

FILES, V.S. and CRAM, E.B.: J. Parasit. *35:* 555 (1949).

KAGAN, I. G. and GEIGER, S. J.: J. Parasit. *51:* 622 (1965).
McQUAY, R. M., jr.: Exp. Parasit. *1:* 184 (1952).
NEWTON, W. L.: J. Parasit. *38:* 362 (1952).
NEWTON, W. L.: Exp. Parasit. *2:* 242 (1953).
Pan American Health Organization-World Health Organization: A guide for the identi-
    fication of the snail intermediate hosts of schistosomiasis in the Americas. Scientific
    Publ. No. 168 (1968).
PARAENSE, W. L. and CORRÊA, L. R.: Rev. Inst. Med. trop., S. Paulo *5:* 15 (1963a).
PARAENSE, W. L. and CORRÊA, L. R.: Rev. Inst. Med. trop., S. Paulo *5:* 23 (1963b).
RAMOS, A. DA SILVA; PIZA, J. DE T., and CAMARGO, L. S. VIEIRA DE: Arq. Hig., S. Paulo *26:*
    121 (1961).
RICHARDS, C. S.: Amer. J. trop. Med. Hyg. *12:* 26 (1963).
RICHARDS, C. S. and FERGUSON, F. F.: Trans. amer. micros. Soc. *84:* 580 (1965).

Future Trends

It is difficult to predict the course of a disease such as schistosomiasis in which little control has been achieved in the past, even though more effective measures are now available to combat it.

From a long-term view, certain general factors will have an influence in gradually limiting the disease. Economic development of backward areas will eventually come about and will play a decisive role in promoting education, the expansion of health services and the extension of sanitary facilities.

It is possible that present and future research will provide new mollus-cicides which will retain a highly potent activity under all conditions, and will not be affected by physical and chemical factors in the environment. It is conceivable also that a new, attractive and highly efficient snail bait may be developed and that a truly effective chemotherapeutic treatment may appear at some future time. Any, or all, of these possibilities would greatly enhance efforts to control the disease.

On the debit side of the ledger, one must consider that genetic and physiological changes take place in schistosome strains as well as in molluscan intermediate hosts. Such changes have occurred in the past and there is no reason to suspect that they are not now taking place or that they will not take place in the future. Any long-term delay in controlling the disease may well permit human schistosomes in some localities to become adapted to new snail hosts. On the other hand, species of snails which at present demonstrate some resistance to schistosome infection could become so altered that they may serve as efficient hosts.

The introduction of an intermediate host into a new area is another possibility, as is the influx of a sufficient number of infected persons into a non-endemic area already known to harbour susceptible snails.

The question of lower animal reservoir hosts has not been settled and their exact role in the maintenance of infection in many areas needs to be determined.

Future trends in schistosomiasis will no doubt vary from country to country and from area to area. For this reason, it would seem best to consider such trends on a regional basis.

Africa

Future trends in Africa are much more difficult to predict than for any other area, because of the many varied factors which are concerned in the epidemiology of the disease in most parts of that continent.

Changes in Behavioural Characteristics of Hosts

As time goes on, the habits of the human host will change but at present such habits are not changing rapidly, except for that part of the population which migrates to the cities, where there is less opportunity for transmission. In parts of Africa, exposure to schistosomiasis is definitely linked to occupation. For instance, in an area in the United Arab Republic (Egypt), FAROOQ *et al.* [1966] found that in total numbers infected, the main burden of infection is borne by farmers and farm labourers, although the infection rates were highest among fishermen and boatmen. In the four divisions of the population surveyed, differences in prevalence rates were explainable, at least in part, by the occupational make-up. The Muslims, because of their religious ablutions, had more than twice the infection rates of the Christian population. Occupational and ablution hazards will remain unless effective control measures are introduced for the population at large. Since children usually show the highest infection rates, it may be possible to alter habits by educational methods. In fact, an encouraging feature of the report by FAROOQ *et al.* concerned lower infection rates in children who attended school.

The discussion on the schistosome-intermediate host complex for Africa (p. 210) has already indicated the immeasurably delicate physiological balance which exists between the two. Under these circumstances, it is possible that changes may occur in this complex and that molluscan hosts, which are now believed to be of minor importance, may assume a more dynamic role in transmission.

Reclamation and Rehabilitation of Lands

The increase in irrigation in parts of Africa has been the means of spreading schistosomiasis. For example, KHALIL and AZIM [1938] reported that in the Aswan Province of Egypt the amount of infection with *S. haematobium* increased from 4- to 40-fold in three years following the substitution of the perennial type for basin irrigation.

The extension of irrigation has taken place mainly in East and South Africa and in the United Arab Republic (Egypt) and Sudan. There has been less similar activity in West Africa.

OLIVIER and McMULLEN [1963] have reported that the United Nations Special Fund had approved 286 projects since it was founded in 1958 and, of these, 50 refer to large irrigation schemes; 25 of the schemes are in endemic areas of schistosomiasis. The Managil extension of the Gezira and the Roseires Dam in Sudan are examples, as well as the High Aswan Dam in Egypt. Other large projects, projected, in the course of construction, or just completed, include the Volta Dam in Ghana, the Somoto River Valley in Northern Nigeria, the Sabi-Lundi area of Rhodesia, the Limpopo scheme in Mozambique, the Elephant Marsh area in Southern Malawi, and the Kafue River polder scheme in Zambia. The Orange River project in South Africa, while situated on the fringe of an endemic area, may create problems associated with the water transfer to areas south and east of the Drakensberg mountain range.

In addition to the huge engineering projects mentioned, water conservation of other types is greatly on the increase in parts of Africa. These types consist of the damming of streams and the construction of small reservoirs which enable more intensive farming to be undertaken in areas that experience long months of drought each year. As with the larger projects, many of these less imposing ones are located in East Africa, although similar trends are current elsewhere. Some of the small schemes are financed by land owners themselves while others receive government support. BLAIR [1964] has indicated the extent to which these smaller conservation projects have grown in Rhodesia; from December 1958 to December 1963, the number increased from 3,562 to 6,143 (excluding the Kariba Dam), and the capacity was more than doubled from 194,317 to 575,813 million gallons. In Kenya, schistosomiasis is spreading into regions which were formerly regarded as being above the level of transmission. This is because the recently constructed artifical dams are warmer and more favourable habitats for transmission than the natural streams [NELSON, 1965].

BLAIR [1964] foresees that the introduction of large scale irrigation into Africa may well herald a turning point in the drift of the rural population to the towns and cities. This is already being witnessed in Rhodesia, where the former migrant to the town now finds better living conditions and more security in the newly irrigated areas. If this trend becomes more general, the impact on the epidemiology of schistosomiasis will be considerable.

In summary, land reclamation in Africa will undoubtedly augment rural health problems and especially promote the transmission of schistosomiasis, unless there is full awareness of the potential dangers involved and unless adequate preventive measures are instituted.

Migrations

In the past, migration of various peoples has no doubt materially influenced the distribution of schistosomiasis in Africa. GAUD [1955] pointed out that the sharp demarcation of S. haematobium in former Ubangi Shari is linked to the northern Islamized peoples who have come into the territory from the north (Sara and Kaba tribes), while the pattern of S. mansoni has been influenced by southern tribes of animistic civilization (Nadja and Banda tribes) originating from the Great Lakes region. AZEVEDO [1956] attributed the introduction of S. haematobium into Northern Cameroon to invasion by Islamized peoples. He equally correlated the introduction of S. mansoni into these regions with the Bantu invasion from the Upper Nile in the 10th century.

GILLET and WOLFS [1954] reported on the southward spread of S. mansoni from the north-eastern Congo along the transportation lines of the mining companies, which is in part also due to the return of fishermen from Lake Albert to the Beni region. The spread has also been westward from Wele along the Wele-Ubangi fluvial axis. A northward advance of both forms of schistosomiasis has been noted along the Lualaba River in Katanga, where S. mansoni prevalence has been heightened by immigration from the Lomani-Kasai and into which S. haematobium was introduced within this century from Zambia and Malawi. AYAD [1956] called attention to the former movements of troops and labour from Egypt into the Sudan as having contributed materially to the extension of the disease in the latter country.

The results of mass movement of populations into an endemic area of schistosomiasis are well illustrated by the transference of Portuguese settlers en masse into the Limpopo River Valley irrigation scheme in the Gaza District of Mozambique, an area endemic for both urinary and intestinal forms of the disease. The first settlers began to arrive in 1955; all had originated in parts of Portugal in which the disease is not endemic. In 1956, 2.86% had acquired S. haematobium and by 1958, the prevalence rate had increased to 29.9%; 3% had acquired S. mansoni infections [MORAIS, 1958].

With large scale plans for increased water conservation projects through-out many parts of Africa, population movements can be expected to continue and to have an influence on the spread of the disease and on prevalence rates in already known endemic areas. Religious pilgrimages may also play a role in the dissemination of the disease, although it is difficult to pinpoint their exact influence in this regard.

Itinerant Labour

Despite the lack of adequate transportation facilities in many parts of Africa, the movement of itinerant labour takes place on a vast scale. The establishment of diamond mining in Sierra Leone has resulted in the move-ment of tens of thousands of persons and the introduction of schistosomiasis into areas formerly free from the disease. The migratory labourers of West Africa and former French Equatorial Africa have no doubt contributed to the intensity of the disease in Sudan. This is particularly true during certain seasons of the year, such as the cotton picking season. Other seasonal move-ments concern the labour force from Mali which goes to Senegal to harvest ground nuts and the extensive labour exodus from Mali, Upper Volta and Niger to pick coconuts in the Ivory Coast, Ghana, Dahomey and Western Nigeria. On the other hand, migrant labour to the mining and industrial areas of Katanga Province, Zambia, Rhodesia and South Africa and to the industrial and commercial areas of Uganda, Kenya and the East African coast is not seasonal but occurs all year round. PROTHERO [1961] has discussed the problem of migratory labour as related to malaria eradication in Africa and has mapped the routes of migration. Much of this information has a bear-ing on the distribution of schistosomiasis. These large scale movements of temporary labour have traditionally occurred in Africa and will continue to occur on a continental basis.

South-West Asia

Changes in Behavioural Characteristics of Hosts

In most of this region, transmission patterns are well defined and are characteristic of the habits of the human population and the nature of the intermediate host environment.

In Saudi Arabia, schistosomiasis is largely a disease of oases with marked focal distribution. Nomads play an important role in transmission and are least subject to control. Exposure in Yemen takes place mainly in the ablution pools of the mosques and in the rainwater reservoirs or magils. There is little or no association of the disease with agricultural activites. The transmission season in Turkey and Syria is limited to the period July to October and infection is related, in part, to irrigation. Nomads are also concerned. Infection is high in children.

Schistosomiasis in Iraq is extensively associated with irrigation. In Iran, infection is usually acquired near villages in the normal course of village activity. Water for drinking and household use is taken from irrigation canals or pools. Children are exposed to the same sources and the male population acquires infection from washing animals and in agricultural activity. In Israel, schistosomiasis has declined rapidly with changes in the composition of the population, and the disease is now a rarity. *S. haematobium* hosts are numerous but human carriers are few; on the other hand, human infection with *S. mansoni* is common but the snail host is limited to a restricted part of a single watercourse which is not used for bathing. The disease is not a problem in Lebanon, where it is limited to a single focus, which probably resulted from the installation of an irrigation system in 1952. Schistosomiasis is widespread in the western areas of Southern Yemen [WRIGHT, 1963a]. In part, infection is associated with irrigation. As far as is known, lower animal reservoir hosts are not concerned in the epidemiology of schistosomiasis in South-West Asia.

Little is known concerning the interrelationships of intermediate hosts and potential hosts in this region. WITENBERG and SALITERNIK [1957] were unable to obtain infections in *B. (B.) truncatus* from Israel with strains of *S. haematobium* from Morocco and Yemen. WRIGHT [1963a] regarded this failure to be due to the fact that the highland form of *B. (B.) truncatus*, which he regards as *B. (B.) sericinus*, is probably the host of *S. haematobium* in Yemen. WRIGHT [1963b] found that two Southern Yemen strains of the parasite would not experimentally infect *B. (B.) truncatus*.

In view of the marked aridity of South-West Asia, it cannot be expected that the human population in endemic areas of schistosomiasis will quickly change habits closely linked with religious practices, nomadism and irrigation, which lead to exposure.

Reclamation and Rehabilitation of Lands

Irrigation is an essential part of land reclamation in South-West Asia. Public and private systems are in use in Central and Southern Iraq. A number of government-financed schemes are in operation, and others are planned. The Dujaila scheme has been in operation since 1945, the Latafia scheme since 1954 and the one at Musayeb since 1956. The first two, if not the last, are infested with host snails. The Diyala and Gharraf projects are in the planning stage. In addition to government supported schemes, many private systems are in operation.

A large scale irrigation project is now under construction in the Khuzestan area of Iran. An environmental health programme is being pursued and will no doubt reduce, or even eliminate, exposure to schistosomiasis.

As previously indicated, land reclamation has taken place in other parts of the region, although on a smaller scale.

Migrations

The major migrations within the area have been to Israel. Within recent years, many of the immigrants have come from countries, such as Morocco, Yemen, Iraq, etc., where schistosomiasis is endemic. As indicated previously, however, there has been no increase of the disease in Israel. Hejjaz with its holy Moslem cities attracts pilgrims in very large numbers from 34 different countries. However, infection is not present at Mecca, the nearest focus being at Wadi Fatima, 45 km distant.

Itinerant Labour

This is not a major factor in the spread of schistosomiasis in South-West Asia. Labourers and domestic servants from Yemen are employed in large numbers in Saudi Arabia. A considerable movement of labour from Turkey into the endemic areas of Syria is reported to take place during the harvest season in the Syrian Jezireh (June to October), which coincides with the schistosomiasis transmission season in that area. WRIGHT [1963a] reported that labour employed in picking cotton in Abyan in Southern Yemen comes from Zabeed in Yemen. It is probable that many of these people carry a strain of S. haematobium suited to the snail hosts in Abyan.

The Orient

Changes in Behavioural Characteristics of Hosts

In the main endemic areas of schistosomiasis japonica in the Orient, exposure is intimately linked with daily human activity. In China (Mainland), wet rice cultivation provides one of the chief means of infection. While the molluscan intermediate host, O. hupensis, does not ordinarily inhabit rice fields, it finds ideal conditions in natural and man-made irrigation canals and in low, marshy sites which, in many parts of the endemic areas, are flooded during the wet season of the year. The canals serve as a source of household water supply and as play areas for children. The practice of applying night soil for the fertilization of rice and other crops also contributes to the spread of infection. Boatmen are exposed through frequent contact with infested waters. Strenuous efforts are being made to change age-old habits and to control snail infestation in canals and other foci. No doubt progress has been made in this regard.

In Japan, the transmission pattern is not materially different. *O.noso-phora*, the intermediate host, is found chiefly in the moist soil of the banks of the irrigation ditches and in marshy areas. Along the Tone River, the snail is limited to the marshy ground between levees and the river channel. Here, transmission is at a low level and is mainly associated with the cutting of marsh reed and grasses. In other types of endemic foci, exposure is related to agriculture and household tasks. While it cannot be said that the habits of the population have altered materially, a marked reduction has taken place in prevalence of infection because of long continued control measures, such as the lining of irrigation ditches and the employment of molluscicides. No doubt this trend will continue.

In the Philippines, the endemic areas are mainly rural and, in the majority, wet rice cultivation is practised. The snail host, *O. quadrasi*, favours moist lowland and sluggish streams. In marshy areas, the snail survives the dry season through cover provided by thick grass. Many people of all ages and both sexes have frequent contact with infested water in the course of farming activities, household chores and recreation. While some progress has been made in control, especially in experimental areas on Leyte, there is no indication of any change in habits on the part of the population in general.

The four geographical races of *Oncomelania*, serving as intermediate hosts of *S. japonicum* in the Orient, have been successfully interbred. However, uniform susceptibility to all strains of the parasite does not necessarily follow. Strains from certain geographical locations may or may not be susceptible to *S. japonicum* from other areas, although serving as efficient intermediate hosts for the local strain of the parasite. Future changes may occur in this parasite-intermediate host complex.

*Reclamation and Rehabilitation
of Lands*

There is no considerable movement in this regard in endemic areas of schistosomiasis in the Orient. In China (Mainland), control efforts include the installation of better drainage in order to obviate snail habitats and probably also to convert low-lying land to agriculture, but details as to the extent of the effort are not available. In Japan, improved drainage has been one of the schemes associated with the control programme. A vast marsh near Ukishima in Shizuoka Prefecture has been reclaimed for rice production. In the Philippines, land reclamation on an experimental basis in Leyte has proved to be an important contribution to control. It remains to be seen whether initial costs and subsequent maintenance will be such that the programme can be extended to other endemic areas.

Migrations

These have not figured materially in extending the distribution of schistosomiasis in the Orient, with the exception of the Philippines. Here, the opening of virgin lands in Mindanao has resulted in the creation of new endemic foci and will probably continue to do so.

Itinerant labour

This factor is of little importance in the epidemiology of the disease in the Orient.

Lower Animal Reservoir Hosts

S. japonicum commonly infects a large variety of domestic and feral animals. In some parts of the Orient, these reservoir hosts no doubt contribute to the maintenance of infection and must be reckoned with in efforts to control the disease.

In China (Mainland), more than 30 species of lower animals have been found infected, including cattle, water buffaloes, horses, donkeys, mules, mice, wildcats, badgers, etc. Heavy mortality has been recorded in certain instances from S. japonicum infection in cattle and goats. Cattle, goats, dogs and various rodents are infected in Japan. In the Celebes, dogs and deer are reported to carry the parasite. S. japonicum occurs in dogs, swine, carabao, cattle, goats and rats in the Philippines. PESIGAN et al. [1958] indicated that the cow had the highest relative transmission index and the rat the lowest. The dog index was higher than that of the human and second to that of the cow. The authors believed that it was imperative to keep the cow and the dog population in check in endemic areas. LEE and WYCOFF [1966] failed to find S. japonicum in rodents in two endemic localities in Thailand. In China (Taiwan) where human schistosomiasis does not occur, the parasite infects dogs, water buffaloes, pigs, goats, wild rats and other small mammals.

The Americas

Changes in Behavioural Characteristics of Hosts

A significant reduction in intestinal schistosomiasis has taken place in Venezuela within the past two decades. In 1946, in the Municipality with the highest infection rate (Tejerias, Aragua), the percentage of infected children below 10 years of age was 71.4 and persons above that age 70.4. In 1963, 6% of the children under 10 years of age and 16.3% of individuals above that age were infected. Part of the decrease can be attributed to molluscicides and to chemotherapy. In addition, a considerable role was played by an intensive sanitary programme to avoid contact of people with infested waters. It is apparent that the populations in endemic areas have learned to utilize the new facilities and to this extent their habits have changed materially.

In Surinam, there is no marked evidence of change of host characteristics as regards exposure. Rice culture is probably one of the most important causes of infection; recreation is also involved. The level of sanitation is relatively low and canal water is used for household purposes and for bathing. Population pressures and concentration near the coastal area, which is better adapted to farming, tend to aggravate the schistosomiasis situation.

Snail intermediate hosts of *S. mansoni* in Brazil are distributed in various kinds of habitats. *B. glabrata* is found in sluggish streams, ponds, borrow pits, vegetation-clogged irrigation canals, rivers and lakes. *B. straminea* occurs more frequently in seepage areas, small ponds, low marshy tracts and borrow pits. *B. tenagophila* is found in the southern parts of Brazil and in much the same habitats as *B. straminea*. Contact of the people with one or more of these types of infested waters is a daily occurrence. There is no evidence that human habits have changed materially in any of the endemic areas in Brazil. Geographical strains of snail hosts in Brazil vary considerably in their susceptibility to schistosome strains. Evolutionary changes in this regard may influence future transmission patterns.

Changes are taking place in the prevalence of schistosomiasis in some of the Caribbean Islands. Human infection has apparently disappeared from St. Kitts [FERGUSON et al., 1960]. A considerable reduction has occurred in Puerto Rico. Some of this is probably due to sporadic control procedures but probably more to the economic rehabilitation of the Island and the higher living standards of the people. Industrialization has removed a portion of the population from the rural areas, while emigration has resulted in many infected individuals leaving the Island. The past three decades have witnessed a material reduction in the extent of the disease, and changes in behavioural practices of the people have no doubt contributed to this result. Schistosomiasis seems to have declined in Antigua, although the reasons for this are not clear. In St. Lucia, the disease is still a problem, as it is in the French Islands.

Reclamation and Rehabilitation of Lands

In endemic areas in the Western Hemisphere, this factor has little influence on schistosomiasis, except in reverse order. The opening-up of virgin lands in Southern Brazil has brought many infected persons from the northeastern part of the country and has resulted in new foci. However, elaborate plans are being made for land reform in the north-east. No doubt, new irrigation projects will be instituted, thus creating favourable conditions for the spread of the disease, unless adequate preventive measures are taken.

Migrations

The extensive migration to the south of Brazil has been mentioned. In other endemic areas in the Americas, migration has played little part in the extension of schistosomiasis.

Lower Animal Reservoir Hosts

Natural infection with *S. mansoni* have been found in a considerable number of lower animals in Brazil, including a number of wild rodents, an opossum and cattle. The precise role of these animals in the transmission pattern has not been determined but should be taken into consideration in connexion with control campaigns.

References

AYAD, N.: Bull. Wld Hlth Org. *14:* (1956).

AZEVEDO, J. FRAGA DE: Rapport sur les bilharzioses humaines au Cameroun français. WHO unpublished document, WHO/Bilh. Conf./49 (1956).

BLAIR, D. M.: The relation between economic development schemes and bilharziasis. WHO unpublished document, Bilh./Exp. Com. 3/WP/22 (1964).

FAROOQ, M. *et al.:* Bull. Wld Hlth Org. *35:* 281, 293, 319, 331 (1966).

FERGUSON, F. F.; RICHARDS, C. S.; SEBASTIAN, S. T., and BUCHANAN, I. C.: Publ. Hlth, Lond. *74:* 261 (1960).

GAUD, J.: Bull. Wld Hlth Org. *13:* 209 (1955).

GILLET, J. and WOLFS, J.: Bull. Wld Hlth Org. *10:* 315 (1954).

KHALIL, M. and AZIM, M. A.: J. Egypt. med. Ass. *21:* 95 (1938).

LEE, H. F. and WYKOFF, D. E.: J. Parasitol. *52:* 323 (1966).

MORAIS, T. DE: in Proceedings of the Sixth International Congresses on Tropical Medicine and Malaria, vol. 2, p. 183 (1958).

NELSON, G. S.: Personal commun. (1965).

OLIVIER, L.J. and MCMULLEN, D.B.: in Proceedings of the Seventh International Congresses on Tropical Medicine and Malaria, vol. 2, p. 24 (1963).

PESIGAN, T.P. *et al.:* Bull. Wld Hlth Org. *18:* 345 (1958).

PROTHERO, R.M.: Bull. Wld Hlth Org. *24:* 405 (1961).

WITTENBERG, G. and SALITERNIK, Z.: Bull. Res. Counc. Israel B *6:* 107 (1957).

WRIGHT, C.A.: Trans. roy. Soc. trop. Med. Hyg. *57:* 142 (1963a).

WRIGHT, C.A.: Bull. brit. Mus. (nat. Hist.) Zool. *10:* 259 (1963b).

Chapter 4

Epidemiology and Control of Schistosomiasis, pp. 250–336
(Karger, Basel and University Park Press, Baltimore 1973)

The Dynamics of Transmission[1]

N. G. HAIRSTON

Introduction

Schistosomes exist through the common presence of their definitive and intermediate hosts, but their transmission consists of a series of events whereby the parasite population perpetuates itself. All of these events involve rates: rates of reproduction in the two hosts, rates of survival within hosts, and rates of survival in the brief periods when the parasites exist away from their hosts. A complete understanding of transmission requires the measurement of these rates, and of the factors in the environment which determine their magnitude. Although the measurements themselves, and the methods devised to obtain quantitative data, may be extremely varied, the focal point of all work on the transmission of schistosomes should be the population of parasites. It is not always easy to view the whole physical, biological, and social environment from the standpoint of a schistosome population, but persistent attempts to do so will give unity to separate studies, which might otherwise yield results whose terms and units are not compatible, and which would thus be of only peripheral interest in terms of the central problem.

Needless to say, no complete quantitative description has yet been made of the dynamics of any schistosome population. It is encouraging to note, however, that attempts are being made [HAIRSTON, 1962, 1965a; MACDONALD, 1965]. The attempt itself, no matter how unsuccessful, helps to identify critical

---

1   While data published after May 1966, when this chapter was last revised, could not be included the basic principles remain unchanged.

observations that remain to be made, and requires that all relevant data be placed in the same framework. It is optimistic, but not impossibly so, to hope that the epidemiology of schistosomes will reach the stage where quantitative predictions are possible, and that is the ultimate goal of any science.

Studies on the transmission of schistosomes may be thought of in terms of three levels of sophistication: the establishment of the fact of endemicity in a given area, the measurement of the level of endemicity, and the measurement of the rates involved in the dynamics of transmission. These levels are not completely separate, but they represent a series of increasing commitments in terms of the requirements for their investigation.

After brief statements of the personnel and material resources needed to carry out investigations at each level, this chapter will continue with descriptions of how such studies are carried out, of the problems that will be encountered, and of the ways in which results may be interpreted.

The primary aim is to present the current knowledge on the epidemiology of schistosomes, rather than to provide a complete set of instructions for conducting research in the field. For the benefit of those readers who are preparing to undertake such studies, descriptions are given of the precautions that have been found to be important. Although these parts of the chapter have been written in the form of instructions, this has been done for convenience of presentation, and it is not intended to imply that the instructions are complete in all aspects. Details of methods and techniques have been specifically omitted, as they have been placed together on pages 620–748.

Requirements for Studies of Transmission

Before studies of the transmission of schistosomes are attempted, it should be understood that the type of study should be commensurate with the resources available to the investigator. Useful information can still be obtained by conscientious individuals working alone, especially in areas where little is known of the distribution of the parasites and their hosts. In many places, however, the endemicity of the disease is thoroughly established, and much background information is already available on the prevalence of the parasite in the human population and on the nature and distribution of the intermediate hosts. In such situations, it is pointless to repeat studies already done, unless there is reason to question the results. The requirements for further progress in knowledge in such places involve a sophisticated approach, and good resources in personnel and equipment.

Adequate Staff

Preliminary Observations

The fact that the disease is endemic in a given locality can be established by one person with a minimum of equipment. He may find, however, that an extraordinary amount of persistence is necessary to obtain the required information. This is especially true with regard to the location of snail hosts and the presence of infection in them.

Staff Requirements
for Measuring the Level of Endemicity

The decision to measure accurately the level of endemicity in any locality represents a serious investment in trained personnel and equipment, and also requires dependable transportation.

In addition to the director of the work, two professionals should be recruited at this stage, because their specialized knowledge will be required for proper completion of the studies. They are a field biologist with training in quantitative methods, and a qualified engineer with special knowledge of water management.

More important than the size of the staff is the attitude of all personnel. Measurement is a quantitative expression, and the numbers obtained must be reliable because of the human tendency to accept them as an exact representation of the facts. Rigorous attention to all details is, therefore, an absolute requirement. The person in charge must be willing to supervise all aspects of the work personally and, if at all possible, he should participate in it. In this way, technicians are constantly reminded that their efforts are important and that the results which they obtain are subject to scrutiny. The director who remains behind his desk will doubtless obtain impressive-appearing tabulations of results, but he has no way of knowing whether they are real or invented.

The number of technicians needed for the measurement of the level of endemicity depends, of course, upon the size of the area to be covered, and especially upon the number of categories into which the human population is to be divided. These categories will be discussed later.

If they are properly trained and equipped, a staff of 4 to 6 technicians could make all necessary observations on a sample of 2,000 people in an area of 50 to 100 km² in one year. They could also obtain reasonably complete data on the distribution of host snails in the area, and carry out minimal studies on seasonal changes in abundance and infection of the intermediate hosts. This estimate is based upon the assumption that the area under investigation is accessible to a laboratory, so that no more than 10 to 25% of the working time is consumed in travel.

It will be most convenient if all technicians are trained in all of the methods used. Such a procedure allows for flexibility of assignment, and has the added benefit of preventing the attitude that some positions carry higher prestige than others.

Staff Requirements for Measuring Factors in the Dynamics of Transmission

The accurate quantitative evaluation of the factors determining the rates of transmission of the parasite requires a major research effort. Not only is it necessary to have a large number of good technicians (15 or more), but the quality of the staff at the professional level must be exceptional. In addition to highly competent professionals of the kinds already specified, there should be an epidemiologist or a population ecologist. Unless a staff member is thoroughly efficient in statistics, the permanent or frequent assistance of a biometrician is essential to success.

It should be obvious from the foregoing statements that few, if any, countries with endemic foci are able to undertake a research project of the magnitude required to obtain all of the needed information. Such a project would almost certainly be international in personnel and support. Certain aspects of the problem can be attacked piecemeal, and valuable information can be obtained by a smaller staff than the one outlined above. This is only true if the quality of the work is high, and if it is planned and carried out with the over-all problem in mind.

Adequate Facilities

Location

Laboratory work plays an important part in all investigations on schistosomes, and if the effort involves more than establishing the fact of endemicity, it is essential that the laboratory should be located in the endemic area. At least 25% of the working day is lost if the laboratory is an hour's drive away from the area where transmission is taking place. The requirement of having a laboratory in the endemic area may pose serious problems of staff accommodations, and may in fact preclude serious studies in some endemic areas. It is an important consideration in selecting an endemic area for epidemiological analysis.

Laboratory Facilities

Requirements for Establishing the Fact of Endemicity

The fact that transmission is occurring in a locality can be demonstrated with a minimum of equipment. A microscope, ordinary laboratory glassware, and some kind of snail-collecting equipment would be needed. A small amount of space in a laboratory with running water would be desirable, but not absolutely essential.

Requirements for Measuring the Level of Endemicity

As will be explained below, many examinations are needed for confidence in the results of a parasitological survey. This means that in order to complete the survey within a reasonable time, a number of examinations must be performed each day. It is estimated that two or more compound microscopes would be required, plus sedimentation glasses and other glassware. For snail studies, two stereoscopic dissecting microscopes are needed, as are specific tools for quantitative sampling of the snail population. Details of requirements will become apparent from a study of the techniques used, as described on pages 620–748.

For such quantitative studies, a laboratory is required, with microscope benches, a chemical bench, and storage facilities. Running water is a necessity. It is estimated that not less than 10 m² of floor area is needed for each technician.

Requirements for Measuring Rates
in the Dynamics of Transmission

In the preceding estimates of requirements, the minimum necessary for completion of the work was stated. Measuring the factors influencing transmission requires the complete facilities of a modern parasitological laboratory. These need not be described in detail, because anyone undertaking such a study would be familiar with the equipment and space necessary. It will suffice here to remind the reader of the necessity for dependable supplies of water and electricity, and of the requirement for the maintenance of large numbers of experimental hosts, both mammals and snails.

Transport

Dependable transportation is absolutely essential to all but the simplest type of study.

Establishment of the Fact of Endemicity

Investigation of the Disease in Man

The first step is to search for infected people by means of random stool or urine examinations in clinics, in hospitals, or in occasional surveys among school-children, villagers, or other convenient groups. Records from hospital pathological laboratories are often a valuable source of preliminary information. Some of the newer and more specific serological techniques may be of value for survey purposes.

Determination of Distribution

Before a rational decision as to control can be made or a suitable plan envisaged, the extent of the endemic area must be established. This can be done by examining relatively small numbers of faecal and urine specimens from a large number of localities in the suspected area. Such data need not necessarily be quantitative since their only object is to define more precisely the limits of the infected area. Mapping of the results while this work is in progress will assist in the selection of places to be added to the study.

Investigation of the Snail Host

Usually, the discovery of autochthonous cases leads to the search for, and implication of, the snail intermediate host. In any endemic area one species of snail is primarily responsible for the transmission of each species of schistosome. Occasionally, more than one species is involved. Often, closely related snails which do not serve as intermediate hosts will also be present; differentiation of these forms from the intermediate host or hosts is important.

The control plan depends very heavily on information relative to the snails, since these are to be the object of attack. It will be necessary, at least in the early phases of the snail investigation, to have advice and help from specialists, because snail control involves attacking snails in their habitats with a minimum of disturbance to man, his crops and his animals. Such an attack calls for an intimate and detailed knowledge of the local snails. The usual sequence of investigation is as follows:

Search for Possible Intermediate Hosts

Initially, there must be a widespread search for snails which might be involved. In the Orient the hosts are operculate snails belonging to the genus *Oncomelania*. In other areas the hosts are usually pulmonate snails belonging to the sub-families Planordinae and Bulininae; but *Ferrissia tenuis*, belonging to the family Ancylidae, is said to serve as the intermediate host for *Schistosoma haematobium* in a focus in India. These molluscs and closely related species are found in other endemic areas and should not be ignored. The recognition of the species of snail which is transmitting the disease in a given area requires the skill and experience of a field biologist who must know which snails to seek and where they are likely to be found.

Proof of Involvement

When snails suspected of harbouring the schistosome are found they must be tested to find out whether, in fact, they can convey the infection. Proof that a particular species of snail transmits the disease, by demonstrating that it can pass the infection, requires the expert assistance of an experimental biologist. Three methods of approach are possible:

(a) Examination of wild snails for naturally-acquired infection: Specimens collected throughout the endemic area can be examined for naturally-acquired schistosome infection by the inspection of crushed individuals. The method used in making examinations by crushing snails is given on page 663. This can demonstrate whether schistosome infections are harboured, but will not conclusively prove that the schistosomes found are indeed the species infecting man, since the cercariae of schistosomes infecting domestic and wild animals resemble those of the human parasites.

In searching for naturally-infected wild snail hosts it should be constantly borne in mind that not only may the occurrence of the snails be a seasonal phenomenon but also infection with schistosome larvae may show seasonal fluctuation. Therefore, it might be necessary to search for infected snails through a period of at least one year.

(b) Infection of laboratory animals with wild cercariae: Infection of schistosome-free laboratory animals with cercariae collected from naturally-infected snails permits the rearing of the adult worms, which can be more readily and certainly identified than the larvae and immature forms. It is necessary, however, to have available a stock of schistosome-free test animals, usually rodents, together with the means of maintaining and handling them. Accurate identification of the adult parasites is also required.

(c) Infection of healthy snails with miracidia from human infections: Additional proof that the real intermediate host has been found comes from infection of uninfected snails with miracidia obtained from human infections and the subsequent emergence of cercariae which can be used to complete the life cycle in the laboratory.

Identification

If the trials outlined above indicate that a snail species can serve as the intermediate host, it then becomes desirable to obtain positive specific identification. This may be done locally if a sufficiently skilled malacologist is available. Otherwise specimens should be sent to a central reference laboratory such as the WHO Snail Identification Centres under the direction of Dr. G. MANDAHL-BARTH at the Danish Schistosomiasis Laboratory, Danmarks Akvarium, Copenhagen, Denmark, and under the direction of Dr. W. LOBATO PARAENSE at the Institute of Biology, University of Brasilia, Brazil.

Methods for collecting the snails, transporting them to the laboratory and preparing them for identification, are outlined on pages 658–673.

Specific identification of the suspect or proven intermediate host may not be absolutely necessary to the development of a snail control programme. It is only essential to have adequate proof that a recognizable, but not necessarily identified, species is the host. In any event, positive identification should follow as soon as possible, since the biology of the species incriminated may have some bearing on control procedures.

In some localities incrimination of the snail host is not very difficult since there is only one species belonging to the taxonomic group to which the known hosts belong; and the number of other schistosomes which might be confused with the schistosomes of man is very limited. In other localities, however, the task can be very difficult indeed and may require both the expenditure of considerable time and effort and the aid of specialists.

Measurement of the Level of Endemicity

Once it has been demonstrated that transmission of human schistosomes is taking place in an area, the next logical question to be answered concerns the seriousness of the problem. Obviously, if few people are involved, some other health problem may well take precedence. If, however, a large proportion of the people are infected, serious consideration should be given to means of controlling transmission of the parasite. It is, therefore, important to know, with reasonable accuracy, the number of people in the endemic area and the proportion infected. Measurement of the level of endemicity implies that control of the parasite is being contemplated. It is, therefore, essential that studies be conducted on the distribution and seasonal abundance of the snail intermediate hosts. This information will determine the method and timing of snail control operations.

Some foreknowledge of approximate epidemiological happenings in the area should be sought through an exploratory field survey. The initial survey provides useful information on the variability of the components involved and the rates of infection to be expected in the area, so that sample size and design can be determined. Also, it allows for the testing of techniques, training of technicians, and pre-testing the tentative record forms that have been prepared. It further helps considerably in establishing procedural details regarding a preliminary educational programme to gain the co-operation of villagers in order to reduce non-response to a minimum, in standardizing field procedures in the collection and transport of samples, and in setting up survey schedules.

Prevalence in the Definitive Host

The proportion of hosts found positive on examination is the prevalence of the parasite. It is customarily reported as a percentage, and is usually thought of as representing the percentage of the population that is infected at the time of the survey. In the case of the schistosomes, this is not entirely accurate, and if the concept is extended to include the probability of becoming infected, it can be very misleading, as will be demonstrated below. One reason for these statements is that the prevalence of the parasites is different in different age groups of people, and correct interpretation of the data requires that prevalence be reported separately by age.

Sampling

Examination of the entire population in an endemic area is neither possible nor desirable in the great majority of cases, and the information gained would not compensate for the effort spent. It is only where the population consists of 2,000 people or less that all persons should be examined. In all other cases, a sample of the population will be selected for study. Inasmuch as the situation in the entire population will be evaluated from the findings on the sample, *it is absolutely essential to take great care in the selection of the sample, which must be representative of the population from which it is drawn.* A sample that is taken because the subjects are accessible, co-operative, or under some form of discipline is unlikely to represent the population properly. For example, if school-children are selected as the representatives of their age group in the sample, and if only half of the children in the area attend school, a biased sample has been drawn, and the data may not be used in making conclusions about the relationship between prevalence and age, nor may they be used in determining the incidence of the disease. Bias can be avoided only if sampling is random. This means that each individual has an equal chance of being included among the subjects chosen for examination. It is clear that true random sampling requires a census. In most cases, the available census figures will be outdated, even if they are available, and the investigators will have to conduct a census for themselves. Each person in the population should be assigned a number, and a sample of predetermined size selected by the use of a table of random numbers.

In some areas, the principal obstacle to carrying out a census is the fact that few, if any, people know their own ages. This is particularly true of older people, who often estimate their ages to the nearest five years. In such situations, it may be possible to obtain reasonably accurate estimates of age by relating each individual's birth to one of a series of significant and easily remembered local events.

a) The Size of the Sample to Be Examined

The size of any sample used to estimate a proportion may be determined in advance by the accuracy demanded of the estimate. The larger the sample, the more accurately the prevalence in the sample reflects the prevalence in the whole population, a relationship that is shown in figures 1, 2, and 3 for actual observations that have been reported. The data for *Schistosoma japonicum* are taken from PESIGAN *et al.* [1958a]; those for *S. haematobium* come from FAROOQ *et al.* [1966]. Study of the graphs shows that there must be an optimal number of examinations. Where the number is low (50 or less), the confidence

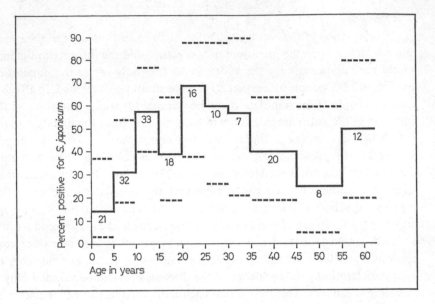

Fig. 1. Age-prevalence histogram for *S. japonicum* in Bagahupi, Leyte, Philippines. The upper and lower 95-percent confidence limits for each age group are shown as broken lines above and below the histogram. Numbers indicate the number examined in each age group.

interval is so wide that the observed percentage is not meaningful. On the other hand, the examination of very large numbers does not achieve a compensatory reduction in the width of the confidence interval. The reason for this is that the width of the interval is related inversely to the square of the number of examinations, so that in order to reduce the interval to half its width, it is necessary to examine four times as many people. The numerical relationship between sample size and the 95-percent confidence limits for various observed percentages is given in table VIII, on page 732.

The characteristics of the age-prevalence histogram can be demonstrated adequately if no fewer than 125 to 150 people are examined in any age group. It appears that around eight age groups are necessary to describe the relationship between prevalence and age, and therefore between 1,200 and 1,600 examinations should be made if the investigator is to have confidence in the results.

Because the number of people available for examination declines with age, it may be necessary to use wider age bands after the age of 30 years. However, where sudden ecological changes are occurring as the result of the intro-

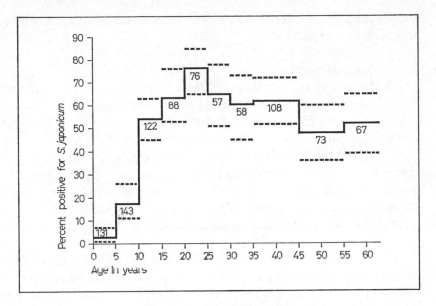

Fig. 2. Age-prevalence histogram for *S. japonicum* in Coastal Division of Palo, Leyte, Philippines. The symbols are the same as for figure 1.

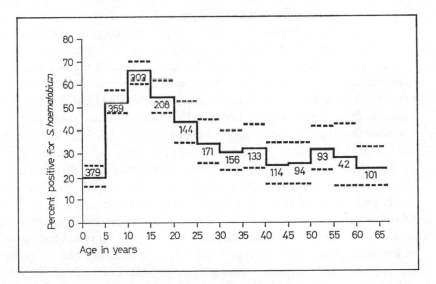

Fig. 3. Age-prevalence histogram for *S. haematobium* in Control Division of Egypt-49 Project Area. The symbols are the same as for figure 1.

duction of irrigation schemes there may be an increased incidence in older age groups requiring special study.

b) Stratified Sampling

Within nearly all endemic areas, there is reason to suppose that some parts of the population are less exposed to the parasite than others. Prevalence in urban areas, for example, is usually lower than in rural villages. Snails may also be much more abundant and widespread in part of the whole area than elsewhere, and this factor also causes heterogeneity of prevalence data. In cases where such areas of differing endemicity can be recognized and determined with reasonable accuracy, it is best to sample the population separately for each area. It is undesirable to pool data from obviously heterogeneous groups, since the results would be without meaning.

The process of sub-dividing the total population on the basis of prior knowledge is called stratified sampling. Each group so defined is then sampled independently of the other groups. It is obvious that many other possible sub-divisions can be made in addition to those already mentioned, and additional to the well-known variations in prevalence between the sexes and between persons of different ages. Occupation, recreational habits (swimming), religious practices, and level of education have all been shown to influence the prevalence of schistosomes [PESIGAN et al., 1958a; FAROOQ et al., 1966]. A simple exercise in geometrical progression will show that complete stratification before sampling would require an impossibly large number of examinations. The preliminary divisions of the population must, therefore, be made with care, so that the confounding of factors influencing the observed prevalence is kept to a minimum. By 'confounding' is meant the determination of a result by two or more factors, each to an unspecifiable extent. For example, if persons following a certain occupation live mostly within a single area, and it is found that they have an unusually high or low prevalence, it is not possible to state to what extent the occupation or the area inhabited influenced the prevalence. If the decision is important epidemiologically, it may be necessary to design a new series of observations to resolve the matter.

In general, it is satisfactory to sub-divide the endemic area geographically into obviously different divisions, and then to make certain that sufficiently large random samples are taken from each division. The data from each sample may then be broken down to reveal differences between age and sex groups, and probably between some other groups as well. For each geographical division, the sample should contain 1,200 to 1,600 persons, as indicated in the foregoing section.

c) Cluster Sampling

The ideal sampling procedure described in the foregoing sections may prove to be very difficult to execute, especially where the area and the total population are large. Moreover, selecting individuals completely at random requires a large amount of extra effort in visiting different households in different villages, and in obtaining the co-operation of widely scattered individuals. In the Egypt 49 Project Area, these problems were overcome by using two-stage cluster sampling [FAROOQ and NIELSEN, 1966]. After the delimitation of area boundaries, the first stage consisted of drawing a random sample of the villages in each area, so that 20% of the population was included. The probability of drawing a village was proportional to its size. Within each village drawn in this manner, all households were assigned numbers, and a 25-percent sample of these households was taken at random. All members of each randomly selected household were then examined. In this way, a 5-percent sample of the entire population was obtained, and the subjects were grouped in households, a fact which permitted the concentration of effort in relatively few places. The method is not free from pitfalls, as the authors have pointed out; for example, small villages were under-represented in the sample, and moderately large ones were over-represented. Subsequent analysis of the data showed that this bias did not affect the prevalence figures that were obtained.

d) Sampling Reservoir Hosts

In areas where *S. japonicum* or *S. mattheei* is endemic, reservoir hosts play an important role in maintaining the level of parasitism. *S. mansoni* has also been found in a number of non-human mammals. It is important, therefore, to have information on the extent to which these animals are infected. Domestic animals may be sampled in much the same way as their owners. The most effective method would be to examine all domestic animals belonging to randomly selected households. Data on the total population of domestic animals are collected most efficiently by including appropriate questions at the time of the census of the human population [PESIGAN *et al.*, 1958a].

Wild mammals present great difficulties in the estimation of population size, and this should not be attempted in studies to establish the level of endemicity. Some of the smaller species, especially species of rodents, may be caught in appropriately baited snap-traps. Trap lines should be set shortly before dusk, and the traps picked up early the next morning. This timing takes advantage of the period of maximum activity of small mammals and also avoids, as much as possible, disturbance by people and most of the domestic animals. Specimens caught during the night should be examined immediately for the presence of schistosomes and their eggs. The method will not obtain all species in the area, and gives no indication of their true abundance. It does provide an estimate of the extent to which these animals are infected, and also reveals seasonal changes in transmission, since most small mammals have short average life spans. 'Live' traps for rodents may be preferred because this allows better examination for adult worms using perfusion methods.

Methods of Establishing Prevalence

Examination of persons selected for the sample may be carried out by either parasitological or immunological techniques. The details of techniques are given on pages 622–642. It is important to realize that no technique will reveal all cases, and the proportion detected on a single examination varies from one species of schistosome to another. With good sedimentation concentration methods of detecting eggs in stool or urine samples, the following proportions of all positives have been obtained on the first of a series of examinations: S. japonicum 93.5%, S. haematobium 88%, and S. mansoni 80% [PESIGAN et al., 1958a; FAROOQ et al., 1966]. In areas where both parasitological and immunological tests can be carried out on the sample people, the combination of results will reveal information that could not be obtained by either technique alone [HAIRSTON, 1965b].

The figures quoted for S. japonicum, S. haematobium and S. mansoni are mentioned as an indication of what might be found in heavily infected, endemic areas. In areas of low endemicity with low density infections, the technique will be less reliable.

It should be emphasized that immunological tests are of value in preliminary screening but that prevalence data for studying the dynamics of transmission must be based on the demonstration of eggs in the urine and faeces.

Whatever technique is chosen, it should be standardized before the sampling begins, and should be adhered to *rigorously* throughout the survey, and in all subsequent surveys, to determine the effect of control efforts. It is imperative to resist the temptation to adopt a new technique because it is claimed to be more sensitive than the one already in use. Failure to heed this warning can result in the invalidation of much work. The precaution should be carried to the point of using the same technicians throughout the study, if this is at all possible. Regardless of the thoroughness of their training, poeple vary in their ability to carry out routine duties, and any factor which could increase the variability of results may lead the investigator to make false conclusions. Programmes which were executed in excellent fashion from other

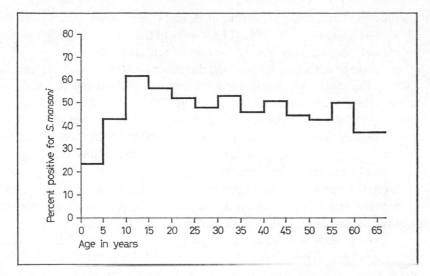

Fig. 4. Age-prevalence histogram for *S. mansoni* in Control Division of Egypt-49 Pro-
ect A rea. Note differences from histogram for *S. haematobium* in same area.

standpoints have yielded inconclusive data because sampling procedures were
changed by new technicians.

The Interpretation of Prevalence Data
a) The Relationship with Age

A complete set of prevalence data can yield valuable information on the
epidemiology of schistosomes, provided that the data were taken from an area
that is reasonably homogeneous in snail abundance and in human habits.
Under these conditions, the relationship between prevalence (as determined
by the examination of excreta) and age forms a histogram, the shape of which
reflects characteristics for each of the common species of human schistosomes.
In areas where the endemic situation has remained essentially unchanged for
many years, the prevalence of all three species rises usually to a maximum
between the ages of 10 and 25 years. Thereafter, prevalence decreases with
age, and frequently reaches a more or less constant value above the age of 35
to 40 years. Typical age-prevalence histograms for *S. japonicum, S. haematobium*, and *S. mansoni* are shown in figures 2, 3, and 4, respectively. The fact
that prevalence declines with age after reaching a peak can only mean that
parasitological evidence of infection is lost among at least part of the infected

population. Thus, if the prevalence at 10 to 14 years of age is 65%, and that at 40 to 44 years of age is 25%, at least 40% of the older age group have lost their infections, in many cases in the face of repeated exposure.

The shape of the histogram must, therefore, be determined by at least two factors: the rate at which infections are acquired and the rate at which they are lost [HAIRSTON, 1965b; MUENCH, 1959]. The combination will determine the height of the peak prevalence and the age at which it is reached. There is some evidence that the two rates are inversely related, so that infections result-ing from frequent exposures are lost less rapidly than are those resulting from occasional exposures which presumably give lighter worm loads. Thus, the younger the age of maximum prevalence and the higher this peak is, the greater the rate of transmission in the area. Such comparisons apply only within a species of schistosome, as will be discussed below.

These observations lead to the important conclusion that it is not necess-ary to invoke differential susceptibility to account for the failure of the histo-grams to rise to 100%. By appropriate calculations, it can be shown that under the interpretations made, all negative persons over the age of 25 to 30 years can be accounted for as having been positive at an earlier age and as having lost their infections. Confirmation of this conclusion comes from data on skin-test surveys, which show a continuous rise in percent positive with age, until a very high proportion of persons over 25 years old give a positive reaction.

A simple report of the over-all prevalence for an area, therefore, will be likely to give the impression that the situation is less serious than the true picture indicates.

The preceding comments apply to areas where transmission has been more or less constant for a number of years. The interpretations do not apply in places where this is not the case, where large numbers of uninfected immi-grants have moved into an endemic area, or where changes in land use, as by increased irrigation, have greatly increased the extent of snail habitats. These areas may be considered epidemic in nature probably for many years. In such places, the prevalence may not decline with age, since the decline implies long previous experience with the parasite. Stratified prevalence data from epidemic situations are likely to reflect differential exposure to snail-inhibited water, and may provide indications of the most urgent needs for safe water supplies, or for priorities in snail control efforts.

b) Comparisons between Species

In hyperendemic areas *S. haematobium* usually yields age-prevalence histograms having a characteristic difference from those seen in the other two species. There are exceptions in areas of low endemicity and it has been suggested that the histogram characteristics vary with different strains of the parasite in East Africa. The decline in prevalence after the age at which it is highest is much more marked for *S.haematobium* than for *S.japonicum* or *S.mansoni*. Parasitological evidence of infection is therefore lost by far the most rapidly in the case of *S.haematobium*. The basis of this phenomenon is not known, but it could be related either to the difference between the normal locations within the host, or to intrinsic differences between the parasites. Whatever the cause, even in areas of high endemicity, the proportion of older people who pass eggs of *S.haematobium* tends to be much lower than is the case with other species. One result of this fact is that in areas with similar transmission rates, the over-all prevalence of *S.haematobium* is lower than that of *S.mansoni*. In fact, even in the same area, *S.mansoni* may have a higher total prevalence than *S.haematobium*, though its incidence is appreciably less [FAROOQ *et al.*, 1966; FAROOQ and HAIRSTON, 1966]. Incidence, as will be described later, is the rate at which negative people become positive.

   c) Prevalence in Reservoir Hosts
   The prevalence of schistosome species in various mammal hosts is an important piece of information, for two reasons. The first reason is that these animals may act as important reservoirs for infecting snails, particularly where *S.japonicum* is the parasite. The demonstration of importance of reservoir hosts would have a serious influence upon plans for a control campaign, since it would lessen the value of treatment and of sanitation, and place more importance on snail control and on the provision of safe water supplies. The second reason for determining the prevalence of schistosomes in non-human mammals is in the interpretation of infections in snails. It is not feasible to distinguish the cercariae of many of the species of mammalian schistosomes, including human ones, and some species not parasitizing man use the same species of snails as do the human schistosomes in the same area. Their presence thus complicates the interpretation of snail infections, since seasonal changes would mean less in terms of planning a control campaign.

   Changes in prevalence among wild animals are difficult to interpret. It has been suggested that such changes might provide a sensitive index of epidemiological events, and might give early indications of success of control operations. Several observations in the case of *S.mansoni* have shown that marked decreases in prevalence among wild mammals may occur in the absence of control effort. It appears, therefore, that it will be necessary to know the population dynamics of the species of wild mammals involved before changes in prevalence are understood. This requires a specialized research effort, and is not recommended in connexion with studies of the type described in this section.

Intensity of Infection in the Definitive Host

Ideally, the intensity of infection refers to the actual worm load in the vertebrate host. In most instances, direct observation through counts at autopsy will not be possible without a specific research effort, as is discussed later.

Egg-Counts in Human Excreta

It is generally agreed that there is a definite relationship between the intensity of infections and the amount of disease in the population. It is thus important to attempt to assess intensity by any means available. If all other factors were equal, there would be an easily specifiable relationship between prevalence and the intensity of infection [HAIRSTON, 1962, 1965a]. The relationship depends upon the assumption that the distribution of worms among hosts is similar in all areas endemic for a given species of schistosome. This assumption does not appear to be tenable, except under very similar conditions of human habits and snail distribution. The difficulty can be illustrated with a hypothetical and somewhat exaggerated example. If 50% of a single age group is positive, and if the worms are distributed completely at random among the population, the average load of reproductive female worms would be about 1.4 per positive person [HAIRSTON, 1965a]. The situation may be such that some people are much more likely to be exposed than others, either because of their habits, or through residence near concentrations of snails. In such a case, the mean worm load could be much higher, as much as 10 to 20 reproductive females per positive person, with the same prevalence of 50%. Such a distribution would also indicate very high worm loads in at least part of the population.

Since prevalence does not appear to be completely satisfactory as an index of intensity, much attention is being given to the use of egg-counts as a more accurate reflection of the worm load. Up to the present, it has not been possible to establish a direct relationship, and the value of egg-counts is in comparing one area with another. Comparisons between age groups are hazardous, especially among those ages which include and follow the age of maximum prevalence.

If egg-counts are used to assess the level of endemicity, rigorous care must be taken in selecting the subjects for examination. They must be drawn at random from the entire age group in the particular area under study. It is not valid to select only those persons known to be passing eggs, because counting techniques are uniformly less sensitive than the concentration techniques used in establishing prevalence. This means that the zero values that are inevitably obtained for some people known to be passing eggs cannot be handled statistically unless the known negatives are added to them.

In calculating statistics from egg-counts, the actual counts themselves should be the starting point, rather than the number of eggs per unit volume of urine or the number of eggs per unit weight of stool. It is advisable to make each count as a constant fraction of the person's daily output of urine or faeces, because of the variability in output by different people, especially where there is a reasonable amount of variation in ages among the subjects, as among children up to 4 or from 5 to 9 years of age.

Because of the large variance among egg-counts, it has been found advisable to compare geometric means, rather than arithmetic means. The appropriate techniques of making egg-counts are given on pages 622–634, and in the papers of BELL [1963] and BRADLEY [1965]. The method for statistical treatment of the data is to be found on pages 731–733.

Worm Loads in Reservoir Hosts

The abundance of worms in non-human mammals can, of course, be observed directly by killing the animals and searching the appropriate blood vessels. In addition to searching in the hepatic portal system, where most of the worms are located, the liver and lungs should be cut into pieces, crushed between glass plates, and examined for worms and their eggs. Perfusion is advisable for smaller animals.

This procedure is, of course, impractical for domestic animals. For the smaller ones, such as dogs, cats and pigs, purchase of as many as possible is advisable. Each individual should be followed for at least three days with careful egg-counts. The animals should then be killed and searched for worms. It is possible that a regression of mean egg-count on the number of reproducing female worms can be established from a reasonably small series of animals of each species, although the variation around the regression line is almost sure to be great. Such data would help in the interpretation of more extensive egg-count data.

In all data on reservoir hosts, care should be taken to keep separate records for each species of host. For wild animals, the assistance of a mammalogist will be required. The staffs of museums of natural history are ordinarily very helpful in such matters, provided that they are approached in advance.

Incidence

In contrast to 'prevalence', which is static, the term 'incidence' carries the dynamic implication of a change in time. The distinction has not been made as regularly as it should be in the literature on schistosomes, and some authors have used the two terms interchangeably. Incidence should mean the rate at which uninfected people become infected per unit of time. It is conventionally expressed as percent per annum in work on schistosomes [PESIGAN et al., 1958a; FAROOQ and HAIRSTON, 1966].

It is most appropriate to carry out the observations on young children, because most of them have not been infected previously. It has been found that incidence increases with age in this group, and a large series of children from infants to 8- or 9-year olds should be followed in making the necessary observations. Examinations should be made at one-year intervals on the same individuals. When intervals other than 12 months are used, the data can be converted to an annual basis by the use of the formula

$$I = \left(1 - X^{\frac{12}{y}}\right) 100,$$

where I is the annual incidence in percent, and X is the proportion remaining negative for y months. The formula assumes a constant monthly incidence, and is, therefore, the less reliable the more transmission is restricted to a short season.

Measures of incidence are affected by two unavoidable factors: the fact that not all positives are detected by a single examination, and the fact that a surprisingly high proportion of cases becomes negative spontaneously, especially among children up to 4 years of age. In Egypt, it was estimated that the effect of these two factors, especially the latter, was to cause an underestimate of the incidence by 21% of the true value in S. haematobium, and by 30% in S. mansoni [FAROOQ and HAIRSTON, 1966].

Despite the difficulties, incidence is a much more sensitive index of changes in transmission than is prevalence, and will yield evidence of success of control measures within one year, as opposed to the two to five years required for prevalence to change by a convincing amount.

Studies on the Intermediate Host in Assessing Endemicity

Few scientific subjects are likely to seem so esoteric or to be so far removed from the ordinary experience of public health officials as the distribution and population dynamics of snails. These factors must be determined, however, because snail control is so important in efforts to combat the disease, and is the chief method that has so far yielded scientifically acceptable evidence of success in arresting transmission of the parasite.

The Distribution and Ecology of Snails

As the evidence implicating the intermediate host accumulates, the distribution of the suspected snails should be plotted on the basis of widespread collections. If the prevalence or severity of human infection seems to warrant it, all potential or known habitats for the snails should be mapped. Such information will not only assist in evaluation of the magnitude of the problem but will also be needed should snail control be attempted later.

It is essential to discover the exact distribution of the snail hosts, since this will indicate the true limits of the zone in which transmission can occur. This information is required in order to select the control methods giving the best cost-efficiency ratio, and to determine the feasibility of a control programme. The distribution of the snails is established by systematic search of all potential snail habitats. Usually, it is necessary to bring sample collections to the laboratory for confirmation of field identification. It is not necessary to measure accurately the density of the snail populations at this time, although it is valuable to record a rough estimate of the snail density for each habitat detected in order to gain a useful impression of the habitat preferences of the snails, which can be taken into account later when reliable population density studies are planned.

These snail searches for the purpose of establishing the geographical limits of the intermediate host must be carried out at regular intervals throughout at least two years, since there may be considerable variation in distribution of the snails from season to season. In some areas snail distribution may also vary from year to year.

Study of bionomics. Before any valid decisions can be taken in connexion with a substantial programme of snail control, a systematic study of the bionomics of the snails must be instituted, since anti-snail measures can only be effective and efficient if they are based on sound and thorough knowledge of snail habits and ecology. Here again, the expert assistance of a field biologist is necessary, since the investigations required involve familiarity with the snail life cycle and a broad understanding of freshwater biology and ecology. Included in the study should be the reproductive habits, life-span, seasonal cycle and population trends, capacity to withstand drying or life out of water, habitat preferences and other characteristics of the snails; the impact upon them of seasonal, climatic, topographic and hydrographic conditions, and the variations in prevalence of snail infections from place to place and from season to season.

Such evidence gives important indications as to the time and places of transmission, and can assist greatly in the selection of points and seasons at which the snails can be attacked. It also provides a rational foundation upon which assessment of the prospects of successful control through a campaign directed against the snail host can be based.

It is not possible to specify all the procedures to be used in obtaining this information concerning the snails, but some further details regarding procedures and techniques are given on pages 658–674. As already stated, it is necessary that the investigations be directed by a trained biologist.

In addition to the biological studies involved, it will be necessary to have detailed information on certain other factors. The amount, distribution and types of all bodies of water and damp and marshy areas within the endemic region should be investigated and mapped. Seasonal variation in rainfall and annual amount of rainfall are both important in relation to snail control measures, their chances of success and the time at which they should be attempted. Other climatic factors, such as the amount of solar radiation, daily and seasonal temperature variations, and humidity may be important.

Abundance of Snails

A study of the snail populations must be carried out with as much care and as much attention to statistical precautions as is the study of the parasite in the human population. After the general search for snails described above, it will usually be found that the habitats have certain characteristics which will allow them to be grouped into categories. Lakes, permanent ponds, temporary ponds, flowing natural streams, pools in intermittent streams, irrigation canals, drains, spring seeps, swamps, and rice-fields are among the types of habitat that are commonly recognized. In planning studies on the snail population, it is important that representative examples of the different kinds of habitats in the area be selected for study. This preliminary selection is as important as is the preliminary stratification of the human population, since it has been observed that populations of the same species may show marked differences in seasonal abundance in different situations. For example, *Bulinus (B.) truncatus* in Egypt reaches a very high peak of abundance in May and June in the irrigation canals. In drains, however, it reaches maximum densities in January, and with less seasonal difference than is found in the canals [DAZO *et al.*, 1966].

Depending upon local circumstances, 5 to 20 habitats should be selected for population studies. It is important that they represent the variety of situations in which snails occur, and that at least two of each kind of habitat be studied. The latter requirement will help the investigator to avoid mistaken interpretations based on atypical events. A final factor which should enter into the choice of habitat is the fact that infections in the snails will also be determined. The habitats should, therefore, include a variety of degrees of probable human contact.

Each habitat selected should be sampled systematically at monthly intervals for at least a year. Sampling techniques and precautions regarding snail sampling are described on pages 668–673. The method used varies widely with the kind of habitat sampled, but it is important that the method chosen obtains a constant proportion of the snails actually present. It is essential that the technique be standardized before the start of data collection, so that all results may be compared.

Interpretation of snail population data. In many areas, snail populations follow an easily demonstrable cycle of abundance over the year. Changes may involve differences of the order of tenfold or more. In the case of such dramatic changes in density, it is unnecessary to resort to statistical analysis of the data. It should be remembered, however, that snails ordinarily have patchy distributions, even in habitats that appear uniform to the human observer, and that this patchiness causes the average density in samples to have very wide confidence limits. It is common for the upper 95-percent confidence limit to be at least 160% of the mean, and for the lower 95-percent confidence limit to be 50% or less of the mean. From these figures, it can be seen that it is difficult to demonstrate the statistical significance of differences that seem superficially to be fairly large. If such differences seem to be important in the investigation, the only method of narrowing the confidence limits is to increase the number of samples.

In this connexion, it should be remembered that even in the field many species of snails are capable of doubling their populations in two to three weeks when conditions are most favourable. The evidence for this is given in some detail in the paper by DAZO *et al.* [1966].

In addition to the large sampling error, there is a precaution involving the under-collection of small sizes of snails. Even the most efficient and exhaustive collecting methods fail to obtain young snails in their true proportions. The loss may amount to 95% or more of the youngest age category (up to 15 days after hatching), and snails a month or more old may still be under-collected to a marked degree. Less precise collecting methods often fail to obtain young snails in any significant numbers at all.

This error has frequently caused misinterpretations in regard to the most favourable season for the snail population. The apparent abundance, as revealed by monthly collections, only reflects the abundance of the sizes that are collectable. If these sizes are of snails whose average age is 6 weeks to 2 months, it is clear that the true maximum population size must occur 6 weeks to 2 months before it is observed in the samples. Such facts have an important bearing on the timing of snail control efforts. The quantitative collection of snail eggs in such cases will help the investigator to obtain a more accurate picture of the timing of changes in population density than will the collection of snails alone. Unfortunately, the collection of snail eggs is not always feasible; this is generally true of the genus *Oncomelania* and is also true of *Bulinus (Physopsis)* species in many habitats in Africa. The identification of snail eggs requires practise. Careful study of eggs of known parentage should be carried out in the laboratory before identification of field material is attempted.

Infections in Snails

The proportion of snails infected with schistosomes at any given time depends upon a complex interaction of factors. The most important of these are the distribution and behaviour of definitive hosts, the relative susceptibility to infection of the strain of intermediate host, and such climatic factors as temperature and rainfall. The complete resolution of this complex requires a research effort that is beyond the scope of most anti-schistosome services. Approaches to this research problem will be described later.

In the present context, the information that should be obtained is the proportion of snails infected in a variety of locations, and at all seasons. Ideally, the snails collected for population studies should provide sufficient data on infections. In practice, it may prove to be difficult or impossible to obtain sufficient numbers of snails under the important requirements for population sampling. A study of table II, page 708, will demonstrate the difficulty. Low percentages are the rule, as shown in table I, and the statistical table shows that 500 to 1,000 snails must be examined in order to keep the 95-percent confidence limits within a factor of two of the observed rate, when

Table I. Seasonal changes in the proportion (%) of snails infected in three different endemic areas

A. Oncomelania quadrasi/Schistosoma japonicum – Philippines

Site	1954			1955/56							
	17 May–4 June	16 Aug–1 Sept.	18 Oct.–11 Nov.	10 Jan.–4 Feb.	22 March–5 April	6 May–8 June	12 July–22 July	15 Aug.–27 Aug.	10 Oct.–9 Nov.	3 Dec.–23 Jan.	15 Feb.–12 March
Colony 1	0	0.89	1.79	1.76	3.36	0.81	0.62	6.43	10.06	4.04	3.40
Colony 2	1.49	1.59	5.00	5.51	5.80	3.69	1.85	0.67	4.55	4.52	5.90
Colony 3	0.29	0.25	0.62	26.76	27.92	7.59	6.09	9.99	4.33	4.46	12.96
Colony 4	0.28	3.09	1.47	1.89	6.27	1.62	1.61	0	0.88	3.95	2.42
Colony 5	0.38	1.41	1.27	4.74	2.36	0.31	0.26	0.87	2.64	1.99	3.69
Av. by snails	0.48	1.21	1.76	14.67	11.64	3.75	3.01	5.33	5.16	3.94	7.61
Av. by colonies	0.49	1.45	2.03	8.13	9.14	2.80	2.09	3.59	4.49	3.79	5.67

B. Bulinus (Ph.) nasutus productus/Schistosoma haematobium – Tanzania

	Year	Jan.	Feb.	March	April	May	June	July	Aug.	Sept.	Oct.	Nov.	Dec.
Number of habitats	1960	6	14	15	17	17	19	17	13	11	9	12	16
	1961	18	16	16	17	17	19	18	15	–	–	–	–
Mean monthly snail density	1960	57.0	25.6	35.2	44.5	86.6	69.3	69.7	51.9	34.4	57.5	36.7	38.7
	1961	40.7	61.2	47.3	58.8	70.5	75.3	66.8	66.5	–	–	–	–
Mean monthly S. haematobium infection rate, %[1]	1960	0.3	0.8	0.9	2.8	6.6	12.5	7.7	12.6	0.8	0	0.5	0.2
	1961	2.0	1.8	2.9	0.8	1.5	3.3	5.1	7.5	–	–	–	–

1 Calculated from the total number of snails taken monthly and taking into consideration the number of habitats holding water and available for sampling each month.

C. *Bulinus (B.) truncatus/Biomphalaria alexandrina* – Egypt
(*Schistosoma haematobium/Schistosoma mansoni*)

Month	Bulinus			Biomphalaria		
	Number of snails collected and examined	Number infected	% infected	Number of snails collected and examined	Number infected	% infected
1962						
March	1,081	2	0.18	786	0	0.00
April	1,922	4	0.21	2,458	2	0.08
May	913	2	0.22	1,248	1	0.08
June	2,095	22	1.05	2,158	71	2.82
July	1,702	20	1.17	16,967	156	0.92
August	1,679	7	0.42	13,831	152	1.10
September	507	7	1.38	10,563	105	0.99
October	1,675	3	0.18	15,248	114	0.75
November	1,485	1	0.07	10,720	92	0.86
December	2,611	21	0.80	4,128	12	0.46
1963						
January	3,382	4	0.12	2,283	22	0.96
February	904	0	0.00	899	2	0.22
March	2,807	0	0.00	7,223	15	0.21
April	2,040	9	0.44	11,815	28	0.24

1 to 2% of the snails are found infected. Except where snails occur in very dense populations, as in the case of *Oncomelania quadrasi* [PESIGAN *et al.*, 1958b], the collections from population studies are unlikely to yield sufficient numbers of snails for the accurate determination of the proportion infected. The amount of effort required to take a large enough number of quantitative samples will frequently exceed the resources of most units.

In such cases, the strict quantitative sampling must be supplemented by methods which yield snails in sufficient numbers. It is necessary to emphasize the fact that the supplementary data should not be used in assessing changes in population density, since the effort required to obtain large numbers of snails will be greater at seasons of low snail density, and the standardization of the effort may be as laborious as direct quantitative sampling. Although the determination of the proportion of snails infected may be performed without quantitative sampling, there remain scientific precautions which must be

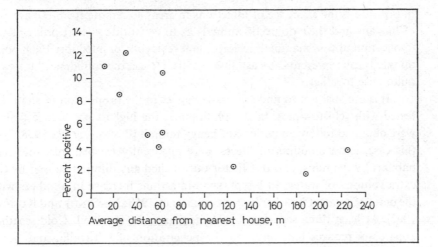

Fig.5. The relationship between proximity to houses and prevalence of *S. Japonicum* in *O. quadrasi* in Palo, Leyte, Philippines [graph constructed from data in PESIGAN *et al.*, 1958b].

taken. Because of the importance of the location of the collecting sites, collectors must avoid expanding or contracting the area of any pre-determined location, and the collections should be taken with as uniform an effort as is possible over the site. A second precaution concerns the part of the snail population that is obtained in non-quantitative collections; the techniques employed uniformly fail to obtain representative numbers of smaller snails and, since these are ordinarily less heavily infected than the larger specimens, the data tend to be biased towards higher prevalence rates. The true prevalence in seasons of intense breeding of snails will, therefore, be over-estimated relative to seasons when breeding occurs less rapidly.

Whatever method is used in assessing infections in snails, the observations should be repeated regularly over at least one full year.

Interpretation of snail infections. Subject to the statistical limitations that have been described, the interpretation of snail infection data is straightforward. An example of the relationship between the location of habitats and the average proportion infected is given in figure 5. The association between high prevalence and proximity to houses is quite clear, especially when it is noted that the habitat most out of line was an area of intense human activity, even though it was more than 60 m from the nearest house. Of equal interest in this case is the existence of infections in areas so remote from the activity of humans and their domestic animals as to constitute virtual proof of the implication of wild mammals as important reservoirs of infection. Each point on this graph represents at least 3,600 snails. Hence, the confidence limits are quite close together.

It is unusual not to find seasonal changes in the proportion of snails infected with schistosomes. In the Philippines, the highest prevalence figures were obtained following periods of heavy rainfall [PESIGAN et al., 1958b]. In this case, extra amounts of faeces were apparently washed into the snail habitats by the rains, and this factor outweighed any dilution caused by the extra volumes of water. In Egypt, snail infections increase in numbers with the onset of summer weather [VAN DER SCHALIE, 1958; EL-GINDY and RUSHDI, 1962]. At least three separate factors appear to be involved. Cold weather apparently reduces hatching and the penetration of miracidia, and warm weather induces much more extensive human contact with water, especially in the form of swimming and bathing. In Lake Province, Tanzania, where S. haematobium is transmitted in small temporary ponds, snail infections increase as long as the ponds hold enough water to make them attractive as sites for bathing [WEBBE, 1962a]. Mention should be made of delayed maturation of pre-existing infections in hibernating snails in cold weather and in aestivating snails in habitats that have dried out in hot weather.

From these examples, it can be seen that information on snail infections is important in planning measures against the parasite. In Egypt and in Tanzania, snail control should be initiated before the annual wave of new infections begin to produce cercariae. In the Philippines, by contrast, location is the most important factor, and attention to snail habitats should begin near houses and work outward, and seasonal factors are less important.

Measurement of the Factors in the Dynamics of Transmission

At the beginning of this chapter, it was pointed out that transmission of schistosomes is best thought of as a series of rates. It is convenient to visualize these rates within the framework of the life cycle of the parasite. Starting at any point in the cycle, the consecutive events would then be described in terms of the successive rates of reproduction and survivorship[2]. There is no ideal starting point in the life cycle, since the determination of each step depends on

2   Survivorship here means the proportion of organisms surviving per unit of time.

knowledge of both preceding and successive steps. Thus, if the cycle is presented as a linear series of events, there must be overlap between the beginning and the end of the series. Starting with the eggs in the excreta, the following are the rates which are known to be involved:

Survival of eggs that reach the excreta of the definitive host
    Hatchability
    Survival of hatchable eggs
        Probability of being deposited in water containing snail hosts
        Survival of miracidia while free in the water
        Probability of locating and penetrating a host snail
        Probability of establishing an infection after penetration
Survival of, and reproduction by, larval stages in the snail host
    Survival of mother sporocysts
    Reproduction by mother sporocysts
    Survival of daughter sporocysts
    Reproduction by daughter sporocysts
    Survival of snail host before the production of cercariae
    Survival of snail host after the start of production of cercariae
    Probability of cercariae escaping from the snail host
Survival of cercariae
    Survival of cercariae while free in the water
    Probability of coming into contact with a definitive host
    Probability of successful penetration of the skin
Survival of young schistosomes in the definitive host
    Survival during migration through skin, lymph glands and lungs
    Probability of finding the appropriate blood vessels
    Survival in appropriate blood vessels until maturity
Survival of, and reproduction by, adult worms
    Probability of locating a mate
    Reproduction by the female schistosome
    Survival of adult worms
    Survival of the definitive host during infection
Probability that eggs will reach the excreta of the definitive host.

A consideration of the foregoing list makes it clear that the three rates of reproduction must compensate for the various death rates, in order for the parasite population to maintain itself.

From a practical standpoint, it is not necessary to consider each of the foregoing rates as a separate entity, and many excellent studies have been carried out by combining several of them. Perhaps the commonest approach has been to regard the events in the mammal host as comprising no more than one or two steps. Thus, the cercariae injected into, or applied to, the skin of the host are counted, and the results are evaluated in terms of the number of eggs reaching the faeces, or of the number of adult worms recovered. The host is thus regarded as an unknown mechanism for converting cercariae into eggs or adults with a discoverable efficiency. For some experimental purposes, this is a legitimate approach, at least in the initial stages of an investigation. For this presentation, however, it seems more appropriate to take each step separately, and to state what is known quantitatively of the probability of success of the parasite, and of the factors influencing the probability. Significant observations that include groups of steps will be included after the steps involved are described separately. As will be evident in what follows, much more is known about some steps than others. In all stages of the life cycle, the available estimates have an unfortunately high variance. Any studies that will reduce this disparity will, of course, be significant contributions to the quantitative description of the dynamics of transmission of the parasites.

The Fate of Eggs in Excreta

From the standpoint of the parasite, the success of eggs is an apparently simple fraction, namely, the proportion of eggs available that succeed in establishing infections in snails. Thus, the average number of snails becoming infected per day is equal to the number of eggs passed in faeces per day, multiplied by the probability that an egg will be able to hatch, the probability that an egg will be deposited in a snail-inhabited area, the probability that the miracidium will succeed in penetrating a snail, and the probability that the infection will succeed in the snail. In mathematical symbols, this would read:

$$\frac{S}{D} = \frac{E}{D} \times h \times d \times p \times i.$$

S is number of snails infected; E is number of eggs in faeces; D is days; h is probability of being able to hatch; d is probability of being deposited near snails; p is probability of penetrating a snail; i is probability of establishing an infection in the snail after penetration.

The equation can be solved for $(d \times p \times i)$ if the available data can be used to estimate the rate at which mammal hosts pass viable eggs, and the rate at which snails become detectably positive for infection. The individual factors in the equation may be difficult and complex.

The Enumeration of Eggs in Excreta

The first requirement for an estimate of the daily output of schistosome eggs in an area is a knowledge of the number of definitive hosts that are present; the second requirement is a knowledge of the prevalence of the parasite in the definitive host; the third requirement is a knowledge of the average number of eggs passed by each infected host per day. The quantitative measurement of these factors has already been described (pp. 258–270). It only remains to discuss the sensitivity of egg-counting techniques. Within limits, sensitivity is not very important in establishing the relative intensity of infection in two or more areas. In making a quantitative estimate of the probability of success of an egg, however, it is important to obtain accurate information on the total number of eggs passed daily in the area under study. Therefore, all positive cases should be detected by the egg-counting technique used. BELL [1963] has estimated that the use of the MIFC technique to concentrate the eggs of *S.mansoni* before filtering the sediment, increases the sensitivity of the examination by a factor of five. The disadvantage of the method is that the MIFC technique has a less than perfect efficiency of extraction, approximately 80 to 90%. With a combination of MIFC with BELL's filtration the passage of 200 to 250 eggs per day is detectable with 95% confidence. By approximately doubling the effort, it is theoretically possible to detect an infection with a single reproductive female *S.mansoni*. This species, as will be described later (p. 300), lays the lowest number of eggs of any of the human schistosomes, and there is thus no necessity for making extrapolations based on dubious assumptions about apparently negative cases.

The Viability and Hatchability of the Eggs that Escape into the Excreta

It is a common observation that eggs of abnormal appearance occur in urine and faecal samples. The abnormality may be obvious, as in the case of calcified and blackened eggs, immature eggs, and those in which internal structure is clearly malformed, or the egg may be of normal appearance with the miracidium showing no sign of life. By visual observation, between 60 and 70% of the eggs of *S. japonicum* passed by humans appear to be normal, in that they contain a mature, moving miracidium [BANG and HAIRSTON, 1946; Dr. A.T. SANTOS, personal commun.]. Not all of the eggs of normal appearance, however, are able to hatch. PESIGAN *et al.* [1958a] found that of 4,608 eggs from the faeces of people of all ages, only 1953, or 42.4%, produced miracidia.

Except for casual comments and for follow-up studies of treatment, quantitative data are scarce on the hatchability of the eggs of *S. mansoni* and

S. haematobium. Two adult cases with the latter parasite yielded 86.6 and 74.1% hatchable eggs [DAVIS, 1966].

If, in any particular area, a serious attempt is made to analyse the dynamics of transmission, it will obviously be necessary to determine the hatchability of eggs for the local species or strain of parasite in different age groups.

Factors influencing hatchability. PESIGAN *et al.* [1958a] give data showing significant differences in the hatchability of *S. japonicum* eggs from people of different ages. Children in the 10- to 14-year age group yielded eggs with a hatching rate of 48.4%. The percentage was lower among both younger and older people, being 40% in young children and 37.7% in people over 15 years old. The decrease after 15 years of age is probably related to immunity; the increase after the age of 10 is more difficult to explain. The authors found more illness among the 10- to 14-year-olds than in any other group, and it is possible that the greater hatchability is related to the physiological state of the host.

Among physical factors, light, temperature and pH have been found to be important influences on hatching [INGALLS *et al.*, 1949].

Survivorship after Hatching

Once a mature, hatchable egg arrives in the excreta, its chances of success are affected by a series of influences of a very different kind from those to which it has been subject since its deposition in the wall of the gut or bladder. As indicated earlier, at least three sets of factors are extraneous to the resources of the egg: the habits of the host, the weather, and the distribution and abundance of the snail host. Two sets of factors depend upon the intrinsic potential of the miracidium: its survival in the water, and its ability to find and penetrate a snail of the correct species.

a) The Probability of Being Deposited in Water

The chance of success of a schistosome egg is dependent upon the place chosen by its host for depositing the excreta. A general consideration of the facts indicates that in most endemic areas the habits of people in this regard are more likely to favour than to hinder the parasite. Concealment is usually sought, especially for defaecation, and the most obvious sources of concealment are high vegetation and moderately high banks. Both high vegetation and banks are very commonly associated with water, and to this attraction is added the general desirability of having the faeces washed away, either immediately or when the water level rises. In the study referred to above, HAIRSTON [1962] calculated that the eggs of *S. japonicum* were one and a half times to twice as successful in reaching snail habitats as they would have been had the faeces been deposited randomly in the area concerned.

These and other considerations have frequently led to attempts to interrupt transmission by campaigns for the construction and use of latrines, or to correlate the prevalence of the parasites with the failure to have or to use latrines. Latrine-building campaigns have been uniformly unsuccessful in producing more than transient effects [CHANDLER, 1954; PESIGAN et al., 1958c]. This does not invalidate their logical desirability, but indicates that they are generally unacceptable to most people who have habitually disposed of their excreta in the open.

It is completely unreasonable, of course, to expect latrines to be effective against S. haematobium. It is generally agreed that for this parasite the most important source of infection of snails is micturition by children while swimming.

Correlations between the absence of latrines and the prevalence of the parasites are suspect, because it is not possible to separate the possession of a toilet from a generally higher economic condition. Thus, the toilet per se may only be an indicator of a series of factors which tend to reduce prevalence.

Studies of a sociological or anthropological nature, when designed to have relevance to the interruption of transmission, should concentrate upon learning enough about the habits, customs and beliefs of the people so that those in charge of control programmes can design acceptable alternatives to the dangerous habits leading to the infection of snails.

In areas where S. japonicum or S. mattheei are endemic, reservoir hosts may be more important than humans in contributing to snail infections. In such cases, careful studies should be made on the local distribution and abundance of these animals, and on the relationship of their distribution to that of snails. Where domestic animals are the principal reservoirs, the studies present no great problems. It is very difficult, however, to obtain accurate estimates of the numbers of wild mammals present in an area. If such studies are important to an understanding of the dynamics of transmission, it is necessary to obtain the assistance of a mammalogist specializing in population dynamics.

The actual method that has been used to estimate the probability of success of eggs in excreta will be presented below.

b) The Survivorship of Miracidia

The free-living stages of schistosomes do not feed, and must rely on energy stored before leaving the hosts. In the case of miracidia, this energy is

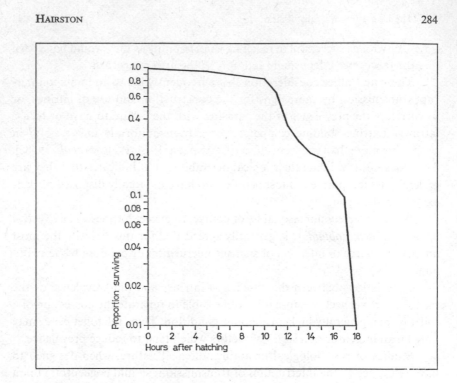

Fig. 6. Survivorship of miracidia of *S. japonicum.*

provided by the female worm before the eggs are laid. Under these conditions, it is to be expected that survivorship will be good until the energy supply is nearly exhausted, and that this more or less fixed period will be followed by one of a high death rate. Figures 6, 7, and 8 show that this expectation is borne out for all three species. All have good survival until between 8 and 10 h after hatching. The miracidium must find and penetrate a snail of the appropriate species during this period, or be lost to the population.

c) The Ability of Miracidia to Establish an Infection

The question of specific attractiveness on the part of the snail host for the miracidium has been studied by a number of workers. Some have failed to perceive any such phenomenon while FAUST and HOFFMAN [1934] thought that the miracidia were attracted by mucus secreted by the snail host. ETGES and DECKER [1963] endeavoured to quantitate experimental results which seemed to indicate a positive chemotaxis on the part of *S. mansoni* miracidia for *B. glabrata.* When the snails were crushed prior to exposure of the mira-

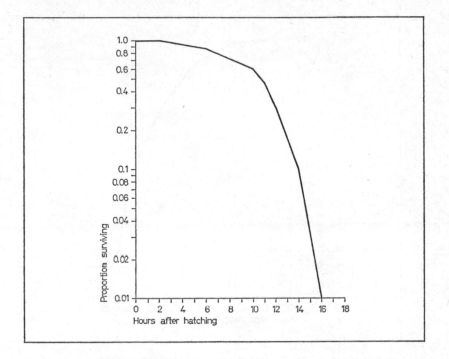

Fig. 7. Survivorship of miracidia of *S. mansoni.*

cidia there appeared to be a slight repulsion, an observation somewhat in accord with the findings of MICHELSON [1964] of miracidia-immobilizing substances in extracts prepared from snails infected with *S. mansoni*. BARBOSA [1965] stated that penetrating trophism in the miracidia of *S. mansoni* is by no means specific, since they will penetrate freshwater snails of the families Physidae and Ampullariidae and eagerly attack and enter the skin of tadpoles. PESIGAN *et al.* [1958b] thought that miracidia of *S. japonicum* appear to be stimulated occasionally by some substance emanating from the snail. However, CHERNIN and DUNAVAN [1962] could not accept evidence that snails attract miracidia. Thus, direct orientation towards the snail appears to be lacking. However, contrary to such evidence, WEBBE [1966] considered on the basis of experimental data that water velocity may enhance the effective scanning capacity of miracidia so that snail hosts may be located and infected under conditions of high water velocity and low miracidia pressure. The somewhat contradictory evidence appears to be reconcilable by separating the phenomenon of attraction from that of stimulation [DAVENPORT *et al.*, 1962].

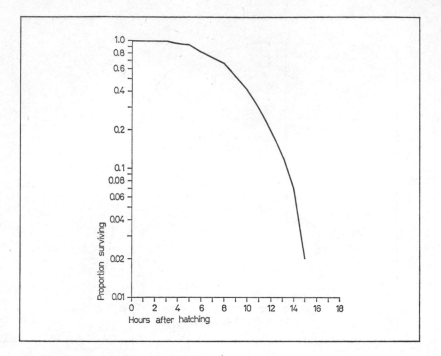

Fig. 8. Survivorship of miracidia of *S. haematobium.*

They present photographic evidence that the miracidium of *S. mansoni,* while not showing directional movement towards the host extracts, undergoes a rapid change of direction in swimming. This change in behaviour would keep the miracidium in the vicinity of the snail.

In spite of apparent inefficiency, miracidia in the immediate vicinity of snails usually appear to succeed in penetrating the tissues of the intermediate host. PESIGAN *et al.* [1958b] found that one third of the miracidia of *S. japonicum* placed with one or two snails had penetrated the tissues within 20 min. If it can be assumed that the success rate is constant up to the 10-hour duration of good survival, virtually all miracidia coming within the appropriate distance from snails will be successful in penetrating them.

Successful penetration does not guarantee the establishment of an infection. In the experiments of PESIGAN *et al.* [1958b], only 44 to 68% of the snails entered by a single miracidium ever produced cercariae. Similar figures were obtained by PERLOWAGORA-SZUMLEWICZ [1964] for *S. mansoni.* In order to improve on the percentage, many workers expose snails to five or more miracidia. This seems unrealistic from the low percentages of snails that are found infected in nature, although both sexes of cercariae have sometimes been recovered from single naturally-infected snails, thus demonstrating that they had been infected with at least two miracidia.

d) The Influence of Weather on the Success of Schistosome Eggs

Unless the eggs of schistosomes are deposited directly into snail habitats, their fate depends very largely on their immediate physical environment. If the excreta are exposed to direct summer sunlight or to strong desiccation, the chances of the contained eggs are very slight. If the excreta are deposited near snail habitats in moist, shady places during cool or wet weather, the eggs have a much better chance of eventually reaching the water. Seasonal changes in the proportion of snails infected are the rule, and it seems likely that the weather is directly responsible for many of the seasonal differences. In the Philippines, heavy rains are followed by increases in snail infections [Mc-MULLEN, 1947; PESIGAN et al., 1958b].

Weather may also determine the availability of snails to become infected. This is particularly true in areas where the habitats dry out completely between rainy seasons, as in Lake Province, Tanzania [WEBBE, 1962a], or in northeastern Brazil [BARBOSA, 1962].

The weather also has an indirect effect on the fate of schistosome eggs through its influence on human activity. Warm weather induces much greater contact with water, especially in the form of bathing and swimming, during which occupation micturition releases the eggs of S. haematobium directly into the water. This is generally agreed to be the cause of increased snail infections during the summer months.

Analysis of the Fate of Schistosome Eggs

The equation presented on page 280 provides a convenient framework for obtaining an estimate of the proportion of eggs passed that succeed in infecting a snail. The methods of obtaining the terms E/D, h, p, and i have already been given. In the village for which the analysis was actually performed, (E/D × h was found to be 8.32×10^5; p was estimated as virtually 1.0; and i as 0.44 to 0.68. Therefore, if an estimate can be made of the number of snails becoming infected per day (S/D), it will be possible to calculate the one term for which no direct observation is possible. This is d, the proportion of eggs actually reaching a snail habitat.

The number of snails becoming infected daily can be calculated from the following information:

The average number of positive snails present. This information came from repeating sampling of all snail habitats, and was found to be 4.38×10^5, of which 2.80×10^5 were females and 1.58×10^5 were males.

The average length of life of an infected snail, estimated from laboratory and field studies as 51.3 days for females and 37.6 days for males.

The survival of infected snails during the 30 days between becoming infected and becoming demonstrably positive. From observed death rates, this was estimated as 0.557 for female snails and 0.446 for males.

The standing crop, divided by the mean length of life, gave estimates that 5,464 females and 4,193 males became positive daily. Dividing these numbers by the respective survival figures gave the estimates that 9,801 females and 9,401 males became infected per day, as an average figure. Thus, $(d \times p \times i)$ can be calculated to be

$$\frac{1.92 \times 10^4}{8.32 \times 10^5}, \text{ or } 0.0231.$$

A hatchable egg, then, would have a probability of

$$\frac{0.0231}{1.0 \times 0.68} \text{ to } \frac{0.0231}{1.0 \times 0.44}, \text{ or } 0.034 \text{ to } 0.053,$$

of being deposited in a location where it could succeed in infecting a snail. The numerical values apply only to *S. japonicum* in an inland village in Leyte.

This approach gives a more reliable estimate where snail populations are essentially stable than in areas where the population and the proportion infected show wide fluctuations. In the latter case, intensive sampling would be required during the season of transmission in order to reach a satisfactory level of confidence in the results.

The Survivorship of Larval Stages in the Snail Host

As shown by the observations cited above (p.284,c), successful penetration of a snail by a miracidium does not mean automatically that cercariae will be produced. Some loss of larval stages, then, occurs during the period when the infection in the snail is still immature.

Survivorship in the Snail

Unfortunately, most of the data on the success of immature stages in the snail do not permit the distinction between successful penetration by the miracidium and survival in the tissues of the snail. This is frequently compounded by the use of five or more miracidia per snail. The latter practice provides a larger proportion of infected snails than does the use of a single miracidium per snail, but also seems to reduce the average success per miracidium. Thus, PITCHFORD and VISSER [1965], using five miracidia of *S.mattheei* for each specimen of *Bulinus (Physopsis)* spp. obtained cercariae from an average of 66.5% of the snails. The 33.5% not successfully infected represent the combined failures of five miracidia (and the sporocysts arising from them). It can be calculated that each miracidium had an average probability of failure of 0.8035, since $(0.8035)^5$ is 0.335. Thus, the average success of a miracidium up to maturity of infection was around 20%, not including the deaths of infected snails. The success rate per miracidium of both *S.mansoni* in *Biomphalaria pfeifferi* and *S.haematobium* in *Bulinus (Physopsis)* spp. was 8.6% in the same type of experiment.

The most complete data are those of CHU *et al.* [1966] from Iran. Their data, on the proportions of *Bulinus (B.) truncatus* becoming positive for *S. haematobium* following exposure to various numbers of miracidia, give the following estimates of average success:

Number of miracidia to which each snail was exposed	Proportion of surviving snails cercaria-positive	Average probability of success per miracidium
1	0.244	0.244
2	0.578	0.350
5	0.614	0.173
10	0.834	0.164
20	1.000	

Their text indicates that unfavourable conditions existed for the group of snails exposed to one miracidium each. Thus, the increase in success rate from one miracidium to two may have been an artifact caused by laboratory conditions. The decrease above two miracidia per snail appears to be valid, and is of interest. These estimates are all lower than the success rates of 41.5% obtained by PERLOWAGORA-SZUMLEWICZ [1964], using one miracidium of *S.mansoni* in *Biomphalaria glabrata*, or the 44 to 68% obtained by PESIGAN *et al.* [1958b] using one miracidium of *S.japonicum* in *Oncomelania quadrasi*.

After the infection in snails is mature, the proportion of snails producing cercariae rises rapidly to a peak or plateau, and gradually declines, sometimes over a long period, especially in cool weather [PITCHFORD and VISSER, 1965]. It is a common observation that during this period, cercarial production may be interrupted for days, weeks, or months. Under these conditions, it is almost impossible to be certain that the parasite has died or exhausted its reproductive capacity completely. PESIGAN *et al.* [1958b] found that spontaneous cure, if it occurred at all, was negligible in the case of *S. japonicum* in *Oncomelania quadrasi*, and McCLELLAND [1965] stated that there was no record of a cure of *Bulinus* infected with *S. haematobium*. Spontaneous cures of *B. glabrata* and *B. straminea* infected with *S. mansoni* have been reported [STIREWALT, 1954; BARBOSA, 1962], as have cures of *S. haematobium* in *Bulinus nasutus*.

The population of parasites is affected much more by the decreasing number of cercariae produced and by the death of the molluscan host, than it is by the actual loss of infections in the snails.

The Survivorship of Infected Snails

Schistosome infections are commonly observed to cause increased death rates in snails, although there are a few observations in which the survivorship was similar for infected snails and uninfected controls. Observed death rates in the laboratory are almost universally lower than are death rates in the field, where the latter have been estimated. The presence of an infection causes the death rate to be higher by a factor of from 1.3 to 3.5 in a variety of species (table II). The rates are, of course, much higher than would be expected in the laboratory.

The Rate of Reproduction in the Snail

Cercarial output has been studied in at least 18 species of snail hosts, infected with one or another of the three major species of human schistosomes [McCLELLAND, 1965]. The number of cercariae produced is related directly to the susceptibility of the snail to infection but, among more or less equally susceptible snails, the most important factor determining cercarial output is the size of the host. Thus, *B. glabrata*, the largest host of any human schistosome, has been recorded as yielding as many as 17,600 cercariae of *S. mansoni* in one day, and an average of 2,000 per day for three months. The African species of *Biomphalaria* are somewhat smaller than *B. glabrata*, and estimates of 250 to 600 cercariae per day encompass the range of values that have been obtained from them.

The hosts of *S. haematobium* do not equal the largest species of *Biomphalaria* in cercarial output, but average numbers range as high as 1,068 per day from *B. (Ph.) nasutus* [McCLELLAND, 1965].

CHU *et al.* [1966] obtained an average of 1,180 *S. haematobium* cercariae per day from one infected *B. (B.) truncatus* for a brief period, but their over-all means were only as high as 213 per day for the shedding life of the snail. The smallest host of *S. haematobium, Ferrissia tenuis*, is reported to shed only four or five cercariae at a time [GADGIL and SHAH, 1956].

In the case of *S. japonicum*, the snail hosts are much smaller than are most of the hosts of the other species. Under special conditions of forcing, PESIGAN *et al.* [1958b] were able to obtain an average of 160 cercariae in one day from *Oncomelania quadrasi*, but when the infected snails were allowed to shed cercariae naturally, the average was only 15 per day of shedding. Cer-carial production was not continuous in this species, and late in the infections there were many days in which none was produced at all. *O. quadrasi* is the smallest species of snail host for *S. japonicum*. Infected *O. nosophora* from Japan have been found to produce several times as many cercariae as *O. quadrasi*.

Table II. Calculated instantaneous death rates per day of uninfected and infected snails of various species in the field[1]

		Uninfected	Infected
Oncomelania quadrasi	females	0.010	0.019
	males	0.017	0.027
Bulinus (Ph.) nasutus		0.025	0.042–0.089
Biomphalaria sudanica		0.036	0.064
Bulinus (B.) truncatus		0.040	0.055
Biomphalaria alexandrina		0.043	0.056

1 Data for *O. quadrasi* from PESIGAN *et al.* [1958b] and HAIRSTON [1965a]; for *Bulinus (Ph.) nasutus* and *Biomphalaria sudanica* from WEBBE [1962a, b]; for *Bulinus (B.) truncatus* and *Biomphalaria alexandrina* from HAIRSTON [1965a] and DAZO *et al.* [1966].

The Net Reproductive Rate in Snails

The actual contribution of the average successful miracidium to the parasite population is usually considerably less than might be supposed from the quoted figures for daily cercarial output. This is partly because of a nat-urally greater interest in maximum than in minimum or mean numbers, and partly because survival of snails in the laboratory is nearly always better than that estimated for field conditions.

Table III. Ecological life tables for S. japonicum in the snail host[1, 2]

Age of infection	Survival of infected female snails (l_x)	Cercariae produced per infected snail (m_x)	$l_x m_x$ (females)	Survival of male snails (l_x)	$l_x m_x$ (males)
0	1.000	0		1.000	
5	0.907	0		0.875	
15	0.746	0		0.668	
25	0.614	0		0.510	
35	0.505	0		0.390	
45	0.416	12.98	5.400	0.298	3.867
55	0.342	55.50	18.981	0.228	12.654
65	0.282	54.09	15.254	0.174	9.412
75	0.232	37.84	8.779	0.133	5.033
85	0.191	30.77	5.877	0.102	3.139
95	0.157	15.80	2.481	0.078	1.232
105	0.129	11.34	1.463	0.059	0.669
115	0.106	22.27	2.361	0.045	1.002
125	0.087	7.43	0.646	0.035	0.260
135	0.072	3.77	0.271	0.026	0.098
145	0.059	1.27	0.075	0.020	0.025
155	0.049	3.80	0.186	0.015	0.057
165	0.040	9.39	0.376	0.012	0.113
175	0.033	17.29	0.571	0.009	0.156
185	0.027	15.93	0.430	0.006	0.095
195	0.022	7.74	0.170	0.004	0.031
205	0.018	0	0	0.002	0
215	0.015	0	0	0.002	0
225	0.012	0	0	0.001	0
235	0.010	0	0	0.001	0
			$\Sigma = 63.321$		$\Sigma = 37.843$

1 Differential survival of male and female snails requires separate life tables for the parasite.
2 HAIRSTON, N.G.: On the mathematical analysis of schistosome populations. Bull. Wld Hlth Org. 33: 45 (1965a).

The net reproductive rate is calculated as the sum of the products of the proportion of infected snails surviving to the mid-points of successive time intervals and the number of cercariae shed by the average snail during the same time intervals [BIRCH, 1948]. This is conveniently done as in table III. A column was prepared showing the mid-points (x) of successive 10-day intervals. The estimated proportions of infected snails surviving to these mid-points (l_x) are then entered in the adjacent column. The mean cercarial ouput per infected snail during each 10-day interval (m_x) is entered in the third column, and the fourth column contains the successive products ($l_x m_x$). The sum of the $l_x m_x$ entries is the net reproductive rate, which thus includes the deaths of infected snails before cercariae are produced, but does not include losses of miracidia which penetrate but fail to establish infections in the snails.

The table shows some important points. The first of these is the significance of survival in the estimation of the net reproductive rate. An average daily output of 500 to 1,000 cercariae sounds impressive, but if the daily death rate is only 0.05, the net reproductive rate will be only 1,500 to 3,500. There-fore, the actual contribution of the average successful miracidium is much less than is frequently assumed from observations of the gross reproductive rate (the sum of the m_x column), which is most frequently cited in the literature.

A second point worth noting is the importance of producing large num-bers of cercariae early in the infection. Not only does the parasite take advan-tage of a higher probability of survival, but the cercariae have an important advantage in time. A cercaria produced at the peak of the $l_x m_x$ column (50 to 60 days after infection) would, if successful, have grown to maturity and laid nearly, 45,000 eggs within two months. Some of these would have infected snails and be well on the way to producing cercariae of their own before the original infection was more than half way to its termination. This property is known as the reproductive value of an organism [FISHER, 1958; SLOBODKIN, 1961], and is strongly dependent upon its age and the shape of a curve de-scribing the $l_x m_x$ column. The parasite, therefore, gains greatly by a rapid in-crease to maximum cercarial output. Findings similar to those shown above have been reported by PITCHFORD and VISSER [1965] for snails infected with S. mansoni, S. haematobium and S. mattheei. The cercarial output data of CHU et al. [1966] are somewhat different, and indicate a more prolonged increase in output per snail. Their data showing the proportion of snails shedding, however, are in agreement with those of PITCHFORD and VISSER [1965].

The Fate of Cercariae

The probability of success of a cercariae is the ratio between the number infecting mammals in a given area and the number shed into the water in the same area per unit of time. Stated in terms similar to those on page 280, the number of flukes successfully infecting mammals per day is equal to the number of cercariae shed per day multiplied by the probability that a cercaria will reach a mammal, and the probability that the infection will succeed in a mammal, or

$$\frac{F}{D} = \frac{C}{D} \times c \times m.$$

F is number of flukes infecting mammals; C is number of cercariae shed; D is days; c is probability of reaching a mammal; and m is probability of maturing in a mammal. The equation is solved for (c × m), after which m is calculated as a separate term (p. 298).

The Survival of Cercariae in the Water

Like the miracidia (p.283,b), the cercariae are dependent upon their stored energy for survival, and curves describing their survivorship are similar in shape (fig. 9 and 10). The cercariae of both *S. japonicum* and *S. mansoni* have low death rates during the first day of their existence; thereafter the rates increase sharply, until virtually all are dead after two days. Survival has been shown to be adversly affected by a temperature of 36 °C, and by ultra-violet light.

STIREWALT [1964] reported a decrease in penetration by cercariae after only 8 h, and OLIVIER [1966] showed that in the laboratory under favourable conditions the infectivity of *S. mansoni* cercariae fell to one-half in eight hours and to one-tenth of the maximum in 14–15 hours.

The Influence of the Habits of the Definitive Host on the Success of Cercariae

In any consideration of the epidemiology of schistosomes, it must be borne in mind that while the snail is, by definition, the intermediate host, man himself is a true vector [WRIGHT, 1962]. For *S. haematobium* and *S. mansoni*, man is by far the most important definitive host. This fact gives exceptional importance to the behaviour of people in any attempt at a complete understanding of the dynamics of transmission. In the present context, it is the habits bringing people into contact with water that must be considered, their habits in connexion with the disposal of excreta having been discussed earlier (p. 282, a).

The multiple human uses of water lead to a variety of types of exposure, and these have been discussed at length in the literature, with much stress being placed on the type of occupation and its relation to water use. The majority of these comments have been based upon either deduction or ques-

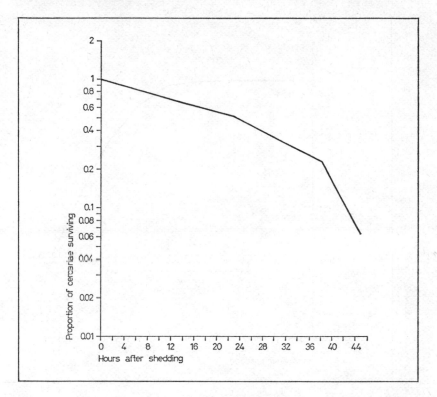

Fig. 9. The survival of the cercariae of *S. japonicum* [data from WHO Philippines-9 project].

tioning, rather than upon direct observation. Such methods can be misleading, or yield contradictory results. For example, the gatherers of palm wine in Leyte showed consistently higher prevalence rates than the average for adults [PESIGAN *et al.*, 1958a]; yet the most conspicuous feature of their occupation is the amount of time spent in the tops of coconut palms.

Direct quantitative observations of the actual water contact by a human population has been attempted occasionally, with interesting results. In a village in Leyte, a team of 15 men made an attempt to record all cases of contact with water during a single day between 5.00 a.m. and 7.00 p.m. [HAIRSTON, 1959]. The sex and approximate age of each person exposed were recorded. Two essentially different kinds of water body were recognized, the snail habitats themselves and the river into which all of the habitats drained. The conditions were such that most, but probably not all, exposures were observed. The population consisted of 752 people, and 653 separate exposures

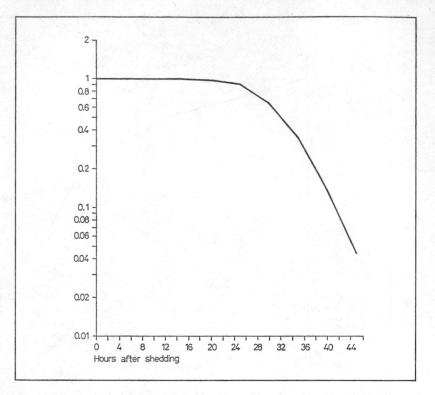

Fig. 10. The survival of the cercariae of *S. mansoni* [data from DAZO *et al.*, 1964].

were noted, varying in duration from less than 1 min to nearly 1 h; the average was 9.5 min. The results are summarized in table IV. When these are matched against prevalence data, some interesting points can be found. In this and similar inland villages, prevalence rates are significantly higher for boys than for girls. However, women have slightly higher prevalence rates than men, and the over-all difference between the sexes is not significant. Females, however, spent 2.5 times as many hours in contact with water as did males, and age made only a little difference in this ratio. The kind of water in which the exposures took place, therefore, appears to be especially important. Males of all ages had more exposures in snail habitats than did females, and the average exposure there was longer for males. The extra time spent by females in water was all in the normally less dangerous river, over 90% of their total exposure time being in that location, as compared with 55% for males. Mouse exposures in both locations subsequently yielded comparable recoveries of flukes only

Table IV. The exposure of people to water during one day in an inland village in Palo, Leyte, Philippines

	Exposure in snail habitats			Exposure in river			Total exposures		
	number of exposures	total time min	average time per exposure	number of exposures	total time min	average time per exposure	number of exposures	total time min	average time per exposure
Children									
Males	49	159	3.24	100	707	7.07	149	866	5.81
Females	44	101.5	2.31	169	1,875.5	11.10	213	1,977	9.28
Adults									
Males	52	644	12.38	63	289	4.59	115	933	8.11
Females	26	296	11.38	150	2,190.5	14.60	176	2,486.5	14.13
Totals									
Males	101	803	7.95	163	996	6.11	264	1,799	6.81
Females	70	397.5	5.68	319	4,066	12.75	389	4,463.5	11.47
Total	171	1,200.5	7.02	482	5,062	10.50	653	6,262.5	9.59

under exceptional conditions. Similar observations have been made in Egypt [DAZO et al., 1964]. The preliminary observations reported, however, did not include activities associated with farming, which prevents the data from being strictly comparable with those from Leyte. Thus, in spite of repeated demonstrations that viable cercariae can be carried long distances in flowing water [SULLIVAN and FERGUSON, 1946; PESIGAN et al., 1958b; RADKE et al., 1961; DAZO et al., 1964], the proximity of exposure to the snails is a factor of great quantitative importance.

The nature of the exposure obviously affects the success of cercariae in several ways. Swimming and bathing expose the entire surface of the body; most other activities involve only a small area of skin. Laundry and dishwashing may be less dangerous than might be supposed, particularly if soap is used.

The habits of reservoir hosts may also influence the success of cercariae. Among domestic animals, the avoidance of water by cats and the affinity of pigs to mud are proverbial. The ecological distribution of wild animals may be taken as evidence of their importance in maintaining *S. japonicum.* The wild rat of the Philippines reaches its maximal abundance in the swampy, low-lying situations that are ideal habitats for *O. quadrasi*.

Analysis of the Fate of Cercariae

The proportion of cercariae that succeed in infecting definitive hosts can be estimated by the use of the equation presented above (Cp. 294), provided that the number present and the number reaching maturity can be determined. The number of cercariae presents no great difficulty, if adequate snail population samples are available, combined with the proportion with mature infections and the mean number of cercariae shed per snail. For example, in the study on *S. japonicum*, it was found that the area produced 9.77×10^5 cercariae as a daily average. This number was obtained by dividing the net reproductive rates of the parasite in female and male snails by their average life-spans, respectively, and multiplying the results by the number of infected snails estimated to be present.

The number of flukes reaching maturity in the area is much more difficult to determine, especially with respect to the human hosts. The approach to the problem was through the rate at which young children were observed to become positive. The incidence was found to be 0.5425 per year. This, of course, represents the combined probabilities of acquiring both male and female worms. The mouse exposures referred to above showed male and female cercariae to be equally abundant, and the product of the two probabilities (0.5425) should, therefore, be equal to the square of either one. Thus, 0.737 of the children acquired female worms, and 0.737 acquired male worms. The assumption was then made that worms are randomly distributed among people. If true, this assumption permits the easy calculation of the mean number of female worms acquired per year. It would follow from the proportion not acquiring females, since

$$(\text{proportion without females}) = e^{-m},$$

where e is the base of natural logarithms and m is the mean number of female worms per child, or 1.335. The number of males would be the same, giving an average of 2.67 worms acquired per child per year. After minor corrections for lower exposure at the extremes of age, and for over-estimates of the rate of becoming positive [HAIRSTON, 1962], the average number of cercariae estimated to succeed in infecting people was 4.2 per day. Thus,

$$4.2 \quad = 9.77 \times 10^5 \times (c \times m),$$
$$(c \times m) = 4.30 \times 10^{-6}.$$

This estimate is minimal, since the assumption of a random distribution of flukes among people is unlikely to be correct, and non-randomness of distribution would cause an increase in the estimated rate of acquisition of parasites.

For the reservoir hosts, it was possible to use more direct methods. The number of flukes found in animals killed for examination, the estimated or counted populations, and the estimated age of the animals gave approximate values for F/D. The calculated values for $(c \times m)$ for reservoir hosts were:

rats 1.04×10^{-3},
dogs 1.64×10^{-6},
pigs 9.82×10^{-6}.

All of the values, of course, include losses of cercariae in penetrating the skin, in migrating to the definitive location, and in growing to maturity. It is worthwhile to examine these losses separately.

The Survivorship of Cercariae after Reaching the Definitive Host

Once the cercaria has reached a suitable host, it has a long, complex, and incompletely known route to follow before arriving in its final location. At all stages, the parasites face problems, and sustain some losses.

Losses in Penetration and Passage through the Skin

Very few cercariae appear to be lost in the skin. STIREWALT [1964] reported that under favourable conditions, 92 to 98% of *S. mansoni* cercariae were able to penetrate the tails of mice; VOGEL and MINNING [1953], using *S. japonicum* in monkeys, found very little evidence of death of schistosomules in the skin, even in animals showing a high degree of functional immunity. Similar studies in man would be of very great interest.

Losses during Migration

The proportion of parasites reaching maturity after entering the body of the host depends upon a number of factors. In experimental infections, one of the most important of these is the species of parasite. The usual experimental hosts are fully susceptible only to *S. japonicum*. Although various rodents are acceptable hosts for maintaining *S. mansoni* in the laboratory, percentage recoveries as adult worms are generally lower than is the case with *S. japonicum*, 20 to 40% being normal for *S. mansoni*, and 50 to more than 70% for *S. japoni-*

cum. S. haematobium is less tolerant of laboratory hosts. This is especially true of the strain from north of the Sahara, which has *B. (B.) truncatus* as an intermediate host. This strain gives very low recoveries in mice, but hamsters are usually satisfactory. PITCHFORD and VISSER [1965] reported that the South African rodents *Mastomys natalensis* and *Saccostomus campestris* are good laboratory hosts for the local strains of *S. mansoni, S. mattheei* and *S. haematobium.*

The well-known fact that *S. japonicum* is regularly found in a greater variety of mammal hosts than are *S. mansoni* and *S. haematobium* makes it appear likely that these species achieve as great a success in man as can be demonstrated for *S. japonicum* in experimental animals. It is possible, therefore, that in normal hosts, schistosomes are at least 70% successful in reaching maturity after once arriving on the skin.

Immunity seems to play its most important role in the destruction of schistosomules during migration. In experimental animals which have recovered from one or more previous infections, very few worms can be found even after massive challenge doses of cercariae. VOGEL and MINNING [1953] found in monkeys, which had been immunized to *S. japonicum* and killed a few days after a massive challenge, that most of the schistosomules recovered were in the lungs where they were surrounded by infiltrations of eosinophils, in contrast to the situation in non-immune animals where the schistosomules made their way rapidly through the lungs, with no eosinophil infiltration. Search in the skin and lymph nodes revealed few parasites in the immunized animals. From these and other observations, VOGEL and MINNING concluded that the lungs are the principal site of action of the immune mechanism.

The relevance of these findings to the dynamics of transmission lies in the implications for the probable worm loads in people in age groups past the age of peak prevalence. It is a common observation that even when passing eggs in the excreta, their egg-counts are notably less than those of younger people. It is thus likely that their worm loads are lower, in spite of continuing exposure.

The Rate of Egg Laying by Female Schistosomes

Although quantitative knowledge of reproduction is essential to an understanding of the population dynamics of schistosomes, relatively few attempts have been made to obtain direct quantitative data. Experimental infections in small mammals have been used for estimating the daily egg production of both *S. japonicum* and *S. mansoni*. The estimates range from 1,400 to 3,500 for *S. japonicum*, and from 250 to 350 for *S. mansoni*. Thus, although there is less than perfect agreement between the estimates for the same species, it is clear that *S. japonicum* lays 6 to 10 times as many eggs each day as does *S. mansoni*. This observation must have important implications concerning differences between the two species in the dynamics of the remainder of their life cycles.

Unfortunately, comparable observations have not been reported for *S. haematobium*. If, as seems likely, there is a relationship between the size of the female and the number of eggs produced, *S. haematobium* should have an egg laying rate intermediate between those of the other two species. The lengths of females are: *S. mansoni* 7–17 mm, *S. haematobium* 16–20 mm, and *S. japonicum* 16–28 mm.

Factors Influencing the Rate of Egg Laying

Egg output has been the subject of numerous studies, but with few exceptions these have used counts of eggs in faeces or urine as the relevant data. Such information does not distinguish between the actual rate of egg laying and the proportion of eggs reaching the excreta. They will be discussed under that factor (p. 304).

It has been shown that in *S. japonicum* the reproductive rate is a function of the age of the parasite [PESIGAN *et al.*, 1958a]. During the first two to three weeks of maturity, the rate rises from 100 to 1,400 eggs per female per day. There is also some suggestion from experimental infections that old females (2–5 years) may produce fewer eggs than those of younger ages. VOGEL and MINNING [1953] found that worms 3 months old contained an average of twice as many eggs in their uteri as did worms 1–5 years old. These observations were on *S. japonicum* in monkeys. The evidence from other studies, however, does not distinguish among the effects of age of females, survivorship of females, and increasing host reaction, since the data consist of egg-counts in faeces.

It is possible that the strain of the parasite and the species of host used, affect reproduction. MOORE and SANDGROUND [1956] obtained an estimated 3,500 eggs per female per day, using the Formosan strain of *S. japonicum* in hamsters. This may be contrasted with the estimate of 1,400 made, using the Philippine strain in white mice.

In many helminth infections the number of eggs laid per female per day is inversely proportional to the number of worms in the host. This may also be true with schistosome infections.

The Survivorship
of Adult Worms

Schistosomes are commonly stated to live for many years, a belief that is based on finding viable eggs in the excreta of patients who have resided away from any endemic area for prolonged periods. Some individual worms have been demonstrated to survive for 20 or 30 years, but recent information indicates that such a statement may be as misleading as claiming that humans live for 120 years.

The most convincing evidence for a relatively short life-span, at least for female schistosomes, consists of the observed rates at which positive people become negative. Thus, FAROOQ and HAIRSTON [1966] found that in Egypt children under the age of 5 years became negative for S. haematobium at a rate of 48% per year, and became negative for S. mansoni at a rate of 58% per year. Older children lost their infections less rapidly, presumably because of the larger average number of worms harboured. For 5- to 7-year-olds, the estimated rates of loss were 5% per year for S. haematobium and 33% per year for S. mansoni. Similar figures have been obtained indirectly by analysing the age-prevalence data. HAIRSTON [1965b] estimated the instantaneous rates of loss in children in the same part of Egypt as 0.30% per year for S. haematobium and 0.34% per year for S. mansoni. Strictly similar data are not available for S. japonicum; very indirect methods yield the estimate that female worms have a death rate of around 25% per year [HAIRSTON, 1962].

Information of this kind indicates that if becoming negative reflects the death of female worms, the death rates must be higher than has been supposed in the past. Regardless of the maximum possible, the mean length of life of female schistosomes may be as short as 2 years, and is probably not greater than 5 years.

In addition to the death rates of worms in their hosts, the deaths of the hosts themselves may be an important source of loss to the parasite population. For human hosts, this seems to constitute a minor addition to the total death rate of flukes, but where reservoir hosts are important, as in areas endemic for S. japonicum, the death rate of the host may be as high as, or higher than, the death rate of the parasite in the host [HAIRSTON, 1962].

It can, therefore, be concluded that the survival of adult worms is less than has been supposed, and that death rates of adults are important in the population dynamics of the parasite. More work is obviously needed on this point, since the estimates that have been made are far from exact.

Factors Influencing Survivorship of Adult Worms

It is possible that many factors influence the survivorship of adult worms in the host. The most obvious of these are the species of mammal and the state of immunity. Unfortunately, there are no data available which permit the distinction between survival prior to reaching maturity and the survival of the adults. Since most of the information relates either to the proportion of cercariae reaching adulthood or to the number of eggs appearing in the excreta, the topic will be discussed more fully under those headings.

The Survivorship of Eggs after Being Laid

In order to be effective in maintaining the parasite population, an egg must, of course, reach the excreta. Those remaining in the tissues of the host are wasted.

Eggs may remain in the tissues because they die in the gut or bladder wall, or because they are carried away from the site of egg laying by the blood stream. Some cases have been recorded in which the parasites themselves have reached ectopic locations and deposited eggs directly into such tissues as lungs, brain and skin, but the great majority of eggs that fail to stay in the walls of the gut are trapped in the liver, where they are carried by the portal circulation. There is evidence that the female worms occasionally depos't eggs in the larger mesenteric veins, with the result that none remain in the normal location, but it is probable that the more usual situation is for a more or less constant loss to the liver of eggs laid in the normal manner. The proportion of eggs reaching the liver is not known with certainty, but various observations indicate that it is probably 15% or higher. PESIGAN *et al.* [1958a] presented data showing that during the first three weeks of reproduction by *S. japonicum* in mice, 19% of all eggs found were in the liver. Similar estimates can be deduced for *S. mansoni* from various sources. In the case of *S. haematobium* infections, the location of the parasites in the pelvic veins of the vesical plexus permits a more uniform dissemination of eggs than is usual with *S. mansoni* and *S. japonicum*. Accordingly, the eggs of *S. haematobium* are found no more commonly in the liver than they are in the appendix, lungs, rectum, or uterus [ALVES, 1958b].

The eggs of all species can nearly always be found in the tissues of the specific organ infected. The proportion of these eggs that reach the excreta is unknown, but some remain in the gut or bladder wall. This is shown by the fact that even early in experimental infections of dogs with *S. japonicum*, one third of the eggs found in mucosal scrapings are degenerate [BANG and HAIRSTON, 1946].

The total loss to the reproductive output from eggs stranded in various tissues is not known with accuracy, but the observations cited above suggest that at least 25% of the eggs remain in the body of the host, and the figure may be much higher, perhaps 70% or more.

Factors Influencing the Retention of Eggs in Tissues

Egg output studies in humans and in experimental infections have shown a great amount of variation with a number of factors. Among these are the age of the host, the immunological state of the host, the stage of the infection, and the species of host. Many observations are made in such a way that it is not possible to distinguish the proportion of eggs escaping into the excreta from the proportion of cercariae that survive to maturity or the survivorship of worms after the start of egg laying. Nevertheless, there are data which suggest strongly that some of the factors enumerated have an effect on the proportion of eggs retained in the tissues of the host.

a) The Age of the Human Host

Data from various studies show that the average output of eggs in the faeces of stool-positive individuals increases greatly during the early years of life [PESIGAN *et al.*, 1958a; KLOETZEL, 1963]. The increase in egg-count up to the age of 15 is much greater than can be accounted for on the basis of any reasonable assumptions or calculations of the increase in average worm load [HAIRSTON, 1962]. Although it is possible that some of this is due to an increase in egg laying by the worms, it seems more probable that the changing physiological state of the host permits a higher proportion of eggs to escape in the faeces of older children. Similar comparisons have been made for *S. haematobium*, but the results are not always in agreement. They suggest, however, that the phenomenon observed for *S. japonicum* and *S. mansoni* is less pronounced for *S. haematobium*, if it exists at all.

After the age of 15 years, or even earlier in some areas, the number of eggs in excreta declines to levels well below those found in younger age groups. Since it is not always possible to attribute this decrease to decreased exposure, it seems most likely to be related to the phenomenon of immunity.

b) The Immune State of the Host

Previous experience with the parasite appears to restrict the release of eggs through the tissues and into the excreta. VOGEL and MINNING [1953] showed that in monkeys that had recovered from an initial attack of *S. japonicum*, subsequent exposures led to decreasing proportions of cercariae reaching adulthood, but they also showed that although it was possible to recover normal adult females with normal eggs *in utero*, very few eggs could be found in the faeces. The difference between the numbers of eggs in faeces early and late in the same infection was much greater than the twofold difference in the number of eggs in the uteri of female worms recovered during the two stages of infection.

c) The Species of Host

Apart from experimental infections in small laboratory mammals, many of which are abnormal hosts, there are no convincing data showing significant differences in the number of eggs passed by different species of hosts, if the egg output is computed in terms of the number of female schistosomes recovered at autopsy. The important differences in total egg output that exist among the various hosts of *S. japonicum* [PESIGAN *et al.*, 1958a] appear to be attributable to differences in worm load. Experimental infections in dogs and pigs, for example, showed a much higher recovery of cercariae as adults in dogs.

The Net Reproductive Rate in the Definitive Host

The calculation of the average contribution of a female schistosome to the next generation proceeds in much the same way as the calculation of the net reproductive rate of the parasite in snails. In the case of the adult, however, the fact that only females produce eggs requires that the reproductive rate be calculated in terms of only the female eggs. In the absence of contradictory evidence, an equal sex ratio is assumed, and there is some evidence that this is indeed the case.

There are two possible methods of approaching the problem of calculating the net reproductive rate of the female parasite. One of these would be to accept the egg laying rates that have been observed in experimental animals, as described above (p. 300). The numerical description of the population dynamics of the parasite would then have to contain a separate loss rate for eggs that do not escape into the excreta (p. 303). The alternative to this approach is to count as reproduction only those eggs which actually leave the body. This approach has been taken by HAIRSTON [1962, 1965a].

In the case of net reproduction in human hosts, the greatest uncertainty lies in estimating the number of worms actually present. The calculation can be made from the estimates of the rate of acquisition of schistosomes by people (p. 298) and the death rate of female worms (p. 302). The mean number of mated females per person in any age group, and the egg-counts in excreta, can be used to make calculations for the m_x column (see p. 292). The combined death rates of female worms and their hosts provide the l_x column.

For the data on *S. japonicum* in Leyte, it appeared that the reproductive rate of female worms declined with the age of the human host after the age of 10 to 15 years. This required the calculation of net reproductive rates for flukes assumed to have entered the host at different ages of the latter. A weighted mean of these was found to equal 9.05×10^4.

The net reproductive rate of *S. japonicum* in reservoir hosts was also calculated. Worm loads could be determined directly from naturally infected animals, and are, therefore, not subject to the uncertainty that is involved with humans. The net reproductive rates of flukes in these animals were: in dogs 5.03×10^3, in pigs 6.40×10^2, and in field rats 63. The lower values, as compared with that for humans, are brought about both by the higher death rates of the hosts, and by the lower output of eggs per female worm present.

An Ecological Life Table for the Parasite

The estimates of the different elements of reproduction and survivorship that have been made can be combined to give the over-all net reproductive rate of the parasite [HAIRSTON, 1962, 1965a]. Since the net reproductive rate of an organism is the number of female progeny produced per female per generation, it can be regarded as the ratio of increase or decrease of the population during an average generation. If the population is at equilibrium, it should equal 1.0. Equilibrium conditions appear to be common in many endemic areas, inasmuch as the relationship between age and prevalence does not change in a significant way over periods of 15 years or more. This is the case with the endemic area of eastern Leyte [HAIRSTON, 1962]. Therefore, the combined products of survivorship and reproduction should equal 1.0, as follows:

$$d \times p \times i \times T \times c \times m \times Q \times f \times h = 1.0$$

In this equation, T is the net reproductive rate of the parasite in snails, Q is the net reproductive rate in mammals, f is the proportion of eggs reaching faeces, and h is the proportion of eggs that are hatchable. The other terms are defined on pages 280 and 294. As explained above (p. 305), $(Q \times f \times h)$ is estimated as a single term. The great variations in the success of cercariae in reaching different mammals, and in the net reproductive rates in these mammals, require separate values of $(c \times m)$ and $(Q \times f \times h)$ for each host. The products of these are then summed for the final calculations of the net reproductive rate of the parasite, thus:

$(d \times p \times i) \times T \times \Sigma[(c \times m) \times (Q \times f \times h)]$ should equal 1.0,

in fact

$$(0.023) \times (54.15) \times \Sigma \left\{ \begin{array}{l} 4.30 \times 10^{-6} \times 9.05 \times 10^4 \\ 1.04 \times 10^{-3} \times 63 \\ 1.69 \times 10^{-6} \times 5.02 \times 10^3 \\ 9.82 \times 10^{-6} \times 6.40 \times 10^2 \end{array} \right\} = 0.59.$$

In the case of *S. japonicum* in eastern Leyte, then, the equation fails to balance by a factor of 0.41 of the theoretical net reproductive rate. The equation is useful as a check upon the accumulated assumptions and observations that were made. The potential error in this array is, of course, very large, but it is considered that the survivorship and reproduction of *S. japonicum*, under the conditions observed, are reasonably well known. Equally complete data do not exist for *S. haematobium* or for *S. mansoni*.

The inland village in which the observations were made is in an area of intense transmission. There are nearby areas in which transmission is less rapid, yet in which the parasite population remains in equilibrium. A lower level of transmission implies that the terms d and c are lower; therefore, if the equation is to balance under these conditions, other terms must be proportionally higher. One of these is $(Q \times f \times h)$ for humans, which has been estimated as 1.47×10^5, an increase of nearly 63% over the 9.05×10^4 for the inland village. The range of values over which such compensatory mechanisms are effective is not known, but there is in principle a lower limit below which they fail. The most important cause for the failure is the increasing probability that single parasites which succeed in entering the definitive host will remain unmated. The point at which this phenomenon becomes self-accelerating is critical for the parasite, and the ability to predict it would be extremely useful. By finding solutions for the terms in the equation above, for three or more situations involving a wide range of transmission rates, it should be possible to establish the upper limits of the net reproductive rates in the two hosts, and from these could be calculated the minimum probabilities of successful trans-

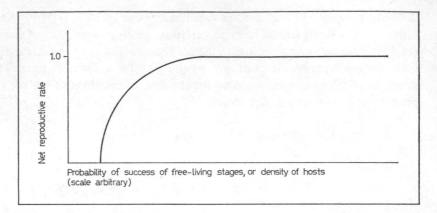

Fig. 11. Graphic representation of the dynamics of schistosome populations, as described in the text.

mission that would permit the continued existence of the parasite population. Once these facts were established, a definite prediction could be made of the degree of effectiveness of any control measure or combination of measures that would be necessary to cause the population to fall to zero. The situation can be expressed graphically, as in figure 11. Over a wide range of transmission rates, the net reproductive rate of the parasite remains constant at 1.0. At some low level of transmission, not yet specifiable numerically, reproduction can no longer compensate for the decreased chances that the few successful parasites will find a mate. When this level is reached, the net reproductive rate of the parasite will decrease more and more rapidly until none is left.

Special Methods Used in the Measurement of the Dynamics of Transmission

In order to make quantitative estimates of the rates involved in the dynamics of transmission, it is necessary to obtain a large amount of data in a careful manner. For a few of the parameters, the information obtained by experimentation or by observation may be used directly, but for most of them the data must be manipulated in various ways, sometimes with the help of simplifying assumptions. The methods have been described for some of these, but for others the lengthy discussion of methods would have interrupted the general description of the dynamics of transmission. This section will be devoted to a description of the data required at the remaining steps, and to a discussion of the assumptions and manipulations of the data that are necessary.

Methods for the Analysis of the Fate of Schistosome Eggs

In order to estimate the fraction of eggs that succeed in establishing the infection in snails, it is necessary to have extensive information about the population dynamics of snails. The first requirement is the total population of snails in the area under study; to acquire this information it is essential to have a sampling method that obtains at least a known fraction of the snails present, and that is repeatable at all seasons. Some of the precautions regarding snail sampling are given on pages 272–278. The actual technique used will depend upon local conditions. Various examples are given on pages 668–673, but it is necessary to state that for present purposes, methods that give relative snail densities are not satisfactory. These include the number of snails collected per unit of time and the number collected per pass of a dip net. Sampling should continue until any seasonal pattern of abundance is known quantitatively. With each sampling, the number of infected snails must be determined. The methods for detecting infections are described on pages 662–664.

Infected snails. Whatever method is selected, the time required for the development to the youngest detected stage must be determined. In areas with marked seasonal changes in temperature or rainfall, this incubation period may vary greatly. Observed minima are 4 or 5 weeks in *S.mansoni*, 5 or 6 weeks in *S.haematobium* and 6 to 7 weeks in *S.japonicum*. Maxima of 20 to 30 weeks have been observed in winter, and the survival of sporocysts over periods of drought has also been reported. From these data, it is possible to calculate the average number of infected snails within the area under study. This number is the average standing crop of snail infections. Its magnitude is determined by the rate at which snails become infected and the rate at which infections are lost. Infections are lost to the parasite population primarily through the death of infected snails, the instances of 'self-cure' being uncommon during the average life of the snails in the field, except in the case of a few species.

The death rate of infected snails in the field may be estimated by two different methods; neither method is exact. The first is to observe the death rates of infected and uninfected snails in the laboratory, estimate the death rate in the field of all snails, most of which are uninfected, and assume that the proportionality observed in the laboratory also takes place in the field. Methods

of estimating snail death rates in the field are given on page 322. The second
method is to select the steepest decline in the observed proportion infected in
the field, and assume that this represents the death rate of infected snails. The
method yields a minimal estimate, since it requires the assumption that no
new infections appeared during the interval. In principle, the method could
be improved by selecting a highly infected natural habitat and fencing it off
from further sources of infection. This refinement has not been attempted.
Once the death rate of infected snails has been estimated, the mean length of
life is easy to establish, since it is the reciprocal of the finite death rate. The
calculations are as follows:

$$1_x = e^{-ax}, \text{ and (mean length of life)} = \frac{1}{1 - e^{-a}},$$

where 1_x is the proportion surviving x days, e is the base of natural logarithms,
and a is the instantaneous death rate per day.

The mean length of life, divided into the average standing crop, gives the
number of snails becoming positive per day. This number represents the
number becoming infected minus the number dying between the time of infection and the time of becoming positive. The proportion surviving the
incubation period can be calculated from the first of the foregoing equations.

Methods for the Analysis of the Fate of Cercariae

By far the most difficult information to obtain on the proportion of
cercariae that are successful, is the number of parasites in the human host.
With a single exception to be described below, the only data available are egg-
counts from people of different ages, and observations on incidence. With
sufficient data on egg output, combined with numerous carefully performed
autopsies on a random sample from the same population, it is possible that
a direct relationship could be established between egg-count and worm load.
Such information is not available, and it is necessary to attack the problem
from the rate of becoming positive (see p. 298).

The relationship between the rate of acquisition of parasites and the rate
of becoming positive on examination depends very strongly upon assumptions
about the distribution of worms among hosts. The point can be readily visualized from figure 12. In constructing the figure, the Negative Binomial Distribution has been used, but the same pattern would be found with any contagious
distribution. The constant k in the Negative Binomial is inversely related to
the degree of non-randomness of the distribution.

Thus, if the same number of worms is visualized as being distributed in

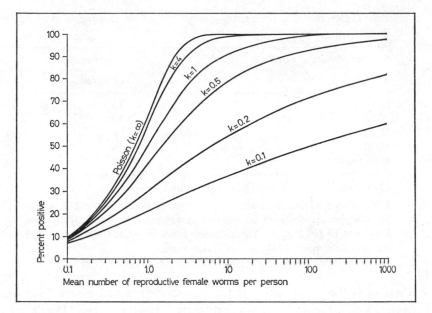

Fig. 12. The relationship between the proportion positive and the mean load of mated female worms, under various assumptions about the extent of non-randomness of distribution of worms among people. The indicated values of 'k' are from the Negative Binomial Distribution.

different ways among a certain number of people, a truly random distribution would mean that each person would have an equal chance of becoming infected by each worm. The operation of chance in this system is such that some people would acquire more than others, and unless the average number of worms was large, a finite proportion of the population would escape infection. This proportion can be calculated as: e^{-m} where e is the base of natural logarithms and m is the mean number of worms per person. This relationship was used previously (p. 298), where the proportion not becoming infected was known and the mean number of worms was required.

If, however, each person does not have an equal chance of becoming infected, as where the area is heterogeneous with respect to exposure, the relationship between the proportion not infected and the mean number of worms per person can be expressed as follows:

$$(\text{proportion negative}) = \frac{1}{\left(1 + \frac{m}{k}\right)^k},$$

Table V. Observed distribution of *S. mansoni* adults from 45 autopsies in a hospital in Brazil[1]

Number of pairs of worms	Number of cases	
	observed	expected
Less than 6	13	18.60
6–10	10	5.87
11–20	6	6.04
21–40	6	5.69
More than 40	10	8.80

Chi-square $= 4.77$; d.f. $= 3$; $0.20 > p > 0.10$.

1. The data are from cases without symptoms obviously attributable to *S. mansoni*. The observed distribution is compared with a Negative Binomial Distribution having a mean of 10 and k of 0.1. The difference is not significant. The data are presented through the courtesy of Dr. ALLEN W. CHEEVER.

where m is the mean and k is the constant discussed above [BLISS and FISHER, 1953]. Figure 12 shows that where k is 4.0 or larger, the difference from a random distribution is not great, and the assumption of randomness under these conditions does not lead to many inaccuracies. In the case of the data being analysed, the egg-counts in children [PESIGAN *et al.*, 1958a] can be reconciled with a Negative Binomial Distribution of mated female worms with a value of k of around 4 [HAIRSTON, 1965a]. In other areas the non-randomness of distribution may be much greater, as suggested by the fact that egg-counts for any age group commonly conform to a lognormal distribution, rather than to a Poisson [BRADLEY, 1963; FAROOQ *et al.*, 1964]. Such distributions provide for the possibility that some people are heavily infected, while others have few worms or escape infection entirely.

The only example of a carefully examined series of worm-counts is that of CHEEVER [WHO, 1967], who has devised a special perfusion technique for the recovery of schistosomes at autopsy. Careful counts from 45 autopsies at a hospital in Brazil gave the data in table V, where they are compared with an expected distribution based on a Negative Binomial with a mean of 10 and k of 0.1. The departure from a random distribution is very great, doubtless because of the variety of situations from which hospital cases are ordinarily drawn. It would be expected that epidemiological studies would be conducted separately on such different areas (see p. 262), and these valuable data give an indication of the maximum degree of non-randomness that could ever be anticipated.

Since some non-randomness of exposure is sure to exist, the probable distributions of worms among people will occur between the uppermost and the lowermost lines in figure 12.

The Ecology of the Intermediate Host

Certain aspects of the ecology of the snail hosts of schistosomes are important to the dynamics of transmission of the parasites. These aspects have been discussed earlier in the chapter. In the planning of control operations, the whole ecology of the snail species involved must be thoroughly understood. Ecology is used here in the broad sense of including local distribution, seasonal changes in distribution and abundance, and population dynamics.

The Ecological Distribution of Snails

The intermediate hosts of schistosomes are almost never found in all bodies of water in an area. In some cases, the difference between potential habitats which do and do not contain the appropriate species is clear, and with experience it may be possible to predict in advance whether a given habitat is a likely source of transmission. For example, in Lake Province, Tanzania, *B. (Ph.) nasutus* is virtually confined to small ponds which dry completely between rainy seasons [WEBBE, 1962a]; streams and permanent ponds in this area are thus never dangerous for the transmission of *S. haematobium*. In most other areas, long experience and detailed research may fail to make analogous predictions valid.

Physicochemical Factors

The fact that snails have special habitats has stimulated the imagination of many investigators, and has prompted them to attempt correlations between the presence of snails and a tremendous array of physical and chemical factors [SIOLI, 1953; ALVES, 1958a; DE MEILLON et al., 1958; GOHAR and EL-GINDY, 1960; HARRY et al., 1957; MALEK, 1958; MARILL, 1958; PESIGAN et al., 1958b; PIMENTEL and WHITE, 1959a; SCHUTTE and FRANK, 1964; WEBBE, 1962a]. The results of all of these studies indicate that the chemical composition of water does not permit the prediction of the presence or absence of the intermediate hosts of schistosomes. Laboratory experimentation on the tolerance by the snails of various conditions has shown that limits of tolerance are well beyond the usual conditions found in the field. Much more sensitive than tolerance tests is the determination of the intrinsic rate of natural increase [BIRCH, 1953; SHIFF, 1964; WILLIAMS, 1963; SEVILLA, 1965]. This population parameter is discussed in more detail below. It includes both reproduction and survival, and has been shown to be very sensitive to small differences in temperature, and to differences in concentration of calcium and bicarbonate ions. In many cases, however, the snails continued to have a positive rate of increase under conditions outside those in the area in which they are found. For example, SEVILLA [1965] found that *B. pfeifferi* from Tanzania reached its greatest rate of increase at 25 °C, a temperature characteristic of the annual mean for coastal East Africa, where the snail does not occur naturally. In this case, climate is obviously not the direct factor determining the geographical distribution of the species.

STURROCK [1966] has also shown that the optimum temperature for rapid population expansion of *B. pfeifferi* appears to be close to 25 °C. At other temperatures population expansion was much slower, but whereas at 19 °C survival was good, at 30 °C it was poor. STURROCK stated that the maximum temperature tolerated by *B. pfeifferi* appears to be about 32 °C, but he considers that under field conditions it is doubtful whether colonies would survive temperatures much above 28 °C, and concluded that high temperatures are a major barrier to the colonization by this snail of suitable natural habitats on the coastal plain of Tanzania; in certain circumstances he thinks that artificial habitats created by irrigation schemes could support colonies of the species at least seasonally. However, temperature may be only indirectly responsible for the pattern of *Biomphalaria* distribution in East Africa.

Physiography

The distribution of the snail hosts of schistosomes has frequently been related to certain topographical features of the landscape. *B. (B.) truncatus* does not occur in rapidly flowing water; a rate of 20 to 30 cm/sec is approximately the maximum in which it is found [WATSON, 1950, 1958; WITENBERG and SALITERNIK, 1957]. *B. alexandrina* is apparently even less tolerant of a high rate of flow. Stream gradient has been found to have an important influence on the distribution of *B. glabrata* [HARRY and CUMBIE, 1956; PIMENTEL and WHITE, 1959a]. The snail population does not maintain itself where the gradient is steeper than 20 m fall per 1,000 m of length. As might be expected, the snails do occur in pools and eddies, even in streams which are otherwise too swift to support them.

The general topography has been found to be important in the distribution of the amphibious *O. quadrasi* [PESIGAN *et al.*, 1958b]. The snails are found only in very flat areas, regardless of elevation or other topographical features.

Biological Factors

In contrast to the chemical composition of the water or soil, the biological constituents of potential habitats have frequently been found to be correlated with the distribution and abundance of the intermediate hosts of schistosomes.

a) Aquatic Vegetation

Many studies have shown that snails are associated with aquatic plants. As far as the intermediate hosts of schistosomes are concerned, these studies have been concentrated on *B. (B.) truncatus* and *B. alexandrina*. There can be little doubt that these species are most abundant in the presence of certain plants [DAZO *et al.*, 1966], but are certainly not confined to them [WATSON, 1958]. The plants, especially certain species of *Potamogeton*, provide good surfaces for both feeding and egg laying [WITENBERG and SALITERNIK, 1957], but it is also likely that a large part of the association is due to the common cause of generally favourable aquatic habitats, rather than to cause and effect [WATSON, 1958]. The complexity of this relationship is shown by the differential abundance of *Bulinus* and *Biomphalaria* in the presence of the water hyacinth, *Eichornia crassipes*. *Bulinus* was no more abundant in the presence of this plant than it was on bare silt, whereas *Biomphalaria* was as abundant with *Eichornia* present as it was in any other situation, including *Potamogeton crispus* [DAZO *et al.*, 1966].

B. *glabrata* also has a high degree of association with aquatic vegetation [PIMENTEL and WHITE, 1959b].

In Africa south of the Sahara, only *B. (B.) truncatus rohlfsi* has been found to be related to the vegetation [McCULLOUGH, 1962]. Reproduction in this case was strongly related to the seasonal availability of *Nymphaea*. Other snail hosts of schistosomes in this region do not appear to be associated with any plants [TEESDALE, 1962; DE MEILLON *et al.*, 1958].

In general, the snails do not appear to be associated with emergent vegetation, except as this may influence water currents or wave action [WITENBERG and SALITERNIK, 1957], or provide attractive surfaces in the form of leaves falling into the water [ZAKARIA, 1954, 1955; WATSON, 1958].

The food of schistosome-bearing snails is either algae or a combination of these and decaying vascular plants. Accordingly, it might be supposed that a high correlation would exist between snail abundance and the abundance of microflora. One study in which such a correlation was attempted was that of DAZO and MORENO [1962], who found a positive relationship between the presence of green algae and the occurrence of *O. quadrasi*. Corroborative evidence consisted in the common occurrence of green algae among the gut contents of this species. Furthermore, a negative correlation was found between the presence of blue-green algae and the occurrence of *O. quadrasi*. In a similar study on the stomach contents of *B. (B.) truncatus*, *B. alexandrina* and *Lymnaea caillaudi*, GOHAR and EL-GINDY [1961] found algae to be most abundant, especially diatoms; they observed no important differences between the three species.

b) Aquatic Animals

Attempts to correlate the ecological distribution of the intermediate hosts of schistosomes with that of other aquatic animals have generally been unsuccessful. Weak correlations, both positive and negative, have been found between the presence of *B. glabrata* and the presence of some other snail species in Puerto Rico [PIMENTEL and WHITE, 1959b]. Certain mayfly species are also fair indicators of the habitats of *B. pfeifferi* and *B. (Ph.) africanus* in South Africa [DE MEILLON *et al.*, 1958].

c) Pollution

One of the most widely held beliefs about the ecology of aquatic hosts of schistosomes is that they are most abundant in waters polluted by human or animal excrement or by decaying vegetable matter. Some investigators have carried this correlation to the point of concluding that the relationship of snail distribution to human excreta is obligatory [GORDON *et al.*, 1934; RANSFORD, 1948]. Such extreme claims have not been substantiated in other studies [see MALEK, 1958; and WATSON, 1958, for reviews]. The ability and willingness of these snails to eat almost any organic material offered to them is largely responsible for the correlation found between human pollution and refuse, and number of snails; in other words, mild pollution has an enriching effect on the general environment rather than a specific effect on the snails.

Heavy pollution from sewage or industrial sources is inimical to the snails.

Changes in Abundance

Very few species of snail hosts of schistosomes have stable populations It is usual for marked fluctuations in density to occur, especially in populations of aquatic snails. The two factors cited as being responsible for marked changes in abundance are temperature and rainfall. In the sub-tropical and temperate regions, the low temperature in winter reduces reproduction or stops it entirely. With the onset of warmer weather, reproduction is resumed, and the population increases to a maximum. This pattern has been observed for *B. (B.) truncatus* in Egypt and Iraq, for *B. alexandrina* in Egypt, and for *O. nosophora* in Japan. In some areas, high temperatures also appear to reduce breeding. In Egypt, March is the month of maximal breeding, and both *B. (B.) truncatus* and *B. alexandrina* show reduced reproductive rates thereafter [WATSON, 1958; DAZO et al., 1966]. This results in decreasing populations before the arrival of the Nile Flood in August, although the silt-laden flood waters are often stated to be responsible for the low numbers. They may, of course, be partly responsible for further reduction in snail abundance after their arrival. In Sudan, it is only the high temperature of summer that appears to reduce reproduction. MALEK [1962] presented data showing the greatest abundance of *B. (B.) truncatus, B. (B.) forskalii* and *B. pfeifferi rüppelli* in March and April. This probably represents maximum reproduction in January or February (see p. 273). Seasonal temperature changes may also be responsible for changes in the local pattern of distribution of snails. This has been observed with *B. (B.) truncatus* in Iraq [NAJARIAN, 1961].

Tropical populations generally tend to be influenced most strongly by rain which may have the effect of stimulating an increase in the snail populations, or it may have the opposite effect of flushing snails out of habitats where they had been abundant. WEBBE [1962a, b] has reported both types of effect in Tanzania: *B. (Ph.) nasutus* is dependent upon the rain to fill the temporary ponds which are its habitats and populations increase rapidly after the start of the rainy season; *Biomphalaria sudanica*, in the same area, was flushed out of its stream habitat by rains, and the species reached high densities only during the dry season. Both kinds of effect have been reported elsewhere. *B. (Ph.) globosus* in Rhodesia responds to rainfall by very active breeding [SHIFF, 1964], as do *B. glabrata* and *B. straminea* in North-Eastern Brazil [BARBOSA and OLIVIER, 1958], *B. (B.) truncatus rohlfsi* in Ghana [McCULLOUGH, 1962], and many other species in areas with seasonal rainfall. The reduction of stream-dwelling populations of *B. glabrata* through high rainfall has been reported from Puerto Rico (PIMENTEL and WHITE, 1959a).

Snail populations may show great fluctuations for reasons which are unknown, but which do not appear to be related to changes in the weather [McMULLEN et al., 1951; RITCHIE et al., 1962; WEBBE, 1962b].

In areas where seasonal changes are minor, or where the habitats consist of large bodies of water that are relatively unaffected by such changes as occur, snail populations may be remarkably stable. *O. quadrasi* in the Philippines showed very minor changes in density over a two-year period, and the changes observed were not synchronous in different habitats [PESIGAN *et al.*, 1958b]. Small and irregular fluctuations in the population of *B. pfeifferi* in Nairobi Dam, Kenya, were observed by TEESDALE [1962], although major changes occurred in stream-dwelling populations of the same species.

Population Dynamics

It is a truism that the abundance of any species is the result of a combination of reproduction and death rates, and many observers have recorded periods when snails appeared to be producing eggs or when they appeared to be dying. Only recently, however, have attempts been made to use the techniques and principles of population ecology for accurate quantitative descriptions of the parameters of snail populations. One of these parameters, the net reproductive rate, has been described and used above in connexion with the parasite population. The method of obtaining this and other parameters can best be described from a hypothetical experiment in which a large number of newly laid eggs are observed through hatching, growth, reproduction and survival, until all are dead or until reproduction has ceased completely. Since the hosts of all human schistosomes except *S. japonicum* are hermaphroditic, all eggs laid are counted in calculations of reproduction. In the case of the dioecious snails of the genus *Oncomelania*, however, only female snails and their female progeny enter into the calculations.

The data from such an experiment are cast into an ecological life table [LESLIE and RANSON, 1940; BIRCH, 1948; EVANS and SMITH, 1952; SHIFF, 1964; SEVILLA, 1965]. The form of the table and the method are given above (pp. 291–293 and table III). There are fundamental differences between the use of the life table in the context of part of the life cycle of the parasite as given in the preceding section and its use in the population dynamics of snails, where the complete life history is encompassed by the table. In the present usage, the reproductive products in principle start the life table over again. Therefore, the net reproductive rate, which is the sum of the $l_x m_x$ column, is the ratio of increase per generation. In laboratory experiments, this ratio, symbolized by R_0 in population ecology, is very large under most circumstances. In the field, however, the ratio should be unity for data taken over one or more years, since under ordinary conditions the snail population fluctuates around a more or less constant mean value, and on average does not show long-term trends

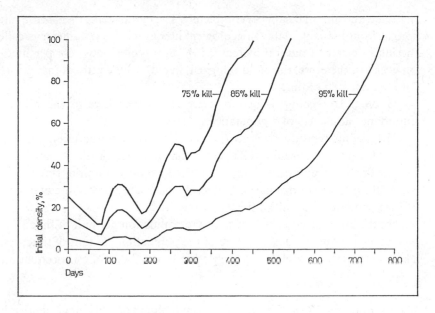

Fig. 13. Calculated repopulation curves of *O. quadrasi,* based on observed survival and reproduction rates.

[HAIRSTON, 1965a]. The net reproductive rate would provide an excellent basis for comparing the favourability of different sets of experimental conditions, were it not for the fact that it is based upon a generation, rather than upon absolute time, and the mean time per generation varies widely under different conditions [see SHIFF, 1964].

It is necessary, therefore, to introduce a different parameter, which expresses the rate of increase of a population per unit of time. This presents certain difficulties, which can be visualized by considering the history of an unrestricted population starting from a group of uniform age (fig. 13). The waves in the population curves represent successive generations, and this prevents the population from growing at the uniform rate which it is necessary to calculate for purposes of comparison. The difficulty has been solved mathematically through the proof of the theorem of the stable age distribution [SHARPE and LOTKA, 1911; LOTKA, 1922]. This theorem states that any population growing with constant age-specific death and birth rates will eventually reach an age distribution, each part of which is increasing at a constant rate r; thereafter, the age distribution and the rate of population growth, r, will be constant. Figure 13 provides an empirical demonstration; the waves diminish in height, and almost disappear completely. The parameter r, then, is the value sought from life table data. In ecological literature, this parameter is called the intrinsic rate of natural increase; it is an instantaneous rate per unit of time, and is, therefore, the natural logarithm of the finite ratio of increase (R) for the same unit of time.

From the foregoing discussion, it can be seen that there are the following important parameters of a population:

R_0: the net reproductive rate (ratio of increase per generation);

T: the mean generation time (in the time units for the life table);

R: the finite reproductive rate (ratio of increase per unit of time);

r: the intrinsic rate of natural increase (the instantaneous rate of increase of the population per unit of time);

b: the instantaneous birth rate of the population per unit of time;

d: the instantaneous death rate of the population per unit of time.

These parameters are related to each other through the following equations:

$$R_0 = R^T; \quad R = e^r; \quad r = b-d.$$

The calculation of R_0 as the sum of the $l_x m_x$ column of an ecological life table has already been described. The calculation of the other parameters requires the use of the theorem of the stable age distribution, and is accomplished by the trial and error solution for r in the following equation:

$$\Sigma l_x m_x e^{-rx} = 1.0.$$

The rationale for this equation can be found in SLOBODKIN [1961].

The intrinsic rate of natural increase has been determined under various conditions for a number of different snail species (table VI). The sensitivity of this parameter to minor differences in the environment is well illustrated by the figures for *B. pfeifferi*. The strain from Tanzania has a very sharply defined optimum temperature at 25°C, a difference of 2.5°C reducing the value by a factor of two to six, and a difference of 5°C in either direction results in a negative value, which means that the population would die out. The strain from Rhodesia, which has a more variable climate, has the same optimum temperature, but r is positive at a constant temperature at least 4.5°C below that at which the strain from Tanzania can maintain itself.

This parameter also reflects the natural stability of the population. Where the population goes through important fluctuations, the selective advantage of a high value of r is obvious, since it permits the population to recover rapidly with the return of favourable conditions [SMITH, 1954; SHIFF, 1964]. On the other hand, a high rate of increase entails a high cost in energy, and

Table VI. The intrinsic rate of natural increase of various snail species under different conditions. All rates calculated per day

Snail species and strain	Experimental temperatures in the laboratory, °C						Field	Authority
	18	20	22.5	25	27.5	30		
O. quadrasi (Leyte)	–	–	–	–	0.013	–	0	PESIGAN *et al.*
B. glabrata (Puerto Rico)	–	0.063	–	0.123	–	0.048	–	SEVILLA
B. alexandrina (Egypt)	–	0.028	–	0.082	0.056	0.014	0.044	SEVILLA (lab.) DAZO *et al.* (field)
B. pfeifferi (Tanzania)	–	neg.	0.015	0.085	0.039	neg.	–	SEVILLA
B. pfeifferi (Rhodesia)	0.016	0.033		0.034	0.031	–	–	SHIFF
B. (B.) globosus (Rhodesia)	0.016	–	0.034	0.047	0.043	–	–	SHIFF
B. (B.) truncatus (Egypt)	–	–	–	–	–	–	0.048	DAZO *et al.*
B. (B.) truncatus (Iran)	–	–	–	0.065	–	–	–	data of CHU, SABBAGHIAN and MASSOUD

would not be favoured by natural selection in populations which are not decimated from time to time. This is reflected in the low value of r for *O. quadrasi*, which has the most stable populations of any schistosome-bearing snail yet investigated.

Population parameters calculated on the basis of field data are useful in two different ways. The first of these is the use of the net reproductive rate as a check upon the observations on reproduction and survival, as previously discussed for the parasite population (pp. 306–308). The second use for a population parameter from field data is in the prediction of the maximum possible rate of repopulation following a control measure. Thus, given age-specific reproduction and survival at different seasons, r can be calculated for the most favourable conditions encountered in the field [DAZO *et al.*, 1966]. The maximum expected average rate of repopulation can then be calculated from the equation of exponential growth:

$N_t = N_0 e^{rt}$,

where N_0 is the starting population, N_t is the population expected after time t, and e is the base of natural logarithms. A graph representing N in time will then cut through the waves of successive generations shown in figure 13.

Life tables based on field data have been constructed for *O. quadrasi* [HAIRSTON, 1965a], and for *B. (B.) truncatus* and *B. alexandrina* [DAZO et al., 1966]. The life table for *O. quadrasi* is based on average values of reproduction and survival over a long period in a stable population, and the net reproductive rate is calculated as 0.997, almost exactly the theoretical 1.0. The life tables for *B. (B.) truncatus* and *B. alexandrina* are based on the rates during the most favourable month (March), and lead to the calculation that the population of either species could double in 14 to 16 days. Given an estimate of the percentage killed by a mollusciciding, an arbitrary level could be established at which the snail population would again require attention. From this and the foregoing kind of calculation, it is possible to specify the greatest frequency with which the habitat would have to be re-examined for evidence of recovery of the population.

It is not possible to observe directly the necessary age specific rates of reproduction and death under field conditions. They must be calculated from observations which it is possible to make in the field, and their accuracy depends upon the accuracy of sampling the populations of snails, and upon the validity of the assumptions required for the calculations.

The Estimation of Survival of Snails in the Field

Survival, or its complement, the death rate, can be calculated from the age distributions of collections made at successive times. It should be noted that all collections are subject to an unavoidable sampling error and, therefore, large numbers of repeated observations are needed before confidence can be placed in the calculated death rates. The distribution of ages among a collection of snails may be derived from the size distributions, if an accurate growth curve can be constructed. Methods of obtaining growth curves are given by McMULLEN [1947], PESIGAN *et al.* [1958b], WEBBE [1962a], and SHIFF [1964]. Once the age distributions are known for two successive collections taken in the same habitat in exactly the same way, the survival of the snails present at the time of the first collection can be estimated. The total snails older than age x in the first collection are represented in the second collection by the total snails aged (x + y), where y is the time between collections. The ratio between the two numbers is l_x in the equation appearing on p. 310. The method,

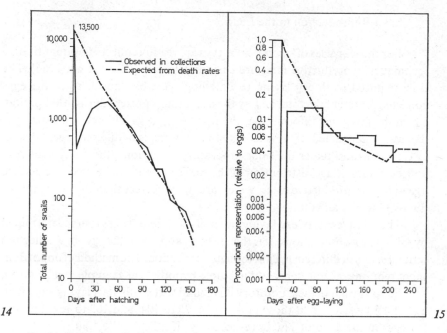

Fig. 14. Estimates of observed and expected age distributions of *B. (B.) truncatus* over a three-year period in Egypt [from DAZO *et al.*, 1966].

Fig. 15. Estimates of observed and expected age distributions of *O. quadrasi*. Expected line (broken) is based on observations over two years. Observed distribution (histogram) is based on a single large collection [data of PESIGAN *et al.*, 1958b].

of course, assumes a constant death rate during the interval. In using the rates to construct a life table, the same equation can be solved backwards to find l_x for any time after egg laying. Since the rates change at different ages, attention must be paid to when they change. In general, it is only possible to estimate three different rates from field data: during incubation, during immaturity, and after the snails become reproductive. It is emphasized that even the best quantitative sampling techniques fail to obtain young snails in their true abundance (fig. 14 and 15). This means that snails younger than 45 to 50 days old may not be used in the estimations of survivorship in the field. Survivorship during the first six weeks after hatching must come from collections of eggs and of snails at least 45 days old. It is also noted that in the data for *O. quadrasi*, a quantitative but less exhaustive technique resulted in inadequate collection of snails up to 100 days old. Further comments on this subject can be found on pages 272–274.

Snail Reproduction in the Field

For those species of snails whose eggs are readily collected by quantitative techniques, reproductive rates are easy to calculate [DAZO et al., 1966]. The time required from egg laying to hatching must be known, since the eggs collected represent the total laid by the adult snails present during that period. From the foregoing information, the number of eggs laid per adult snail per day can be calculated. If, as is usually the case, snails of different ages lay eggs at different rates under the same laboratory conditions, the number of eggs collected and the age distribution of the snails present can be used to calculate age specific reproductive rates, which are more correct than the crude reproductive rate for all adults.

The relative rate of egg laying by snails of different ages is first determined by laboratory observations. It is then used to apportion the eggs in a collection among snails of different ages in the same collection. The method of apportionment requires several steps, and a simple hypothetical example will be given.

Suppose that in the laboratory it is found that snails start laying eggs at an age of 45 days, and that those of 45 to 74, 75 to 104, and 105 to 134 days old lay eggs in the ratio of 1:4:5, respectively; if a field collection is made at a time when the incubation period is 20 days, and 1,000 eggs are collected, this represents 50 eggs per day for the adult snails present in the same area as the 1,000 eggs. Assume that along with the eggs, there were collected 67 snails 45 to 74 days old, 25 snails 75 to 104 days old, and 8 snails over 104 days old, for a total of 100 adults. The distribution of the daily egg production among them could be calculated as:

Age days	Proportional reproduction	Proportional representation	Proportion of eggs laid by snails of indicated age	Total eggs per day available to be apportioned	Total eggs laid per day by age group
45– 74	0.1	× 0.67 = 0.067	(× 4.831) = 0.324	50	16.20
75–104	0.4	× 0.25 = 0.100	(× 4.831) = 0.483	50	24.15
105–134	0.5	× 0.08 = 0.040	(× 4.831) = 0.193	50	9.65
		$\Sigma = 0.207$		total =	50.00
		(1/0.207 = 4.831)			

The daily production per snail 45 to 74 days old would be 16.20/67, or 0.242. For those 75 to 104 days old, the figure would be 24.15/25, or 0.966 eggs per snail per day. The group 105 to 134 days old would have produced 9.65/8, or 1.207 eggs per snail per day. In order to use these figures in an ecological life table they must, of course, be multiplied by the number of days that it has been found convenient to use as time units. HAIRSTON [1965a] used 20-day intervals for *O. quadrasi*; SHIFF [1964] used fortnights for *B. (Ph.) globosus*, *B. pfeifferi* and *Lymnaea natalensis*. In general, the shorter the life-span, the shorter the time units should be, since the use of too few time units in a life table can lead to serious inaccuracies in calculating the parameters.

Human Customs and Practices

Man's position as the vector in the life cycle of schistosomes makes his behaviour exceptionally important in their transmission. The direct results of human behaviour in promoting transmission have been discussed earlier (pp. 282 and 294). Many habits of various peoples are indirectly important to the parasite, in addition to the obvious habits relating to exposure to water and to the disposal of excreta. These other practices are mostly those affecting the extent of the habitats and the size of the populations of the intermediate hosts, but some special customs relating to exposure require elaboration.

Practices Affecting the Snail Population

Except for the few remaining primitive food-gathering societies, humans everywhere have an overwhelming effect upon their surroundings. The ways in which man modifies the natural environment are innumerable and, in general, the more complex his own society the more profound are the modifications. These modifications cannot fail to affect the populations of all other species of animals and plants, among which are the intermediate hosts of schistosomes.

Agriculture

From the standpoint of the area covered, of all of man's activities agriculture has the greatest effect on the environment. In relation to schistosomes, agricultural communities are those in which the parasite has the best chance of flourishing. Agriculture may have the effect of reducing snail populations through control of streams, drainage and proper cultivation, but it may also bring about great increases, especially through the requirement of irrigation, and also through certain improper practices, such as permitting the land to become waterlogged and inadequate cultivation.

a) Rice Farming

The best example of the influence of agriculture on snail populations is that of *O. quadrasi* in the Philippines [PESIGAN *et al.*, 1958b]. The original habitat of these species appears to have been swampy, flood-plain forests [McMULLEN *et al.*, 1954]. As these are cleared for rice farming, snails may persist for a few seasons, but ordinarily the repeated disturbance of ploughing and weeding renders the area unsuitable as a habitat. In the islands of Leyte and Samar, however, a primitive form of rice culture is practised in which the seedlings are planted close together and without pattern. This precludes any weeding, and combined with over-irrigation, permits the area to remain a permanent snail habitat. Some of these fields are several square kilometers in area, a fact which virtually precludes the use of molluscicides as an initial control measure.

b) Fish Culture

Fish ponds provide ideal habitats for many species of aquatic snails. The necessity of pisciculture as a means of relieving protein deficiency requires the presence of these potential snail habitats, but experience in various areas has shown that strict vegetation control, combined with proper fish culture, prevents the establishment of snail populations [McMULLEN, 1962]. In the Philippines, it has been shown that existing snail habitats can be eradicated by the construction of fish ponds, since these do not provide conditions suitable for the amphibious *O. quadrasi* [PESIGAN *et al.*, 1958c; HAIRSTON and SANTOS, 1961].

Irrigation

No human practice has had as much direct effect in increasing snail populations as irrigation. Virtually every important species of intermediate host of human schistosomes has been found to be able to take advantage of the extra water introduced into an area in the form of canals, drains, storage dams, and reservoirs. The unfortunate relationship between this aspect of economic development and the increase in disease has been stressed repeatedly [see McMULLEN *et al.*, 1962, for a general review]. Irrigation does not automatically mean an increase in snail populations; proper regulation and use of water may prevent the establishment of snail populations in some areas. These are principally situations where the water can be shut off completely when it is not being applied to the fields, or where it is feasible to use piped water throughout the system. Where water supplied for irrigation must also be used for household purposes, the situation is much more difficult, since the canals contain water practically all of the time.

Irrigation systems which are poorly designed or improperly managed, or which do not provide for adequate removal of excess water, are especially favourable for snails, and in addition do not permit acceptable crop yields [GIL, 1960].

Water Storage

In semi-arid regions, the catchment and storage of rain is necessary. The problem is, of course, related to that of irrigation but the practice is more widespread and is often carried out in multiple catchments, such as the hafirs of Africa, each of which is quite small but in the aggregate provide a large potential for snail habitats and which, for logistic reasons, are as difficult to deal with as an irrigation system.

Catchments vary in size from what is no more than a large puddle to hydro-electric and irrigation works covering many square kilometers. Regardless of size, these impoundments nearly always provide good snail habitats, and in some cases they raise the water table at downstream locations, thereby further increasing the snail-inhabited area.

Schistosomes derive a dual profit from both irrigation and water storage as these are usually practised. The success of these parasites appears to be a simple function of the product of the abundances of the intermediate and definitive hosts [HAIRSTON, 1962]. Irrigation and water storage increase the productivity of the land, and lead to denser populations of people as well as snails. The parasites are fully adapted to take advantage of the increasing development of many parts of the world.

Careless Engineering and Construction

Throughout the world, construction projects involve a disturbance of natural drainage. It is customary for water to be left standing in borrow pits, and for culverts to be built only as low as is necessary to protect a roadway or other construction. The universal reason given for this dangerous practice is the cost of doing otherwise, but engineering which does not provide for proper drainage is bad engineering to begin with and, in addition, creates new habitats not only for snails but for mosquitoes as well. As the various endemic areas become more and more developed economically, this problem is sure to become more acute.

Practices Directly Affecting the Success of the Parasite

It has already been pointed out in a general way that the normal behaviour of many peoples in rural areas is such as to enhance the transmission of schistosomes (p. 282, a). This applies to habits affecting the success of both eggs and cercariae of the parasite.

Habits Affecting the Success of Schistosome Eggs

Humans are not indiscriminate in the means whereby they dispose of their excreta, whether or not they avail themselves of structures that might be called latrines. As discussed with reference to the fate of schistosome eggs, the general desire for concealment results is an improved likelihood that the eggs will reach the water. In some cultures, the habits of people in this regard are quite specific in helping the life cycle along. FAROOQ and MALLAH [1966] are the most recent to call attention to the relationship between customs of Muslims and the improvement of the chances for the parasites. As far as the contamination of snails is concerned, the religious requirement of ablution following defaecation or urination means automatically that excreta will be deposited near water. The injunction is upon adult males only, but it may well have a more general effect through the establishment of customary places for disposal of excreta.

People whose occupation keeps them in the water, whether fishermen boatmen, or children swimming, are very likely to urinate directly into the water. A more effective means of assisting the transmission of *S. haematobium* could scarcely be devised.

Habits Affecting the Success of Cercariae

Human contact with water is, of course, universal, and such contact increases in rural versus urban areas and also increases directly with the temperature. Some occupations mean certain contact with water for long periods; other instances may be casual or unintended. In the description of exposure in the Philippines (p. 295), emphasis was placed on the nature of the water in which exposure occurred, i.e. whether in snail habitats or in the river into which the habitats drained. The actual activities were also noted; these included, in order of decreasing average duration, ploughing, washing clothes, bathing, swimming, obtaining water, and wading across the river or the snail habitats.

The studies in Egypt [DAZO et al., 1964; FAROOQ and MALLAH, 1966] contain a detailed breakdown of the age and sex of the persons involved, the frequency and duration of each kind of activity, an estimation of the fraction of skin surface involved, and diurnal and seasonal changes in all of these variables. The information is summarized in tables VII–X. The term 'wadu' may not be familiar to all readers; the authors describe this custom as follows:

'Wadu' is ritual washing enjoined by religion on all Muslims before 5-times-a-day prayers (dawn, noon, afternoon, dusk and night). This is an exclusively male activity, in which mostly adults are engaged. It involves washing mostly three-times, all exposed parts of the body (hands, forearms, face, neck and feet), throat gargling and rinsing nares. 'Wadu' is usually preceded by urination and ablution.

The data are very interesting from a number of standpoints. Like the Philippine study, observations in Egypt indicated that girls and women had more frequent contact with water than did boys and men, although the parasitological data [FAROOQ et al., 1966] show a greater prevalence for males of all ages except the youngest. Exposure during farming and irrigation are not included, but it seems unlikely that they would completely resolve the apparent paradox, especially for ages below 15 years. The most plausible explanations appear to lie in the type of activity and the time of day during which it is likely to occur. It will be observed that the nearly exclusively female activities of washing clothes and utensils and drawing water account for 1,241 of 1,538 female contacts with water. These are shown to be primarily morning activities, approximately two thirds of them occurring before noon, when the principal danger of infection is just beginning. By contrast, the primarily male activities of washing animals and vegetables, swimming, ablution, wadu, and fishing took place largely in the afternoon, 40% of them in the most dangerous period, between noon and 3.00 p.m.

In at least one study on human exposure, it has been shown that the frequency of daily contacts with fresh water in Puerto Rico is related to the prevalence of schistosomes [PIMENTEL et al., 1961]. The estimates of frequency of contact were determined by questioning, and not all possible types of contact were included. Nevertheless, the results are clear, as shown in table XI.

The General Economic Level

It has been stressed repeatedly in the literature that the transmission of schistosomes is associated with impoverished rural populations. It must be emphasized that it is the general economic level of the community that influences transmission, more than the status of individuals within the community. Certain occupations and other indications of prosperity have been correlated

Table VII. Frequency of outdoor social and religious water contact activities at four observation posts by sex and age groups during a total period of observation of 164 hours (March 1964 to February 1965)

Activities	Males						Females						Total both sexes
	0–4	5–9	10–14	15–24	25+	all ages	0–4	5–9	10–14	15–24	25+	all ages	
Washing clothes	–	–	–	–	3	3	–	3	31	57	63	154	157
Washing utensils	–	–	2	–	–	2	37	230	173	192	236	868	870
Washing animals	1	2	11	33	18	65	–	1	3	6	10	20	85
Washing vegetables	–	–	2	5	4	11	–	1	1	–	–	2	13
Bathing, playing	194	129	20	7	6	356	208	39	–	3	7	257	613
Swimming	–	12	9	–	–	21	–	–	–	–	–	–	21
Urination	5	3	–	10	16	34	4	–	–	–	1	5	39
Defaecation, urination	7	10	–	4	26	47	10	1	–	–	–	11	58
Ablution	3	–	1	8	40	52	2	–	–	–	–	2	54
'Wadu'	–	–	2	15	71	88	–	–	–	–	–	–	88
Taking water	–	1	1	–	4	6	–	14	30	70	105	219	225
Angling	–	13	9	–	1	23	–	–	–	–	–	–	23
Fishing	–	–	–	–	2	2	–	–	–	–	–	–	2
Total observations	210	170	57	82	191	710	261	289	238	328	422	1,538	2,248

Table VIII. Frequency of outdoor social and religious water contact activities by sex and by season

Activities	Males					Females					Total both sexes
	spring	summer	autumn	winter	total	spring	summer	autumn	winter	total	
Washing clothes	–	–	3	–	3	25	51	43	35	154	157
Washing utensils	–	–	2	–	2	199	265	202	202	868	870
Washing animals	7	24	22	12	65	1	15	–	4	20	85
Washing vegetables	3	–	2	6	11	1	1	–	–	2	13
Bathing, playing	59	110	115	72	356	71	67	58	61	257	613
Swimming	2	15	4	–	21	–	–	–	–	–	21
Urination	3	14	9	8	34	2	–	3	–	5	39
Defaecation, urination	8	20	12	7	47	–	5	2	4	11	58
Ablution	7	21	12	12	52	–	1	1	–	2	54
'Wadu'	15	31	23	19	88	–	–	–	–	–	8
Taking water	6	–	–	–	6	44	56	49	70	219	225
Angling	1	17	5	–	23	–	–	–	–	–	23
Fishing	1	–	1	–	2	–	–	–	–	–	2
Total observations	112	252	210	136	710	343	461	358	376	1,538	2,248

Table IX. Duration of exposure involved in the different activities during *winter* (observed between 26 November 1964 and 17 January 1965)

Type of activity	Number of persons observed	Total exposure period min.	Average duration of exposure min.	Range of exposure min.
Washing clothes	34	950	27.9	10–55
Washing utensils	33	660	20.0	5–40
Washing animals	8	69	8.6	3–35
Washing vegetables	2	25	12.5	10–15
Bathing, playing	36	650	18.1	5–30
Swimming	3	35	11.7	10–15
Urination	4	9	2.3	2–3
Defaecation, urination	5	32	6.4	5–10
Ablution	3	3	1.0	1–
'Wadu'	7	25	3.6	3–5
Taking water	8	28	3.5	2–5
Angling	3	75	25.0	15–40
Fishing	1	35	35.0	35–
Total	147	2,596	17.6	–

Table X. Duration of exposure involved in the different activities during *summer* (observed between 6 June and 27 July 1965)

Type of activity	Number of persons observed	Total exposure period min.	Average duration of exposure min.	Range of exposure min.
Washing clothes	73	2,291	31.4	10–35
Washing utensils	75	1,648	21.9	5–45
Washing animals	29	246	8.5	3–30
Washing vegetables	8	180	22.5	10–40
Bathing, playing	60	1,225	20.4	5–40
Swimming	17	378	22.2	3–35
Urination	13	21	1.6	1–3
Defaecation, urination	12	76	6.3	4–10
Ablution	13	11	0.8	0.5–1
'Wadu'	19	59	3.1	2–5
Taking water	30	99	3.3	2–6
Angling	10	410	41.0	30–55
Fishing	3	115	38.3	35–55
Total	362	6,759	18.6	–

Table XI. The relationship between the prevalence of *S. mansoni* and the number of daily contacts with water in three watersheds in Puerto Rico [from PIMENTEL *et al.*, 1961]

Number of contacts with infected water	Number of persons examined	Number of persons positive	% positive
0	69	22	32
1	100	51	51
2	24	18	75
3	79	68	86

with relatively lower prevalence rates [FAROOQ *et al.*, 1966], but water teeming with cercariae is dangerous to the well-to-do and to the poor alike. Moreover, children everywhere have a remarkable affinity for water, and they exercise very little discrimination as to its quality.

Sanitation is a highly desirable goal, but it is so closely tied to the economy that to advise sanitation as a principal means of interrupting transmission of schistosomes is tantamount to asking less developed areas to tolerate the disease for another generation or more.

The ancient interlocking combination of poverty, ignorance, and disease has always appeared impregnable until it has been attacked by men determined to succeed and willing to persist with all their energy in applying the knowledge at hand. The complexity of the life cycle of schistosomes, requiring as it does an absolute minimum of 11 weeks for completion, is an advantage to be pursued. It cannot continue in the face of well-planned persistent attack, as has been demonstrated in various parts of the world. Surely it is better to make intelligent use of the weapons at hand than to assume an attitude of helplessness while awaiting a hypothetically perfect method of the future.

References

ALVES, W.: Bull. Wld Hlth Org. *18:* 1071 (1958a).
ALVES, W.: Bull. Wld Hlth Org. *18:* 1092 (1958b).
BANG, F.B. and HAIRSTON, N.G.: Amer. J. Hyg. *44:* 348 (1946).
BARBOSA, F.S.: Aspects of the ecology of the intermediate hosts of *Schistosoma mansoni* interfering with the transmission of bilharziasis in north-eastern Brazil; in WOLSTEN-HOLME and O'CONNOR Bilharziasis, pp. 23–35 (Churchill, London 1962).
BARBOSA, F.S.: Rev. Inst. Med. trop., São Paulo *7:* 112 (1965).
BARBOSA, F.S. and OLIVIER, L.: Bull. Wld Hlth Org. *18:* 895 (1958).
BELL, D.R.: Bull. Wld Hlth Org. *29:* 525 (1963).
BIRCH, L.C.: J. anim. Ecol. *17:* 15 (1948).

BIRCH, L. C.: Ecology *34:* 698 (1953).

BLISS, C. I. and FISHER, R. A.: Biometrics *9:* 176 (1953).

BRADLEY, D. J.: E. afr. med. J. *40:* 240 (1963).

BRADLEY, D. J.: Bull. Wld Hlth Org. *33:* 503 (1965).

CHANDLER, A. C.: Amer. J. trop. Med. Hyg. *3:* 59 (1954).

CHERNIN, E. and DUNAVAN, C. A.: Amer. J. trop. Med. Hyg. *11:* 455 (1962).

CHU, K. Y.; SABBAGHIAN, H. and MASSOUD, J.: Bull. Wld Hlth Org. *34:* 121 (1966).

DAVENPORT, D.; WRIGHT, C. A., and CAUSLEY, D.: Science *135:* 1059 (1962).

DAVIS, A.: Effect of CIBA 32644-Ba on *Schistosoma haematobium.* Acta tropica, suppl. 9, pp. 132–144 (1966).

DAZO, B. C. and MORENO, R. G.: Trans. amer. microsc. Soc. *81:* 341 (1962).

DAZO, B. C.; FAROOQ, M., and MALLAH, M.: WHO unpublished document BILH/Exp. Com. 3/WP/20 (1964).

DAZO, B. C.; HAIRSTON, N. G., and DAWOOD, I. K.: Bull. Wld Hlth Org. *35:* 339 (1966).

EL-GINDY, M. S. and RUSHDI, M. Z.: The variability in morphology and anatomy of the bulinid snails in Egypt, with special reference to their transmission of *Schistosoma haematobium*; in WOLSTENHOLME and O'CONNOR Bilharziasis, pp. 81–102 (Churchill, London 1962).

ETGES, F. J. and DECKER, C. L.: J. Parasit. *49:*114 (1963).

EVANS, F. C. and SMITH, F. E.: Amer. Nat. *86:* 299 (1952).

FAROOQ, M. and HAIRSTON, N. G.: Bull. Wld Hlth Org. *35:* 331 (1966).

FAROOQ, M. and MALLAH, M. B.: Bull. Wld Hlth Org. *35:* 377 (1966).

FAROOQ, M. and NIELSEN, J.: Bull. Wld Hlth Org. *35:* 281 (1966).

FAROOQ, M.; NIELSEN, J.; SAMAAN, S. A.; MALLAH, M. B., and ALLAM, A. A.: Bull. Wld Hlth Org. *35:* 293 (1966).

FAUST, E. C. and HOFFMAN, W. A.: Puerto Rico J. publ. Hlth *10:* 1 (1934).

FISHER, R. A.: The genetical theory of natural selection; 2nd rev. ed. (Dover Press, New York 1958).

GADGIL, R. K. and SHAH, S. N.: Indian J. med. Res. *44:* 577 (1956).

GIL, N.: Unpublished report to the Government of the Philippines on land use and bilharziasis control. FAO/60/G/4846, Report No. 1267 (1960).

GOHAR, H. A. F. and EL-GINDY, H. I.: Proc. egypt. Acad. Sci. *15:* 70 (1960).

GOHAR, H. A. F. and EL-GINDY, H. I.: J. egypt. med. Ass. *44:* 976 (1961).

GORDON, R. M.; DAVEY, T. H., and PEASTON, H.: Ann. trop. Med. Parasit. *28:* 323 (1934).

HAIRSTON, N. G.: Assignment report, Philippines-9 project. WHO unpublished document (1959).

HAIRSTON, N. G.: Population ecology and epidemiological problems; in WOLSTENHOLME and O'CONNOR Bilharziasis, pp. 36–62 (Churchill, London 1962).

HAIRSTON, N. G.: Bull. Wld Hlth Org. *33:* 45 (1965a).

HAIRSTON, N. G.: Bull. Wld Hlth Org. *33:* 163 (1965b).

HAIRSTON, N. G. and SANTOS, B. C.: Bull. Wld Hlth Org. *25:* 603 (1961).

HARRY, H. W. and CUMBIE, B. G.: Amer. J. trop. Med. Hyg. *5:* 921 (1956).

HARRY, H. W.; CUMBIE, B. G., and MARTINEZ DE JESUS, J.: Amer. J. trop. Med. Hyg. *6:* 313 (1957).

INGALLS, J. W., jr.; HUNTER, G. W.; MCMULLEN, D. B., and BAUMAN, P. M.: J. Parasit. *35:* 147 (1949).

KLOETZEL, K.: Amer. J. trop. Med. Hyg. *12:* 334 (1963).

LESLIE, P.H. and RANSON, R.M.: J. anim. Ecol. *9:* 27 (1940).

LOTKA, A.J.: Proc. nat. Acad. Sci., Wash. *8:* 339 (1922).

MACDONALD, G.: Trans. roy. Soc. trop. Med. Hyg. *59:* 489 (1965).

MALEK, E.A.: Bull. Wld Hlth Org. *18:* 785 (1958).

MALEK, E.A.: Bull. Wld Hlth Org. *27:* 41 (1962).

MARILL, F.G.: Bull. Wld Hlth Org. *18:* 1064 (1958).

McCLELLAND, W.J.R.: Bull. Wld Hlth Org. *33:* 270 (1965).

McCULLOUGH, F.S.: Bull. Wld Hlth Org. *27:* 161 (1962).

McMULLEN, D.B.: Amer. J. Hyg. *45:* 259 (1947).

McMULLEN, D.B.: The modification of habitats in the control of bilharziasis, with special reference to water resource development; in WOLSTENHOLME and O'CONNOR Bilharziasis, pp. 382–396 (Churchill, London 1962).

McMULLEN, D.B.; KOMIYAMA, S., and ENDO-ITABASHI, T.: Amer. J. Hyg. *54:* 402 (1951).

McMULLEN, D.B.; BUZO, Z.J.; RAINEY, M.B., and FRANCOTTE, J.: Bull. Wld Hlth Org. *27:* 25 (1962).

McMULLEN, D.B.; HUBENDICK, B.; PESIGAN, T.P., and BIERSTEIN, P.: J. Philipp. med. Ass. *30:* 615 (1954).

MEILLON, B. DE; FRANK, G.H., and ALLANSON, B.R.: Bull. Wld Hlth Org. *18:* 771 (1958).

MICHELSON, E.H.: Amer. J. trop. Med. Hyg. *13:* 36 (1964).

MOORE, D.V. and SANDGROUND, J.H.: Amer. J. trop. Med. Hyg. *5:* 831 (1956).

MUENCH, H.: Catalytic models in epidemiology (Harvard University Press, Cambridge, Mass. 1959).

NAJARIAN, H.H.: Bull. Wld Hlth Org. *25:* 435 (1961).

OLIVIER, L.: Amer. J. trop. Med. Hyg. *15:* 882 (1966).

PERLOWAGORA-SZUMLEWICZ, A.: Bull. Wld Hlth Org. *30:* 401 (1964).

PESIGAN, T.P.; FAROOQ, M.; HAIRSTON, N.G.; JAUREGUI, J.J.; GARCIA, E.G.; SANTOS, A.T.; SANTOS, B.C., and BESA, A.A.: Bull. Wld Hlth Org. *18:* 345 (1958).

PESIGAN, T.P.; FAROOQ, M.; HAIRSTON, N.G.; JAUREGUI, J.J.; GARCIA, E.G.; SANTOS, A.T.; SANTOS, B.C., and BESA, A.A.: Bull. Wld Hlth Org. *19:* 223 (1958c).

PESIGAN, T.P.; HAIRSTON, N.G.; JAUREGUI, J.J.; GARCIA, E.G.; SANTOS, A.T.; SANTOS, B.C., and BESA, A.A.: Bull. Wld Hlth Org. *18:* 481 (1958b).

PIMENTEL, D. and WHITE, P.C., jr.: Ecology *40:* 533 (1959a).

PIMENTEL, D. and WHITE, P.C., jr.: Ecology *40:* 541 (1959b).

PIMENTEL, D.; GERHARDT, C.E.; WILLIAMS, E.R.; WHITE, P.C., jr., and FERGUSON, F.F.: Amer. J. trop. Med. Hyg. *10:* 523 (1961).

PITCHFORD, R.J. and VISSER, P.S.: Bull. Wld Hlth Org. *32:* 83 (1965).

RADKE, M.G.; RITCHIE, L.S., and ROWAN, W.B.: Exp. Parasit. *11:* 323 (1961).

RANSFORD, O.N.: Trans. roy. Soc. trop. Med. Hyg. *41:* 617 (1948).

RITCHIE, L.S.; RADKE, M.G., and FERGUSON, F.F.: Bull. Wld Hlth Org. *27:* 171 (1962).

SCHALIE, H. VAN DER: Bull. Wld Hlth Org. *19:* 263 (1958).

SCHUTTE, C.H.J. and FRANK, G.H.: Bull. Wld Hlth Org. *30:* 389 (1964).

SEVILLA, J.Z.: The effects of temperature on the intrinsic rate of increase of three species of pulmonate snails; unpublished PhD Thesis, University of Michigan, Ann Arbor, Mich. (1965).

SHARPE, F.R. and LOTKA, A.J.: Philosoph. Magaz. *21:* 435 (1911).

SHIFF, C. J.: Ann. trop. Med. Parasit. *58:* 94 (1964).

SIOLI, H.: Arch. Hydrobiol. *48:* 1 (1953).

SLOBODKIN, L. B.: Growth and regulation of animal populations (Holt, Rinehart & Winston, New York 1961).

SMITH, F. E.: Quantitative aspects of population growth; in BOELL Dynamics of growth processes, pp. 277–294 (University Press, Princeton 1954).

STIREWALT, M. A.: Exp. Parasit. *3:* 504 (1954).

STIREWALT, M. A.: WHO unpublished document, BILH/Exp. Com. 3/WP/28 (1964).

STURROCK, R. F.: Ann. trop. Med. Parasit. *60:* 100 (1966).

SULLIVAN, R. R. and FERGUSON, M. S.: Amer. J. Hyg. *44:* 324 (1946).

TEESDALE, C.: Bull. Wld Hlth Org. *27:* 759 (1962).

VOGEL, H. and MINNING, W.: Z. Tropenmed. Parasit. *4:* 418 (1953).

WATSON, J. M.: J. Fac. Med. Baghdad *14:* 148 (1950).

WATSON, J. M.: Bull. Wld Hlth Org. *18:* 833 (1958).

WEBBE, G.: Bull. Wld Hlth Org. *27:* 59 (1962a).

WEBBE, G.: Population studies of intermediate hosts in relation to transmission of bilharziasis in East Africa; in WOLSTENHOLME and O'CONNOR Bilharziasis, pp. 7–22 (Churchill, London 1962b).

WEBBE, G.: Ann. trop. Med. Parasit. *60:* 85 (1966).

WHO: Philippines-9 project. Quarterly reports for the quarters January–March and April–June. Unpublished document (1955).

WHO: Measurement of the public health importance of bilharziasis; report of a WHO Scientific Group, Geneva 1965. Wld Hlth Org. techn. Rep. Ser. 349 (1967).

WILLIAMS, N.: in University College of Rhodesia and Nyasaland, Zoology Department, Snail Ecology Research Unit, Annual Report for the year ending December 1963. Document (1963).

WITENBERG, G. and SALITERNIK, Z.: Bull. Res. Coun. Israel B *6:* 107 (1957).

WRIGHT, C. A.: in WOLSTENHOLME and O'CONNOR Bilharziasis, p. 156 (Churchill, London 1962).

ZAKARIA, H.: Bull. endem. Dis. *1:* 46 (1954).

ZAKARIA, H.: Bull. endem. Dis. *1:* 123 (1955).

Chapter 5

Epidemiology and Control of Schistosomiasis, pp. 337–353
(Karger, Basel and University Park Press, Baltimore 1973)

The Public Health and Economic Importance of Schistosomiasis

Its Assessment

G. MACDONALD and M. FAROOQ

Introduction

Two hundred million people are estimated to be affected by schistosomiasis. The disease is widespread in the tropical world. It has substantially increased in prevalence and intensity in some countries during the last half-century as a consequence of the development of water resources for irrigation and industrial purposes. Nevertheless, and despite the considerable amount of published work on the various morbid manifestations of the disease, the importance of schistosomiasis from the public health standpoint has long remained an open issue.

That heavy infection with *Schistosoma mansoni* or *S. japonicum* can produce severe disease is now generally recognized but schistosomiasis caused by *S. haematobium* was held in some countries, such as Egypt, to be one of the major public health problems while it was denied practically any significant role in the morbidity and mortality recorded in other countries of the African continent and of the Eastern Mediterranean region. This latter view was, however, disproved recently by community and group studies conducted in Tanzania, Nigeria, and Senegal which revealed a high incidence of severe lesions – calcified bladder, deformity of the ureter, hydronephrosis – in the youngest age groups (45% of school-children in some localities) [FORSYTH and BRADLEY, 1964, 1966; FORSYTH and MACDONALD, 1965; GILLES *et al.*, 1965a, b; GELFAND, 1965; FORSYTH and MACDONALD, 1966; FORSYTH, 1969]. While these studies are being pursued to establish the prognosis of these lesions [LUCAS *et al.*, 1966; LUCAS and COCKSHOTT, 1966; CHAPMAN, 1966; DAVIS, 1966; EL BADAWI, 1966; MACDONALD and FORSYTH, 1968], the evidence thus gathered suggests that schistosomiasis may be the cause of considerable morbidity, unsuspected so far, in adolescents and children, as well as in adults.

For the above reasons, schistosomiasis ranks among the most important public health problems of the tropics and subtropics, and is recognized today as second only to malaria in importance as a parasitic disease. However, in areas where schistosomiasis is endemic, this disease is not the only problem. Poverty and disease notoriously form a vicious circle so ably described in WINSLOW's study and defined by MYRDAL [1952]: 'Men and women were sick because they were poor; they became poorer because they were sick, and sicker because they were poorer.' In the circumstances, policy-making bodies must decide which of the problems they are being faced with require first attention. In the public health field there is, however, a general tendency to single out acute dramatic conditions at the expense of chronic ones, in particular parasitic diseases, although some of the latter affect much greater numbers of people and have far deeper repercussions on the economy. Policy decisions would, therefore, be facilitated if the people vested with authority were provided with as correct as possible an assessment of the public health significance of schistosomiasis. When such an assessment has shown that schistosomiasis needs to be controlled, an attempt should then be made to estimate the cost of the proposed control programme and the returns which it is likely to bring in terms of human welfare and economic benefits, taking into account the socio-economic level of the population.

To provide guidelines for the relevant investigations, WHO convened two scientific groups in 1960 and 1965. The main substance of the present chapter and of the chapter on pages 354 to 387 is derived from their consolidated report [WHO, 1967].

Approaches to the Assessment of the Public Health and Economic Importance of Schistosomiasis

Basically, the evaluation of the public health importance of any disease is difficult. The first attempts to assess the extent of morbidity due to chronic conditions (mostly respiratory and cardiovascular diseases) were made recently in the past 10 to 15 years and in economically advanced countries enjoying the highest level of medical services. Considering that the methodology for such studies is still far from being perfected, the difficulty is increased when the condition is not solely characterized by acute readily-recognizable episodes of disability which can be counted and measured, and it is worsened when the disease typically occurs in places not well served by hospitals and pathological services. In the case of schistosomiasis, an additional complication is that there is often an association with other parasitic infections, malnutrition, poverty and poor hygienic conditions, the relative importance of which is difficult to evaluate.

In developing countries the annual vital statistics form an inadequate basis for valid assessment of mortality caused by schistosomiasis, and estimates from different countries in which the infection is widely endemic may vary from 5% to practically nil. Morbidity rates are of similarly limited value. Numerous reports in the literature quote the number of cases of schistosomiasis seen in hospitals, clinics or private practice. Sometimes these data are broken down into types and degrees of severity, and related to the total number of patients admitted. Occasionally, an attempt is made to relate such data to the population which the institution serves, but the sampling problems are almost always insuperable and the results of doubtful value.

To the individual concerned, the importance of an infection turns upon its actual or potential severity, and the degree to which it is going to detract from his normal enjoyment of life, and is not affected by the question of whether the condition is rare or common. By contrast, a consideration of the public health importance of an infection takes into account its community aspects: its frequency, the common range of ill-effects, and their severity and frequency; the distribution of the disease amongst various age, sex, occupational or other groups of the population; the social or economic effects of the disease; and the total contribution of the infection to the load of morbidity and premature mortality carried by the population.

The economic importance of an infection depends largely on the prevailing economic, social and industrial conditions which inevitably vary from country to country and from area to area. In a community dependent on subsistence farming, ill-health at one season of the year may be economically unimportant whilst at another season its economic consequences may be dramatic. Reduced work output in diseased people is meaningless when there is no available occupation on which the individual could have profitably engaged himself. This is often one of the reasons given to explain why loss due to illness is regarded as small in many areas, although illness may be common. Nevertheless, it is the objective of governments in both developing and developed countries to provide an opportunity for fruitful employment for all people at all times, and the economic importance of a disease must, therefore, be assessed in relation to the way in which it detracts from the working potential capacity of the population and the extent to which it impedes utilization and development of the country's natural resources.

For investigation purposes, the public health and economic importance of schistosomiasis may be broken down into the following components:

(1) the prevalence of infection;

(2) the intensity of infection;

(3) the magnitude of resulting disease in clinical and pathological terms;

(4) the consequent disability in social terms; and

(5) the economic expression of such disability.

In the following sections, the organization and types of investigations required in the study of the above components will be discussed rather than the procedures and working criteria which are dealt with in the chapters on pages 354 to 387 and 609 to 748.

Prevalence and Intensity of Infection

Prevalence Surveys

There is a large number of records of surveys of the prevalence of schistosomiasis in numerous countries. Many of these surveys concern only limited areas. Occasionally, they were planned so as to cover samples more or less representative of the entire population, but in most surveys particular groups have been deliberately chosen for examination, either because these groups were of special interest or because they were more accessible.

Observations on the detailed distribution of *S. haematobium* in East Africa and Nigeria and on *S. mansoni* in Northern Egypt indicate that it is sometimes unwise to consider large areas as being more or less homogeneous for studies of either prevalence or intensity since, if accurately measured, they would be found to be a patchwork with widely varying prevalence between places only small distances apart. For an over-all figure of the proportion of people infected in a country or large region, it is reasonable to take the findings of a mass survey covering very many areas. For most other purposes, it may be found best to identify the small foci in which the principal transmission occurs and measure prevalence within such foci. However, although prevalence data form the basis for extrapolation of local results to a region or country, the prevalence rates give no indication of how much harm is caused by the parasite.

Measurement of the Intensity of Infection

In a number of prevalence surveys, there has, therefore, been an attempt to make an associated determination of the intensity of infection, using excretal egg-counts. Good correlation has been found between egg output and the prevalence of various ill effects. For *S. japonicum*, clinical severity was related to egg output; for *S. mansoni*, the prevalence of splenomegaly; and in the case of *S. haematobium*, the prevalence and severity of specific urological lesions. It is becoming increasingly clear that egg output may provide an index of disability and should be measured in prevalence surveys concerned with public health assessment. Methods have been developed that decrease the amount of labour and technical skill required (see pages 622 to 634 and pages 729, 730).

The Magnitude of Resulting Disease in Clinical and Pathological Terms

The lesions and syndromes resulting from schistosomal infection in different people are numerous and varied. Assessment must, therefore, be based on certain of the more objective clinico-pathological phenomena lending themselves to quantitative evaluation (see chapter on pages 354 to 387). Care must be taken to follow, as far as possible, uniform quantitative clinical, pathological and epidemiological techniques not only to ensure reproducibility of the results but also to allow comparison between different areas. This is of particular importance where the lesions may not be entirely of schistosomal origin. Quantitative data will be useful in evaluating the morbidity and mortality due to schistosomiasis and will also yield information on the development of the disease and the relation of lesions to the intensity and duration of infection. Moreover, they will give insight into apparent differences in the severity and types of lesions encountered in various geographical areas such as the low prevalence of severe intestinal and hepatosplenic schistosomiasis in some *S. mansoni* areas in contrast to the frequency of these conditions in Egypt.

One site for study is an endemic area where conditions have been little disturbed over a number of years, and in which the water, snails and people constitute a reasonably static ecological complex, all of which can be examined. Equally important from the public health standpoint is the investigation of the disease under conditions wherein the ecological complex has undergone material change.

Ideally each member of the community, or a random sample, should be studied throughout the duration of infection and its after-effects, using elaborate diagnostic and sociological procedures. This is technically so difficult, time-consuming and expensive as to be impossible. The form of survey depends, therefore, on its objectives. Two main types exist: (a) the cross-sectional study in which a group of individuals is studied at a specified point in, or segment of, time, and (b) the longitudinal survey whereby a specified group of individuals is observed and examined over a relatively long period of time, usually several years. Considerable progress has recently been made in the former field for S. haematobium and the manner of its execution has been formulated and tested. Many problems remain which can only be studied longitudinally, and the need for studies of this type is very great indeed. In the case of S. mansoni, cross-sectional community studies have been carried out by BARBOSA [1965] in Brazil. Apart from these field investigations, useful indications on the severity of deep lesions and their relation to intensity of infection may be provided by autopsy and viscerotomy studies.

Cross-Sectional Surveys

A population is selected for study and either the whole of it or a random sample is investigated. In the selection of the sample, note must be made of the characteristic uneven distribution of schistosomiasis in nearly all areas.

Since the urological lesions of S. haematobium cannot be assessed adequately from simple field studies, cross-sectional surveys are sometimes organized in two stages; in such a study, a representative sample of the field group is investigated in hospital. Such studies have shown a close correlation between the load of infection as measured by egg output and the pathological changes that were shown on radiological examination. Thus, simple parasitological studies in the field may provide estimates of the frequency of urological lesions.

Simple focal survey procedures will determine the prevalence of S. mansoni and S. japonicum infections. However, the relative lack of pathognomonic and obvious symptoms and signs necessitates detailed clinical investigation. Even in cases showing hepatosplenomegaly, differential diagnostic procedures are required. Assessment of the public health significance of S. mansoni and S. japonicum is, therefore, relatively difficult.

Special Features of S. haematobium Studies

One of the most striking findings of recent studies on the lesions produced by *S. haematobium* in the urinary tract is the co-existence of gross anatomical lesions and apparently unimpaired health. The lesions cannot, therefore, be reliably detected by history and physical examination alone, and brief hospitalization may be required. The cardinal procedures are simple radiography of the abdomen and pelvis, followed by intravenous (excretion) urography to detect calcification of the bladder or ureters, calculi, and abnormalities of the renal pelvis, ureters or bladder. Because of the florid changes produced in the urine by uncomplicated schistosomal infection, urinary examination for abnormal cellular constituents provides equivocal information. Cystoscopy, though surprisingly acceptable to communities as an investigational procedure, carries dangers of introducing bacterial infection, but it provides data on the prevalence of bladder growths, benign and malignant. Cystometrography and micturating cystography have been little used in studies so far. They may prove to have considerable potential in ascertaining the mechanism by which renal changes are produced, and as such are primarily suitable for individual rather than community studies. Renal function has been little studied in relation to the anatomical lesions. Blood urea determination is an obvious procedure, though it has yielded only negative information in surveys carried out so far. If practicable under the circumstances of survey, more sensitive measures such as phenolsulphonthalein (PSP) excretion may be attempted.

Special Features of S. mansoni and S. japonicum Studies

In the case of *S. mansoni*, there are certain physical signs that appear strongly correlated with severe internal lesions, so that some separation of cases in the field is possible. History and physical examination constitute, therefore, the first stage of examination, though internal checks are essential to demonstrate that the history taken has some degree of reproducibility. Stratified sampling is then used, bearing in mind that the greatest single need at present is to clarify the public health meaning of hepatosplenomegaly in endemic areas of schistosomiasis, that is, its importance as a clinical finding, its correlation with infection intensity, and its ultimate effect on morbidity and mortality in the infected population. Since coincident factors such as malnutrition and alcoholism may possibly affect the course and prognosis of schistosomal hepatic lesions, it is necessary to attempt to assess these as well.

Longitudinal Surveys

The Community

Cross-sectional studies of communities will provide data on the nature and prevalence of certain lesions. In many cases the precise significance of these lesions for public health is still uncertain. Such uncertainty can only be resolved by longitudinal studies, in which cases presenting such lesions are observed over a period of years to determine their fate in terms of morbidity and mortality. There is no substitute for prolonged observation to determine the prognosis of many specific lesions. Among such lesions, our need to clarify the consequences of schistosomal ureteric deformity and hydronephrosis is outstanding. Although much of the information collected by cross-sectional studies will remain inconclusive in the absence of adequate follow-up, the very great effort needed for longitudinal studies will be of limited value unless they are planned from basic cross-sectional data.

Certain precautions, desirable in any study, become imperative in work of this type. They include clear definition of the purpose of the study, expert statistical advice at the planning stage, adequate allowance for loss of people from the study by emigration, transfer, withdrawal of co-operation and means of coping with the changes of name customary in some cultures. The detection of uncommon occurrences may necessitate extremely large samples; for example, a million person-years have been estimated to be necessary in cancer studies.

Since longitudinal studies of patients with schistosomiasis are in their infancy, no firm recommendations can be made on the frequency of periodic re-examination. It is tentatively proposed that detailed clinical review should be repeated at intervals of one to two years. Methods comparable with those for cross-sectional surveys should be used. However, an additional mechanism is needed to ensure early notification of any major illness that may affect the patients, and deaths within the study population should be reported at once. The value of autopsy data from any member of a longitudinal study who dies cannot be over-estimated and the effort needed to obtain such data would be more than repaid.

Longitudinal studies have additional uses. An infected population group may be followed to discover the rate of onset of specific lesions or complications whilst a sample of the population may be followed to elucidate the natural history of the infection. A method for compressing a lifetime's follow-up into less than a decade is to follow the whole of a community, considered in five-year age groups, for five years and to consider the end point of each group as the starting point of the next older age group. Such a study demands a reasonably stable epidemiological pattern.

The effect of treatment on prognosis can be studied by careful controls in the same endemic area. Yet the inclusion in the investigation of two additional control groups sampled from an area of interrupted transmission, one receiving treatment, the other not, would answer many of the problems that incipient control schemes are likely to pose for assessment of the expected changes in public health importance following chemotherapy.

The Individual

Studies of individuals over a long period, even with only limited knowledge of their history of exposure to infection, can provide data of value to understanding the consequences of schistosomiasis. Many infected people have migrated to areas where schistosomal infection is not endemic, where medical facilities are more extensive, and where developed postal systems make follow-up less arduous. They may be studied to provide information of value to assessing the likely public health importance of schistosomiasis after transmission control schemes have been instituted, though care must be exercised in the interpretation of such data since the patient's nutritional status and general medical care may also have improved.

Although complete autopsies on all individuals dying in infected communities are almost impossible to obtain, clinico-pathologically correlated studies on even a few are most valuable. They make it possible to bridge the gap between measurements obtained in surveys and their underlying basis in morbid anatomy, and between egg excretion in the living and worm burden and egg load of organs in the dead, and the resulting pathology.

Autopsies

As in the study of any disease, the use of autopsy as the final examination in follow-up of a patient is of enormous value and greatly to be encouraged.

The direct use of autopsy surveys in assessing the public health importance of schistosomal infection is less clear. Any autopsy population is biased, and the limited number of autopsies possible in most regions where schistosomiasis is endemic may be very highly selected, so that it would be almost impossible to relate these to the general population. Quantitative conclusions are, therefore, rarely possible in a direct manner, but more qualitative deductions may be made. In Nigeria, deaths directly attributable to schistosomiasis have not been found to be in proportion to the high prevalence of anatomical lesions in the living [EDINGTON, pers. comm.] while in Ghana a prevalence of 2% of deaths of schistosomal etiology suggested that the infection was an important cause of death there [EDINGTON, 1957]. Such discrepancy clearly points to the need for further investigations.

Autopsies done for verification of the cause of death in non-hospitalized patients (medico-legal autopsies) are likely to be more representative, but the data obtained are usually fragmentary, and clinical data are seldom available.

It is also clear that present knowledge of many aspects of the pathogenesis of schistosomiasis is so inadequate that further basic information is a necessary prerequisite to assessing the public health importance of the infection. The two main sources of such basic data are longitudinal studies and careful autopsies. (As mentioned earlier and subsequently, when these two can be combined on the same population the resulting information is of still greater value.)

Many of the places where schistosomal patients come to autopsy have limited facilities and staff, and only a limited number of cases can be dealt with. If the resulting data from several centres in contiguous areas could be combined, their value would be greatly increased. The types of control necessary for such a study can only be defined in relation to the hypotheses under test, but it is felt that at the present time more descriptive information is needed before even hypotheses can be clearly formulated. A general consensus among pathologists on definitions and descriptions of lesions is the first step. To this end attempts have been made to devise standard methods for autopsy of schistosomal patients (see pages 375 to 376; and page 744). It is hoped that comparability of data may be facilitated by exchange of material.

The specific objectives of autopsy studies on schistosomiasis are three in number:

(1) to verify the cause of death and how far schistosomal infection is contributing to it;

(2) to evaluate schistosomal lesions and assess the factors that modify them; and

(3) to investigate the relationship between worm and egg load, pathological lesions and the *ante mortem* clinical state of the patients.

The first of these requires thorough rather than standardized procedures; the second requires standard techniques, and comparability between centres to permit valid comparison between areas, as also does the third. This last necessitates measurement of egg load in the tissues as well as study of the lesions by histopathological means.

Enumeration of Worms at Autopsy

The enumeration of worms in human cadavers has posed many problems and is still not practicable except by laborious empirical searching in the case of *S.haematobium*. For *S.mansoni* and *S.japonicum*, perfusion of portal and mesenteric veins of cadavers for worms can be performed with apparently reliable results though it is still slow (chapter on pages 652 to 656). A quantitative *post mortem* study of *S.mansoni* in man indicated that nearly all worm pairs were recovered with such a technique, and that the number of eggs per gram of faeces and the total egg burden in the tissues (liver, intestines, and lungs) showed strong positive correlations with the number of worm pairs recovered [CHEEVER, 1968].

In the course of autopsy, press preparations from various parts of the intestine will detect most cases of schistosomiasis infection, so that digestions may be carried out on them. The sites are detailed in the chapter on page 656. Several are necessary because of variation between patients in the localization of eggs in the intestinal tract. In recent studies, cases with more worm pairs had larger numbers of eggs in the mucosa and as the number of worm pairs increased, larger numbers of eggs were found at higher levels, i.e., in the transverse colon, caecum and small intestine. Cases of Symmers' fibrosis showed a unique distribution, with few or no eggs in the specimens of rectal mucosa and a maximum in the jejunal mucosa. In all other groups the largest number of eggs was in the rectosigmoid.

Quantitative study of the relations between egg output and the organ load of eggs will provide a basis for relating infection to pathology so that excretal egg counting may be more precisely used in assessment of the importance of schistosomiasis.

Viscerotomy

This procedure may be resorted to in population surveys of remote communities, where personnel or facilities for *post mortem* studies are not available, or where autopsy permission is denied but viscerotomy is tolerated. It can also be offered as an alternate proposal for obtaining vitally needed information from cases previously studied by clinical means, and whose families do not consent to *post mortem* study.

Thus far, viscerotomy experience in schistosomiasis studies has been limited to the liver and to *S.mansoni*, where it has provided data on prevalence as well as on the cause of death. Although its use in field surveys appears very attractive, its acceptability to communities has been found to be limited.

The sampling error inherent in blind puncturing of the liver is less in viscerotomy than in hepatic biopsy, but it is obvious that localized lesions (tumours, gummata or abscesses) may be missed. On the other hand, there is usually sufficient tissue not only for establishing the presence and degree of liver fibrosis, but also for its classification.

Viscerotomy may have value in *S.haematobium* areas for renal biopsy when autopsy is refused, but has so far not been tried in practice. Since renal change may be rather localized several samples may be needed to establish a diagnosis.

A form of drill biopsy instrument capable of removing small cores from numerous sites may be used in hospitals. It comprises a steel needle adapted to a dental drill engine which can rotate at 5,000 rpm. There is no danger of damage of tissue by heating or distortion of the material. Specimens can be obtained in one minute and the size of the biopsy is adequate for histological techniques (up to 0.5 cm × 0.2 cm).

The Economic Effects of Schistosomiasis

Health is so important that it has to be maintained even at a considerable financial sacrifice. No economic pressure should prevent right action in this respect. However, although the final decision on control primarily rests upon epidemiological considerations, it will inevitably be affected by economic factors. To support a request for funds for a control campaign, it would be desirable to be able to provide the funding authority with information to show that the cost of a particular programme was a reasonable investment because it removed from the community a considerably greater economic burden due to the disease.

The economic importance of a disease may be assessed from: (a) the loss of potential wealth owing to death and temporary or permanent inability to work; (b) the direct costs of medical care; and (c) losses due to failure to take advantage of opportunities for economic development, in particular for agricultural and animal production. Health economics is a new science and it is realized that any assessment of these or other components will suffer from the basic deficiencies due to the present lack of an accepted standard methodology. Until such a methodology is found, economic evaluations will, however, provide useful broad indications [WRIGHT, 1961, 1968].

Mortality and Disability

As long as appropriate longitudinal studies have not been carried out in endemic areas, an estimation of the number of deaths resulting, directly or indirectly, from schistosomiasis will remain difficult. However, it has been shown that up to 12% of the people autopsied after dying in hospital in parts of South America died of the consequences of schistosomiasis. In parts of Tanzania around 20% of people have what in Western countries would be considered serious damage to the urinary tract and a proportion of these would be expected to live only a few years. These changes, in Tanzania, Zanzibar, Nigeria and Egypt, are seen commonly in children and would be expected to produce their most serious results in adolescent and early adult life. Indirect evidence suggests that deaths at this age from schistosomiasis do occur and such people, at the end of training and schooling and about to begin their productive life, are the very ones a developing country can least afford to lose. It could, therefore, be of interest to compute the saving in productive years of life that the control of schistosomiasis will bring about.

A number of studies has been made elaborating the method for the computation of the corresponding gains in productive years added to each life. This involves the concept of life tables and reference should be made in this connexion to 'Years of Life Lost' in B. BENJAMIN's book 'Elements of Vital Statistics' [1959].

Reduced work output due to illness is hard to measure where continuous industrial employment is not the rule. In industrialized countries where almost everyone's attendance at work is recorded, the loss due to temporary illness can be fairly estimated, but even so there is no recognized system of allowing for premature retirement from work, and for death. Serious efforts to find an objective physiological criterion of fitness have been quite fruitless, and surveys based on using measures of this type have almost always failed to secure acceptance of their findings as representative of health. Disability measurement can be based on subjective histories, clinical assessment and observations of work done by the patients, and these three approaches need evaluation against each other to produce a valid method of study.

In a few studies it has been shown that absenteeism from work is greater in those infected than in apparently uninfected controls [FOSTER, 1967]. Such studies under-estimate the true morbidity to an uncertain extent since anyone seriously and overtly unwell is excluded from employment in the first place.

In rural communities, disability due to disease cannot be appreciated on the basis of absence from work. In one of the first field investigations of this problem (see chapter, page 371) which was carried out in the Philippines [FAROOQ, 1963] in an area where most men were subsistence farmers, an attempt was made to calculate the frequency of periods of sickness and the average duration of each such period. The product of these two components gave the duration of sickness in man-days lost yearly. A clinical gradient scale permitted the recognition of degrees of disability. The disability in man-days per year was then converted into economic terms on the basis of the standard minimum wage for the area. This tentative assessment suggested that schistosomiasis was less important than malaria to the country as a whole but that this was mainly due to the more widespread distribution of malaria. The cost per exposed or per infected person was almost the same for the two infections.

While there is need for further studies, in particular among closed groups of people such as industrial employees and plantation workers, it can be stated with reasonable confidence that a major achievement of any public health programme is the increased working capacity it imparts to masses of diseased individuals who, instead of being a drain on society, are in a position to prove an asset.

Cost of Medical Care

The infection remains largely untreated in most of the countries where schistosomiasis is endemic. However, the cost of such treatment as is actually given can be derived from the expenditure on drugs (these are rarely used for other conditions) and by surveys of dispensary attendance and bed occupancy in hospitals.

On an enterprise basis, costing of medical care is relatively easier to estimate. In Tanzania, for instance, in one irrigated estate employing 2,300 people, a sample study revealed a prevalence of schistosomiasis of 84% on an average among cane cutters and irrigation workers who have extensive contact with the irrigated waters. For medical care alone, schistosomiasis cost the estate an estimated annual total of £4,866 (£3,686 for direct treatment; £922 for additional in-patient treatment; £258 for additional out-patient treatment), i.e. more than the combined annual cost of a snail control scheme and treatment of new labour and dependents, which was estimated at £3,533 [FOSTER, 1967].

Other Effects on the Economy

Loss to agricultural production also results from infection with schistosomes affecting domestic animals, such as *S. japonicum*, *S. mattheei*, and *S. spindale*. Since criteria here are purely economic, co-operation with veterinarians and data from abattoirs should allow estimation of the financial loss involved.

In the rainy areas of the Far East, it has been demonstrated that environmental control of schistosomiasis, through water management and better utilization, results in a parallel increase in food crop production [PESIGAN *et al.*, 1958].

Much of the needed increase in food production and improvement of living standards in developing countries depends on the implementation of water-resource conservation and hydro-electric schemes, as well as on the reclamation of land for agricultural purposes. However, the presence of schistosomiasis may well constitute a serious obstacle in the way of attaining these objectives if the necessary preventive measures are not taken. For this reason, it has now become a regular practice for WHO and FAO to investigate the health implications of economic programmes, in particular schistosomiasis, in connexion with requests submitted to the United Nations Development Programme for technical assistance to planned, economic development programmes.

The Cost of Disease versus the Cost of Control

The schistosomiasis situation in the world is by no means static. Recent surveys have revealed the existence of foci not previously reported, the spread of the infection among immigrants to newly developed areas, and an increased prevalence and severity of the disease in some known endemic areas. In parallel with this worsening of the situation, control has become more tractable with the advent of improved or new snail control techniques and drugs. Nevertheless, the cost of control schemes acts sometimes as a deterrent as it is not infrequently assumed to be prohibitive.

Cost is undoubtedly an essential factor in disease control, and it should be predicted with reasonable accuracy in budgetary estimates. The comparison of programmes in different areas may be extremely difficult, if not impossible, because of inherent epidemiological and other differences between the areas.

As indicated at the beginning of this chapter the benefits expected to accrue from a control programme should also be taken into account as they may not only reduce but even more than offset the ultimate costs. One such instance where rough estimations of the economic loss due to schistosomiasis were compared with the cost of control may be quoted to illustrate this point. In the Philippines a long-range plan for the control of schistosomiasis has been formulated at an estimated cost of a million pesos (US $ 166,670) per annum for a period of 15 years. This figure compares with the 13 million pesos (over 2 million US $) estimated as the annual cost of the disease. The plan was considered a profitable investment since the cost of control was less than 10% of this figure.

There is, however, a limit to the accuracy usefully attainable in an economic analysis. It is the view of experts that schistosomiasis constitutes a serious public health problem, and experience in its control shows that the cost involved is normally comparable to that of other major public health programmes.

References

BARBOSA, F. S.: Morbidade na esquistossomose. Estudo em quatro localidades no estado de Pernambuco, Recife; Thesis, Recife (1965).

CHAPMAN, D. S.: Brit. J. Surg. *53:* 544 (1966).

CHEEVER, A. W.: Amer. J. trop. Med. Hyg. *17:* 38 (1968).

DAVIS, A.: Lancet *ii:* 546 (1966).

EDINGTON, G. M.: West afr. med. J. *6:* 45 (1957).

EL BADAWI, A. A.: Brit. J. Urol. *38:* 24 (1966).

FAROOQ, M.: Ann. trop. Med. Parasit. *57:* 323 (1963).

FORSYTH, D. M.: Bull. Wld Hlth Org. *40:* 771 (1969).

FORSYTH, D. M. and BRADLEY, D. J.: Lancet *ii:* 169 (1964).

FORSYTH, D. M. and BRADLEY, D. J.: Bull. Wld Hlth Org. *34:* 715 (1966).

FORSYTH, D. M. and MACDONALD, G.: Trans. roy. Soc. trop. Med. Hyg. *59:* 171 (1965).

FORSYTH, D. M. and MACDONALD, G.: Trans. roy. Soc. trop. Med. Hyg. *60:* 568 (1966).

FOSTER, R.: J. trop. Med. Hyg. *70:* 185 (1967).

GELFAND, M.: Cent. afr. J. Med. *11:* 14 (1965).

GILLES, H. M.; LUCAS, A.; ADENIYI-JONES, C.; LINDER, R.; ANAND, S.; BRABAND, H.; COCKSHOTT, W. P.; COWPER, S. G.; MULLER, R. L.; HIRA, P. R., and WILSON, A. M. M.: Ann. trop. Med. Parasit. *59:* 441 (1965a).

GILLES, H. M.; LUCAS, A.; LINDER, A.; COCKSHOTT, W. P.; ANAND, S. V.; IKEME, A., and COWPER, S. G.: Ann. trop. Med. Parasit. *59:* 451 (1965b).

LUCAS, A. O. and COCKSHOTT, W. P.: Lancet *ii:* 697 (1966).

LUCAS, A. O.; ADENIYI-JONES, C. C.; COCKSHOTT, W. P., and GILLES, H. M.: Lancet *i:* 631 (1966).

MACDONALD, G. and FORSYTH, D. M.: Trans. roy. Soc. trop. Med. Hyg. *62:* 766 (1968).

MYRDAL, G.: Chron. Wld Hlth Org. *6:* 203 (1952).

PESIGAN, T. P.; FAROOQ, M.; HAIRSTON, N. G.; JAUREGUI, J. J.; GARCIA, E. G.; SANTOS, A. T.; SANTOS, B. C. and BESA, A. A.: Bull. Wld Hlth Org. *18:* 345; *19:* 223 (1958).

WINSLOW, C. E. A.: The cost of sickness and the price of health. Wld Hlth Org. Monogr. Ser., No. 7, Geneva (1951).

WORLD HEALTH ORGANIZATION: Report of a Scientific Group on Research in Bilharziasis (Assessment of medical and public health importance), Geneva. WHO unpublished mimeographed document MHO/PA/125.60 (1960).

WORLD HEALTH ORGANIZATION: Measurement of the public health importance of bilharziasis. Report of a WHO Scientific Group, Geneva 1965. Wld Hlth Org. techn. Rep. Ser. 349 (1967).

WRIGHT, W. H.: Amer. J. trop. Med. Hyg. *10:* 119 (1961).

WRIGHT, W. H.: Bull. N. Y. Acad. Med. *44:* 301 (1968).

Chapter 6

Epidemiology and Control of Schistosomiasis, pp. 354–387
(Karger, Basel and University Park Press, Baltimore 1973)

Measurement of the Clinical Manifestations of Schistosomiasis

G. MACDONALD

General Aspects of Measurement

Measurement of clinical manifestations of an infection only has point in relation to some specific objective, which is here taken to be the estimation of its public health and economic importance (chapter, pp. 337–353). Analysis is no mean task to be approached lightly, or as if there were some well-founded set of established criteria. Measurement of the public health importance of conditions other than acute infections with immediate dramatic consequences, is a very new discipline even in highly developed countries and has rarely been attempted in others. It demands careful preliminary examination of the meaning of the various concepts involved, and of the way in which deviations from normal health in the individual can come to have significant consequences to the public well-being and economy. It is perhaps, particularly difficult to make this assessment in the case of schistosomiasis: it may be very long-standing in the individual so that ill-effects may be very far removed in time from the original infection; ill-health may be the product of *sequelae* rather than of immediate infection, and the picture may be modified by concomitant conditions such as malnutrition. For this reason, an effort is here made to provide a review of the course of an infection and its possible bearings on public health, before considering the specific manifestations of this infection.

Ill-Health

Ill-health may be defined as the physical or mental state in which there is some detraction from normal well-being, physical or mental capacity, enjoyment of life and normal social, occupational and other relationships, or which is likely by its persistence or consequences to imperil these conditions during a normal span of life.

This definition elaborates the standard one and, in particular, it covers conditions which may be minor at the time though they have major complications in the future. As an example, it covers precancerous conditions of the uterine cervix which would not be discoverable except by special examination and which, at the time of examination, do not detract in any way from physical or mental capacity or the enjoyment of life. This inclusion is significant in relation to any chronic infection and particularly schistosomiasis, which may have greater implications for the future than actual present ill-effects.

Principles of Measurement

Which clinical manifestations should be measured for the objective stated? The answer turns very largely on the system to be used in assessing the public health importance of the condition, developed pages 337 to 353, but the following general considerations are relevant.

An acute infection may result in immediate unquestionable incapacity, or in death, and these manifestations can be measured in simple statistical terms. As a chronic infection, such as schistosomiasis, cannot be quantified in this manner, there must be some selection of the manifestations to be measured, and usually there must be a considerable subjective element in estimations of their significance. Very common consequences of infection, such as pain or weakness, cannot be measured precisely but are subjectively experienced by the individual who reacts to them by action, such as abstention from work, which can be measured objectively. This type of effect, and reaction to it, may well be used in assessment of public health importance and has been developed in the case of schistosomiasis by Farooq [1963]. The problems of measurement involved are not so much those of the clinical manifestations as of potential and actual working capacity. This method has certain limitations and is imprecise, but it is to be remembered that it accurately reflects the opinions of the sufferer of the importance of his infection.

On the other hand, there may be a fully objective assessment of the pathological lesions present. If the individual is examined, he is found to have certain abnormal features, usually of a recognized pathological type and, for the most part, these can be readily measured and classified. The method gives an objective measurement of the number of abnormalities. However, their importance has still to be assessed, and usually in a subjective manner. The only way of substituting an objective measurement is by collateral evidence, proof of associated incapacity or mortality, or by the establishment of a long-term follow-up mechanism which, in the case of schistosomiasis, might have to operate for many years before it can produce decisive results. This approach has substantial advantages in that it can be precise, but it also has limitations. Its value very largely depends on the observer's preliminary judgement of the type of abnormality likely to be found and its importance, and on the manner in which he organizes his examination in relation to this judgement.

There is no generally accepted single measure of health by which the effects of infection can be calibrated. Physiologists have no set criteria by which to measure well-being or ill-health. The examination of individuals or groups of individuals by a general physical examination may well result in an important, or potentially fatal, lesion being completely overlooked through not being sought. There have been many studies of the significance of schisto-somiasis in which the clinical examinations have been established on this principle, and the general outcome has been to cast doubt on the significance of urinary schistosomiasis and, to a lesser extent, of other forms. A notable example of such study is the work by FORSYTH and BRADLEY [1966] who made a cross-sectional survey of a population in Tanzania covering 2,338 persons, of whom 42% had *Schistosoma haematobium* eggs in the urine. The exami-nations were careful: they covered a detailed history of previous symptoms, treatment or evidence of infection; an elaborate general physical examination; examination for the enlargement of the liver and spleen; the taking of blood pressure and of haemoglobin values; record of heights and weights, and examination of the urine. Apart from immediate and purely symptomatic happenings, such as haematuria, no evidence could be collected in this way showing any correlation between ill-health and infection with either *S. haema-tobium* or *S. mansoni*. However, when examinations were carried out on the basis of a hypothesis that infection might cause significant damage to the urinary tract discoverable by radiological means, important pathological ab-normalities were seen in 79 of 647 successful urograms. The generalized examination was therefore useless and wasteful of time for this purpose, as most previous studies of the same nature had been, whereas the specialized examination based on a preliminary hypothesis was very rewarding.

Principal reliance should, therefore, be placed on a search for specific lesions or effects which are thought to occur. The range of examinations may be considerably broadened during the preliminary and experimental stages of the survey in order to check the original assumptions, but once this has been done, effort may be concentrated on the lines suggested by the hypothesis.

Immediate interpretation of the significance of the lesions found is usually subjective, though it may be made objective by a parallel or subsequent examination. One of the ways in which such evidence might be collected turns on the permanence of any particular lesion and its age prevalence. An irreversible lesion can only become rarer in old people than in young, either by having been associated with a differential mortality or as the result of a change in the incidence in previous years. Measurement of clinical manifestations should, therefore, include an attempt to estimate the permanence of the lesions, their age prevalence, and any past changes in local epidemiology of infection.

In making assumptions as to the nature of lesions to be sought, it should not be forgotten that a chronic infection such as schistosomiasis may die out, but leave behind it *sequelae* or complications which may continue to be detrimental and which may be the ultimate cause of death. Possible *sequelae* should, therefore, be considered in arranging this study.

Parasitological Aspects

Normal Development

Schistosomiasis is the state of infection with worms of one or more of the species of *Schistosoma*, usually *S. haematobium*, *S. mansoni* or *S. japonicum*. Infection takes place through the skin by invasion of cercariae. Cercariae shed their tails on contact with the skin and then penetrate as schistosomules, usually via a sebaceous gland. They penetrate down to the cutaneous capillary bed, on being aided by the secretion of a proteolytic enzyme. They may cause a local allergic reaction, which is more commonly observed with animal cercariae that are destroyed *in situ*, producing 'swimmer's itch'.

The schistosomules then enter the venous circulation, are carried through the right heart to the lungs and, after passing through the pulmonary capillaries or directly through the diaphragm, ultimately gain the portal circulation. Growth of the schistosomules takes place in the intrahepatic portal vessels, within which they feed and grow. *S. haematobium* takes a subsequent migration through the inferior mesenteric veins, ultimately reaching the vesical and pelvic plexuses, while *S. mansoni* and *S. japonicum* remain within the portal circulation. The reasons for this location are not known with certainty, though there are some indications that *S. mansoni* has a tropism to indole and some related compounds, which may explain its location. Maturation of *S. haematobium* usually takes place in 10 to 12 weeks, of *S. mansoni* in 7 to 8 weeks, and of *S. japonicum* in 5 to 7 weeks.

The whole of this stage from completion of penetration of the skin to maturation of the adult worm is usually asymptomatic, but may not be so, in heavy invasions. The first symptoms are generally associated with maturation and oviposition and resemble a non-specific allergic reaction to foreign protein which, in laboratory infections of non-immune animals, is proportionate to the numbers of invading cercariae. These reactions have on many occasions been recorded in man, sometimes of a very severe nature, and there are several examples of even fatal reactions following massive primary infection. In most people, however, the original invasive stage is marked by no more than a mild febrile attack, often with some degree of enteritis or haematuria.

The following pathological reactions are principally associated with the deposition of eggs around which granulomata are formed, and the immediate symptoms are referred to the site of their deposition. The sites of choice for oviposition by *S. haematobium* are in the walls of the bladder, the ureter and rectum. The immediate reactions are discomfort or pain, dysuria and frequency of micturition, often associated with systemic effects such as headache, backache and lethargy.

The comparable happenings of the same stage of development of *S. mansoni* and *S. japonicum* are at first 'schistosomiasis dysentery' with blood and mucus in the faeces, which may slowly subside and give way to diarrhoea.

Invading worms may continue to lay eggs for long periods of time but subsequent invasion by others may be modified by immunity, development of which has been substantiated in experimental animals [VOGEL, 1949; VOGEL and MINNING, 1953]. There is little doubt about the occurrence of this immunity in man but it is as yet impossible to put any quantitative values of the degree of stimulus needed or the extent of reaction to it. Immunity takes the form of stunted development of invading schistosomules, reduction in numbers of such as may mature, and reduction in their egg output. In communities subject to intensive heavy exposure there may be some signs of this partial immunity in children from the age of about 10 years upward, though in those subject to lesser invasion the first apparent signs may be long delayed. In neither case, however, does the immunity come in time to prevent the development of infection.

Many past conceptions of the normal course of schistosomiasis have included the belief that, after some long period of egg deposition with granuloma formation around them, there was a gradually increasing development of fibrous tissue which ultimately became manifest as a general fibrosis in the organs concerned, causing functional failure through mechanical interference. The general outline of this is correct but observations by POLAK *et al.* [1959] and NEVES and RASO [1965] on the development of fibrosis in *S. mansoni* infections indicate that fibrosis may occur in the liver at a very early stage of infection. Other observations by FORSYTH and MACDONALD [1965, 1966] and by GILLES *et al.* [1965] on *S. haematobium* have shown that great distortion of the ureters occurs in young children aged no more than six years, and within a year or two of the first infection.

While the time scale of the above concept may be wrong, its general principle is sound; there is one group of effects which can be attributed to the direct reaction of the body to the deposition of eggs, and there is another group of effects which are more indirectly caused in that they are the result of disturbance of function following local allergic reactions, growth of fibrous tissue, or distortion of organs in other ways. Lesions and associated symptoms are, therefore, usually progressive, though the occasional development of compensatory mechanisms may prevent this, and treatment may arrest further development and give the compensatory mechanisms a chance to operate. However, once deformity of an organ has occurred through the extensive development of fibrous tissue, it must be assumed that there is some associated loss of function which at first diminishes safety margins and may later cause functional incapacity.

Ectopic Infections of Lesser Importance

While most symptoms and signs can be fitted within this framework, it does not cover all possibilities. It was shown by GELFAND and ROSS [1953] that eggs might be found in virtually any organ or tissue of the body, to which symptoms and signs may in consequence be related. Eggs are commonly deposited in all parts of the genital as well as urinary tracts, and infections of the cervix, fallopian tubes, vulva, and vagina are common. Spinal schistosomiasis is well known [GELFAND, 1965; BARNETT, 1965; BIRD, 1965]; spinal locations have usually been discovered in association with, and as a result of, a clinical myelitis causing paralysis, but the condition may be quite silent [BUDZILOVICH *et al.*, 1964]. While the ova of *S. haematobium* and *S. mansoni* tend to be localized in the spinal cord, those of *S. japonicum* have a peculiar predilection for the brain, viz. basal ganglia, cortex, and internal capsules, and for involving motor rather than sensory tracts [MOST *et al.*, 1950]. Dermal schistosomiasis with indurated papules composed basically of granulomata containing eggs follows a well-established pattern [EL-MOFTY and CAHILL, 1964]; invasion of the prepuce has been associated with a development of squamous-cell carcinoma [KOVI, 1964], appendicitis has been caused, together with innumerable other lesions in all parts of the body.

Intensity of Infection

The detection of schistosomiasis gives no indication of the numbers of worms involved. There is, however, mounting evidence on the pattern of egg output in communities, on variations between communities and individuals, and in individuals from time to time. It seems probable that the relative egg output in different individuals would be an indication of the relative worm load carried, provided that the individuals were immunologically similar, as might be expected if they came from the same age group and the same locality. In consequence, the prevailing intensity of infection can best be described in terms of egg output, provided that examination is restricted to a standard age group of people, preferably that typical of primary school-children, 4 to 14 years. Whatever the relationship to worm load, the egg output varies enormously; FORSYTH and BRADLEY [1966], using a standardized technique, produced records of from 1 to 8,000 S. haematobium eggs in a 10-ml sample of midday urine, and comparable variations have been found in the number of eggs of S. mansoni in the stools.

The association between egg output and the severity of effect of S. mansoni infection was amply documented by SCOTT [1937]. The relationship between the output of S. haematobium eggs and the prevalence of lesions detectable by radiology has been demonstrated by FORSYTH and MACDONALD [1965]. The prevalence of these lesions in children with egg outputs less than 250/10 ml of midday urine was 22.7%, and those with higher output 45%. The greatest differences were in the presence of calcified bladder and deformed ureter, both of which were twice as common in the children with heavy infections as in those with light infections, there being less difference in the prevalence of hydronephrosis in the two groups. Later studies by the same authors [FORSYTH and MACDONALD, 1966], however, show that hydronephrosis is very much more common in children in heavily infected areas than amongst those from lightly infected areas. Being a sequel, rather than an immediate result of infection, hydronephrosis occurs some time after the acute infection so that the association with heavy output of eggs may be somewhat blurred.

Clinical and Pathological Aspects

The Early Stages: All Species

The symptoms and signs during the early stage of infection before maturation of the worms are so similar in infection by the different species of parasites that they may be described together. Invasion may produce a dermatitis which by analogy with experimental animal work is believed to be more severe in re-infections due to sensitization by previous ones.

The clinical manifestations of cercarial dermatitis are itching and pricking sensation related to the sites of penetration of cercariae, local erythema, and papular eruption, with systemic manifestations. Fever, weakness and other symptoms may occur after the skin changes. Blood examination may show a moderate early eosinophilia, which increases later.

Because the symptoms of this stage, when present, are relatively non-specific, they have been missed in many endemic areas and their importance for the public health is unknown. Presently available immunological tests – the intradermal test, the complement-fixation test and the fluorescent antibody test – have proved to be excellent screening tools in epidemiological surveys but they cannot be considered as having a true diagnostic value. With increasing diagnostic facilities and interest in pyrexias of childhood, studies of the maturation stage and its consequences should be possible [WHO, 1967].

Later Stages: *S. haematobium*

Manifestations

The urological changes in *S. haematobium* infection have been fully described by HONEY and GELFAND [1960], by MAKAR [1955], by EDINGTON *et al.* [1970] and by others. In the early stages there is a marked hyperaemia of the bladder wall, proceeding to the formation of tubercles or polypoid patches representing small and large collections of granulomata. These may be associated with diffuse inflammatory infiltration and oedema of the bladder wall. There may be interference with bladder function, and perhaps one of the important aspects of this interference is the symptomless incompetence of the ureteric orifice facilitating back-pressure effects in the ureter and later the kidney. There is commonly massive deposition of eggs within the bladder wall, and the collections of calcified eggs may become so great as to form the 'sandy patches' which are a characteristic cystoscopic and autopsy feature of schistosomiasis due to *S.haematobium*. Basically they consist of large quantities of eggs and some fibrous tissue visible through the overlying mucous membrane. Although the trigone is most frequently involved, prominent patches occur commonly on the fundus of the bladder. In many persons the deposition of calcified eggs is visible on an X-ray plate as a thin line encircling the bladder, typically of 2 to 3 mm thickness, but on occasion up to 5 mm across. GELFAND [1950] found this in 17% of Africans passing *S. haematobium* eggs in the urine. FORSYTH and BRADLEY [1966] found it in 17% of children and adolescents but only in 6% of adults, indicating the possibility of resolution in some cases, and a marked association with heavy infections has been shown in later studies. Schistosomal papillomata are a common sequel in Egypt, less commonly in other endemic foci; they usually occur near the ureteral orifice, may lead to haemorrhage, and possibly to stone formation, but are not thought to be precancerous.

Vesical cancer occurs in association with *S.haematobium* infection; a causal relationship is strongly suspected but cannot be established beyond doubt because there are marked variations in the reported prevalence of carcinoma from different endemic areas of schistosomiasis. The commonest form is a squamous-cell carcinoma, though columnar-celled and other types occur. It seems very probable that there is some association but perhaps a metabolic factor in addition to infection is needed to complete the stimulus required.

Eggs are laid in the wall of the ureter as in the wall of the bladder, involvement of the lower ureter being most common. The pathological consequences, though less studied, are the same in principle. Much of the relevant study has been by urographic examination and depends on the interpretation of X-ray findings, although GELFAND [1950] and HONEY and GELFAND [1960] record considerable series of autopsy findings. The commonest radiographic finding is dilatation, usually from the lower third upwards and often immediately above the bladder, but it may extend throughout the length of the ureter in 'drain-pipe' form. The dilatation is usually irregular, and may be saccular. It has been shown that dilatations occur in very young children not long after their original infection with schistosomiasis, whence it would seem that chronic fibrosis is an unlikely cause, and they are attributed by HONEY and GELFAND [1960] to disturbance of the muscular function of the ureter by massive deposition of eggs between the muscle bundles. This dilatation may be exaggerated by distortion of the ureteric orifice facilitating back-pressure from the bladder.

Hydronephrosis may develop, presumably as a sequel to these ureteric deformities. In Tanzanian studies it is much more common in boys than in girls, despite the equality of load of infection and other lesions in the two sexes. The reason for this is not understood and it is presumed to be due to difference in physiological functioning between the two sexes. Hydronephrosis may first consist of a simple dilatation of one or more calices, but may continue until the kidney tissue is restricted to a narrow fibrous envelope from which it is very difficult to discern the excretion of any dye on intravenous pyelography.

In *S. haematobium* infections, deposition of eggs in the liver may lead to the development of a focal portal fibrosis, though this takes place later and in a less severe form than the comparable occurrence in *S. mansoni* and *S. japonicum* infections and is rarely, if ever, of clinical significance. The syndrome of cor pulmonale which is common in *S. mansoni* infections, has been described but is certainly not a regular concomitant of *S. haematobium* infection. The radiographic and electrocardiographic examination of several thousands of people infected with *S. haematobium* in Rhodesia or Tanzania, many of them coming from places where infection is intense, has not revealed this syndrome as associated with *S. haematobium*. An interesting recent finding by EDINGTON *et al.* [1970] is an augmented frequency of lymphoreticular neoplasms in *S. haematobium*-infected Nigerian patients compared with uninfected patients found at autopsy.

Measurement

Methods of selection of a community for study are set out on pages 340–344. Whatever the form of clinical examination the records should include identification, location of residence, age, sex and, where appropriate, occupation or other information. The examinations should include a parasitological examination for the presence and intensity of infection. Urine samples should be examined by the techniques described on pages 622–629 and, if possible, this should be repeated on those found negative until three successive negatives are recorded. Findings in Tanzania in children, strongly suggest that if three successive examinations are negative the probability of significant lesions due to *S. haematobium* can be excluded. When urines are found to be positive an egg-count should be performed, preferably by the method described on pages 628–629. General examination may include a number of subjects according to the specific interest of the observer, and a classification of how this may be undertaken is set out in table I.

It would not usually be necessary to undertake all these examinations. In the absence of specific indications, the patient should be given a general physical examination, including palpation and inspection of the abdomen,

Table I. S. haematobium – Tabular form of working criteria for assessment of lesions

Stage of disease	Phenomenon for assessment	Phase 1 techniques (all patients studied)	Phase 2 techniques (stratified sample)	Limit
1	dermatitis	clinical history	–	immersion. Later oviposition or FAB or CFT conversion
2	pulmonary fever syndrome	clinico-pathological	–	fever-eosinophilia ≥ 800 mm³. Chest X-ray abnormal. Later oviposition or FAB or CFT conversion
3	(a) ova urine	quantitative count	–	enumerate
	(b) ova stool	qualitative	rectal snip	presence
	(c) haematuria	–	Hb extraction from 24-hour urine	in g/24 h (or limiting level)
	(d) proteinuria	–	Esbach	in g/24 h (or limiting levels)
	(e) early bladder lesions:			
	(i) nodular granulomata	radiography	cystoscopy or biopsy	–
	(ii) others	–	cystoscopy or biopsy	–
	(iii) calcified bladder wall	radiography	–	observer agreement test
	(f) calcified ureter	radiography	–	–
	(g) abnormal ureter	excretion urography	retrograde pyelography diuresis pyelography micturation cystography cystoscopy – biopsy radioisotope studies (renal function tests)	

Table I. (continued)

Stage of disease	Phenomenon for assessment	Phase 1 techniques (all patients studied)	Phase 2 techniques (stratified sample)	Limit
3 (continued)	(h) genital lesions:			
	(i) vaginal papilloma	clinical (speculum)	biopsy	
	(ii) cervical papilloma	clinical (speculum)	biopsy	
	(iii) vulval papilloma	clinical (speculum)	biopsy	
	(iv) seminal vesicle lesion	rectal palpation and radiology	} radiology	
	(v) prostatic lesion			
4	(a) bladder polyps	clinical – excretion urography	cystogram, cystoscopy	
	(b) bladder neck obstruction		cysto-urethrogram	
	(c) ulcerative cystitis	clinical – pyuria	cystoscopy	
	(d) hydronephrosis	clinical assessment	cystoscopy	
		excretion urography	diuresis pyelography	
			biochemistry	
			renal function tests	
	(e) non-functioning kidney	clinical assessment	diuresis pyelography	
		excretion urography	retrograde pyelography	
			renal biopsy	
			radioisotope renography	
	(f) calculus of urinary tract	radiography		
	(g) urinary infection	MSA plated MacConkey or Kass method (state which)		apparent significant growth or $\geq 100,000$ organisms/ml (specify)

Table I. (continued)

Stage of disease	Phenomenon for assessment	Phase 1 techniques (all patients studied)	Phase 2 techniques (stratified sample)	Limit
4 (continued)	(h) fistulae of urinary tract	clinical	biopsy	
	(i) uraemia	blood urea	renal function tests biochemistry	blood urea >40 mg/100 ml
	(j) bladder cancer		cystoscopy – biopsy	
	(k) pulmonary hypertension and cor pulmonale	ECG	chest x-ray. Pulmonary artery catheterization and angiography	either to give negative, both to give positive
	(l) systemic hypertension	blood pressure. ECG	Full renal investigations	diastolic >100 mm Hg
	(m) liver enlargement	clinical	liver function tests liver biopsy	

From WHO, 1965a.

examination for enlargement of the liver and spleen, examination of the chest to exclude marked cardiac or pulmonary disability, manometry recording systolic and diastolic blood pressures. The most profitable form of specific examination has been by intravenous pyelography, which is best carried out in conjunction with radiography of the chest and electrocardiography after admission to hospital on the previous day, purgation and restriction of food. Acceptable techniques are described in annex 1.

Full safety techniques should be adopted and, in particular, care should be taken to exclude from examination any women who are, or might be, pregnant. This inevitably excludes a large proportion of the young adult age group amongst whom findings must be inferred from other collateral evidence.

Urography may be supplemented by direct radiography of the pelvis, principally for the purpose of identification of calcification of the bladder or ureters.

Table II shows radiological findings among children passing eggs in their urine, from two groups in Tanzania. The distinction between them is that the one comes from an area where all are infected and the prevailing infection is heavy, while the other comes from an area where 30% were infected and the majority of these lightly. The groups are in other ways comparable.

Table II. Radiological findings in two groups of children from neighbouring and highly endemic and mildly endemic areas

	Highly endemic	Mildly endemic
Examined	106	109
Pathology found, %	43	17
Calcified bladder, %	20	5
Deformed ureter, %	42	11
Hydronephrosis, %	19	8
Non-functioning kidney, %	0	1

Analysis of findings such as these, classified according to the associated egg output found, to age, sex, occupation and other characteristics of the individuals, can throw much light on the prevalence of significant happenings.

Measurement of the frequency, and to some extent of the intensity, of pulmonary hypertension may be made by systematic chest radiography and by electrocardiographic findings. The diagnostic indications of right ventricular hypertrophy are set out by an Expert Committee [WHO, 1961]. Some of their conclusions are reproduced in annex 2.

Some of the difficulties inherent in taking sterile urine samples on which to carry out bacteriological culture for the measurement of the prevalence of significant bacteriuria, can be overcome by accepting the criterion that significant bacteriuria is characterized by the presence of 100,000 bacteria or more per mm³. For this purpose it is adequate if specimens of mid-stream urine are taken which may be cultured by the dilution plating method of KASS [1956]. An alternative method is the TTC (triphenyl tetrazolium chloride) test of SIMMONS and WILLIAMS [1962], which depends on the reduction of the colour of this material within 4 h at 37°F by actively respiring bacteria. However, FORSYTH and BRADLEY [1966] found both of these tests difficult to apply with limited technical assistance and attained their most reproducible results by direct plating on MACCONKEY's agar with inspection after 24 and 48 h aerobic incubation. Urines giving a heavy, pure culture or an extensive mixed growth on more than one sample were considered infected, and identification to bacterial genus level was then carried out. These authors found no difference between prevalence of bacteriuria in persons with and without eggs in the urine. Considerable care should be used in interpreting the relationship particularly because bacterial infection could be a late sequel occurring at a time when schistosome infection was burnt out.

Despite the great value of cystoscopy in the evaluation of the conditions in an individual, it is neither practical nor desirable to adapt this technique to the epidemiological appraisal of the prevalence of vesical lesions in a population as a whole. It was attempted by FORSYTH and BRADLEY [1966] but the proportion of people on whom it was impossible for one reason or another to get an adequate examination was such as to invalidate the statistical application of their findings to the community as a whole. This, together with the dangers of introducing secondary bacterial infection make cystoscopy inapplicable in even an elaborate field survey.

Later Stages: *S. mansoni* and *S. japonicum*

Manifestations

The pathology and symptomatology of these two infections may be considered together as they are similar, except that developments in *S. japonicum* infection tend to occur earlier and to a more severe degree than in *S. mansoni* infections and are due, apparently, to the greater number of eggs laid. Up to the stage of maturation, symptoms and signs are similar to those of *S.haema-tobium* infection. Pathological changes are at first mainly in the intestinal wall with later development of hepatic fibrosis and its possible *sequelae*.

In the early stage of dysentery there may be congestion and micro-ulceration of the rectal mucosa with resultant bloody diarrhoea, abdominal pain and cramps. In the later stages, there may be changes in bowel habits, including constipation alternating with bouts of diarrhoea. However, absence of intestinal symptoms is common. This stage may last an indefinite time, depending probably on the load of infection. In severe infections, particu-larly in Egypt, inflammatory polyps of the colon are commonly seen. These are far less frequent in Latin America. Other changes occasionally found are focal, exuberant fibrosis, also called 'pseudotumour' or 'bilharzioma', and focal ulceration of the colon.

Fibrosis of the liver develops in some, but not in all, patients, usually 3 to 15 years after initial exposure in *S. mansoni* [PRATA and BINA, 1968], though it is at first asymptomatic. It usually takes the form of a portal fibrosis of Sym-mers' type in which the hepatolobular pattern is preserved. There is no great disturbance of cellular function, but obstruction to portal flow is consider-able. POLAK *et al.* [1959] have given a detailed description of the course of its development, as followed from early to late cases by laparoscopy, biopsy, and other forms of examination. In marked cases, portal hypertension follows, with associated enlargement of the liver and spleen, sometimes to a great extent, as in Egyptian hepatosplenomegaly, and with the usual signs of portal obstruction, with varices in the oesophageal veins and other sites of possible anastomoses.

Pulmonary complications may follow, usually in the form of obstructive pulmonary vascular disease with chronic endarteritis, resulting in pulmonary hypertension or cor pulmonale. The basic cause is embolism by eggs passing from the portal system to the caval system through venous communications dilated by portal hypertension. Eggs may then also begin to reach the periph-eral organs in substantial numbers through shunts associated with the pul-monary arteritis. Symptoms are those of right heart inadequacy; dyspnoea, general weakness, cough, giddiness and fainting, with palpitation, thoracic pain, precordial pains and, perhaps, haemoptysis. Radiographical signs were classified by ERFAN *et al.* [1949] in three grades (on this subject, however, see annex 2): *Grade I*, with focal arterial changes with intensification of the shad-ows of one or more of the second or third degree arteries, mostly the basal. They are wider than normal, give a markedly denser shadow, have a moder-ately tortuous course and sometimes irregular and hazy outline. *Grade II* lesions, when active, are more widely distributed throughout the lung fields, especially the bases. Marked intensification of the arterial shadows, tortuosity and beading, with large hilar shadows, obliteration of the subaortic notch, and hypertophy of the right ventricle. *Grade III* is met in long-standing, neglected cases with repeated infections, the lesions are widespread in both lungs, but more marked in the bases and medial zones, the perivascular mottlings are so dense and widespread that patches of localized opacities may appear here and there, the pulmonary conus and trunk of the pulmonary artery are ballooned, perhaps reaching aneurysmal size, and the heart is increased in size with the typical configuration associated with dilatation.

A second pulmonary syndrome, formerly known as Ayerza's disease, was fully described by DE FARIA *et al.* [1957, 1959] and consists of cyanosis, clubbing of the fingers and toes, and deficient arterial oxygenation but with normal pulmonary artery pressure. The syndrome has been further described by WESSEL *et al.* [1965] and there is little doubt from the original description and the work of ZAKY *et al.* [1964] that it is due to the presence of arteriovenous shunts.

Measurement: Background

An epidemiological study of the effects of disability due to *S. mansoni* or *S. japonicum* should be subject to the same qualifications concerning examination of an appropriate cross-section of a community, or a complete ecological community, as in the case of *S. haematobium* infections. Equally, for all individuals data should be collected on identification, age, sex, etc., together with an estimate of the presence and intensity of infection. Quantitative faecal examinations should be included. See pages 629 to 634 for recommended techniques.

Alternative methods of examination are by rectal snip and by oögram on the basis of a rectal snip. Although these techniques are sensitive and the oögram can be made precise, they are not acceptable in all communities, they entail some risk of haemorrhage and, therefore, cannot be of general utility in field studies.

Measurement: Severity and Disability

These infections differ from *S. haematobium* in that the effects which are attributable to mature infections characterized by intensive oviposition, tend to be more severe and to produce more incapacity and subjective illness. This is so marked that it is wise to include some measurement of these effects in any assessment. Their very severity makes measurement possible despite the frequent subjective nature, because of the patient's reaction to it. It, therefore, becomes desirable to devise a method of systematic analysis of the frequency and degree of symptoms and the patient's reaction to them, as well as to devise techniques for the objective measurement of known pathological processes.

FAROOQ [1963] developed this subject considerably, originally in association with study of *S. japonicum* infection reported by PESIGAN *et al.* [1958]. The analysis relates to two viewpoints, the static one, or condition as seen on a single examination, and the dynamic one, or condition as revealed by analysis of developments over a period of time and, in his case, following periodic examination.

For the static viewpoint, infections were classified as mild, moderate, severe or very severe and a 'Clinical Gradient' established, illustrating the prevalence of the different degrees of severity in the community. For dynamic purposes, disability was defined as meaning a day of inability to work or to pursue normal activities, and the amount of disability per individual was calculated over a period of time as a frequency rate (number of spells of sickness per person), a severity rate (mean duration per spell), and a disability rate (number of sick days per person). He used these measures for the purpose of assessing the economic importance of *S. japonicum* infection in the Philippines and they would be useful for study of contrasting communities elsewhere, though great care is needed to ensure comparability of findings based on subjective assessment.

The classification of severity is as follows:

Class I: mild: occasional abdominal pain, occasional diarrhoea or dysentery; no absence from work.

Class II: moderate: anaemia (haemoglobin less than 10 g/100 ml, as recorded by the Haden-Hausser haemoglobinometer) or weakness; reduced capacity for work.

Class III: severe: recurring attacks of diarrhoea and dysentery; frequent absence from work.

Class IV: very severe: ascites, emaciation; total absence from work.

The Clinical Gradient is a record of the prevalence of the different degrees of severity within a community and, for instance in the Philippines study, a Clinical Gradient was established as 62% asymptomatic carriers and 38% with manifest signs of symptoms. Of these latter, 57% were mild, 39% moderate, and 4% severe or very severe.

Disability was defined as meaning inability to pursue work or normal activities but this needed further classification which was carried out as follows:

	Assumed loss of working capacity, %
Non-disabling sickness	
Class I: no absence from work	25
Disabling sickness	
Class II: absence from work but not classified under III or IV	50
Class III: confined to house	75
Class IV: confined to bed	100

It will be noted that 25% loss of working capacity is attributed to the 'non-disabling' sickness. In these people the ailment was insufficient to prevent work though there was interference with normal activity and some sickness, which was assumed to cause some loss of working capacity.

In the particular study described, periodic examinations were carried out on 278 individuals chosen by random numbers as a 20-percent sample of the stool-positive individuals in the project area. They were examined in their own homes by an interviewing team consisting of two physicians and a technician, who on average examined three to four patients each afternoon. Their results were classified by age groups and could, if appropriate, have been equally well classified in other ways. They recorded a disability rate (number of sick days per person) due to schistosomiasis of 14.2 days per annum, of which 72.6% were class I, and 9.2, 11.5 and 6.7% classes II, III and IV, respectively. This is clearly a set of figures which can be used for comparative purposes providing that a sufficiently strict definition has first been made of the classification to be used and the ways in which it is to be utilized.

Measurement: Pathological Changes

The techniques which may be used in the study of a community for this purpose are set out in table IV. Wherever possible there should be a careful history of past relevant illnesses and, with reference to some specified period of time, a record of the number of periods of illness, their duration and associated disability, and of diarrhoea or constipation. General examination should include examination of the abdomen with special record of the size of the spleen and liver, and the presence or absence of distended veins or other signs of portal hypertension with, where appropriate, an examination for ascites. There should be a full examination of the chest, particularly for any signs of right ventricular hypertrophy or dilatation, with a record of systolic and diastolic blood pressure. Special attention should be paid to the possible

Table III. S. mansoni and S. japonicum – Tabular form of working criteria for assessment of lesions

Stage of disease	Phenomenon for assessment	Phase 1 techniques (all patients studied)	Phase 2 techniques (stratified sample)	Limit
1	dermatitis	physical examination history		immersion, later oviposition or FAB or CFT conversion
2	acute febrile phase	physical examination history	(all patients) stool and blood examination	fever, dysentery eosinophilia, stools negative to positive
3	egg deposition	faecal examination	proctoscopy and rectal biopsy	presence and enumeration of eggs
	(a) diarrhoea, constipation, abdominal pain	history		self-evident
	(b) rectosigmoid congestion, oedema, ulcers or polyps	history and physical examination	proctoscopy barium enema	self-evident
4	(a) hepatomegaly	physical examination	X-ray of abdomen (of limited use) needle biopsy of liver (to help rule out cirrhosis, malaria, leukaemia, kala-azar) thick blood film (to evaluate role of chronic malaria)	by PE-palpable
	consistency surface left lobe			
	(b) splenomegaly	physical examination	X-ray of abdomen (of limited use)	
	(c) liver function		liver function tests	

Table III. (continued)

Stage of disease	Phenomenon for assessment	Phase 1 techniques (all patients studied)	Phase 2 techniques (stratified sample)	Limit
4 (continued)	(d) portal hypertension and portal systemic collateral circulation	physical examination	wedged suprahepatic vein pressure and segmental venography barium swallow oesophagoscopy splenic pulp pressure and splenoportography	characteristics differ from cirrhosis observer agreement one or two observers numerical values
	(e) dyspnoea cardiomegaly	history physical examination chest X-ray		observer agreement
	right ventricular hypertrophy	physical examination chest X-ray	ECG	observer agreement
	pulmonary hypertension	physical examination	chest X-ray, pulmonary artery catheterization, angiography	(i) either to give negative, both to give positive (ii) pulmonary artery heave, heart sounds, prominent pulmonary conus, peripheral vasculature
	(f) ascites	physical examination		observer agreement
	(g) dwarfism and lesser degrees of retarded development		various (bone age, endocrine evaluation)	reversal by splenectomy

From WHO, 1965a.

presence of dyspnoea, cyanosis and clubbing of the fingers. These examinations should be amplified by an electrocardiogram and X-ray of the chest with particular reference to possible hypertrophy or dilatation of the heart.

The interpretation of enlargement of the liver and spleen may be confused by the presence of other conditions having these effects, though this decreases with the diminution of malaria. An effort should be made to define a combined set of findings representing probable schistosome infection. The latter causes a pipe-stem fibrosis, in distinction to the more usual type of cirrhosis, and is marked more by interference with portal circulation than of hepatocellular function. Usually the liver is enlarged with a firm left lobe, there is gross splenomegaly and in later stages distension of superficial abdominal veins. The occurrence of oesophageal varices may be marked by occasional haematemesis, often in a moderately young subject and without associated jaundice or other signs of failure of liver function. Diagnosis may be confirmed in individual cases admitted to hospital by liver biopsy or by splenic puncture and by measurement of portal pressure. However, although these latter studies are of considerable interest in connexion with individual patients, they may not throw great additional light on the prevalence or severity of clinical manifestations, and it is only justifiable to undertake them on a small section of the group studied.

On the basis of these examinations, it should be possible to provide an approximate analysis of the prevalence and, to some extent, of the degree of portal fibrosis, of pulmonary hypertension and of the cyanotic syndrome of DE FARIA et al. [1957, 1959]. All of these are believed to be progressive, and longitudinal studies involving repeat examinations of the same individuals at intervals are much needed. For instance, GREANY [1952] attempting to trace 100 patients two to three years after treatment, was able to trace 77, of whom 43 were in good health, 21 were ill and complaining of handicap, 4 were weak, bedridden and incapacitated, and 9 were dead. Similar investigations have been carried out [KLOETZEL, 1964; KATZ and BRENER, 1965] but amplifications and repetition of this type of study is greatly needed.

Autopsies

The objectives of autopsy studies on schistosomiases have been indicated in the chapter on pages 345–347. In practice, if autopsies are to be carried out in most of the institutions in the areas of endemicity, the protocol must be of simple design in order to obviate interference with the frequently heavy service routine and to avoid excessive demands on the time and clerical duties of the personnel. Yet it should include all procedures necessary to ascertain the intensity and distribution, both of schistosomal infection and of schistosomal lesions. The protocol provided in form¦ 4 (on pages 744 to 748) is intended to be complementary to the routine *post mortem* report utilized in the various investigating centres. An attempt has been made to keep to the minimum the investigations and information required. It is sufficient to make digests of only four organs, although other organ digests are included in the protocol and can be made if facilities permit. Suitable techniques are suggested on pages 652 to 658.

Organization of Studies

Selection of a Group for Study

The principles to be followed in selecting a group for study depend entirely on the objective of the study, and may vary considerably in different circumstances. If the objective is to obtain a picture of the over-all impact of schistosomiasis on the health of the people of a country, it will be desirable to get a cross-section which includes all types of epidemiology and all degrees of prevalence which occur within that community. If, however, the objective is to study the relationship between local epidemiology and ecology on the one hand, and the effects which it produces on the other, then it is desirable to select a group which is epidemiologically and ecologically homogeneous, with as little variation in prevalence and intensity as possible, though it may be desirable to choose two or more such areas for comparison.

The objective and the principles which flow from it should first be carefully defined, and after that careful statistical impartiality should be maintained. An illustration of an effort to get a cross-section covering all relevant degrees of prevalence is given by the procedure employed in obtaining base-line data on the frequency distribution of schistosomiasis in the area covered by Egypt-49, a pilot project sponsored jointly by the Government of the United Arab Republic, UNICEF and WHO.

'Each division of the area is divided into sections, on a topographic and hydrographic basis, that are utilized as strata for purposes of sampling within each division. The sampling procedure is designed to provide every individual in the area with an equal chance of being included in the sample. A 5-percent two-stage cluster sample is taken from each stratum of each division, with villages constituting the natural first-stage units and households the second-stage units. A random sample of villages (first-stage units) representing 20-percent of the population of each section is selected, with probability proportional to the size of their populations. A 25-percent sample of households (second-stage units) is randomly drawn from each selected village with all individuals in the selected households eligible for examination. This provides a stratified over-all fraction of 0.05 (0.25 of 0.20) probability sample, from each section of the three divisions.

The need is emphasized for an exploratory field study to gain fore-knowledge of appropriate epidemiological happenings in the project area and to pretest diagnostic and organizational procedures.

The sample drawn adequately represents typical cross-sections of the populations in the project area. A close measure of approximation between age groups and sex composition of the sample examined and those of the project population has been reached, which eliminates the necessity for the application of any correction procedures for interstratum or interdivision comparisons of the rates obtained. An under-representation of smaller villages in the sample surveyed has, however, occurred owing to the fact that the first-stage units (villages) are selected with probability proportional to their population size. But there is no evidence to show that this method of sampling has introduced any bias in the frequency rates calculated, since there is no clear relationship between prevalence of bilharziasis and size of village – at any rate in the project area where the sampling was carried out.' [WHO, 1965a].

An example of selection with the second type of objective, examination of a homogeneous community, can be derived from the method successfully used for the study of *S. haematobium* in Tanzania. Preliminary studies had indicated that infection was probably highly focal in character and it was decided to select one or more of these foci for intensive examination. All children attending a school were examined, and the data recorded included information on the place of residence. All findings, both positive and negative, were then entered on a map, thereby producing a spot map of prevalence. On this spot map it was then possible to define the foci, certain areas which could be outlined on the map in which all children were found to be infected. A census of both houses and people within them was undertaken within the focus. Examination in this particular case covered all residents within the focus, though where appropriate a cross-section of inhabitants could have been taken by examining a 25-percent (or other) proportion of households within it.

Cross-Sectional and Longitudinal Studies

Studies may be either static (cross-sectional) describing the amount and severity of effect at a given time, or dynamic (longitudinal) describing the incidence of effects over a period of time and the changes in them. Both have their advantages and disadvantages. The static survey can be made reasonably precise, free from major sources of statistical error, so that a true picture of the population is obtained at one moment. However, it leaves the interpretation of findings to the examiner, who must still decide what significance is to be attached to an observed pathological lesion which may not at the time be serious but which is thought to have potential influence on the patient's health. Some part of this confusion can be eliminated by careful analysis of prevalence, particularly by age, but it must in some degree remain. A longitudinal study is intended to be free from this difficulty, in that it should be possible to trace the history of individuals over a period of time and thus to measure the changes in the actual clinical effects following observed pathological lesions. Such longitudinal studies may be very valuable, covering either untreated cases, or those which have been treated. However, they always contain the weakness that usually not all cases are traced, and it is difficult to apply proper significance to those remaining untraced, particularly where it is suspected, but not confirmed, that there may have been a considerable mortality related to the condition, as in the series quoted by GREANY [1952]. Moreover, they involve subjecting the individual to repeated examinations, which may be inconvenient, troublesome or distasteful and there is consequent risk of refusal, particularly if too short an interval is chosen between the examinations.

Ideally both methods should be combined, as in the studies by FAROOQ [1963] already described. The best course is to make the most thorough static survey that is possible and appropriate to the objectives of the project; then, on review of its findings, to decide exactly what would be the purpose of a longitudinal study and what data it would be desirable to collect. In most cases it may well be found that a restricted later examination or series of examinations are suitable; if they involve complete physical examination of individuals they should be spaced as far apart as is justifiable within the terms of the scheme, usually at 2- to 3-year intervals. The intention to make a later examination should be explained at the time of the original study and every effort should then be made to secure arrangements for tracing individuals.

Records

Case histories and findings must be kept in systematic form and preferably in a manner suitable for analysis by punch-card techniques. The temptation to include items which might perhaps be useful in a standard form, should be firmly resisted; if succumbed to, the form soon becomes prolix, a source of wasted time and annoyance to both subject and examiner, and a definite impediment to the programme. The principle should be to decide what items are confidently expected to give useful information bearing on the subject of the study; the record form with its associated punch-card system should be restricted to these items only, except for provision of a space for 'other information' in which incidental observations may be noted. Should it later transpire that some of these types of observations are going to produce valuable information they may be incorporated in a revised card, and some preliminary trials may be run with this in mind.

A great deal of valuable information bearing on the effects of *S. haematobium* infection has been collected on postcard-size forms. The significant entries concerned the identification of the school or other centre at which examinations were carried out, together with the date, and for each individual: name, age, sex, school standard, place of residence, results of each of three urine examinations, and stool examinations, egg-counts classified into 12 intensity groups, satisfactory intravenous pyelography plates obtained, satisfactory straight radiography plates, pathology found or not, and lesions found, classified under six headings. This provided information which was hand-punched on to record cards and analysed by the workers themselves. It might well be necessary to add to, or radically change, this list, but the principle of maintaining a concise list should be followed if the findings are to be manageable with the techniques available to most workers.

Study Unit

The nature of the study unit also will vary with the objective. An effective study will usually require the establishment of a special unit for the purpose staffed by one or two medical officers, one nursing sister, one administrative assistant, four or more technical and clinical assistants, one radiographer, one clerk, one driver and a field liaison officer.

The fullest co-operation of government and medical authorities will be necessary for a survey of this type. This should include not only the provision of laboratory space and facilities for examining the community but also facilities in associated hospitals to which patients requiring further study can be taken and treated. It is very desirable that processes such as pyelography should be carried out under hospital conditions, though they have been practised successfully in out-patient circumstances. The first activity of the unit should be one of public relations, to explain its objectives to the population and to secure the maximum degree of co-operation. This may well involve a considerable effort and expenditure of time but without it much effort may be totally wasted. A logical explanation of what is to be done, why it should be done, what forms of co-operation are requested and what type of result is expected will generally secure public support.

The explanation should include an offer to supply every available form of treatment for any abnormalities found during the course of the survey, thereby making the special provision of drugs and other apparatus necessary. People cannot be expected to submit themselves to medical examination possibly leading to the discovery and study of an ailment, which is not then treated with a similar degree of care and understanding.

Annex 1. Radiographic Methods for Community Surveys [WHO, 1967]

Schistosoma haematobium Infection

Excretion Urography

As a field method of cross-sectional study of the community, this examination will show gross structural changes in the urinary tract. A six-step technique that has proved satisfactory is as follows:

(1) Admit the individual to the clinic the night before the examination, administer a purge and deprive of fluids.

(2) The following morning, take a full-length preliminary film of the urinary tract.

(3) Immediately inject intravenously a suitable contrast medium, such as sodium amidotrizoate (20 ml of the 76-percent solution or 40 ml of the 45-percent solution; no diminution of dose need be made for age).

(4) Lower-abdominal compression is applied and films taken of the kidneys at 5 and 10 min after injection.

(5) If these are satisfactory, compression is released and full-length films of the urinary tract taken at 15 and 20 min.

(6) Further films may be taken if indicated (e.g., a prone film in hydronephrosis).

In longitudinal studies, where the individual may be subjected to more than one such examination over a period of years, the technique needs to be modified in order to cut down X-ray dosage. The following four-step technique is proving satisfactory:

(1) A preliminary film of the bladder is taken.

(2) After injection of the contrast medium, compression is applied and a 15-min film of the renal area taken.

(3) Compression is released and a full-length film of the urinary tract taken at 30 min.

(4) Further films are taken as indicated (e.g., a prone film in hydro-nephrosis).

It is considered that no more than four such examinations should be carried out over a 10-year period. Further, it is important that gonad protection should be provided in all examinations, as far as is practicable. Pregnant women should not be subjected to this examination.

Chest Examination

This examination should be carried out on all subjects in community studies to exclude other disease and to demonstrate or exclude pulmonary vascular changes. It is preferable to use a high-output X-ray apparatus with a short time-factor (e.g., 0.05 sec or less per exposure). Miniature film (100 mm) is satisfactory, but 70-mm film is unsatisfactory.

If this type of X-ray apparatus is not available, it is still possible to exclude the presence of diseases other than schistosomiasis, and this is important, but demonstration of the presence or absence of pulmonary vascular changes is not possible.

The interpretation of the development of pulmonary hypertension must be made by experienced radiologists.

The diagnosis of cor pulmonale is described in annex 2.

Diuresis Pyelography

This is a technique employed for the further investigation of hospitalized subjects in whom structural change in the urinary tract has already been diagnosed.

For an adult, a mixture of 150 ml of contrast medium and 150 ml of dextrose is infused intravenously through a wide-bore needle as rapidly as it will flow (e.g., in about 4 min). No compression is applied. Full-length films of the urinary tract are taken at 5, 10 and 15 min after infusion, and others as indicated. By this method, good nephrograms can be obtained and also good pyelograms, ureterograms, and cystograms.

A post-micturition film of the bladder shows the ability of the bladder to contract.

Micturating Cystography

This procedure is carried out when there is a suspicion of ureteric reflux. It should be performed by a radiologist, using high-output X-ray apparatus and fluoroscopic control. It should preferably be performed using an image intensifier to reduce X-ray dosage.

The bladder is filled retrogradely to capacity with contrast medium. With the subject in the erect position, micturition is observed by fluoroscopy. Shot films are taken to demonstrate any reflux.

Schistosoma mansoni and S. japonicum

Plain Film of Abdomen

The film is taken of the upper abdomen and diaphragmatic region. Its object is to provide a graphic record of liver and spleen size. This is a complement to clinical examination and is for future comparison.

Chest Examination

The procedure is the same as that described for S. haematobium.

Barium Swallow Examination

This technique is not a screening procedure for field work. It must be carried out with high-output X-ray apparatus by an experienced radiologist. It will demonstrate oesophageal varices in 75–80% of cases of portal hypertension in which the collateral circulation has produced such varices. It is a time-consuming procedure, which must be carried out in both the erect and supine postures, possibly employing the Valsalva and Müller manoeuvres.

Portal Venography

This is a complex procedure that can be carried out only in major hospitals under the direct supervision of a radiologist.

Barium Enema Examination

In the individual studies following community surveys, it seems likely that more use will be made of this investigation.

By the modern technique of barium and air examination of the colon, it is possible to demonstrate mucosal changes. It is known that granulomatous masses occur in S. mansoni infections, and many of these have been demonstrated radiologically. By the application of this technique to suspected cases, earlier diagnosis and the extent of the disease may be established.

This is a hospital procedure and is not applicable to field studies.

Wedge Hepatic Venography

This is a complex procedure that can be carried out only in major centres. It is at present applicable only to the full investigation of selected cases and is not suitable for community studies.

Annex 2. Clinical Recognition of Chronic Cor Pulmonale [WHO, 1961]

Recognition of chronic cor pulmonale rests upon the demonstration of right ventricular hypertrophy in the presence of (various diseases). In some of these diverse clinical conditions, the abnormal signs indicative of right ventricular hypertrophy may be readily apparent during life. In other conditions, right ventricular hypertrophy may be unrecognizable in life though demonstrable at autopsy.

The anatomical diagnosis of right ventricular hypertrophy has been considered by the Committee, but it is suggested that further observations using standardized techniques are desirable. For this reason no recommendations concerning this aspect of the problem have been formulated, ... Similarly, the anatomical diagnosis of the various lung diseases, and particularly of the common condition of emphysema, requires further study by standardized techniques. ...

The clinical manifestations and criteria of diagnosis on which the clinical recognition of cor pulmonale in life depends are reviewed in the following sections ....

Diagnostic Indications of Right Ventricular Hypertrophy in Pulmonary Diseases

Clinical Findings

There are no symptoms specifically related to the presence of right ventricular hypertrophy. The cardiac signs are often concealed by distension of the overlying lung, but may include a systolic thrust. This is indeed the only physical sign directly related to right ventricular hypertrophy. Its exact position varies, being sometimes to the left of the sternum, sometimes over the sternum itself and sometimes in the epigastrium. Other physical signs, including a loud pulmonary second sound, a gallop rhythm and jugular venous pulsation are related either to the severity of the pulmonary hypertension or to right heart failure.

Radiological Findings

There may be no observable cardiac abnormality in the chest radiograph. The heart may be small even in the presence of right ventricular hypertrophy. Enlargement of the right ventricle indicative of dilatation and not necessarily of hypertrophy may be seen in the lateral, though invisible in the postero-anterior (PA), position. Enlargement in the transverse diameter of the heart in the PA film is indicative of dilatation and not necessarily of hypertrophy. An alteration in contour of the pulmonary conus with filling-in of the normal concavity or actual convexity seen particularly in the right oblique position may be a manifestation of hypertrophy of the outflow tract of the right ventricle.

Changes in the size of the main pulmonary arteries or of their branches are related to altered haemodynamics of the pulmonary circulation rather than to hypertrophy of the ventricle. Dilatation of the stem and main branches of the pulmonary artery, and a contrast between the enlarged hilar and the diminished peripheral vascular shadows are common radiological findings in pulmonary hypertension. In this respect they may indicate indirectly the existence of right ventricular hypertrophy.

Electrocardiographic Findings

It must be appreciated that there may be no alterations in the electro-cardiogram in cases of chronic cor pulmonale in spite of the presence at autopsy of right ventricular hypertrophy. There are, however, many observed deviations from the normal electrocardiogram, some of which are related to changes in the position of the heart and others of temporary phases of illness. Amongst all these deviations the changes usually accepted as those indicative of right ventricular hypertrophy appear and remain in a proportion of cases and, therefore, constitute important criteria in life.

The presence of a qR pattern with delayed R wave in V1 (onset of intrinsicoid deflection more than 0.03 sec) is not commonly seen in cor pulmonale but, if present, may by itself be considered to be highly suggestive of right ventricular hypertrophy. It is often better observed in V3R and V4R which should thus be recorded in patients in whom right ventricular hypertrophy is suspected. In the absence of a qR pattern a combination of at least two of the following changes must be present for these alterations to be indicative of right ventricular hypertrophy:

(1) alteration in the ratio R/S in the left chest leads with R/S less than 1 in V5;

(2) predominant S wave in standard lead I;

(3) presence of an incomplete right bundle branch block with QRS less than 0.12 sec.

The significance of a P pulmonale in which the P wave in lead II is 2.5 mm or more in height, though considered to be suggestive of hypertrophy of the right atrium and seen in some patients with cor pulmonale, cannot be regarded as diagnostic of cardiac involvement. Right axis deviation of an extreme degree (110° or more) accompanies extreme rotation of the cardiac axis and so may be found in association with right ventricular hypertrophy. Inversion of the T wave in the precordial leads V1 to V4 or in leads II and III may also occur, but may be transitory. A combination of one or more of these alterations in the P or T waves or the QRS complex, together with those mentioned in relation to right ventricular hypertrophy, reinforces the indication of cardiac disease.

Haemodynamic Findings

The most accurate method of defining the altered state of the pulmonary circulation in cor pulmonale is that of cardiac catheterization which permits measurement of blood flow and pressures. Although the demonstration of pulmonary hypertension does not necessarily imply right ventricular hypertrophy, its presence implies strain upon the right ventricle, and persistent hypertension will certainly cause hypertrophy. Catheterization is needed, however, for diagnostic purposes in only very few patients. When performed, both cardiac output and pressure measurements should be made and it is important that the patient should be in a steady state. The technique requires standardization, and catheterization should be performed only by well-trained and well-equipped observers.

The following are regarded as the upper limits of normal values with the reference point[1] 10 cm above the level of the back in the supine position:

---

[1] A more customary reference point 5 cm below the sternal angle is also used with approximately the same normal values. This is not recommended.

	Systolic mm Hg	Diastolic mm Hg	Mean mm Hg
Right atrium	–	–	6
Right ventricle	25	6	–
Pulmonary artery	25	12	15
Pulmonary arteriolar wedge pressure	–	–	9

The total pulmonary resistance lies between 150 and 300 dynes sec cm^{-5}

Pulmonary hypertension is usually considered to be present when the mean pressure in the pulmonary artery exceeds 25 mm Hg at rest. In many instances of pulmonary heart disease this value will not be exceeded at rest. The effects of exercise on the pulmonary artery pressure, though considerable in the presence of pulmonary heart disease, will depend on the amount of work and on the stage of disease. Actual values for the normal mean pressures on exercise are not quoted because of lack of standardization of available figures.

The clinical, radiological, electrocardiographic and haemodynamic findings should be considered together, since the diagnosis of right ventricular hypertrophy becomes increasingly probable with increase in the number and severity of abnormalities demonstrated. It is not possible at present to state any simple definitive criteria which would command general acceptance.

References

BARNETT, A. M.: Sth afr. med. J. *39:* 699 (1965).

BIRD, A. V.: Sth afr. med. J. *39:* 158 (1965).

BUDZILOVICH, G. N.; MOST, H., and FEIGIN, I.: Arch. Path. *77:* 383 (1964).

EDINGTON, G. M.; LICHTENBERG, F., VON; NWABUEBO, J.; TAYLOR, J. R., and SMITH, J. H.: Amer. J. trop. Med. Hyg. *19:* 982 (1970).

EL-MOFTY, A. M. and CAHILL, K. M.: Derm. trop. *3:* 157 (1964).

ERFAN, M.; ERFAN, H.; MOUSA, A. M., and DEEB, A. A.: Trans. roy. Soc. trop. Med. Hyg. *42:* 477 (1949).

FARIA, J. L. DE; CZAPSKI, J.; RIBEIRO LEITE, M. O.; OLIVEIRA PENNA, D.; FUJIOKA, T., and ULHÔA CINTRA, A. B.: Amer. Heart J. *54:* 196 (1957).

FARIA, J. L. DE; VALENTE BARBAS, J.; FUJIOKA, T.; LION, M. F.; ANDRADE SILVA, U., and DÉCOURT, L. V.: Amer. Heart J. *58:* 556 (1959).

FAROOQ, M.: Ann. trop. Med. Parasit. *57:* 323 (1963).

FORSYTH, D. M. and BRADLEY, D. J.: Bull. Wld Hlth Org. *34:* 715 (1966).

FORSYTH, D. M. and MACDONALD, G.: Trans. roy. Soc. trop. Med. Hyg. *59:* 171 (1965).

FORSYTH, D. M. and MACDONALD, G.: Trans. roy. Soc. trop. Med. Hyg. *60:* 568 (1966).

GELFAND, M.: Schistosomiasis in South Central Africa. A clinico-pathological study (Juta, Cape Town 1950).

GELFAND, M.: Cent. afr. J. Med. *11:* 75 (1965).

GELFAND, M. and ROSS, W. F.: Trans. roy. Soc. trop. Med. Hyg. *47:* 215 (1953).

GILLES, H. M.; LUCAS, A.; ADENIYI-JONES, C.; LINDNER, R.; ANAND, S. V.; BRABAND, H.; COCKSHOTT, W. P.; COWPER, S. G.; MULLER, R. L.; HIRA, P. R., and WILSON, A. M. M.: Ann. trop. Med. Parasit, *59:* 441 (1965).

GREANY, W. H.: Ann. trop. Med. Parasit. *46:* 298 (1952).

HONEY, R. M. and GELFAND, M.: The urological aspects of bilharziasis in Rhodesia (Livingstone, Edinburgh/London 1960).

KASS, E. H.: Trans. Ass. amer. Phycns *69:* 56 (1956).

KATZ, N. and BRENER, Z.: Rev. Inst. Med. trop. S. Paulo *8:* 139 (1966).

KLOETZEL, K.: Amer. J. trop. Med. Hyg. *13:* 541 (1964).

KOVI, J.: Ghana med. J. *3:* 84 (1964).

MAKAR, N.: Urological aspects of bilharziasis in Egypt. Société Orientale de Publicité, Cairo; reviewed in Trop. Dis. Bull. *54:* 365 (1957).

MOST, H.; KANE, C. A.; LAVIETES, P. H.; SCHROEDER, E. F.; BEHM, A.; BLUM, L.; KATZIN, B., and HAYMAN, J. M., jr.: Amer. J. trop. Med. Hyg. *30:* 239 (1950).

NEVES, J. and RASO, P.: Rev. Inst. Med. trop. S. Paulo *7:* 256 (1965).

PESIGAN, T. P.; FAROOQ, M.; HAIRSTON, N. G.; JAUREGUI, J.J.; GARCIA, E. G.; SANTIS, A.T.; SANTOS, B. C., and BESA, A.A.: Bull. Wld Hlth Org. *18:* 345 (1958).

POLAK, M.; MONTENEGRO, M. R.; MEIRA, J.A.; CONTE, V.P.; ESPEJO, H.; FRANCHINI, F., and PONTES, J. F.: Rev. Inst. Med. trop. S. Paulo *1:* 18 (1959).

PRATA, A. R. and BINA, J. C.: Gaz. méd. Bahia *68:* 49 (1968).

SCOTT, J. A.: Amer. J. Hyg. *25:* 566 (1937).

SIMMONS, N. A. and WILLIAMS, J. D.: Lancet *i:* 1377 (1962).

VOGEL, H.: Zbl. Bakt., I. Abt. Orig. *154:* 118 (1949).

VOGEL, H. and MINNING, W.: Z. Tropenmed. Parasit. *4:* 418 (1953).

WESSEL, H. U.; SOMMERS, H. M.; CUGELL, D. W., and PAUL, M. H.: Ann. intern. Med. *62:* 757 (1965).

WHO: Expert Committee, Chronic cor pulmonale. Wld Hlth Org. techn. Rep. Ser. *213:* 11–14 (1961).

WHO: Expert Committee on Bilharziasis; 3rd report. Wld Hlth Org. techn. Rep. Ser. *299:* 56 (1965).

WHO: Measurement of the public health importance of bilharziasis; Report of a WHO Scientific Group, Geneva 1965. Wld Hlth Org. techn. Rep. Ser. *349:* 74 (1967).

ZAKY, H. A.; EL-HENEIDY, A. R., and KHALIL, M.: Brit. med. J. *i:* 1021 (1964).

Chapter 7

Epidemiology and Control of Schistosomiasis, pp. 388–421
(Karger, Basel and University Park Press, Baltimore 1973)

Review of National Control Programmes

M. FAROOQ

Introduction

In spite of the widespread nature of schistosomiasis, national programmes for the control of the disease have been developed in only a few countries. The development of methods employed and progress attained in countries where major efforts have been made are reviewed at some length in the following sections, classified according to the species of the parasite or parasites concerned. This has been done in order to provide background information on the course of events in the development of control programmes in different parts of the world, and will also meet the expressed need for providing illustrations from the field of the methods employed and the successes or failures encountered. In the latter case there is no intention whatsoever of discrediting the noteworthy attempts made.

It is interesting to note that in dealing with the same species of parasite, different countries have emphasized different approaches. These include ecological control of snail habitats through water management, and improved land use and agricultural practices; mass therapy; chemical, physical and biological control of snails; environmental sanitation; or a combination of two or more of these, with varying degrees of emphasis placed on the different aspects. Even an omnibus approach has been made by applying everything indiscriminately, without judging to what extent the cost involved by each is justified by the results obtained.

In the adoption of these methods very little attention appears to have been given to benefiting from the success or failures of others. In most cases mistakes have been repeated while achievements have been ignored. It is partly to correct this serious deficiency that the World Health Organization since 1949 has been increasingly bringing together experts from the different countries to exchange views through Committees, Scientific Study Groups and Conferences, and at the request of Governments has assisted by sending advisory teams and experts and by establishing pilot projects for the study of the problems and the development of effective and economical methodology for dealing with the disease under local conditions. Training Courses and fellowships and research grants have been provided. A good measure of success has been attained in inviting attention to gaps in the existing knowledge and in co-ordinating the activities of research workers on the different aspects of this complex problem.

Schistosoma haematobium

Iran

Urinary schistosomiasis has existed since ancient times in Khuzestan Province in the south-western part of Iran. Since 1949 short surveys have been undertaken periodically in the country by the Institute of Malariology and Parasitology of the University of Teheran. In 1957, a permanent laboratory centre was established in Ahwaz and a team organized to carry out more extensive surveys. It was confirmed that the distribution of S. haematobium was confined to isolated foci in Khuzestan [ANSARI, 1958].

Two WHO consultants [GAUD and OLIVIER, 1959] visited Iran in late 1958 and, based on their report, WHO assisted in setting up a pilot project in the Dez-Shahpur-Karkheh River basin, with its headquarters in Dezful in Khuzestan, with the specific objectives of conducting studies on epidemiology, snail ecology in relation to water management, studies designed for the prevention and control of schistosomiasis, training of national staff and to plan for an expanded inter-departmental programme for the control of the disease.

The eight isolated foci in Khuzestan were estimated to have 50,000 infected individuals in 1959 at the time the WHO-assisted project started. A step-by-step programme has been followed, first in the project area at Dezful and then in the endemic foci in Khuzestan:

(1) fact-finding phase 1959–1961;

(2) experimental control studies 1963–1965;

(3) operational and evaluation phase 1965-onward in the endemic foci.

Base-line data on prevalence of infection and ecological studies on Bulinus (B.) truncatus were gathered in the first phase. In the second phase, five molluscicides were field-tested and niclosamide, 2 ppm/10 h in flowing waters and 1.5 ppm for stagnant waters, was considered adequate. Ecological control of snail habitats, including drainage, filling and drying, was used. Sanitary measures were taken in certain villages and field trials of drugs were carried out. The drug of choise was niridazole given 30 mg/kg body-weight, for four days, morning and evening, without untoward effects.

Control operations dealt with ecological control of snails and molluscicid-ing of residual colonies by niclosamide. It was only in villages where there was evidence of interruption of transmission for three years that therapy was used.

The carry-over value of this WHO-assisted project was extremely good. The project was taken over by the Government and since 1967 it is run as a national control programme without WHO assistance.

Evaluation of the data [FAROOQ, 1968] shows that transmission has been blocked in the satellite foci and that the infection is in an unstable state in the two main foci. There are now no more than 8,000 active cases of S. haemato-bium in Khuzestan.

However laudable the achievement of the project may be, the picture is not as propitious as it would appear at first sight. There are several unfavour-able circumstances at work in Khuzestan and these should be taken into ac-count before dismissing schistosomiasis as being of no consequence in Iran. Irrigation under Dez dam is expanding in the area and it is proposed to have a system of 14 major multi-purpose dams that will harness the five rivers that traverse the province, a year-round intensive cultivation and the utilization of many resources in the region to make it the granary of the Middle East.

WHO has been sceptical about the possibility of eradicating schistoso-miasis, except in very limited foci and under exceptional circumstances. It is believed that Khuzestan falls under these exceptional circumstances which call for an operational methodology for eradicating S. haematobium. It would be wise to assess the cost-benefit of the programme and to measure the impact of control and eradication of S. haematobium in socio-economic terms in Khuzestan.

The Plan Organization in Iran, the Khuzestan Water and Power Auth-ority, and the Near-East Foundation, have great interest in Khuzestan and have been actively supporting the schistosomiasis project in Iran.

Iraq

Interest in the study and control of schistosomiasis in Iraq was aroused by three epidemics, one among the Indian troops at Basrah during the First

World War, and two among the British troops stationed at Minaidi and Kufa during 1921 and 1924. The latter outbreaks were attributed to the presence of *B. (B.) truncatus* in bodies of water in which the soldiers bathed. Control measures employed included periodic drying out of canals, increased rate of flow of water and application of cresol and copper sulphate. This, together with the elimination of contact with natural waters, prevented the further occurrence of cases amongst the troops.

Although isolated attempts to study the problem in Iraq were made by HALL in 1925 and CHADWICK in 1936, no control measures were considered until WATSON was invited to study and report on the situation to the Government in 1948. He found the infection to be widespread and serious, not only in the area of the middle and lower Euphrates but throughout the country except in the extreme north. In 1949, a Bilharzia Section was established in the Directorate General of Public Health 'to carry out further research and to apply the results thereof in practical measures in the form of a national scheme for the control of the disease'. This Section originally consisted of headquarters and field staff. The work of the headquarters staff in Baghdad consisted of surveys, research and control. The staff in the field was divided into 'anti-snail units', at least one in each of the 10 southern and central liwas where prevalence was high. Each unit consisted of four labourers and an overseer, working under the supervision of the technician for the liwa. The units visited heavily infected areas and carried out anti-snail measures, consisting of clearing aquatic vegetation from water channels, drains, small pools and swamps, followed by the application of copper sulphate or cresol. Treatment for schistosomiasis cases was made available at the State hospitals and dispensaries.

The staff and activities of the Bilharzia Control Section expanded with the promulgation and application of the 'Law of Bilharziasis Control and Control of Snail Vectors' (No. 38 of 1952) which first became operative in Baghdad Liwa in 1953. The budgetary provisions of the Section increased from I.D. 57,000 to I.D. 70,000 by 1957. Bilharzia Control Units were assigned to 10 provinces where the disease is endemic. The main molluscicide used was copper sulphate, though some copper carbonate and sodium pentachlorophenate were also used. A critical evaluation of this programme has yet to be made and its effect on the prevalence of schistosomiasis in Iraq is unknown. On the other hand, the extension of irrigation systems and the development of new schemes of land reclamation have considerably accentuated the possibility for the spread and intensification of the disease. Recognition of the complexity of the problem has been shown by the organization of a committee composed of representatives from the Ministry of Agriculture, Irrigation and Health.

The Government of Iraq requested the assistance of WHO in the establishment of a Bilharziasis Control project, and project Iraq-15 came into existence in 1956. The first project area selected was situated in the district of Tarmiah 45 km north of Baghdad covering 550 km² with a population of about 15,500.

All work since 1963 has been concentrated in the Horr Rajab area 30 km south-west of Baghdad. The area covers about 16,000 ha and has a population of approximately 21,000 people. The programme outlined was ambitious and included an intensive study of the epidemiology of the disease, the socio-economic conditions of the area, a sanitation survey, the snail life cycle, parasite life cycle and snail control. Control activities were, however, limited to the demonstrations of the application of molluscicides (copper sulphate, sodium pentachlorophenate and niclosamide).

Schistosoma mansoni

Puerto Rico

Initial Experiment in Control
Except for a general educational programme and chemotherapy provided to cases coming voluntarily to public health units and to private and government hospitals in Puerto Rico, no definite programme of schistosomiasis control was undertaken until the beginning of 1947. OLIVER-GONZALEZ and associates from the School of Tropical Medicine [OLIVER-GONZALEZ *et al.*, 1950] initiated a study of multi-factor control in an endemic area, Barrio 'Los Peña' situated alongside Sabana Llana Creek near San Juan, in 1947. The community consisted of 112 houses and 655 inhabitants.

The methods of control applied were: (a) treatment of infected persons; (b) health and medico-social education; (c) installation of sanitary privies; (d) provision of improved supply of water; and (e) biological control of the snail. The last consisted of releasing 40,000 *Lebistis reticulatus* in the bordering creek.

Infection prevalence fell from 44.6 to 4.5% by the end of 1949. The rates of infection in children, 6 to 15 years of age, went down from 60 to 8.9%. This decrease was attributed chiefly to treatment (Stibophen) and to health education activities.

After snail surveys, OLIVER-GONZALEZ and FERGUSON [1959] reported that the snail intermediate host species, *Biomphalaria glabrata*, had a precipitous population decline. This apparently was due to the accidental introduction and establishment of a phenomenally large colony of an ampullarid snail, *Marisa cornuarietis*, first seen in the stream in 1952. During March 1956, this highly competitive species was successfully transplanted to all upstream stations in the watershed, and during a period of 1.5 years, it almost eliminated the host species in these areas.

Two successive annual surveys of the creekside families indicated that in 1959 no new infections had appeared in the statistically sensitive pre-school age group. The community prevalence in all ages and both sexes has levelled off at a rate of about 6 or 7%. This is the first instance of probable biological control of schistosomiasis transmission.

The organizations concerned in schistosomiasis control were:

(1) The Commonwealth of Puerto Rico Department of Health;

(2) Communicable Disease Center, Puerto Rico Field Station (US Public Health Service), and

(3) The US Army Tropical Medicine Research Laboratory.

The various control projects that have so far been undertaken in Puerto Rico are to be regarded largely as extended experiments. Their main purpose has been to gather experience and information regarding the efficiency of the various control measures and their costs. These projects incorporated a combined approach of chemical and biological snail control, chemotherapy, soil sanitation, improved water supply, and health education. Each project covered one or two naturally defined watersheds. The projects were designed to answer certain operational questions.

Planning and Development of Control Projects

Before any control measures were undertaken the whole area was thoroughly surveyed and mapped with regard to the occurrence of *B. glabrata*. The surveying also included other epidemiologically important features. This was planned for each of the 52 principal watersheds of the island and priority determined according to the severity of its problem. The planned anti-schistosomiasis programme then proceeded from watershed to watershed on the aforementioned priority basis as funds were made available. Each control project was run by one supervisor, one foreman and at least five labourers.

Since control measures were not carried out on an island-wide basis and have over the years been of a more or less sporadic nature, it is not possible to evaluate their over-all effect. There is evidence, however, that the prevalence rate has decreased. Economic advances, increased sanitation, general health improvement and other factors have undoubtedly played a role in whatever reduction has taken place in the disease.

Venezuela

The possibility of control of the local intermediate host of schistosomiasis, B. *glabrata* in Venezuela, was first investigated during the period 1940 to 1943. In the Caracas Valley it was found that the removal of vegetation from the waterways and the improvement of drainage and waterflow, followed by applications of freshly slaked lime or copper sulphate reduced the number of B. *glabrata*. In 1942, these measures were adopted by the Venezuelan Ministry of Health and a campaign was started on a modest scale in the suburbs of the capital city, Caracas. Methods of snail control were gradually improved and this, coupled with the concurrent physical changes in the valley due to road-building, new aqueducts and services, landscaping, and development of sub-divisions, all contributed to the reduction in the incidence of schistosomiasis.

A control programme of gradually increasing scope and intensity has since been in progress in Venezuela, though the campaign on a national scale really began with the organization in 1946 of the Antibilharzia Section of the Ministry of Health. The campaign has emphasized, in order of importance, snail control, permanent sanitary improvements, health education and chemo-therapy.

Snail Control
The copper sulphate and lime first used as molluscicides were replaced in 1953 by sodium pentachlorophenate. In 1956, copper pentachlorophenate was adopted as the molluscicide of choice.

The molluscicide is applied whenever any snails are found in the habitat without regard to population density or their probable importance in the transmission of infection. Treatment of some habitats is repeated as often as six times a year, though in most habitats two to three times a year suffices.

Sanitation Programme
The sanitation programme has also been given important emphasis in the control campaign; 46 town water supplies have been installed in endemic foci, and 97 public laundry places with attendant bathing and toilet facilities have been built. Since 1947 up to 4,000 latrines have been built each year in

the States where schistosomiasis is endemic. The Ministry not only gives advice to householders interested in the construction of a latrine but, depending on the local situation and on the ability to pay, it may defray a large part of the cost of the latrine.

Health Education

The health education programme has been extensive and has included the use of the usual audio-visual and other techniques.

Chemotherapy

Chemotherapy was early employed as a control measure in certain localities. However, it became an integral part of the programme in 1954 with the establishment of a field clinic but did not become very intensive until 1959. It is believed in Venezuela that the treatment campaign has further reduced prevalence in areas where snail populations have been brought under control by molluscicides.

Lucanthone hydrochloride has been the drug of choice for the field treatment campaign. In 1961, follow-up faecal examinations were made on 316 treated persons three months or more after completion of treatment. The records suggest that 99% of these persons were cured since no eggs were found in the faeces.

It is significant to note that although the anti-snail campaign has apparently succeeded in reducing snail populations very drastically in many localities, repeated treatment of numerous bodies of water has not resulted in eradication and it has been necessary to treat these places several times a year. Some streams have been treated systematically for six years, yet snails still appear from time to time.

Data on the prevalence of infection among children aged from 1 to 10 years is available for 1947 and 1960 in four localities of the area. Although these data were not collected according to standardized procedures and the populations sampled may not be strictly comparable, the data do seem to indicate a substantial fall in prevalence in all four localities.

There is evidence to show that the schistosomiasis control programme in Venezuela has achieved substantial reductions in snail populations and infection rates. This success has been made possible by the systematic and determined effort of competent personnel, the provision of adequate funds and the sustained support received from the Department of Environmental Sanitation, the Agricultural Extension Services, Department of Hydraulic Works and the National Institute of Agriculture.

Over a period of some 20 years, practically all known methods for the control of schistosomiasis have been persistently employed. Continuation of these methods is expected to maintain the downward trend in both prevalence rates and snail populations. Authorities now believe that this is an opportune period in the Venezuelan control campaign for evaluation of the methods used and for consideration of possible modifications to present practices that may result in reduced costs and greater efficacy.

Schistosoma haematobium and Schistosoma mansoni

Egypt

Early Developments

Professor LEIPER worked out the basis for prophylactic work in Egypt in 1915, to which detailed reference has been made earlier. Until then, the authorities in Egypt had hoped that the preventive measures applicable to ancylostomiasis, namely mass treatment, introduction of conservancy and dissemination of the knowledge of the disease, would also prove efficacious in dealing with schistosomiasis.

Mass Treatment

Following the introduction of tartar emetic by CHRISTOPHERSON in the Sudan in 1918, Egypt started a campaign of treatment through a few mobile units in 1920, gradually increasing in number until 1928, when the Endemic Diseases Section was created to organize a country-wide programme. The treatment provided by the 'Ancylostoma and Bilharzia' units consisted of tartar emetic given intravenously in 6% solution every other day, in doses of 2 grains three times a week for four weeks, to able-bodied adults, and a reduced dose to children according to body weight.

In 1929, working at the Research Institute in Cairo, SCHMIDT of Bayer developed stibophen for intramuscular administration. Stibophen was given as $1/12$ ml/kg body weight for nine injections daily or every other day. Intensive treatment methods were experimented with, and treatment on a mass scale was initiated in 1940. However, stibophen was found to be more toxic than tartar ematic.

A Law (No. 58 of 1941) for compulsory treatment of all schistosomiasis cases was promulgated and, by an order of the Ministry (5 July 1941), it was made compulsory for children entering schools and colleges to produce a certificate of freedom from infection.

In 1943 a non-antimonial compound, lucanthone hydrochloride, became available. It was tried with enthusiasm, but was found to be less effective than tartar emetic.

Snail Control

Following CHANDLER's demonstration of copper sulphate as an effective molluscicide in 1920, KHALIL carried out the first field trials in Egypt in 1924. In April 1927, he applied the chemical in Rashda Village in Dakhla Oasis for the first time, and reported, 'At a cost of £1 of copper sulphate all the Bilharzia snails were killed, and no harm accrued to man, animal or plant' [KHALIL, 1927].

BARLOW, of the Rockefeller Foundation, on the basis of his investigation at the Farm of the Royal Khassa at Mostorod in 1937, recommended that clearing the irrigation canals every two months should be 'a prime factor in a scheme for the control of human schistosomiasis in Egypt because it is efficient, inexpensive, and required no teaching of new methods for its execution'.

Sanitation

SCOTT and BARLOW [1938] conducted controlled experiments jointly sponsored by the Government of Egypt and the Rockefeller Foundation in 1933–1935 to evaluate the effect of installation of bored-hole latrines and treatment, not only on hookworm and ascariasis but also *S. haematobium* and *S. mansoni* in rural communities in Egypt. Changes occurring over a six-year period were evaluated and the conclusion was reached that the construction of latrines provided no measurable effect on *S. haematobium* or *S. mansoni* infections amongst villagers.

Development of Large-Scale Snail Control Programmes

In 1939, a control programme utilizing copper sulphate on a larger scale was carried out in Kom-Ombo in upper Egypt covering a population of 35,000 and a cultivated area of 39,000 feddans. Two divergent schools of thought, one in favour of repeated canal clearance and the other in favour of the use of copper sulphate as a method of snail control, continued in the country for some time. A Bilharzia Snail Destruction (or Eradication) Section was created in 1939. An 'eradication' programme was started in Fayoum Province in 1942 utilizing canal clearance technique. The programme, however, did not progress as planned and canal clearance was reduced from six times to once or twice a year and was later combined with the use of copper sulphate. Happily, the controversy over these procedures died down.

AZIM in 1940 proposed the diversion of watercourses running through villages to a point not less than 500 m form habitation or covering them in case their diversion was impracticable [Ministry of Public Health Annual Report, 1940].

Without a suitable evaluation of the work in Fayoum, similar Programmes of clearing bank weeds and sulphation were started, under the newly established Bilharziasis Control Section, in Giza Province, and Dakhla Oasis in 1943, in Kharga Oasis and Aswan Province in 1944, in Baharia Oasis in 1945, and in Quena, Qualyoubia and the southern part of Beheira Province in 1946. This was soon extended over 10 of the 15 provinces and three oases in the western desert.

Experimental work carried out in Fayoum resulted in the so-called 'open' or 'shore' method of application of copper sulphate to large watercourses, in which only the shallow and weedy marginal strips are treated. Each of a group of men posted 50 m apart dissolved 4 kg of copper sulphate contained in a hessian bag, suspended from a stick, by walking to and fro along the length of the canal bank allotted to him. The men worked towards the intake, at the highest water level. This has mainly replaced the 'closed' method of sulphation, in which copper sulphate in a concentration of 15 to 30 parts per million is left to act for at least three or four days after damming the streams cleaned of vegetation.

In 1945, only canals showing an infestation rate of over 8 snails in 100 dips were treated and the rest were watched until infestation rose. The treatment of drains was restricted to those near villages or those harbouring snails infested with schistosomes [Ministry of Public Health Annual Report, 1945].

The programme was modified in 1948 and it then aimed at the treatment, at least twice a year, of branch canals with over 10 snails per 100 dips. Drains were treated only when they were passing through or near villages, or when infected snails were found in them; main streams were treated when possible. These limitations were due to the 'limited budget, very limited amounts of copper sulphate, and also to the impossibility of obtaining closure of main streams for sulphation on account of agricultural and other necessities, together with general difficulties of co-ordination with the Irrigation Department' [Ministry of Public Health Annual Report, 1948].

In 1950, however, the programme was intensified in certain areas, and the Bilharzia Snail Destruction Section was asked to intensify its snail control activity in watercourses within a radius of 3 km around the villages [Ministry of Public Health Report, 1950].

Existing Programme

The present-day programme in Egypt as evolved over the past half century, rests on the concept of a four-pronged attack of *mass treatment* (with tartar emetic), *snail control* (by use of copper sulphate), *health education* and *sanitation*. These activities are conducted under different sections of the Ministry of Health and it is estimated that the first two activities cost approximately US $3,000,000, 2,000,000 on treatment and 1,000,000 on snail control.

The standard treatment since November of 1961 is based on a dosage of 0.5 ml of a 6-percent solution of tartar emetic per 15 kg body weight, given intravenously once weekly for 12 weeks. If the patient still passes viable eggs he is given two further injections at weekly intervals and re-examined. If eggs are still being passed after the 14th dose, the routine is carried out for two further weekly injections, to a maximum of 16 injections. This is carried out at 148 Endemic Diseases Hospitals, 264 Rural Health Hospitals, 303 Combined Units, 862 Rural Health Units, 101 Social Centres, 43 School Health Centres and 45 Mass Treatment Units. Cure rates are reported to range from 26 to 100% by the different units.

The molluscicide programme consists of 'radius control', i.e. all irrigation and drainage canals within a radius of 500 m around villages are surveyed monthly and snail-infested waters are treated with copper sulphate. It is reported that this method of snail control could be established in only about half of the area as yet covered by snail control activities which in turn constitutes only half of the cultivated area in the country. In the rest of the area under snail control, molluscicide application is restricted to stretches of 250 m on either side of the point at which infected snails are discovered – 'focal control'.

Health Education and Rural Sanitation

These are conducted under the Director of Health Education in the Ministry of Health. They are carried out through schools and health committees formed in rural communities. Posters, pamphlets and other audio-visual aids are employed.

During the past 10 years nearly 60% of rural communities have been provided with access to a protected water supply by the installation of water stand-pipes at convenient locations in villages. It was planned to provide complete coverage by 1970. However, the water supply is not adequate for all domestic purposes, but meets the essential needs for drinking and cooking.

A general programme of good housing, with modern sanitary facilities is in progress for all newly established communities on reclaimed lands.

Organization

The Director of Bilharziasis Control Section of the Endemic Diseases Department of the Ministry of Health, is in technical and administrative control of the snail control programme. The organization consists of peripheral *units* each covering a zone of about 1.6 km²; four of five such *zones* constitute a sector in charge of a field technician with a small laboratory for the examination of snails. Five such sectors constitute an irrigation *district*, supervised by an agricultural engineer. Four irrigation districts form an *inspectorate* under the care of two agricultural engineers. The Director of the Section is assisted by two Supervisory Inspectors and a small staff in charge of a central laboratory and a museum. A school for training of personnel and a workshop are also provided.

Extensive health legislation has been promulgated since 1914 in Egypt to strengthen the hand of the Bilharziasis Control Section. This relates to compulsory treatment, prevention of pollution, and maintenance of watercourses in good condition.

Evaluation

Referring to the treatment programme it was observed by SHOUSHA [1949] that

'Extensive treatment carried out by the units was successful in diminishing both the number and the severity of the complications, and it is now fully acknowledged (1947) that they are of much rarer incidence. Statistics collected from the in- and out-patients of general and district hospitals are available from 1925 to 1933. They show that surgical schistosomiasis cases, which in 1925 amounted to 50.7 per 10,000 fell to 2 per 10,000 in 1933. The incidence of vesical calculus dropped from 10.4 to 6 per 10,000 and that of urinary fistulae from 3.1 to 1 per 100,000.'

HALAWANI [1957] claimed that schistosomiasis had declined in recent years; *S. mansoni* infection by about 70% and *S. haematobium* by about 40% in comparison with the 1937 figures [SCOTT][1].

It should be noted that for such comparisons to be valid, details of sampling techniques employed, age and sex compositions of the populations surveyed and methods used in establishing diagnosis should be clearly stated and remain indentical in all relevant aspects. Any comparisons made between

---

1   SCOTT's epidemiological surveys and studies over the period of 1930–37 in Egypt carried out under the joint auspices of the Government and the Rockefeller Foundation undoubtedly constitute the most comprehensive cross-sectional surveys conducted in the country and provide a firm base-line on human infection with *S. haematobium* and *S. mansoni* and *mixed infections*. The sampling design, laboratory techniques and statistical methods employed in arriving at the conclusions were clearly laid down.

the earlier data and of subsequent surveys, not duly weighted for these variables, are inadmissible.

Recent statistics do, however, indicate a shift in the age at which prevalence is greatest. In SCOTT's survey, the age of peak prevalence for *S. mansoni* in the Nile Delta was 15 to 19 years for both sexes; for *S. haematobium* in
basin-irrigated areas it was 15 to 19 years for females and 20 to 29 years for
males; and for *S. haematobium* in perennially-irrigated areas it was 10 to 14
years for both sexes. Surveys conducted 20 years later by the Ministry of
Health show that the age of peak prevalence is 10 to 14 years for all areas,
for both infections and for both sexes. This shift to a younger age indicates
that the rate of transmission has increased, in spite of the over-all decrease in
prevalence claimed. Confirmation of this shift is also obtained from the
limited area of the Egypt-49 project [FAROOQ, 1967].

Regarding the evaluation of the snail control programme in Egypt, AYAD,
the Director of Bilharziasis Control in the UAR, said in 1961:

'Snail control activities were always ruled by the amount of available molluscicide
and the policy followed had often to be changed accordingly. There was, therefore, such a
constant dovetailing of methods, as regards both time and location, as to make proper
evaluation of any particular method impossible. Moreover, no bilharziasis survey of the
human population, satisfying statistical requirements, has yet been done in Egypt. As a
matter of fact, the only two house-to-house surveys made in some villages were SCOTT's
summary survey, several years before snail control activities started on a large scale, and a
parallel survey (unpublished) performed in 1955 by the Egypt Ministry of Public Health,
which showed a definite lowering of the incidence rate. It is planned to make an extensive
survey, employing sampling methods in accordance with more stringent statistical requirements, for the first time in Egypt.'

At the same time he also stated that,

'It was not thought necessary to evaluate "generalised control" as it has already been
evaluated in Dahkla Oasis and in Warraq el Arab.'[2]

Future Trends

Until recently *Biomphalaria* was definitely considered to be absent south
of Cairo; it is now reported to have been recovered from the two contiguous
provinces in the Nile Valley, Giza and Beni Suef. That conditions in Fayoum

2   The Warraq el Arab project jointly sponsored by US International Co-operation
Administration and the Ministry of Health demonstrated in 1954–58 that a single method of
snail control effectively carried out by use of sodium pentachlorophenate would control
transmission under Egyptian conditions at a cost of approximately US$ 2 per acre. The
difficulty of preventing reinfection of treated canal systems in any localized area was
emphasized however [WRIGHT et al., 1958].

are not unfavourable is evident from the experimental plantation of *Biomphalaria* in 1940 in the dead end of a drain and finding there, after two years, a thriving colony of the snails. It was found possible, fortunately, to destroy all *Biomphalaria* by repeated application of copper sulphate to the colony, but it showed very convincingly that ecological conditions in Upper Egypt are favourable for the spread of this snail and consequently to *S. mansoni* infection, should it gain a foothold there.

The construction of the Aswan High Dam, the greatest single economic development scheme in the country, will bring another 1,000,000 feddans of arid land under perennial irrigation and convert 700,000 feddans of basin-irrigated areas, in Qena and Sohag Provinces in Upper Egypt, to perennial irrigation. With this must be considered the control of the annual silt-laden floods and the unpredictable ecological conditions in the Nile Valley, which may produce profound effects. On the basis of past experience alone it is possible to forecast the results to be expected from the changes following completion of the High Dam. One such attempt has been made by the WHO Bilharziasis Advisory Team in 1962. Without the instution of control measures in the converted and reclaimed areas it is expected that 70% of the population will acquire schistosomiasis. Prevalence data from pump schemes in Upper Egypt indicate that, even with careful water management and improvement of agricultural practices, a reduction in prevalence of more than 15% is unusual. Five million additional people will be exposed to the risk of infection, and it is estimated that the resulting addition of 2,650,000 infected individuals will before long swell the present estimates to nearly 17,000,000 infected individuals in Egypt.

The Government of the UAR is fully aware of the implications of the Aswan High Dam project and has set up a High Committee, composed of officials from the Ministries of Health, Agriculture and Irrigation to study the problem. A number of far reaching principles have been agreed upon to prevent the spread of the infection in the areas affected.

WHO-Assisted Pilot Projects

The first WHO-assisted field project in schistosomiasis (Egypt-10) came into operation in Qalyiub near Cairo in 1952 and lasted for a period of two years. In spite of the many practical difficulties encountered, useful work was done and the broad conclusions arrived at were that, despite the thoroughness of the surveying and treatment of snail breeding areas, the snails were not completely eliminated from the area and it was stressed that the high cost of the molluscicide used (copper sulphate) would prohibit its widespread and continued use. It was considered, however, that until such long-term control measures as improved sanitation, better treatment facilities, and health education of the public were perfected, snail control was of the first importance, and determined efforts should be made to find more efficient and cheaper methods of effecting it [VAN DER SCHALIE, 1958].

The need for a revised plan of operation thus became apparent. Therefore the scope of the project was widened and its ultimate objective redefined to include assistance to the Egyptian Government to develop such new knowledge as is needed for the better application of methods of schistosomiasis control, so as to reduce the transmission, incidence and severity of this disease. Mena area in Giza, near Cairo, was selected as the new project area for implementing the revised plan. Unfortunately, assistance in the form of technical advice was limited to the provision of a sanitary engineer for only a part of the period and beginning in 1958 WHO advisory services were not requested by the Government for this Technical Assistance programme.

Following the decision of the UNICEF Board in 1959 to assist pilot projects in schistosomiasis, the first joint UAR-WHO-UNICEF project (Egypt-49) came into being in the Nile Delta, near Alexandria. Though the project officially started in 1961, it did not get fully under way for various reasons until the beginning of 1962. The project was planned on a five-year basis with the main objective of developing an effective and economical methodology for the control of S. haematobium and S. mansoni under conditions existing in the Nile Delta, and to develop the project in due course into a field demonstration and training centre in the region.

The project made orderly progress in obtaining base-line data relating to several factors that enter into the transmission dynamics of schistosomiasis. Future changes in transmission potential of S. haematobium and S. mansoni infections in man and fascioliasis in cattle could be measured from the established base-lines [FAROOQ and NIELSEN, 1966; FAROOQ et al., 1966a, b; FAROOQ and HAIRSTON, 1966].

Preliminary field screening and field trials of a number of promising molluscicides[3] and herbicides[4] have led to the determination of the most suitable formulations, their appropriate annual cycle and methods of application [UNRAU et al., 1965; DAWOOD et al., 1965a, b]. Large-scale trials with sodium pentachlorophenate and niclosamide, for purposes of evaluation of their effects on transmission of schistosomiasis and fascioliasis, have been under-

3   Aqualin; niclosamide; NaPCP; different formulations of ICI 24223 and WL 8008.
4   2,4-D-Amine; Weedazole-TL; Gramozone, Reglone, Dowpon & Gramevin.

taken. Data have been obtained to indicate that two suitably timed applications of NaPCP or niclosamide could control snails and transmission at a reasonable cost in the area [DAWOOD et al., 1966].

Niclosamide is regarded as the molluscicide of choice. Its application has been extended to cover the whole operational zone of the project, providing protection for a population of 183,000 in 425 villages, in an area of 322 km².

In July 1965 scrutiny of the data on the incidence and prevalence of schistosomiasis in children under 7 years of age from two sections, Kom Ishu and Kom el Birka (area of 51.9 km² and a population of 15,396 living in 80 villages) where molluscicides have been applied since May 1963, in comparison with the data from the reference area (Akrisha Section) where no control measures were taken, showed that reduction of transmission of S. haematobium and S. mansoni has resulted from the snail control programme. This was considered to be the first scientifically acceptable demonstration of reduction of schistosomiasis in the Nile Valley or Delta [FAROOQ et al., 1966]. A significant concomitant fall in the prevalence of fascioliasis among livestock has also been demonstrated in the same area.

Careful ecological studies over a three-year period indicated the necessary rhythm of application of molluscicides, and evidence was obtained showing that one mass application during April and May followed by a system of continuous inspection and local treatment during the rest of the year, should prove effective and economical [DAZO et al., 1966].

Israel

The Anti-Malaria Department of the Ministry of Public Health is also concerned with the problem of schistosomiasis in Israel. It deals with the possible breeding places of snails in natural and artificial water sources (fish ponds, water reservoirs and pools) by clearing vegetation and using molluscicides, and also undertakes public health education to avoid infection by bathing in infected water. Screening and treatment of immigrants is provided as a routine measure of control.

Changes in epidemiological factors may occur in the future and the possibility of the spread of infection may increase, calling for precautionary measures especially in relation to water utilization and conservation [WITENBERG and SALITERNIK, 1957].

In view of the above, studies were undertaken in the country and the following measures were recommended:

(1) Constant surveillance of all waters with which people come into contact. Every new case of schistosomiasis should be notified and immediately given a full course of treatment.

(2) Constant supervision of fish ponds by competent personnel should be compulsory and all workers subjected to periodical helminthological examination.

(3) All bathing places should be supervised by public health staff. If intermediate hosts are discovered in a site used for bathing, aquatic vegetation should be removed and copper sulphate applied. All known *Bulinus* breeding places which may possibly be used for bathing should be marked and provided with signs warning of the danger of bathing, or stating that bathing is forbidden.

(4) Systematic removal of plants favouring the establishment and mass breeding of intermediate hosts should be organized. Frequent periodic drying by rapid emptying of reservoirs, canals and ditches should be practised whenever possible. Routine control of *Bulinus* snails by chemicals should be carried out only in limited foci such as bathing places, fish ponds and storage reservoirs.

(5) Water for filling pools should be drawn from sources free from *Bulinus* snails. Constructional adjustments in natural and artificial streams, in order to ensure a velocity of at least 20 cm per second, are desirable.

(6) Domestic sewage must not be introduced into natural watercourses or artificial pools without proper treatment ensuring freedom from viable eggs of schistosomes.

(7) Obligatory instruction on the bionomics of intermediate hosts, the mode of infection with schistosomiasis and its prevention should be included in the curriculum of all schools.

As a result of the timely study of the problem and intensive precautionary measures taken, Israel represents one of the very few countries in which schistosomiasis is definitely on the wane.

Rhodesia

Initial Programmes
The first planned programme of snail control was undertaken in the Mazoe Valley in 1951 as a combined operation with an experiment in malaria control. All water bodies in the valley were treated with copper sulphate. Although surveys indicated that the operations had greatly reduced the snail populations the programme was abandoned. During the years 1952–54, snail

control was limited to the repeated spraying of stream and river crossings and watering and washing points in certain African Reserve areas. Lack of technical personnel prevented adequate assessment of this control effort.

In 1953, an attempt at total elimination of snails from a whole river catchment was made in the Mtoko African Reserve. The whole river system was given two successive treatments with a six-week interval, applying copper sulphate to give a final concentration of 20 to 30 ppm. This project was designed to last for one year only and it was found that reinfestation of the area was slow. Most subsequent control schemes were based on the experience gained from this control experiment.

Sodium pentachlorophenate was used for the first time on a large scale in 1955, when it was applied to the artificial lake that serves as the source of the Salisbury water supply. It was heavily populated with *Bulinus (Physopsis) globosus* and *Biomphalaria pfeifferi*, which proved to have infection rates of 5 to 10%. The molluscicide was applied around the entire 68 km periphery to give a final concentration of 10 ppm in the shallow water. The treatment greatly reduced the snails and reinfestation was slow, in spite of heavy populations in the untreated tributaries. This control scheme was subsequently abandoned in favour of focal spraying of the picnic and boating sites most frequented by the public, a form of control which was reported to be effective in limiting the number of infected snails in the lake.

During the post-war period much attention had been given to soil and water conservation in the rural areas, and a programme of dam building had been initiated in the country. The rural European-owned areas had been divided, according to river catchments, into Intensive Conservation Areas (ICA) each including 80 to 100 farms and each with a local committee which was responsible for superintending the local conservation programme. By 1955 most of the farms in the country had one or more ponds, which resulted in a marked increase in snail populations throughout the country. A widespread increase of fascioliasis in cattle was associated with the increase in snail populations. The latter resulted in enough uneasiness among the farmers to create an interest in snail control. It was early realized that the co-operation elicited from these Intensive Conservation Area committees, having the full support of the farmers, would be invaluable to a schistosomiasis control programme.

Long-Term Snail Control

In 1957, the Sokis ICA and certain ICAs in the Sinoia area decided to attempt snail control entirely at their own expense but with technical supervision from the Ministry of Health. Surveys to assess the snail populations were undertaken and the spraying teams for each area were given brief training in the application of copper sulphate, the only molluscicide used. In the Sokis ICA, the river systems were sprayed methodically, catchment by catchment, with a second application following four to six weeks after the first. Excellent results were obtained and only isolated, small foci of snails persisted.

The results achieved by the Sokis ICA were rather unfortunately given wide publicity and many other ICAs in the country, attracted mainly by the opportunity of controlling fascioliasis in domestic stock, undertook snail control programmes. Too few trained technicians were available for the supervision of these efforts. In some areas control was spectacular, in others there was little effect on the snail populations. The majority of these ICAs used copper sulphate but in two, totalling some 2,000 km², sodium pentachlorophenate was applied under strict supervision of the Ministry of Health, and in both areas the results were satisfactory.

The varied results led to the conclusion that a successful programme could be realized only by co-ordination and with adequate supervision. In 1958, the Ministry of Health selected four areas, including 22 ICAs and 9 African Reserves totalling approximately 20,000 km² for a co-ordinated malaria and snail control programme. This was to be supervised by the Malaria and Bilharziasis Research Laboratory (MBRL) staff.

In each area brought into the new programme the control activity included a 'blanket' application of molluscicide in all manageable bodies of water, 'selective' application in habitats found infested and 'surveillance' with application in habitats found infested. The last of these was simply a long-term follow-up on the first two phases.

The Government supplied the molluscicide for the African Reserves and for the ICAs in the third phase.

As it became practical, it was hoped that the areas under control could be extended in a logical sequence.

In 1961, the Government requested the WHO Bilharziasis Advisory Team to make a complete assessment of the control and research programme on schistosomiasis. A review was made of the epidemiological situation regarding prevalence and importance of schistosomiasis (*S.haematobium* and *S. mansoni*) and other trematode diseases (*Fasciola gigantica*, *S.matheei* and paramphistomes). Types of habitats of the snail hosts involved were classified, and their relation to transmission was assessed.

The control programme of the Ministry of Health consisted of two main parts, chemotherapy and snail control. The Malaria and Bilharziasis Research

Laboratory (MBRL) which became the Bilharziasis Laboratory about this time, was responsible for the latter.

During 1960–61 the Ministry of Health supplied enough lucanthone hydrochloride to treat 32,000 persons. It was expected that in the following years farmers, business organizations and the Ministry of Health would distribute enough of this drug to treat 500,000 persons and it was estimated that the cost of the latter amount of drug would be approximately £100,000 or an average of four shillings per person. The use of this drug was directed against *S. haematobium* only and it was not correlated with the snail control programme carried out in four specific areas. Cure rates mentioned, ranged from 50 to 70% in those who completed the course. These are higher cure rates than reported in Egypt and authorities in Rhodesia ascribe this to greater susceptibility of the local parasite to the drug. The clinical aspects of this programme and its effect on the infections have not really been assessed.

Bilharziasis Research Laboratory (BRL)

This organization is directly responsible to the Ministry of Health. Its effectiveness in the control programme is correlated with its ability to obtain co-operation from the other agencies. In 1961, the staff of MBRL consisted of 122 full-time technical personnel. The annual budget from the Ministry of Health was £14,600, exclusive of salaries for the technical personnel. In addition, the schistosomiasis control effort has been subsidized to a point where the average spent annually on snail control was about £30,000, not including the salaries of the technical personnel.

During the early stages of the programme, an attempt was made to conserve molluscicides by applying them during dry periods when water levels in the habitats were low. It was found later that snails aestivating above the water level soon repopulated the habitats. While the application of molluscicides during the rainy season appeared to give better snail control, data were not available on snail population dynamics and the infection rates at the time the assessment was made.

Cost Estimates

An estimate was made of the cost of the control programme in the Chikwanda and Zimutu Reserves, of the Kyle catchment, based on prevalence surveys made in 1960 and again in 1962 following two years of snail operations.

While the previous information may give some idea of the methods and costs, it does not indicate how much schistosomiasis and fascioliasis transmission has been curtailed by these expenditures. In regard to fascioliasis, none of the data available in the central government agencies was of value in making such an assessment.

The Bilharziasis Advisory Team revisited Rhodesia in 1963 and made the following observations:

'The programme has achieved an excellent balance between control and research activity and the latter is being used effectively to improve the control effort. This close integration of the two activities is unusual and its effectiveness has demonstrated the wisdom of those who have provided for it.

Another noteworthy feature of the programme is that the Bilharziasis Research Laboratory has established a close and effective working relationship with other agencies having an interest, or delegated responsibility, relating to the bilharziasis problem...

Destruction of the host snail seems to be the best means for control of the disease in Rhodesia at present. Bayluscide is a favourable chemical to use. Better dispersal would be desirable, and this may eventually be achieved by improvement in dispensing technique and by better formulation of the chemical by the manufacturer.'

Sudan

Schistosomiasis is fairly widespread in Sudan but because of the economic importance of the area, control of infection has been concentrated in the Gezira, Blue Nile Province, where nearly 2,000,000 feddans are irrigated from the Sennar reservoir, created by the damming of the Blue Nile about 250 km above its confluence with the White Nile. It has a stable population of about 500,000 and a migrant population of 200,000. Relatively little has been done in other parts of the country.

Early Work in the Gezira

Work in the Gezira has attracted considerable attention; for this reason, it would be well to mention the sequence of events. HUMPHREYS [1932] reported that *S. haematobium* had been found in the general area of the Gezira before 1925, the year when the gravity irrigation system went into use; it had been recognized that the installation of this system would probably cause an increase in the prevalence of schistosomiasis in the area. As a result, an attempt was made to examine tenants going into the area, to site villages away from the canals, to provide water supplies, etc. By 1927, *Bulinus* had been found in six canals and, by 1928, both *Bulinus* and *Biomphalaria* were found throughout the irrigation system. In spite of this it was reported that the prevalence of schistosomiasis was low [HUMPHREYS, 1932]. STEPHENSON [1947] reported that *S. haematobium* was common and that *S. mansoni* had been in the area since about 1940; he concluded that the efforts to control these parasites had been ineffective. In a survey of 15 villages he found 45% of the children infected with *S. haematobium*. A general survey of the snails in the area was started in 1946 and completed the following year. It was during this period that CuSO₄ was first used in the area as a molluscicide. It was effective but it was found that canals treated with the compound became repopulated in about three months.

By 1949, a survey had been completed and it was found that 27.5% of the population had schistosomiasis (both types reported together). In 1950–51, 10 of the 44 blocks in the irrigated area were selected for the intensive study of control methods. One of the first experiments was to compare the results obtained from 10 villages where chemotherapy alone was used, with 13 villages where this and snail control had been used. After one year it was found that there had been no change in prevalence in the first group of villages, whereas it had shown a marked decrease in the latter. These results led to a variety of experiments on ways to improve snail control methods. CSuO₄ was applied in different ways but rapid repopulation of the ditches invariably made its use too costly. CuCO₃ was found to be ineffective. The high cost of repeated applications of CuSO₄ at 30 ppm led to experiments with the continuous application of small concentrations. Experiments using 0.5 and 1.0 ppm were started in 1951–52. It was noted that these concentrations not only controlled the snails, but they also had some effect on the weeds. It was during this period that it was thought that weed and snail control might be combined. During the following year initial experiments were made with the continuous application of 2 ppm after 30 ppm had been used. The schistosomiasis control personnel found this too expensive as a control measure and changed to 0.125 ppm in August 1953. It was about this time that the concept of the action of continuous application began to alter. Originally it was thought that the molluscicide was effective only when it circulated through the system. Later the idea developed that the application of 0.125 ppm actually produced a barrier of a stronger concentration near the point of introduction. However, there was a mixture of the two concepts over a period of years in the Annual Reports and in published material. The Irrigation Department personnel made further tests with the higher concentration for weed control in 1954 and concluded that the method was too expensive.

In 18 villages where control measures had been carried out for two years it was reported that the prevalence of *S. mansoni* had dropped from 20.3 to 12.2%, and then to 7.9%. During the same period *S. haematobium* dropped from 13.1 to 2.4%, and finally to 2.3%. In a further analysis of the effect of snail control with 30 ppm CuSO₄ applied twice a year, the data show that in

1951–52, one year after control had been started, the prevalence had dropped to 15.7%; in 1952–53 it was 12%; in 1953–54 it was 10%, and in 1954–55 it was 8%.

Extension of Programme

In September 1954, a WHO team visited the area and suggested that the newly-devised snail control techniques be extended to the entire irrigation system. Before the molluscicide was applied, 18,923 people from 58 villages were examined. The initial application of 30 ppm $CuSO_4$ was started in the major canals and their branches in November 1955 and it was completed before the summer closure began in April 1956. During the early part of the closure period, the main canal and the small amount of water left behind the dam were also treated. Chemical 'barriers' were placed a short distance above the regulator at the head of each major canal. At first, some difficulty was experienced with the mechanical barrier placed at 50 km on the main canal. By 1957–58 an improved design was working well and records were kept on the number of snails caught by the screens.

Mechanical and Chemical Barrier in Managil Extension

In 1957–58, 12,041 persons in the phase I area of the Managil Extension of the Gezira were examined for schistosomiasis to obtain basic data before the new canal system went into operation in 1958. It was found that 6.2% were infected. At the time when the water was turned into the Managil Extension for phase I, mechanical and chemical barriers were placed across the branch from the main canal. Surveillance was maintained throughout the canal system and, if snail colonies appeared, local applications of $CuSO_4$ were made. It was hoped that this method of control would make it unnecessary to treat the entire system with 30 ppm and maintain a 0.125-ppm continuous application of $CuSO_4$.

Evaluation

During the early phase of the control programme the villages surveyed to determine prevalence and those examined for annual evaluation were not always the same and the data are, therefore, not comparable. However, a highly significant fall both in *S. haematobium* and *S. mansoni* infection rates during the first two years of the campaign in the 10 blocks was reported. It should be noted that (in addition to sulphation, 30 ppm along all canals) six mobile teams, 10 dispensaries and 10 dressing stations, carried out intensive treatment of all infected individuals in the area during the period.

A considerable reduction of *S. haematobium* prevalence has been reported. A lesser but significant decrease in *S. mansoni* also occurred within a year. These changes have been brought about by the intensive treatment programme, rather than by an interruption of transmission.

Schistosoma japonicum

China (Mainland)

FAUST and MELENEY [1924] were the first to conduct extensive investigations on schistosomiasis in China. They believed that the problem of control was infinitely more complex than in Japan or in Egypt. The major transmission occurred in children who were exposed while working in rice nursery beds. Another potent source of infection was the small terminal canals and irrigation ditches which were frequently at, or near, the entrance of human habitations. FAUST and MELENEY did not think that the employment of copper sulphate as recommended by CHANDLER [1920] would constitute an effective snail control method. They suggested research on biological control. It was thought unwise to place absolute dependence on therapeutic measures, although therapy could be used to considerable advantage. A general education programme and pilot control projects were suggested.

Present-Day Programme

No concerted efforts were undertaken against schistosomiasis in China until recent years. The problem of control was revived under the new regime, and an ambitious national programme was started in 1956 under the auspices of the Chinese National Research Council on Schistosomiasis, with the objective of 'liquidating' schistosomiasis in the country in 'seven to twelve years' [MAO, 1958].

A medical delegation of Japanese workers led by KOMIYA visited China in the winter of 1956, to advise and assist the Chinese Government in their efforts to eradicate schistosomiasis [KOMIYA, 1957]. The following measures were under consideration by the Chinese Government at the time:

(1) night soil control;

(2) mass treatment of humans and draft animals with tartar emetic;

(3) further research into the value of traditional Chinese remedies;

(4) snail control by application of heat or chemicals; and

(5) environmental control through burial of snails, cementing ditches and reclamation of marshy areas.

The Japanese delegation, however, noted that snail control was less stressed than mass treatment and that emphasis was laid on developing old Chinese herbs as remedies and as molluscicides.

A group of British doctors who, on the invitation of the Chinese Medical Association, visited China during the summer of 1957, noted that there were 70,000 people at work on a campaign to control schistosomiasis, mainly by destroying the snail host using small flame-throwers to burn the banks of the canals. The campaign was assisted by voluntary efforts of many villagers, and even the children were said to be picking up the snails with chop-sticks [JONES, 1957].

Professor MAEGRAITH, who visited China in 1958, reported that the following methods and techniques are being utilized in control:

Faeces and Schistosome Eggs

Emphasis is being laid on controlling promiscuous defaecation and by storage of faeces for up to a week before use in the fields, in order to allow the ammonia generated to destroy the ova; the major problem, however, is the spread of infection by the faeces of domestic animal hosts.

Control of Snails and Cercariae

Mixtures containing Tung oil are used in the field in the form of repeated applications to exposed areas of skin. The molluscicidal action of many substances in the form of solutions, emulsions and powders has been studied. Nearly 600 Chinese herbs have been tested, of which fewer than 20 have any appreciable molluscicidal effect in concentrations of 1% or lower. Infusions and oil emulsions of croton have been proved successful under laboratory conditions but considerably less so in the field. So far no indigenous substance has been found economically satisfactory for use on a large scale.

The burning of grass on the banks of small creeks and ditches is carried out by means of portable petrol flame-throwers. The banks of larger canals and streams are scorched by flame-throwers mounted on punts, and burning carbon-monoxide gas made on the spot. Snails covered with mud escape the action of heat and molluscicides. However, they will not survive if buried to a depth greater than 10 cm. During the winter months, farmers are encouraged to remove and bury snail-containing mud of ditches and irrigation channels. The technique is considered highly efficient, 71% of the snails are said to die within a month and 98% within three months.

Other physical methods of control which have proved valuable in appropriate areas are reclamation of low or flood land by the erection of embankments and the subsequent removal of the overgrowing grass, and in some cases the conversion of reclaimed rice fields for the growth or other crops. Data are not yet available for an evaluation of the programme in China.

Japan

Development of Molluscicides and their Use

The concept of snail control as a method for preventing schistosomiasis was an early development in Japan. NARABAYASHI recommended the use of lime as a molluscicide in 1915. It was initially used in Hiroshima Prefecture in 1918 and extended to Yamanashi Prefecture in 1924. In Hiroshima Prefecture, it was applied annually until 1947, except during the years 1930–36. In Yamanashi, it was applied only once every three years. No records were kept of the effect on the snail population.

MIYAGAWA [1916] demonstrated that calcium cyanamide was molluscicidal; it was used in the field by FUJINAMI and SUEYASU [1919] and its use extended to the endemic areas of Yamanashi, Hiroshima, Saga, Fukuoka, and Chiba Prefectures. The molluscicide was usually applied once a year from April to June. Sometimes the application was repeated in October. Before each application, a snail survey was made in the irrigation ditches to be tested. Records of the effect of these applications were not kept. However, recent experience indicates that the compound and the method of application were not as effective as had been supposed.

Beginning in 1947, in co-operation with the National Institute of Health and the Yamanashi Medical Research Institute, the 406th Medical General Laboratory of the United States Army conducted a series of laboratory and field investigations to develop more effective molluscicides applicable to conditions in Japan. In this programme, MCMULLEN *et al.* [1948] found promising chemicals that were superior to copper sulphate: sodium pentachlorophenate, dinitro-*o*-cyclohexylphenol and its dicyclohexylamine salt.

Later a series of applications of sodium pentachlorophenate and the dinitro compounds were applied on a large scale in Yamanashi Prefecture. At the dosages used, the three chemicals gave similar results but the first two were much less expensive. These two chemicals cost about one half as much as calcium cyanamide. The area treated, more than 29 km of ditches, offered a wide variety of habitats. The molluscicides were least effective in areas where the sides of the ditches had loose rock walls. The reduction in the snail population averaged 81.7% in areas treated in October. When treated in the spring, the average reduction was 87.7%. When the molluscicides were applied in the autumn and the spring, the reduction averaged 95.4%. Surveys conducted the following autumn showed that a few young snails were present in some of the areas.

The project known as 'Operation Santobrite' was begun in the spring of 1950 [HUNTER et al., 1952]. This project was to serve as a basis for determining whether molluscicides were effective and practical for a control programme. A community somewhat isolated by barriers was selected for this purpose in Fukuoka Prefecture on the Island of Kyushu. It supported a population of 1,050 persons on 0.6 km² enclosed by dykes. Sodium pentachlorophenate was applied, during both spring and autumn of 1950 and 1951, to 19 km of ditch comprising the entire irrigation system of the 0.6 km² area of Nagatoishi. The initial application reduced the snails by 98.1%. The residual population apparently had a high reproduction potential since there was considerable repopulation by the end of the first summer. The autumn application in 1950 was apparently less effective than the spring one but snail counts the following spring indicated that there had been a residual effect which augmented the results secured in the autumn.

In the spring of 1951, the pre-treatment snail count was low and some repopulation occurred during the summer, but this was considerably less than during 1950. The fourth application reduced the population by 99%.

When the efficacy of NaPCP as a molluscicide had thus been established, the prefectural authorities gradually adopted this compound in place of calcium cyanamide. This change was first made by Saga Prefecture in 1952 and then followed by Yamanashi, Fukuoka and Hiroshima Prefectures in 1954.

At the termination of the two-year experiment in Nagatoishi in Fukuoka in December 1951, it was realized that the snails had not been completely eliminated from the paddies and irrigation ditches. Certainly, virtual control had been achieved, and apparently there was little, if any, transmission of schistosomiasis taking place in the treated area. Follow-up surveys showed, however, that pockets of viable snails remained and that they would have to be sought out and destroyed. This in itself constituted a challenge, which was readily accepted by the villagers themselves as well as by the public health officials in Kurume-shi and in Fukuoka and Saga Prefectures.

Cementing of Irrigation Ditches

Cementing of irrigation ditches has been carried out in Japan from before the First World War. A 10-year programme was planned and by 1960 approximately one-third of all ditches had been so converted.

Some idea of costs involved in the programme can be obtained from Fukuoka Prefecture, where it was proposed to cement 411,195 m of canal at a total cost of 793,724,000 yen ($2,204,855). The total population protected in this area is 51,621 and the cost *per capita* will be approximately $42.

In justifying the heavy *per capita* cost involved, it is believed in Japan that there are other gains besides schistosomiasis control from such a programme. These are given as: conservation of water, ease in water control, saving in labour involved, extra land released for cultivation due to the small area taken by concrete channels, and increased food production and land revenue from extra lands cultivated. Because of the high price of arable land in Japan any procedure that reclaims land for cultivation receives high priority.

Present Status of Control

It is believed that once transmission of schistosomiasis is reduced to a minimum, then treatment of domestic animals and the human population with drugs becomes mandatory and should result in the virtual elimination of autochthonous cases. One such programme has been in progress in the endemic area along the Chikugo River (Amaki City and Miwa-Mura) of Fukuoka Prefecture since 1953. It consists mainly of antimony injections following mass stool surveys.

The final results of this particular control programme conducted in a group of villages in the endemic area in Fukuoka Prefecture under the auspices of the Kurume University School of Medicine, and the final conclusions reached from these studies indicate that, even with the problem being reduced to a state of residual infection, Japanese workers hope for complete eradication.

Relentless chemical attack on the molluscan host, coupled with environmental changes (elimination of swampy river beds through construction of levees and embankments, reclamation and intensive cultivation of land, and construction of cement-lined irrigation ditches) and the treatment of residual cases, have reduced the distribution of schistosomiasis during the past 50 years to a few residual foci of infection in Japan. That the disease has ceased to be a major public health problem in the country is evidenced by the fact that annual deaths ascribed to this infection (under 100 a year) in 1957 were less than one tenth of the number caused by ascariasis. The infection, therefore, now appears well on its way to ultimate elimination from the country.

Philippines

Initial Work

TUBANGUI's discovery of the intermediate host of schistosomiasis, *Oncomelania quadrasi*, in 1932 in Palo, Leyte, marked the beginning of the fight against the disease in the Philippines. AFRICA and GARCIA, following their reconnaissance of the problem in the Philippines in 1935, drew pointed attention to the need for better understanding and control of the disease. Three small field units of the Bureau of Health conducted systematic surveys of the Islands of Mindanao, Leyte and Mindoro during 1940–41. They started treatment of the cases found, using intramuscular Fuadin, and attempted snail control by use of unslaked lime and fire. AFRICA, TUBANGUI and their associates continued research on the parasite and on treatment until war broke out in the Philippines in 1941, bringing all progress to a standstill.

Paradoxically, the war brought the problem of schistosomiasis to the fore as a result of an epidemic among the US forces in Leyte in 1944 and 1945, and among a unit of the Australian Air Force also in 1945. As a result of this experience, an effort was made to study all the aspects of the disease which had a bearing on the military operations. Studies were conducted by a number of US Army units, including hospitals, malaria control, survey and research units, and the Commission of Schistosomiasis was organized early in 1945 by the US Army Epidemiological Board.

The activities of the various units covered the clinical and pathological aspects of the disease in a group of individuals who previously had never been exposed to the disease. These studies presented data which were in many respects unique because of the large numbers of individuals in this category.

Because of the extension of military operations to other islands, surveys were made of the distribution of schistosomiasis on Samar, Mindoro and Mindanao. Some additional foci were found on Samar as well as on Leyte, and new foci were discovered in widely-separated areas in Mindanao.

Experiments were conducted on protective ointments which could be applied to the skin to prevent the introduction of cercariae, and methods were devised for the impregnation of uniform cloth as a protection against infection. It was found also that certain cloth such as woollen serge uniform material, itself constituted a good mechanical barrier against the entrance of cercariae.

As certain military personnel had developed schistosomiasis after bathing in Leyte Gulf at the mouth of a river, studies were conducted on the effect of sea-water on schistosome cercariae. The effect of chlorine and chloramine on cercariae was also studied as a practical means for the treatment of drinking water.

Initial studies of considerable value were inaugurated on the biology and ecology of *O. quadrasi*, the molluscan intermediate host. Field tests were also conducted in an effort to develop new molluscicides which might be more effective than copper sulphate.

Post-War Surveys and Control Programme

PESIGAN [1948a, b] found new endemic centres in Mindanao and Luzon (Sorsogon) in 1947. Six field units were organized in 1949–50 under the auspices of the research programme established in the Department of Health, which undertook extensive surveys on human prevalence, snail distribution, treatment of patients, an educational programme, and snail control in the endemic areas.

Establishment of the Division of Schistosomiasis and WHO-Assisted Pilot Project in Palo, Leyte

Following these surveys, the importance of the problem of schistosomiasis in the Philippines came to be recognized and the Philippine Government created the Division of Schistosomiasis in the Department of Health in 1951. At the request of the Government, the World Health Organization sent a team of consultants to the Philippines in 1952. The terms of reference of this team were: (1) to study the schistosomiasis problem in the Philippine Islands; (2) to examine the control work that was being done; and (3) to make recommendations for a national programme.

This team, after a careful study of the situation felt that the disease problem had so far been approached almost entirely from a medical viewpoint, which was but a small segment of the whole. In order to control schistosomiasis it was concluded that it was necessary to get basic information on the biology of the intermediate host and the use of engineering and agricultural measures to control it. It was also considered that thinly-spread efforts to deal with the disease would be more or less unrewarding. The team, therefore, recommended the concentration of funds and efforts on a pilot project, with the World Health Organization providing three advisors for the programme and the Division of Schistosomiasis supplying opposite numbers, technicians, assistants and labourers. The main objectives were to make thorough epidemiological and ecological studies, and to evaluate control measures. The team suggested that parts of eastern Leyte, which appeared to be the most important endemic area, should be used for a pilot project of six years' duration.

The Philippine Government and WHO acted quickly on the recommendations and initiated a control project in Palo, Leyte. Assistance was also
received from the Foreign Operations Administration of the USA in the form
of supplies and from the Philippine Council for United States Aid. A project-
centre building, including laboratories, was constructed, equipped and staffed
and the project officially started functioning in June 1953 [PESIGAN et al.,
1958a, b, c; PESIGAN and HAIRSTON, 1961].

Achievement of the Pilot Project in Leyte

This project remained operative, with WHO assistance and to which
FAO and UNICEF also extended support in its final stages, until 1963, when
the responsibility for it was assumed by the Government. This has been considered as one of the two most successful WHO-assisted schistosomiasis
control pilot projects, with its defined objectives fulfilled to a considerable
extent. Detailed knowledge was obtained on the entire spectrum of epidemiological factors and ecological processes involved in the transmission dynamics
of S. japonicum infection. An effective methodology, including water management practices, drainage and reclamation of swamplands, stream channelling
and ponding for pisciculture was demonstrated [HAIRSTON and SANTOS, 1961].
Improved crop yields and economic gains of the recommended programme
were shown to offset the initial expenses involved, resulting in permanent
benefit to the community in increased health and prosperity. It was considered
that the application of molluscicides to residual colonies of snails in the wet
environment of the Philippines would be feasible and economical only after
the initial land improvements were made.

Effectiveness of the programme in controlling transmission and its economic feasibility have been demonstrated and a national programme, which
would control schistosomiasis at reasonable cost, has been suggested.

Integration and Establishment
of Regional Advisory Teams

Towards the end of the period of WHO sponsorship of the project it was
decided to make schistosomiasis control one of the functions of the rural
health units in the Philippines. Each team consisted essentially of a medical
officer parasitologist, a malacologist, an engineer and supporting personnel
which usually included technicians, a surveyor, a draughtsman and drivers.

These regional teams have not been active long enough to permit a definitive judgement as to their usefulness or their accomplishments since, of
necessity, they have had to move slowly.

References

AFRICA, C. M. and GARCIA, E. Y.: Philipp. J. publ. Hlth 2: 54 (1935).

ANSARI, N.: Unpublished report (1958).

AYAD, N.: Bull. Wld Hlth Org. 25: 712 (1961).

BARLOW, C. H.: Amer. J. Hyg. 25: 327 (1937).

CHADWICK, C. R.: in MILLS, MACHATTIE, and CHADWICK, Trans, roy. Soc. trop. Med. Hyg. 30: 317 (1936).

CHANDLER, A. C.: J. agric. Res. 20: 193 (1920).

CHRISTOPHERSON, J. B.: Lancet ii: 325; Brit. med. J. ii: 652 (1918).

DAWOOD, I. K.; DAZO, B. C., and FAROOQ, M.: Bull. Wld Hlth Org. 35: 357 (1966).

DAWOOD, I. K.; FAROOQ, M.; UNRAU, G. O.; MIGUEL, L. C., and DAZO, B. C.: Bull. Wld Hlth Org. 32: 261 (1965a).

DAWOOD, I. K.; FAROOQ, M.; DAZO, B. C.; MIGUEL, L. C., and UNRAU, G. O.: Bull. Wld Hlth Org. 32: 269 (1965b).

DAZO, B. C.; HAIRSTON, N. G., and DAWOOD, I. K.: Bull. Wld Hlth Org. 35: 339 (1966).

FAROOQ, M.: Ann. trop. Med. Parasit. 57: 323 (1963).

FAROOQ, M.: Chron. Wld Hlth Org. 21: 175 (1967).

FAROOQ, M.: Report on the schistosomiasis control project in Iran, 3 September–10 October 1968. WHO unpublished document EM/SCHIS./44 (1968).

FAROOQ, M. and HAIRSTON, N. G.: Bull. Wld Hlth Org. 35: 331 (1966).

FAROOQ, M. and NIELSEN, J.: Bull. Wld Hlth Org. 35: 281 (1966).

FAROOQ, M.; HAIRSTON, N. G., and SAMAAN, S. A.: Bull. Wld Hlth Org. 35: 369 (1966).

FAROOQ, M.; NIELSEN, J.; SAMAAN, S. A.; MALLAH, M. B., and ALLAM, A. A.: Bull. Wld Hlth Org. 35: 293 (1966a).

FAROOQ, M.; NIELSEN, J.; SAMAAN, S. A.; MALLAH, M. B., and ALLAM, A. A.: Bull. Wld Hlth Org. 35: 319 (1966b).

FAUST, E. C. and MELENEY, H. E.: Amer. J. Hyg., Monog. Ser. 3: 1–268 (1924).

FUJINAMI, A. and SUEYASU, Y.: Nishin Igaku (Jap. J. med. Progr.) 9: 433 (1919).

GAUD, J. and OLIVIER, L. J.: Report on bilharziasis in Iran, with special reference to Khuzistan development plans, 11 November 1958–5 January 1959. WHO unpublished document, EM/BIL./10 (1959).

HAIRSTON, N. G. and SANTOS, B. C.: Bull. Wld Hlth Org. 25: 603 (1961).

HALAWANI, A.: J. Egypt. publ. Hlth Ass. 32: 123 (1957).

HALL, A. H.: J. roy. Army med. Cps 44: 1, 92 (1925).

HUMPHREYS, R. M.: Trans. roy. Soc. trop. Med. Hyg. 26: 241 (1932).

HUNTER, G. W., III; FREYTAG, R. E.; RITCHIE, L. S.; PAN, C.; YOKAGAWA, M., and POTTS, D. E.: Amer. J. trop. Med. Hyg. 1: 831 (1952).

JONES, F. A.: Brit. med. J. ii: 1105 (1957).

KHALIL, M.: Rep. Notes publ. Hlth Lab., Cairo 6: 159 (1924).

KHALIL, M.: J. Egypt. med. Ass. 10: 791 (1927).

KOMIYA, Y.: Jap. J. med. Sci. Biol. 10: 461 (1957).

LEIPER, R. T.: J. roy. Army med. Cps 25: 1, 26: 147, 253 (1915).

MAEGRAITH, B.: Lancet i: 208 (1958).

MAO, C. P.: Amer. J. trop. Med. Hyg. 7: 58 (1958).

MCMULLEN, D. B.; ISHII, N., and MITOMA, Y.: J. Parasit. 34: suppl., p. 33 (1948).

MIYAGAWA, Y.: Mitt. med. Fak. Univ. Tokyo *15:* 453 (1916).

NARABAYASHI, H.: Chugai Iji Shimpo (Int. med. J.) *855:* 1381 (1915).

OLIVER-GONZALEZ, J. and FERGUSON, F.F.: Amer. J. trop. Med. Hyg. *8:* 56 (1959).

OLIVER-GONZALEZ, J.; BIAGGI, N.; ACEVEDO, C.; MARIOTTA, D.A.; MORALES, F.H.; STEVENSON. D.S., and PÉREZ SANTIAGO, E.: Puerto Rico J. publ. Hlth *25:* 387 (1950).

PESIGAN, T.P.: J. Philipp. med. Ass. *23:* 23 (1948a).

PESIGAN, T.P.: J. Philipp. med. Ass. *24:* 19 (1948b).

PESIGAN, T.P. and HAIRSTON, N.G.: Bull. Wld Hlth Org. *25:* 479 (1961).

PESIGAN, T.P.; FAROOQ, M.; HAIRSTON, N.G.; JAUREGUI, J.J.; GARCIA, E.G.; SANTOS, A.T.; SANTOS, B.C., and BESA, A.A.: Bull. Wld Hlth Org. *18:* 345 (1958a).

PESIGAN, T.P.; HAIRSTON, N.G.; JAUREGUI, J.J.; GARCIA, E.G.; SANTOS, A.T.; SANTOS, B.C., and BESA, A.A.: Bull. Wld Hlth Org. *18:* 481 (1958b).

PESIGAN, T.P.; FAROOQ, M.; HAIRSTON, N.G.; JAUREGUI, J.J.; GARCIA, E.G.; SANTOS, A.T.; SANTOS, B.C., and BESA, A.A.: Bull. Wld Hlth Org. *19:* 223 (1958c).

SCHALIE, H. VAN DER: Bull. Wld Hlth Org. *19:* 263 (1958).

SCOTT, J.A.: Amer. J. Hyg. *25:* 566 (1937).

SCOTT, J.A. and BARLOW, C.H.: Amer. J. Hyg. *27:* 619 (1938).

SHOUSHA, A.T.: Bull. Wld Hlth Org. *2:* 19 (1949).

STEPHENSON, R.W.: Trans. roy. Soc. trop. Med. Hyg. *40:* 479 (1947).

TUBANGUI, M.A.: Philipp. J. Sci. *49:* 295 (1932).

UNRAU, G.O.; FAROOQ, M.; DAWOOD, I.K.; MIGUEL, L.C., and DAZO, B.C.: Bull. Wld Hlth Org. *32:* 249 (1965).

WATSON, J.M.: J. Fac. Med. Iraq *12:* 120 (1948).

WITENBERG, G. and SALITERNIK, Z.: Bull. Res. Coun. Israel B *6:* 107 (1957).

WRIGHT, W.H.; DOBROVOLNY, C.C., and BERRY, E.G.: Bull. Wld Hlth Org. *18:* 963 (1958).

Chapter 8

Epidemiology and Control of Schistosomiasis, pp. 422–437
(Karger, Basel and University Park Press, Baltimore 1973)

General Considerations in the Control of Schistosomiasis

M. FAROOQ

Introduction

Schistosomiasis is an insidious and chronic disease lacking the drama usually associated with some fulminating infections prevalent in tropical and sub-tropical countries. The parasite in long association with man relies on co-existence rather than the elimination of the host, and this results in chronic debility with underestimated overt morbidity and mortality; but the damage done to the individual and the community is much more than meets the eye.

Compared with many other parasitic diseases, little over-all progress has been achieved in the control of schistosomiasis and in only a few areas have substantial inroads been made on the disease. This lack of accomplishment may be attributed to a number of factors, among which are lack of basic information on the occurrence and importance of the disease, lack of more efficient control procedures, failure to develop better methods because of limited research, insignificant progress in providing sanitary facilities, inattention to proper water management in irrigated areas, insufficient funds, and the dearth of adequately trained personnel. These are the main deficiencies which will have to be overcome in many areas before substantial progress can be made in checking the disease.

Available information in most endemic areas rarely gives an adequate measure either of the true prevalence of schistosomiasis or of its importance as a cause of disability and death. A relatively limited number of severe cases in which heavy infection of long standing has produced spectacular pathological effects often monopolize the picture. The proportion of clinical cases and of serious complications to the number of persons infected is, therefore, an important factor in estimating the direct effect of the disease upon a given population; it is essential in obtaining a quantitative assessment of human incapacity and of the resulting financial burden imposed by the disease. The determination of this requires not only cross-sectional surveys in the endemic areas, but also longitudinal studies of extensive series of clinical cases, in order to determine the progress and prognosis of the disease in relation to the characteristics of the infected persons and the environments in which the infection occurs. Areas representative for all human schistosomes should be included in such investigations. Hospital human statistics are rarely a sufficient guide, since they often list only those with complaints, and the inhabitants of an endemic area will not ask for treatment for conditions such as haematuria, mild diarrhoea and abdominal pain, which often occur in the early stages of the disease.

Infection ratio and hence the apparent severity of schistosomiasis vary considerably, not only from one endemic area to another but also from one locality to another within the same area, where apparently similar human environmental conditions and prevalence obtain. The reasons for this state of affairs are complex and not well understood. The nutritional status of the human host modifies the pathological manifestations, and immune response to the infection varies, sometimes taking the form of increasing adjustment to the infection, and sometimes that of developing hypersensitivity to the antigenic substances produced by the parasite. Strains of the parasite varying in virulence may well exist in different areas. Many other factors no doubt also contribute to this variability [WHO, 1965b].

Within any special group infection can be described in terms of the prevalence of infection, the incidence of new infections, the intensity of infection carried by the individual and the severity of effects. The inter-relationship between these four is not clear, it is, therefore, not possible to infer one of the characteristics from the other, nor is it possible to foretell the degree of improvement which would be produced by any reduction in incidence short of absolute cessation. Any light which can be thrown on this relationship would be of epidemiological value.

Parasitic load or intensity of infection in schistosomiasis consitutes an important aspect of determining its public health importance. Studies have suggested a probable relationship between the output of eggs and the severity of effects, but it is not possible at present to work back from this to the load of infection which has produced them. Egg output is by no means satisfactory but it is the only quantitative measure possible at present.

A major consideration in planning schistosomiasis control is to establish that the disease really constitutes a problem of community proportions to warrant community action. For this purpose, attention to the exact definition of the situation should be the first objective in order to gain sufficient understanding of the epidemiology of infection for the rational preparation of programmes of prevention. This involves seeking answers to a number of fundamental questions, fulfilment of these necessitates field, clinical and laboratory studies: the distribution of the disease and its prevalence both under present conditions and under probable conditions of expected developments in the different areas affected; the incidence of new cases arising in the communities; the intensity of infection and the seriousness of the disease in the individual (case fatality rate); the magnitude of resulting disease; its clinical pattern (clinical spectrum or gradient); demographic status of the population in relation to these measurements (age, sex and occupation; specific rates); the strategic population sectors in which the problem is concentrated; time trend of the diseases (improving or retrogressing); mortality from the disease in relation to deaths from other causes (relative death rates); and the consequent effect in social terms and the economic expression of it for the community [FAROOQ, 1964a].

Finally, to evaluate the social significance of schistosomiasis, it must be known how important the problem is to the community in comparison with other problems, how effective and economical available control measures are, and whether they are within the economic capabilities of the community.

Health schemes are often promoted for economic reasons, and investment in health in the abstract is difficult to justify. It is conceded that the value of human health is not to be measured in monetary terms, but in less developed countries where resources are scarce, choice must be made between alternatives, and 'under such circumstances it is not possible to indulge in decision-making which might be described as purely humanitarian, as contrasted to judgements and actions dictated by the best economic criteria' [HARRAR, 1963]. In their struggle to achieve economic growth, these countries must channel their limited resources to support schemes which most quickly and effectively contribute to over-all economic prosperity. Therefore, the questions which 50 years ago malariologists asked themselves concerning the social consequences of their control programmes must be considered and an indication given of the economic benefits involved. The estimates produced by the malariologists were largely combinations of the tangible and intangible, which provided answers far short of mathematical ideals, but nevertheless served a very useful purpose.

Unfortunately, very few studies of schistosomiasis have gone beyond establishing a general prevalence rate, utilizing sampling and examination techniques which are either not stated or ill-defined. It is true that we lack well-defined standards for measuring the items enumerated, but so far only a few serious attempts have been made to develop them. There are many difficulties, but a beginning should be made with small additions to teams engaged on transmission or control studies in the different areas that would be rewarding in the development of quantitative methods by trial and error in the field, and their specificity and sensitivity tested in a similar manner before they are standardized and brought into general use.

In respect to health service facilities, the concentration of medical and nursing personnel relative to the area of the endemic region and the number of inhabitants, the size of the health service budget, and the occurrence of other endemic diseases, must be taken into account.

In general, the discussions in this chapter and in some other parts of this manual, relate to the employment of moderate or large scale procedures for gathering basic data and the institution of control measures. It is not to be inferred that other less ambitious efforts are not of value. Health officials with only modest budgets at their disposal should not hesitate to consider small-scale activities for the purpose of determining the extent of endemicity of schistosomiasis and its relative health importance. Initial efforts in this regard can be carried out at relatively small cost and will constitute a nucleus, when additional funds become available, for more extensive investigations and a determination for the need of control measures.

Death, disease and disability constitute the familiar criteria used to express the public health or social significance of a disease, but its economic importance lies in (a) loss of potential wealth due to temporary or permanent inability to work, or death, (b) consequential losses, such as failure to take advantage of opportunities from irrigation, or dislocation of industry, and (c) the direct costs of medical care.

The loss in work time owing to illness is best expressed in proportion to the potential time which could have been utilized. The use made of a country's natural resources is related to the effort available, and if part of the effort is diverted, then a part of the potential national income for that year is also lost. In industrialized countries where almost everyone's attendance at work is recorded, the loss due to temporary illness can be fairly easily estimated, but even so there is no recognized system of allowing for premature retirement from work and for death, and any method for use in schistosomiasis studies must take this factor into consideration and must be applicable where registration of work attendance is ineffective. The economic effect of death and disability depends largely on the age and sex of the persons affected, and economic assessment of the effects of any disease must amount to a quantitative natural history of the disease expressed in economic terms.

Factors Determining Desirability and Feasibility of a Control Programme

General Considerations

Discovery of the magnitude and importance of the endemic area will logically be followed by an inquiry as to whether a control programme is desirable and feasible.

It is not possible to consider whether control measures are to be instituted without giving some thought to the nature of the campaign envisaged. To some extent, therefore, the decision discussed here should be taken in the light of the subject-matter of the other relevant chapters.

The data gathered concerning the distribution, prevalence, and severity of the disease, together with the information obtained on the transmission of the parasite from snail to man and man to snail, should not only enable a sound decision to be taken as to whether a snail control programme is a practicable means of reducing the disease in man, but should also assist in planning the control scheme and selecting the measures to be used. Consideration of the latter aspect will be discussed on pages 438 to 457.

The place and the circumstances in which the infection occurs; the recognition both by observation of the habits of the people and by ecological study of the places in which contact with cercariae is commonly established, the seasons of the year at which it occurs, and the reasons which bring people into contact with this kind of location, are essential. The site at which contamination of the water occurs and whether it is diffuse or tends to be localized and, together with this, the possibility of avoiding contamination of water by means which are practicable within the social structure of the community, constitute important general considerations.

The information obtained on the distribution and extent of the endemic foci and the public health importance of the infection is essential in considering problems of logistics. It will indicate the places where control efforts may have to be concentrated and influence the formulation of decisions as to the magnitude and urgency of the problem. Although the decision to undertake control depends primarily upon epidemiological and biological considerations it will, of course, also be profoundly affected by economic factors [WHO, 1965a].

Precontrol Surveys

Basic Factors

Schistosomiasis is a multifaceted problem and can be understood only if seen from several different points of view. Lack of clear appreciation of the various factors involved in the disease mechanism has often led to isolated and disjointed measures against this complex public health problem. Having gauged the significance of the various determinants, it will then become necessary to make an orderly approach with the establishment of priorities in dealing with them.

The multiple epidemiological patterns encountered in schistosomiasis are due to the interplay of certain basic factors involved. Essentially these are a low standard of living which forces frequency of contact with unprotected waters, indiscreet human activity, density, distribution and movement of population, and density of the molluscan host.

The most fundamental human factor involved in the transmission of schistosomiasis is that it is a water-transmitted infection in which water is polluted as a result of the insanitary habits of the people. Their behaviour is partly based on ignorance but is mainly determined by helplessness and the lack of means of avoiding infection in the ecological complex in which they live. With low income, non-availability of a protected water supply and poor housing conditions in villages located in close proximity to open waters, the people are obliged to use natural unprotected waters for domestic, recreational and religious (ablution and 'wadu') purposes. Unless environmental improvements and better living conditions are brought about it is unreasonable to expect any permanent amelioration of the condition, and health education will continue to remain empty advice. In such a milieu, agricultural and industrial development tends to strengthen the basic conditions for the efficient perpetuation of the life cycle of the parasite. Irrigation projects simultaneously attract people and guarantee contact with newly created snail habitats. Pollution with human excrement again requires special attention in connexion with the density and concentrations of the population, since it is one of the principal conditions that render a habitat suitable for host snails. Under natural conditions opportunities for snail-man contact are rare. One of the most important effects of human concentrations is, therefore, to provide enormously increased opportunities for contact between man and water infested with schistosome-transmitting snails. The stage is thus set for the drama that follows the introduction of the parasite.

General Principles

If preliminary consideration of the situation indicates that schistosomiasis actually or potentially constitutes a serious health hazard, the next step is to organize and carry out a series of fact-finding surveys over the whole of the area involved.

A major survey should include both research elements and the collection of qualitative and quantitative data. It should as far as possible include the following general steps [GORDON, 1963]:

a) Field reconnaissance. A general reconnaissance of the area and the collection of any background information that may be available is an important principle in a field investigation. There is no substitute for personal observation. Establishing working relations with local health services and administrative authorities is essential. Census and demographic data and available maps, however deficient, must be collected for a general assessment of the situation to be surveyed.

b) Field organization. The next step is to institute administrative procedures, select a staff and assemble the necessary supplies and equipment. Staff will consist of directional and assessment staff at the field headquarters which forms the base, and staff for the field station which is both the focus of working activities and the residence for the field or the peripheral staff. At an intermediate level, supervisory staff in charge of the peripheral units is needed, consisting of technicians and field helpers. These would constitute the nucleus of the future control organization.

c) In order to indicate the limits of the area of occurrence of the disease and so to avoid unnecessary expense in the subsequent, more costly investigations, a preliminary survey using some of the newer serological methods may be carried out.

d) A sampling design should be worked out providing a representative sample of adequate size to allow differential observations, in the manifold classifications required, to be significant and generalization to be valid. With appropriate techniques, a sample may be chosen so that the probability of sampling error may be in predetermined tolerable limits. Detailed reference to this essential consideration is made on pages 690 to 700 and 729 to 734. A statistician should be consulted at this stage.

e) Exploratory study. The purpose of this activity is to test record forms and techniques, and to train staff members new to the work and often to research methods and principles. This is necessary because in schistosomiasis, procedures involved have not yet developed to the stage of standardization. Tentative forms may be tried out before proceeding with the main investigation. In field research, a preliminary test of methods and procedures and an evaluation of staff members is imperative. The exploratory study may last for one to three months. The results must be sufficiently extensive to determine whether it is necessary to revise forms, procedures and techniques employed and, especially, the reliability of units of measurements used. Identifying the errors of omission is as significant as recognizing those of commission.

f) Pilot study. A pilot study is advisable where the problem is obscure, where epidemiological constants are ill-defined, or methods new. A material saving in time and money usually results. The course of a pilot study, the full-dress rehearsal of the main investigations, will depend on how much experience the investigators have had with previous studies. The pilot study differs from the exploratory study in being an experiment with adequate controls, designed to support the validity of concept and experimental design. It has the advantage of a proven and experienced staff, derived from the preceding exploratory investigation. A small edition of the projected major study, in size of population examined and in duration, it usually lasts for several months or a year in order to take cognizance of seasonal variations. The pilot study may identify enough flaws or difficulties to lead to the conclusion that the experiment is unlikely to produce a definite answer; it may uncover new evidence suggesting a second pilot study with a fresh approach. It may demonstrate that the plan works or indicate the revisions required to make the control programme practical. On rare occasions the results from the pilot study lead to the conclusion that further investigation is unnecessary.

g) Definitive study. Since the definitive study covers a larger area and population than the pilot study, the staff is necessarily increased and further recruits trained. This process is considerably simplified since the needs of the programme are now more definite and an experienced nucleus exists. By judicious mixture of old and new members, field operations usually start with little delay. This is very desirable, in order to avoid interruption in time trends of the previously collected data. At the beginning efficiency may not match that of the pilot study since the original staff commonly includes people ultimately intended for supervisory duties. The definitive studies include: prevalence and incidence relative to personal attributes of the population (population pathology); the relationship to different environmental factors (geographical pathology); and explaining why the observed differences occur, in *time*, *person* and *place*.

The above outlines are to be followed not only in mapping-out the endemicity of the infection and its determinants, but as general principles applicable to assessments of the clinical severity, morbidity and mortality for which it is responsible.

Next, identification of the snail host is necessary, since most areas support numerous species of mollusc that do not transmit the infection. Finally, investigation of the geographical distribution and seasonal fluctuation of the snail host, with regard both to population numbers and to infection rates, must be investigated. Fuller details relating to studies concerning the intermediate host have been dealt with in relevant chapters.

At the end of this stage it should be possible to map both the endemicity of the disease, the distribution and population dynamics of the snail host, the annual transmission cycle and the relative significance of the various transmission sites.

Research elements of the investigation should involve an improvement in the quantitative aspects of several subjects which are already reasonably well understood in a qualitative manner. This work, for which there are good prototypes in studies at the WHO-assisted Philippine-9 and Egypt-49 projects, requires a team mechanism, essential elements being epidemiologist, biologist and irrigation engineer. Research envisaged would demand the development of one or more mathematical models, which can be arranged in collaboration with other workers, and could considerably broaden our understanding of the ecological complex and the dynamics of schistosomiasis transmission [HAIRSTON, 1962, 1965; MACDONALD, 1961, 1965].

It is on the firm basis of the established basic information collected, which would take from two to three years, that a rational methodology for control on a countrywide basis could be planned. Local control within a region should draw on the experience of the detailed investigations and trials under similarly prevailing conditions with identical hosts involved.

Objectives of Schistosomiasis Control

Prevention of Spread

In many areas where the transmission of schistosomiasis might occur, there is too little water for too short a time, under natural conditions, to support extensive human and live-stock populations and thus favour the full development of the agricultural potential. The introduction of water into such areas tends to build up human, animal and snail populations, and this often leads to a marked increase in snail-borne diseases. In still other endemic areas, low-lying poorly-drained terrain which is supplied with too much water, often offers ideal habitats for snails.

In this first type of area mentioned above, water for domestic use and irrigation is essential for development. In the second type of area, land reclamation and water management tend greatly to reduce the extent of the snail habitats and to increase agricultural production.

Irrigation agriculture is a highly specialized type of farming which requires industrious and healthy settlers if the full potential of the areas are to be realized and if it is to form a base for industrialization and improved standards of living. Such a base depends on the extent to which each farm worker is able to produce beyond the point of mere subsistence. Poor health is one of the factors which limits the farmer's production.

Due to the fact that precautions are not usually taken nor control measures instituted during the early phases, most soil and water-resource development programmes in endemic areas cause the spread of schistosomiasis. In rare instances, however, careful planning in the initial stages of schemes and the subsequent use of suitable agricultural methods and strict water management during their operational phase, have reduced the extent of the snail habitats and lowered the prevalence of the disease. These exceptions lead into the discussion of environmental control on pages 533 to 590.

In dry areas of the first type, the intermediate hosts and man are either entirely absent or limited in their distribution. Even if a snail habitat exists, ecological and climatic conditions often sharply limit the length of the transmission period. The introduction of water into formerly inhospitable places often opens them up for invasion and settlement by both snails and people. The resulting association almost invariably also allows introduction and spread of snail-borne diseases of man and his live-stock. When water is supplied to areas where only occasional foci formerly occurred, the following changes usually take place: (1) the area becomes capable of supporting greater snail and human populations; (2) the number and extent of the sites where transmission of snail-borne disease can occur is greatly increased; and (3) the length of the period of such transmission is extended.

In some of the poorly-drained areas on the coastal plain of parts of East and West Africa, intermediate hosts may be very common but the characteristics of the habitats tend to limit human contact. In such areas reclamation by drainage may greatly reduce the extent of the snail habitats. At the same time, however, the advantage gained in this respect may be offset by increased human activity in the area and correspondingly greater human contact with the snail colonies that remain in the drains, canals, and other residual habitats.

In Leyte, in the Philippines, the poorly-drained endemic area had a dense human population; water management and soil-resource development in experimental areas there, without a corresponding increase in the human population density, brought about a decrease in transmission, more or less proportional to the reduction of transmission sites [WHO, 1965b].

Another human factor of importance has been that of population movements which have markedly influenced the propagation of schistosomiasis. Nomadic habits of certain tribes in many territories have undoubtedly seeded the infection in a number of places. Modern traffic and mechanization of transport, together with agricultural expansion and industrial development which creates demand for opportunities of work, have accelerated these wanderings. In the past, movement of troops and concentration of military forces during the World Wars have brought in their train a marked flaring-up of infection. The movements of pilgrims to the Hedjaz from West and Equatorial Africa and, more recently, the search for seasonal work (e.g. cotton picking) in the large irrigation schemes, have disseminated the infection. Similarly military campaigns and the new roads built in the African continent have led to the extension of both forms of schistosomiasis while infiltration and refugee displacements have constituted other possible sources of danger.

The distribution of schistosomiasis and its intensity corresponds to the distribution of the intermediate snail hosts and to their relative density. The latter is determined by such factors as permanence of slow-moving or stagnant, sheltered backwaters, with submerged vegetation ensuring a substratum of rich organic matter, in areas fed by perennial irrigation. However, instances will also be encountered where the potential intermediate hosts of schistosomiasis are present in wider areas than the corresponding infections. This could occasionally be related to snail host-parasite incompatibility but indicates, as a rule, that the parasite has not been introduced or at least that circumstances do not favour transmission at a level of intensity sufficient to produce endemic occurrence, a situation which might well change and trigger-off the appearance of additional schistosomiasis foci in many other areas [WHO, 1965b].

Transmission Reduction

Reducing the risk of acquiring infection or reducing the intensity of infection for the population protected, remains the aim of a control programme.

The transmission of schistosomiasis is affected by seasonal and hydrological changes which influence the life cycle of the snail host, the production of cercariae, and also determine human contact with water. Unless these relationships are understood, control measures are apt to be ineffective and there will be a waste of funds. The factors which affect the combination of circumstances that result in human infection vary in each area. For this reason the discussion which follows cannot be considered as being specifically applicable in every endemic area, but the basic principles are everywhere the same.

In the temperate zones, not only is the number of snails greatly reduced during the winter but also many of them hibernate and do not produce cercariae; the water is cold enough to discourage human contact and snail control measures during this period have been found to be both unnecessary and ineffective. In the spring the surviving snails become active and have a major egg-laying period that extends well into the summer. The number of infected snails and the time of development of the cercariae, are all factors that are related to the intelligent application of any type of control measures that may be considered for such areas. They are more intimately related to the timing of molluscicide application than to habitat control.

In warmer climates the variations in the snail population density and in cercarial production are often as extreme as those in the temperate zone. This is fortunate because it tends to limit the period during which molluscicides must be applied. However, in the areas where temperature and hydrological conditions approach the optimum and are almost constant, conducive to high snail population density together with high cercarial production rates and frequent human contact with infested water, molluscicides must be applied more often or combined with measures that reduce the snail-producing potential of the habitats.

In those warm climates in which changes are sufficient to produce marked differences in the schistosomiasis transmission pattern from season to season, the basic causal factors are usually hydrological. Under these circumstances, the lack of water may produce conditions in many habitats similar to those that occur in the winter of colder climates. The snails aestivate and some of the vigorous members of the colony which are sufficiently protected against desiccation and lethal temperatures, usually survive and repopulate the area when the water returns. In areas where the infections in aestivating populations have been studied, it has been found that the snails with well-developed trematode infections usually die during this period of stress. Those that happen to have young infections may survive, and the parasite aestivates along with the snail. With the return of the water, surviving snails become active and soon begin to lay eggs. Any young larval forms present in the snails continue their development, and may begin to produce cercariae within two to four weeks after the return of the water. The number of snails that will produce cercariae during this period is usually small, therefore, the number of infective larvae in the water tends to be low. The time which elapses between the hatching of the eggs and the development of the new generation of snails to the egg-laying stage depends on conditions in the habitat, but usually involves a period of from 4 to 6 weeks. If the water contains miracidia, the young snails will become infected, but the development of the infection to the cercariae-producing stage requires a similar period of time. A relatively safe period may, therefore, be expected in some habitats, lasting for approximately 6 to 8 weeks after the return of the water. On the other hand, any extension of the period when water is present in the habitats after cercarial production has started, prolongs the transmission period and usually increases the prevalence and intensity of the infection. This has happened in parts of Egypt where basin irrigation has been converted to perennial irrigation.

It must be emphasized that these are general statements. The actual patterns produced by the relationship of the climatic and hydrological factors to those of the parasite-snail cycles cannot be determined without careful study of the population dynamics, with particular reference to the seasonal prevalence of the infections. This latter factor not only varies in different areas but may also vary in the same area from year to year.

In some irrigation schemes where aquatic snails are the intermediate hosts, the water used to initiate irrigation after the summer closure has a very heavy silt load. Studies made in these habitats before the institution of control measures showed that the silt tended to check the growth of aquatic vegetation and the increase of snail populations in the canals for two or three months. As the water became clearer the snail densities steadily increased, finally reaching and maintaining a high level during the following closure period. Certain canals in some systems contain water during the summer or winter closure, to serve as the water supply for the people and their domestic animals. Without control, these serve as the habitats for numerous snails, and the concentration of human activities along them tends to increase their capacity and importance as transmission sites.

A similar pattern occurs in many areas where streams and auxiliary natural bodies of water serve as transmission sites. Flushing after heavy rains or floods usually causes a great reduction in the number of snails present. During the dry periods the snails must aestivate in many of the habitats, with necessarily increased human contact with the bodies of water that remain. If these relationships last long enough to produce an infected snail population, the stage is set for transmission.

Circumstances in some areas allow transmission only occasionally, with periods of a year or more intervening. If the danger signals are known, major control efforts can be concentrated on the elimination of the conditions that produce transmission, and special precautions can be taken when circumstances indicate that they are needed.

In other areas the water-use and the water-contact patterns of the people in the area determine the location of the major transmission sites and the snail habitats that require control measures.

The most rational water usage and agricultural practices contribute materially to the reduction of the snail habitats through the collateral effects of good drainage, weed control, crop management and sound irrigation procedures. This topic is discussed on pages 533 to 591, but it can be mentioned here that any measures of this kind require the co-operation of the irrigation authorities, the agricultural authorities and the farmers; and that in order to obtain such co-operation it is necessary for the person involved to have some understanding of the principles discussed in this section [WHO, 1965b].

Morbidity Control

While prevalence is being determined, an estimate can be made of the relative severity of the infection. This cannot be done precisely since the available criteria of sickness due to schistosomiasis are very difficult to reduce to terms that can be judged by quantitative measures. However, the prevalence of signs and symptoms usually associated with schistosomiasis can be recorded in sample population groups. In addition, clinical records, morbidity data, mortality data and autopsy records can be utilized to estimate the impact of the disease upon the human population. From such information it can usually be deduced whether or not the infection is producing a marked frequency of overt disease. It must be remembered, however, that schistosomiasis is subtle in its manifestations, and that damage resulting from infection may go undetected if only superficial judgements are made.

The quantitative measurement of the intensity of schistosome infection in a given population is a great deal more difficult than the determination of prevalence. For this reason, the evidence available on this point is generally both indirect and incomplete. Nevertheless, it may reasonably be assumed from the known facts that high prevalence is generally correlated with high intensity and severity of infection and vice versa. Thus, in Egypt, it has been stated that schistosomiasis is the most serious public health problem of the country but that, since the institution of control measures, fewer severe cases with serious complications are seen in the clinics. In the Congo, it has been stated that the severity of the cases increased with the prevalence. While it might be expected that this would be so, with apparently greater opportunity for exposure to cercariae and a greater number of worms in each infected individual, statistically valid data proving that high prevalence and high intensity and severity of infection are correlated have not yet been obtained. Schistosomiasis is one of the few widespread communicable diseases for which treatment needs to be considered from two viewpoints; that of the clinician whose main interest is to reduce morbidity and mortality, and that of the epidemiologist whose interest is more fundamental. The aim of the former is to cure the patient of both his disease and his infection, and that of the latter, which seems comparatively easy, is to stop its transmission.

Although there is no evidence on record of an interruption in transmission of schistosomiasis brought about by mass treatment of a community, there is some evidence, not amounting to proof, that treatment carried out persistently over a number of years has caused diminution in morbidity and in the incidence of severe complications.

Eradication

Eradication in schistosomiasis would mean the ending of transmission and the elimination of the reservoir of infection in the definitive host or hosts, in a campaign limited in time and carried out to such a degree of perfection that, when it comes to an end, there is no resumption of transmission. In contrast, control implies the reduction of schistosomiasis to a prevalence where it is no longer a major public health problem.

Control, having to be maintained by continuous activity, carries with it the implication that the programme will be unending. In contrast, expenditure in eradication will represent capital investment and not a constantly recurring cost. While case finding and epidemiological investigation of individual, suspected or imported, cases are of primary importance in an eradication programme, they are of secondary and minor interest in a control programme. It may be feasible to integrate control with the public health programme of the country but, because of the specific objective to be attained within a limited time, eradication cannot be so integrated.

Taking all the basic requirements of eradication into consideration and in the present stage of knowledge, when no more than partial interference with transmission of schistosomiasis can be hoped for in many of the worst affected areas, control and prevention of infection would remain the reasonable goal in most of the endemic areas. Under the circumstances, it appears necessary to avoid over-enthusiastic reference to eradication, except perhaps in relation to very small and isolated foci occurring in arid areas.

Although snail eradication would ultimately eliminate schistosomiasis and obviate the necessity of further snail control measures, in practice it is an objective beyond reach in most endemic areas. The first reason for this statement is that schistosomiasis is not a self-limiting infection; the parasite has a long life-span and the interruption of transmission brought about for a few years will not eliminate the reservoir of infection in the definitive hosts. The second reason is that the tools and the methods now at hand are not adequate to assure snail eradication in any but small isolated foci; one can often kill all but a few of the snails but eliminating the residual ones is difficult and costly, and any remaining snails can repopulate the areas when control is stopped. Since snails can be carried from place to place by man, domesticated and wild animals, and even on inanimate objects, the snails may be re-introduced into a habitat from which they have been cleared. Therefore, any attempt at over-simplification of the problem should be deprecated, because it is feared that undue optimism may ultimately decrease confidence and create repercussions and unforeseen obstacles in the future [FAROOQ, 1964b].

References

FAROOQ, M.: J. trop. med. Hyg. *67:* 105 (1964a).
FAROOQ, M.: J. trop. mcd. Hyg. *67:* 265 (1964b).
GORDON, J. E.: Amer. J. med. Sci. *246:* 354 (1963).
HAIRSTON, N. G.: Population ecology and epidemiological problems; in WOLSTENHOLME and O'CONNOR Bilharziasis, pp. 36–62 (Churchill, London 1962).
HAIRSTON, N. G.: Bull. Wld Hlth Org. *33:* 45 (1965).
HARRAR, J. G.: Amer. J. publ. Hlth *53:* 375 (1963).
MACDONALD, G.: Publ. Hlth Rep. *76:* 753 (1961).
MACDONALD, G.: Trans. roy. Soc. trop. Med. Hyg. *59:* 489 (1965).
WHO: WHO Expert Committee on Bilharziasis, Geneva 1964; Third Report. Wld Hlth Org. techn. Rep. Ser. *299* (1965a).
WHO: Snail control in the prevention of bilharziasis. Wld Hlth Org. Monogr. Ser. 50 (1965b).

Chapter 9

Epidemiology and Control of Schistosomiasis, pp. 438–457
(Karger, Basel and University Park Press, Baltimore 1973)

Planning and Organization of Control Programmes

M. Farooq

Introduction

The accumulation of knowledge in an area where schistosomiasis occurs and the subsequent organization and execution of a control programme should take place in a well-established and logical series of steps. This applies both to the technical and administrative aspects of the programme.

The nature of the procedures to be adopted will depend greatly on the data assembled during the surveys to determine distribution, prevalence and intensity of infection and the species, distribution and bionomics of the molluscan intermediate host or hosts.

The steps necessary for the securing of such data are described in the following paragraphs. Needless to say, careful analysis must be made of all assembled information. Time is a factor here and unnecessary haste in arriving at decisions may lead to technical errors in organization and control procedures, errors which will prove costly by way of dissipating available resources.

Prerequisites

The initial stage consists of establishing the endemicity of the disease and estimating the prevalence of human infection. The distribution of cases is mapped, and analysis is made in relation to personal attributes and environmental determinants. Evidence of severity of infection is obtained from clinical signs in infected persons in the community and from hospital and autopsy records. Since schistosome transmission is always closely bound up with human habits and occupations, study of human water-contact activities relating to irrigation and farming practices, and to domestic, recreational and religious habits, provides extremely useful information in locating important foci of transmission [FAROOQ and MALLAH, 1966].

Later, more detailed information is collected, some of which is quantitative, and involves not only the human but also the molluscan host, the identity of which must now be determined.

A decision is then reached as to whether an attempt at control is necessary and practicable. Sufficient data should be available to enable this to be done with reasonable confidence. If this condition is not fulfilled, further investigations should be undertaken.

With present-day knowledge and methods available, schistosomiasis control at a reasonable cost is feasible if the will to do it exists in a country. Schistosomiasis control is fundamentally an enterprise directed at reducing or eliminating transmission of the disease so that no more new infections, re-infections, or super-infections occur.

If the gravity of the problem justifies further action, the next step is to proceed to the selection of the measures to be used in the control programme. This aspect is dealt with in detail later in this chapter.

The control plan depends very heavily on information relative to the snails. If these are to be the object of attack, it will be necessary, at least in the early phases of the investigations, to have advice and help from specialists, because snail control involves attacking the snails in their habitats with a minimum of disturbance to man, his crops and his animals. Such an attack calls for an intimate and detailed knowledge of the snail host or hosts. The usual sequence of investigation is as follows:

Search for Possible Intermediate Hosts

Initially there must be a widespread search for the snails which might be involved. In the Orient the hosts are operculate snails belonging to the genus *Oncomelania*. In other areas the hosts are usually pulmonate snails belonging to the sub-families Planorbinae and Bulininae; but *Ferrissia tenuis*, belonging to the family Ancylidae, serves as the intermediate host for *Schistosoma haematobium* in a focus in India. This mollusc and closely-related species are found in other endemic areas and should not be ignored. The recognition of the species of snail which is transmitting the disease in a given area requires the skill and experience of a field biologist who must know which snails to seek and where they are likely to be found.

Proof of Involvement

When snails suspected of harbouring the schistosome are found they must be tested to find out whether, in fact, they can convey the infection. Proof that a particular species of snail transmits the disease, by demonstrating that it can pass the infection, requires the expert assistance of an experimental biologist. Three methods of approach are possible:

1. Examination of wild snails for naturally-acquired infection. Specimens collected throughout the endemic area can be examined for naturally-acquired schistosome infection by the inspection of crushed individuals. The method used in making examinations by crushing snails is given on page 663. This can demonstrate whether schistosome infections are harboured, but will not conclusively prove that the schistosomes found are indeed the species infecting man, since the cercariae of schistosomes infecting domestic and wild animals resemble those of the human parasites. In searching for naturally-infected wild snail hosts it should be constantly borne in mind that both snail population density and infection rates usually fluctuate with season. Therefore, it may be necessary to search for infected snails through a period of at least one year.

2. Infection of laboratory animals with field-collected cercariae. Exposure of schistosome-free laboratory animals to cercariae collected from naturally-infected snails tests their infectivity and permits the rearing of the adult worms, which can be more readily and certainly identified than the larvae and immature forms. It is necessary, however, to have available a stock of schistosome-free test animals, usually rodents, together with the means of maintaining and handling them. Accurate identification of the adult parasites and their eggs is also required.

3. Infection of healthy snails with miracidia from human infections. Additional proof that the real intermediate host has been found comes from infection of uninfected snails with miracidia obtained from human infections and the subsequent emergence of cercariae which can be used to complete the life cycle in the laboratory. This is the most certain procedure, but requires that the snails be reared in the laboratory free from infection and maintained up to eight weeks after exposure to miracidia so that the cercariae can develop.

Identification

If the trials outlined above indicate that a snail species can serve as the intermediate host, it then becomes desirable to obtain positive specific identification. This may be done locally if a sufficiently skilled malacologist is available. Otherwise specimens should be sent to a central reference laboratory such as the WHO Snail Identification Centres at the Danish Bilharziasis Laboratory, Danmarks Akvarium, Copenhagen, Denmark, and at the Institute of Biology, University of Brasilia, Brazil.

Methods for collecting the snails, transporting them to the laboratory and preparing them for identification are outlined on pages 658 to 667.

Specific identification of the suspect or proven intermediate hosts may not be absolutely essential to the development of a snail control programme. It is only essential to have adequate proof that a recognizable, but not necessarily identified, species is the host. In any event, positive identification should follow as soon as possible, since the biology of the species incriminated may have some bearing on control procedures.

In some localities, incrimination of the snail host is not very difficult since there is only one species belonging to the taxonomic group to which the known hosts belong, and the number of other schistosomes which might be confused with the schistosomes of man is very limited. In other localities, however, the task can be very difficult indeed and may require both the expenditure of considerable time and effort and the aid of specialists.

Delineation of Area of Occurrence

As the evidence implicating the intermediate host accumulates, the distribution of the suspected snails may be plotted on the basis of widespread collections. If the prevalence or severity of human infection seems to warrant it, all potential or known habitats for the snails should be mapped. Such information will not only assist in evaluation of the magnitude of the problem but will also be needed should snail control be attempted later.

It is essential to discover the exact distribution of the snail hosts, since this will indicate the true limits of the zone in which transmission can occur. This information is required in order to select the control methods giving the best cost-efficiency ratio, and to determine the feasibility of a control programme. The distribution of the snails is established by systematic search of all bodies of water together with all moist areas, if *S. japonicum* is involved, by persons trained in snail detection and recognition of species. Usually it is necessary to bring sample collections to the laboratory for confirmation of field identification. It is not necessary to measure accurately the density of the snail populations at this stage, although it is valuable to record a rough estimate of the snail density for each habitat detected in order to gain a useful impression of the habitat preferences of the snails, which can be taken into account later when reliable population density studies are planned.

These snail searches for the purpose of establishing the geographical limits of the intermediate host must be carried out at regular intervals throughout at least one full year, since there may be considerable variation in distribution of the snails from season to season. In some areas snail distribution may also vary from year to year.

Study of Bionomics

Before any valid decisions can be taken in connexion with a programme of snail control, a systematic study of the bionomics of the snails must be instituted, since anti-snail measures can only be effective and efficient if they are based on sound and thorough knowledge of snail habits and ecology. Included in the study should be the reproductive habits, life-span, seasonal cycle and population trends, capacity to withstand drying or life out of water, habitat preferences and other characteristics of the snails; the impact upon them of seasonal climatic, topographic and hydrographic conditions; and the variations in prevalence of snail infections from place to place and from season to season.

Such evidence gives important indications as to the time and places of transmission and can assist greatly in the selection of points and seasons at which the snails can be attacked. It also provides a rational foundation upon which assessment of the prospects of successful control through a campaign directed against the snail hosts can be based.

It is not possible to specify all the procedures to be used in obtaining this information concerning snails, but some further details regarding procedures and techniques are given on pages 668 to 674. As already stated, it is highly desirable that the investigations be directed by a trained biologist.

In addition to the biological studies involved, it will be necessary to have detailed information on certain other factors. The amount, distribution and types of all bodies of water and damp and marshy areas within the endemic region, should be investigated and mapped. Seasonal variation in rainfall and annual amount of rainfall are both important in relation to snail control measures, their chances of success and the time at which they should be attempted. Other climatic factors, such as the amount of solar radiation, daily and seasonal temperature variations, and humidity, are also important [WHO, 1965a].

The steps just mentioned are discussed more fully and the necessary techniques are described in later chapters.

Animal Reservoirs and
Animal Schistosomes Infecting Man

In the case of *S. japonicum*, the strain of parasite infective to man is equally transmissible to animals, both artificially and in nature. Field rats and domestic animals such as dogs, pigs, goats, cattle and horses, all serve as good reservoir hosts. In a study of the transmission potential of animals in the pilot area of Leyte, Philippines, it has been found that about 25% of the infection is contributed by the animals mentioned above.

S. mansoni has a more restricted range of definitive hosts, but it has been found in several species, while *S. haematobium* has only occasionally been found in animals other than man. In most cases human *S. mansoni* and *S. haematobium* infections reported from such animals have been from areas where there is a relatively dense human population. As it is not known whether the chain of infection maintains itself in these animals and whether man may be infected from snails shedding cercariae derived from them, the part played by these infections in the epidemiology of the human infection is not certain. Although, in the case of *S. mansoni* and *S. haematobium* transmission, these animal infections are generally considered of little importance in the present state of knowledge, it is recognized that with the introduction of schistosomiasis control schemes such animal infections may assume greater significance. More information is needed in this respect.

In addition to infections in animals by the three human schistosomes, many species of animal schistosomes are recognized. Of them, *S. mattheei* has been found to mature regularly in man in South Africa, and *S. intercalatum* in the Congo, and contiguous areas. Animal schistosomes that have been reported in man have been from areas where there is close association between man and his domestic stock and where there is a high stock density.

The possible role that these infections may play in modifying the usual human-host reactions to *S. haematobium* or *S. mansoni* is not at present known [WHO, 1965b].

Basic Plan and Procedure

A team mechanism is essential in planning the strategy and control of schistosomiasis. Close collaboration of epidemiologist, public health administrator, clinician, biologist, sociologist and engineer, each calling on the skills of associates, will become necessary. The epidemiologist and the biologist will draw chiefly from the natural sciences, the administrator from the social sciences, with the clinician giving aid to both. The necessity for such partnerships in schistosomiasis control is clear and should be enthusiastically cultivated. This will facilitate the welding of medical, biological and behavioural sciences with a broad capability for understanding and studying complex disease problems, of which schistosomiasis is an outstanding example.

Prior to the inauguration of any control procedure, it would be advisable to develop and maintain close liaison with other agencies within the government structure whose functions relate to health planning, irrigation and water utilization, agriculture, environmental sanitation, and veterinary medicine. In most endemic areas, it will be advantageous to request help from time to time from such agencies in various aspects of the control programme. Ultimate success of the programme will depend on the extent of such co-operation that is developed and maintained.

The formation of a National Committee on Schistosomiasis, composed of representatives from these agencies and meeting on a regular schedule, will ensure the desired co-operation on a continuing basis.

A schistosomiasis control programme may include use of ecological or biological control of snails, environmental control of human contact with hazardous water bodies, and chemical control of snails. As regards chemical control, the programme resolves itself into two main phases; preparatory and attack.

Preparatory Phase

This phase has three main elements: initial survey, pilot operations and verification of the efficacy of the methods and organization proposed.

Knowledge concerning all the factors that enter into the transmission of the disease, detailed under *Prerequisites* (above), is needed and should be acquired during the preparatory phase of the programme. The surveys will determine the area or areas that receive initial priority and will establish baseline data with respect to the criteria that are to be employed in evaluating the control programme. The information secured should enable a suitable selection to be made of the area or areas most advantageous for the pilot operations, and therefore the ones that will be the first to pass into the attack phase.

The pilot operations start with preparation of schedules and estimates of the activities to be carried out during the attack phase, proceed to the recruitment and training of the personnel that will be needed, and end with the different administrative details required by the unit to enable it to proceed towards an effective control programme.

The verification of the efficacy of the methods and organization proposed should be performed in an area of adequate size to show clear results. In this stage, elaborate methods may be used to understand more fully the dynamics of transmission in the area and to evaluate the effects of the measures applied. At the same time, however, more practical methods of evaluation should be introduced and their results compared with the more elaborate ones, so that the latter may be applied with confidence during the attack phase in the larger areas where the programme will be carried out. During this stage, lacunae in the proposed organization may be discovered and corrected [WHO, 1965b].

Attack Phase

This begins with the application of the snail-control measures found suitable for the effective control in the pilot areas. In most cases, mollusciciding will be the main measure. The objective pursued during this phase is to achieve a reduction in transmission, with a significant decrease in the prevalence and intensity of the disease.

The rhythm of total coverage with molluscicides in the attack phase will depend on the transmission pattern in a given area; this may involve more than one application a year in most situations. When this regimen is maintained for a few years it may reveal that under continued pressure snail populations diminish progressively over the whole area or become localized to certain favoured spots. These areas would constitute strongholds of re-infestation under favourable conditions. When such a state is reached it may be found advantageous to substitute surveillance and localized application of molluscicides for total coverage. Such foci should be carefully mapped, checked periodically, and molluscicides applied whenever it is found that snail density exceeds certain predetermined critical levels. This procedure will result in considerable saving in the cost of molluscicides used, and it marks the beginning of the consolidation phase in snail control. Vigilance would need to be maintained for a prolonged period, as an operational responsibility of the local health services.

Details of measurements and evaluation procedures involved are described on pages 609 to 619.

Planning, Organization and Supervision

General Considerations

Attention to the administrative aspects of a schistosomiasis control programme is as important as its technical aspects. Failure to take cognizance of the basic considerations involved may result in the failure of any health programme, however sound it may be from the technical point of view. Therefore, the statement of some general considerations of this aspect are considered as appropriate for schistosomiasis workers as they are for other health officials.

Administration has been defined as an enabling process and, in the sense in which it is usually understood, it covers the whole art of carrying into effect any policy or plan. It may, however, go further than the simple executive function of applying known rules to a given case, for in its widest form it must embrace leadership, policy-making and planning. Before a policy or plan can be conceived, some attempt must be made to forecast the situation to which the plan is to be applied, and the degree of accuracy in forecasting will be a measure of the success of the plan. Generally speaking, planning is preparing for certain changes within available means, and integrating them into the existing framework of the administrative structure.

The characteristics of a good plan may be summarized as follows:

(1) It should be based on a clearly defined objective. What the plan is intended to accomplish should be set out in terms which are clear not only to the planner, but also to all who may be concerned in the operation of the plan.

(2) It should be simple. If the objective is at all ambiguous there is a danger of the plan becoming so hopelessly involved that it will lead to misdirected effort and unnecessary expenditure. Therefore, the simpler the plan, the more chance it has of success.

(3) It should provide for a proper analysis and classification of actions. Standards must be set in order that quality as well as quantity of performance can be assessed.

(4) It should be flexible. The plan must be capable of adaptation to meet changing situations.

(5) It should be balanced. The successful integration of a plan into the total purpose of the undertaking is possible only if each activity required is operating with equal effectiveness.

(6) It should use available resources to the utmost.

Most of the above characteristics are so simple as to be obvious, yet it is surprising how many are overlooked in the preparation of a plan, and it is prudent to check against them any plan which may be produced before attempting to put it into operation.

The policy or plan having been decided upon, the next step is *organization*; and it is perhaps in this sphere that administration makes its greatest contribution. Briefly, it is the process of organization which finds the means, human and material, to meet the requirements of the plan. To do this it is necessary to carefully determine what jobs are to be done and what workers are required to do them, and to assess the amount of materials, tools and equipment needed for the accomplishment of the work.

The provision of materials and equipment, important though it is, is only a part of the plan. Administration, which carries the responsibility of accomplishing results through the efforts of other people, is concerned not only with the direction, but also with the development, of people. The organization of work is very much a human affair in which results, though visibly depending on materials and equipment, cannot be accomplished except by human effort. The purpose of organization is to verify that effort, and a clear understanding of human relationships is necessary if the desired result is to be obtained.

Modern management now recognizes certain fundamental ideas which apply equally well to the administration of schistosomiasis control programmes as to any other public health activity, namely:

(a) that the quality of the working force is the most vital factor in success;

(b) that initiative is to be encouraged;

(c) that the raising of morale in the working group is more important than the imposition of a rigid discipline;

(b) that training based on careful selection must become a conscious and continuous process; and

(e) that proficiency is not dependent on skill alone, but on the use made of available energy and latent ability, and that potential qualities can be drawn out under favourable working conditions by the proper guidance, direction, and stimulus exercised by those who administer.

All these factors are implied in good organization.

There must be an authority to see that sectional interests do not conflict with the main purpose, and the principle upon which this is based is known as centralization. This does not, however, mean that every order must emanate from the central authority. Once the policy and plan have been laid down, the process of delegation must come into play. If it does not, the central authority will quickly find that it is overwhelmed with details, and the co-ordination of the efforts of the total working force will become impossible. High morale is the most potent factor in that synthesis of effort which is called team-work, and its resultant effect is seen in the stability of the working force, (GODDARD, 1958).

Field Organization and Supervision

Direction of schistosomiasis control should be centralized at the provincial headquarters. The chief of the services should be an epidemiologist with a wide technical knowledge and organizational ability. His staff should

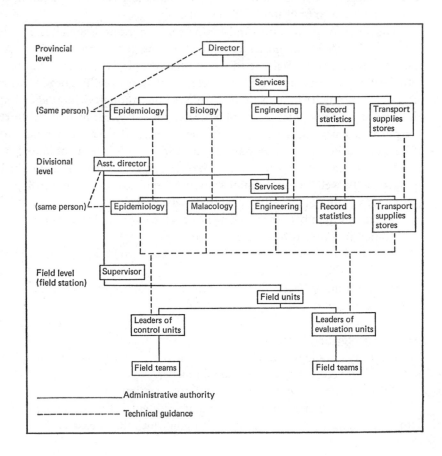

include a senior biologist, with training in malacology, ecology and parasi-tology, and a civil engineer. According to the size of the province and the availability of professional staff in the country, the chief may, at the same time, have to take direct responsibility for the epidemiological assessment of services. A recording service, employing a statistician, should form part of it, as also a section dealing with transport, supplies and stores.

Depending on the extent of the area and the population covered, a number of junior professional or senior sub-professional personnel must be assigned to the provincial services. These staff members can be selected from the best qualified field personnel and be given the necessary technical au-thority to guide and supervise the lower echelons.

A province should be divided into a number of divisions with a replica of the provincial services for each division, staffed with junior professional and senior sub-professional personnel. Each functional unit should be directly responsible for the relevant services at the lower levels. A division should be responsible for a number of field stations under a sub-professional supervisor having control of the field units.

The lines of administrative authority will normally be channelled through the provincial director, the chiefs of services, assistant directors, the super-visors at the intermediate levels, to the field units. Given below are outlines of an organizational chart indicating the lines of technical guidance and admin-istrative authority referred to above.

The chief at the divisional level should be an assistant director who should not only possess sufficient imagination and drive, but should have a marked flair for the outdoors. He should be selected from the level of super-visors with intimate knowledge of field-work.

The activity in the field should be decentralized, as far as possible, and placed in the hands of trained staff at the supervisory level stationed at suitably selected field stations. They should act as supervisors and be respon-sible, not only for the general conduct of field operations, but also for the collection and keeping of records, maintenance and repairs of equipment and establishment of good relationships with the public.

No hard and fast rules can be laid down on the organization and struc-ture of the peripheral (field) units. This will depend on the extent of the operations, on the topography and the climate of the area, on communications and accessibility, the availability of labour, level of literacy and attitude to work. Generally each peripheral unit (a squad or a team) in a mollusciciding programme will be composed of labourers under a foreman, who closely supervises work and collects and records field data. All equipment must be kept in serviceable condition if inefficiency and waste of chemicals and time is to be avoided. At least one man in each team should have received thorough training in the maintenance of equipment.

These peripheral units should each have a pre-determined area of work and itinerary. Details of work should be clearly defined and no ambiguity or room for avoiding responsibility should exist. It is an advantage to have separate evaluation units, distinct from the control units, but the invidious distinction of 'field' and 'laboratory' technicians, as existing in certain countries, should be avoided in schistosomiasis control.

An 'operations manual' in a local language, containing detailed information on the executive and technical aspects of the organization of the campaign, is of great value, and every effort should be made to prepare such local manuals which should not only outline the routine execution of the programme but also mention possible difficulties in the field and means of overcoming them. They should also include detailed instructions for protection against toxic hazards, if any are involved. These manuals should be revised from time to time and any improvements in operational procedures and techniques incorporated.

Supervision. A good organization, providing close and constant supervision of field operations, is a *sine qua non* for a successful control operation. Nothing guarantees failure more than inadequate attention to details and lack of thorough watchfulness and vigilance in field operations. Supervision applies to every echelon and every function and, naturally, it includes also superintending the supervisory staff. At field level, daily contact of the supervisor with every member of the team is advisable. If this is not feasible, the intervals between supervisory visits should not exceed two to three working days; any longer interval must be exceptional. The visits have to be planned in advance but in such a way that the field staff cannot predict the time or day they may expect the supervisor. In general, each staff member should have the feeling that his work is always being reviewed, but to give the impression that he is being instructed must be avoided. The supervisor has not only to look for faults but endeavour to create a spirit of confidence in the people working under him.

It is not sufficient to check that the team leader keeps to his schedule and is actually in the locality in which he is expected to be. Of even greater importance is the supervision of the work performance itself and whether or not the leader has any problem in his routine work which calls for help or advice from higher echelons. Each visit must be of sufficient duration to improve and stimulate the field work when necessary [WHO, 1962].

Programme Evaluation

The term 'evaluation' has been used to describe the administrative and technical procedures by which the value of a planned activity is measured. The process of evaluation should start at the inception of the programme and be recognized as an integral and continuous part of the responsibility for running it. Evaluation procedures have therefore to be built into the plan and should constitute its essential ingredient to be pursued continuously. In evaluation, such elements as reliability, validity, performance, cost, and public acceptance should be studied. This requires meticulous skill and scientific methodology to obtain unbiased results.

Evaluation therefore is not an end in itself, or a means to justify past performance, but rather a powerful tool for improving and reorienting the development of the campaign. It should cover as many of the different activities as possible, the emphasis naturally shifting according to the stage of development reached. Statistical methodology could assist considerably in this task of scientific appraisal. As far as possible, subjective methods, i.e. those based on individual opinions, should be replaced by objective critical indices that provide similar results at the hands of different observers of the campaign [SWAROOP, 1959].

A detailed account of the various measures and techniques to be employed in the evaluation of control are described on pages 609 to 619. General considerations involved are briefly stated here.

During the preparatory phase of schistosomiasis control, evaluation of changes in transmission could be made in terms of age-prevalence data, incidence of new infections among pre-school-children, measurements of the intensity of infection and changes in the severity of the disease in the different age groups. Attempts should be made, as far as possible, to include these parameters in the assessment of change.

Interpretation of results from arbitrarily selected samples becomes extremely difficult in schistosomiasis, therefore detailed requirements of sampling design and sample size for the collection of age-prevalence data have been laid down on pages 690 to 700. Significant changes can be observed over a period of not less than five years by measurable shifts to lower levels of prevalence. On the other hand a change in incidence rates could be detected within a year of the institution of control measures by observing the proportion of negative children in the pre-school age continuing to remain negative during a given interval of time, provided steps have been taken to establish this index in the year preceding the introduction of the control measures [FAROOQ et al., 1966].

In pooling data from different ages, the relative number of children examined in each age year must be kept constant.

It has been shown that, among children having schistosomiasis, the rise in egg output with increasing age is considerably greater than the proportional rise in prevalence rates. This indicates that egg-counts are a most sensitive measure of transmission. A methodology of this kind was utilized in the Egypt-49 project to evaluate control measures. The study was planned on the premise that varying degrees of reduction of transmission will be reflected in the diminution observed in the egg output in young age groups compared with the level predicted on the assumption that transmission continues as before. Scrutiny of the prevalence data suggests that the greatest discernible change in prevalence occurs in the year which separates children aged four and five years. Therefore, it appears that they are the most effective human monitors of transmission. Adoption or modification of this approach is recommended [WHO, 1965b].

In certain circumstances, changes in the severity of disease may occur without the prevalence of infection having changed concomitantly, and it is therefore essential whenever possible to establish a clinical gradient of disease in the community following a defined classification of the stages and severity of the disease; such a classification has been provided on pages 700 to 703. Any shift in the clinical pattern in relation to age, qualitatively and quantitatively, could then be followed from this base-line in subsequent examinations, and should provide important indications of the effects of control on the disease.

Establishment of parallel indices for comparable reference areas is essential so that evaluation could be made with confidence by noting that no significant change, in respect of the parameter used, has taken place as a result of factors unrelated to control activities and not directed specifically against schistosomiasis control, and that they have remained essentially stable during the interval.

At the end of the preparatory phase, when attack starts for practical reasons evaluation must involve simpler procedures owing to practical necessity. Inasmuch as prevention of transmission remains the goal, the primary concern should be with the prevalence in early age groups. Details of exact methods will vary with the number of age groups considered, the initial prevalence in these age groups, and the length of time over which full-scale control efforts have operated. Such details are again to be found on pages 609 to 619.

Age-prevalence data, however, are likely to change slowly and persons in charge of control programmes will wish to have more rapid assessment, and estimates of the snail densities may serve. Only coarse methods are available, but the preparatory phase provides the opportunity to test rapid and inexpensive methods, such as noting the presence or absence of snails in a large number of habitats, and of standardizing these methods against more elaborate ones. Improvements in speed and accuracy should be constantly sought [WHO, 1965b].

Choice of Single or Combined Methods

General Considerations

The information which should, by now, have been amassed will permit a rational plan of control to be made. It is tempting to avoid some of the delays and expense that the collection of such data entails, but there can be no doubt that it is very unwise to proceed without such information. It is extremely important to realize that in the long run schistosomiasis control will benefit by slow progress in the early stages. Methodically-planned collection of basic information and accomplished experiments takes time but will finally permit a much more exact choice of control measures suited to each special situation. Trial and error can be expected to give little additional information and may result ultimately in considerable waste of time and money. All control experience so far has emphasized consideration of this important fact, and failure of some control projects in the past can be attributed in large measure to the inadequacy of such background knowledge and lack of rational choice of method or methods employed.

One thing that retards the development of effective control programmes arises from the classification of the possible approaches as different methods. One often hears of the four-fold control measures: snail control, treatment, sanitation and health education, and that if they are used in combination they will serve as the panacea in the control of schistosomiasis. These are perhaps useful as descriptive terms, but the problem is that, if adopted as basic methods, each approach tends to have proponents who give inadequate or no attention to other methods and, on occasion, oppose and defame them. This retards the development of the best control programmes, which must be based on an objective evaluation of all methods in relation to each situation, which in turn involves regarding control as a unified concept, and not as consisting of a number of disjointed and mutually-exclusive methods. If instead we could consider the epidemiological course of events in schistosomiasis in relation to the definitive host, the first free-living aquatic stage, and think in terms of the dynamics of transmission in an ecological complex, and of ways and means of dealing with them, it would broaden our understanding and throw light on the uncertainties of some present-day control programmes.

Selection of Control Method or Methods

In the choice and application of control measures it is likely to be forgotten that schistosomiasis does not pose a single disease problem. The infection as caused by the different species of the parasite, each species possibly comprising various strains which differ in their geographical distribution and vary in their epidemiology, affects the body in different ways and responds differently to treatment. The bionomics of the intermediate hosts involved and their ecological needs, and the habits of the people and the social environment which determines contact frequency with natural waters, are so varied that different situations and varying problems in the different geographical locations involved are presented. Lack of appreciation of these fundamental facts has led to a 'shot-gun' technique of applying all possible methods indiscriminately in control, without knowing how far the cost of each is justified by results under local conditions. Thus, money and effort are eventually wasted. The need for integrated research before a control programme can be practised effectively deserves careful consideration by workers in schistosomiasis control.

Land reclamation and change of agricultural practices could be very important to certain countries, outstanding examples of which are to be found in the Orient. Irrigation hydraulics in relation to snail harbourages are extremely important in the Middle East and in Africa. Progress made to date in schistosomiasis control has resulted from the integrated action of epidemiologists, biologists and engineers, but its potentialities have not yet been developed to full effectiveness. The complexities of the problem are such that each of these groups must absorb some of the training of the other, and all must adopt the epidemiological viewpoint for maximum effectiveness.

Use of molluscicides, with all its present limitations, and the inherent defects involved in a chemical attack on a disease arising from faulty environment and poor sanitary habits of the people, still provides a most hopeful tool for bringing transmission under control in a number of situations. It should be fully realized, however, that in a larger irrigation system effective appli-

cation of molluscicides becomes an impossibility without the closest partici-
pation of the engineers and the agriculturalists [FAROOQ, 1964]. This is
discussed on pages 533 to 591.

Schistosomiasis endemic areas are remarkably diverse. They range from
the temperate zone to the tropics; from areas where cold or lack of rainfall
confines transmission to very short periods to warm wet areas where it can
occur almost continuously; from flowing water in streams and canals to
static waters in swamps and pools which may dry up during five to seven
months of the year; from habitats where aquatic snails spend their whole life
in the water to those where amphibious snails spend most of their life on
damp soil. It is obvious from these examples that seasonal, climatic and
hydrological changes have marked effects on the life cycle of the intermediate
hosts, on the production of cercariae and on the transmission of the infection.
The changing characteristics of each area will influence the choice of control
methods and the period most suitable for their effective application. The basic
observations needed for making these judgements have been outlined on
pages 499 to 510. Unfortunately, in many areas such observations have often
not been made.

The most effective method used in the control of snails ranges from a
variety of engineering and agricultural techniques to the application of
molluscicides. The selection of the method or methods must depend on an
assessment of the local conditions and the cost of the control measures,
compared with the data obtained from an analysis of the economic stress
caused by snail-borne diseases.

In some circumstances snail populations can be reduced or eliminated
by drainage, filling, water management, modification of agricultural practices
and similar environmental measures. In other circumstances this can be done
only by the application of molluscicides. The more common situations often
involve thousands of square kilometers of difficult terrain which may include
habitats in streams, pools, reservoirs, swamps, irrigation canals, rice-fields,
drainage ditches and similar places. For these reasons, effective control at
reasonable cost in most areas can be obtained only by a combination of
methods, involving both modification of habitats and application of molluscicides to the remaining colonies.

If a combination of methods is to be used, it is necessary to consider the
order in which they should be implemented. For example, in dealing with a
very heavily infested area, or with an outbreak of epidemic proportions, the
intensive use of molluscicides may be required until more permanent measures
can be instituted. On the other hand, in many areas certain measures directed

toward habitat reduction or elimination will be the most logical initial step, followed by the application of molluscicides to residual colonies [WHO, 1965b].

The different approaches to control are discussed in detail in subsequent chapters. Decision on the choice of single or combined methods depends, as stated earlier, on local conditions, therefore it is difficult to generalize on this and aspect. Available methods of snail control are outlined on pages 458 to 532 and 533 to 591 and on therapy on pages 592 to 608. However, recent attempts at developing mathematical formulations for describing the transmission of schistosomiasis have led to basic assumptions and a set of parameters, arbitrarily selected as constants, built into a schistosomiasis mathematical model [MACDONALD, 1965], for subsequent testing of the effect of control, by alteration of their values, over a period of years of transmission. Analysis of the significance of these factors (contamination, snails, exposure, and longevity of the parasite in the vertebrate host) in the maintenance of transmission, according to the model, have indicated, among other things, the following:

(1) Treatment carried out to an extent which does not approach eradication of the infection is of great value to the recipients but is of little value to the general population in reducing infection rates, and cannot therefore be considered as of public health significance.

(2) The only method of limited control which has any public health value within this definition is the control of the snail factor.

(3) Sanitation as a prime measure of control would require an absolute standard of sanitation to attain the 'break point' in the mean worm load below which the infection is unable to maintain itself in a community. The common supposition that 'sanitation diseases' are best controlled by provision of latrines finds very little support.

(4) A very much more effective aspect of sanitation is reduction of the frequency of contact with possibly contaminated water, chiefly by provision of safe water supplies which makes frequent resort to natural waters unnecessary. Therefore safe water supplies are more important than latrines, and sanitation policy in respect of schistosomiasis needs to be reoriented in this way.

(5) A very strong implication of the 'break point' is that schistosomiasis campaigns should be very intensive and, if necessary, limited in extent.

It should, however, be pointed out that in the present state of our knowledge the above indications should at best be taken as tentative, as the existing mathematical models for schistosomiasis transmission [HAIRSTON, 1962; MACDONALD, 1965] cannot be regarded as truly predictive until extensive data, as detailed on pages 250 to 336, become available from intensive *ad hoc* field studies. Such data should enable the two models to predict, in principle, the threshold values of the different variables that determine the dynamics of schistosomiasis transmission, as also the intensity and the duration of individual control measures necessary to bring about its interruption. All the effort and time involved in the collection of such data should, however, be found very rewarding.

In summation this chapter may be concluded by reference to a stimulating discussion of the methods to be considered in financing disease control programmes. In the Seventeenth Charles Franklin Craig Lecture, WOLMAN had the following to say:

'We need not debate, therefore, that scientific knowledge is sufficiently far in advance of application to make it possible for us to reduce or even eliminate many of the environmental diseases, provided we could produce the economic and social climate essential for the introduction of our well understood techniques. Money, therefore, becomes almost the major key to disease eradication in many areas of which we speak. It is not the sole source of hope, because the development of informed professional workers, of improved legislative sanctions and of wider and more efficient administrative machinery are all essential parts of a major effort.'

It is believed that these comments are particularly applicable to schistosomiasis control.

References

FAROOQ, M.: J. trop. med. Hyg. *67:* 265 (1964).
FAROOQ, M. and MALLAH, M. B.: Bull. Wld Hlth Org. *35:* 377 (1966).
FAROOQ, M.; HAIRSTON, N. G., and SAMAAN, S. A.: Bull. Wld Hlth Org. *35:* 369 (1966).
GODDARD, H. A.: Principles of administration applied to nursing service. (World Health Organization, Monogr. Ser., No. 41 (Geneva 1958).
HAIRSTON, N. G.: Bull. Wld Hlth Org. *33:* 45 (1965).
MACDONALD, G.: Trans. roy. Soc. trop. Med. Hyg. *59:* 489 (1965).
SWAROOP, S.: Statistical considerations and methodology in malaria eradication; part I: Statistical considerations. Unpublished document WHO/Mal/240, WHO/HS/102 (1959).
WHO: Manual on epidemiological evaluation and surveillance in malaria eradication. Unpublished document MHO/PA/214.62 (1962).
WHO: Snail control in the prevention of bilharziasis. World Health Organization, Monogr. Ser., No. 50 (Geneva 1965a).
WHO: WHO Expert Committee on Bilharziasis, Geneva 1964; Third Report. Wld Hlth Org. techn. Rep. Ser. *299* (1965b).
WOLMAN, A.: Amer. J. trop. Med. Hyg. *2:* 557 (1953).

Chapter 10

Epidemiology and Control of Schistosomiasis, pp. 458–532
(Karger, Basel and University Park Press, Baltimore 1973)

Chemical Control of Snails

L. S. RITCHIE

With the collaboration of E. PAULINI, W. R. JOBIN, V. DE V. CLARKE and A. E. H. HIGGINS

Introduction

The control of schistosomiasis by molluscicides has advanced more in the past two decades than other measures used to interrupt transmission of this infection. Several chemicals have been found that kill snails at 0.1 ppm, formulations have been improved, and better strategy and methods for applying them have been recognized. The use of molluscicides is costly, but an inexpensive control method is not available. Successful use of molluscicides in sizeable areas has been achieved in Japan, Venezuela, Brazil, Rhodesia, Egypt and Puerto Rico. Current advances and accomplishments appear to warrant greater control efforts with molluscicides.

There are both advantages and limitations to using molluscicides. They stop transmission of schistosomiasis almost immediately. Although eradication of snails has been accomplished only in circumscribed areas where physical and ecological situations are simple, the present status of molluscicides warrants the hope that transmission of schistosomiasis can be interrupted without complete snail eradication.

It is an advantage to have chemical control of snails in the hands of trained personnel and under the control of a single organization, the public health administration. Sometimes other agencies have supervisory control over agricultural lands and irrigation water and, in such cases, their co-operation is essential for an effective molluscicidal programme. However, active co-operation of the general public will not be necessary, although it is essential for other control measures against schistosomiasis and is often difficult to obtain.

Whereas molluscicides are specifically for destruction of snails, certain other methods provide control for additional diseases, improvement in agriculture or betterment of health. However, there is the possibility of dual benefits from herbicidal molluscicides where combined control of schistosomiasis and fascioliasis might be achieved. It is important in planning any control programme to equate cost and over-all benefits of each control measure against each other measure.

Most effective molluscicides are toxic in varying degrees for other organisms. Some must be handled with special care. It is essential to ensure that their application to bodies of water will not cause harm to the human or animal population and crops. Moreover, the over-all balance of nature must receive consideration.

This chapter includes a brief historical review of molluscicides, procedures and results of comprehensive laboratory evaluations and field testing, characterizations of the most effective molluscicides and practical aspects of application. In practice, molluscicides have not always equalled expectations, due to a number of factors: diversity and extent of habitats, inadequate strategy and methods of application, and poor understanding of dispersal patterns have sometimes resulted in the chemical not contacting all the snails; physiological differences, habits and ecology of the various species of snails may have been involved; and characteristics of the chemical may not have been adequately understood. These points fall within the scope of this presentation.

Historical Aspects

Prior to 1945, chemical control of snail hosts of schistosomiasis had been attempted for 25 to 30 years in Egypt and Japan [for historical reviews see KOMIYA, 1961; AYAD, 1961]. The chemicals of choice in the respective countries were copper sulphate [CHANDLER, 1920], calcium oxide [NARABAYASHI, 1915] and calcium cyanamide [MIYAGAWA, 1913].

From 1946 to 1955, about 7,000 compounds were screened in the laboratory, and some were evaluated under field conditions. As a result, sodium pentachlorophenate (NaPCP) and dinitro-*o*-cyclohexylphenol (DNCHP) proved more effective than the above-named compounds. NaPCP, DNCHP and copper sulphate were extensively evaluated in such places as Egypt, Japan, the Philippines, Brazil and Venezuela. In this period, little was done on formulating molluscicides, except to provide a relatively soluble product (e. g. NaPCP vs. PCP), or a wettable powder (DNCHP). The limitations of molluscicides under certain environmental conditions were recognized, particularly in the Philippines [McMULLEN *et al.*, 1954]. This led to emphasis on the importance of biological study of the snail and the host-parasite relationships of the infection, and application of a broad spectrum of knowledge through multiple control measures [McMULLEN, 1952].

During the decade 1956 to 1965, leadership and co-ordination of research on schistosomiasis, including molluscicides, was provided by the World Health Organization. About 12 research agencies throughout the world agreed to co-operate in the evaluation and development of molluscicides, with several chemical companies contributing to the search for additional active compounds. A standardized procedure for definitive laboratory screening was developed [WHO, 1965a] and adapted to tests for comprehensive evaluations. Improvements in field testing were made with suggestions for sequential integration of laboratory and field evaluations and correlation of the results from these efforts. 'Available' molluscicides in 1965 included niclosamide, NaPCP, and copper sulphate. New ideas relative to the use of molluscicides include snail repopulation control by means of prolonged or repeated applications with low concentrations [SHARAF EL DIN and EL NAGAR, 1955; WILLIAMS *et al.*, 1957] and emphasis on transmission control rather than snail killing [McMULLEN and HARRY, 1958]. A practical example of the latter is focal-radial control [AYAD, 1961]. The advantage of herbicidal-molluscicidal compounds became apparent and the inclusion of such in the 'available' group is desirable.

As presently conceived, chemical control of snail hosts of schistosomiasis is based on the assumption that the snail is the weakest link in the parasite cycle and provides the quickest and most efficient means of interrupting transmission. In spite of current limitations of molluscicides, it is generally agreed that studies must be continued to improve their effective use.

Evaluation of Molluscicides

While a snail control programme may not become directly involved in the screening of compounds or in the testing of their molluscicidal potency, its success will be dependent on the fact that this type of investigation must be done by someone. It is essential, therefore, for all of those involved in snail control to have some understanding of how compounds are screened, what has been done in this field, and some familiarity with the conclusions reached. This section will be devoted to these objectives. The 'available' and 'candidate' molluscicides, and methods for their application are discussed later (pages 481 to 492 and 492 to 523).

The evaluation of a compound as a molluscicide includes the following major steps: (1) laboratory screening; (2) comprehensive laboratory evaluation; and (3) field evaluation. The last two become involved in a number of subsidiary investigations. The tests required before a molluscicide can be recommended with confidence will be considered below.

Laboratory Screening

Experience in both the laboratory and the field has confirmed the expressed need [WHO, 1961] for screening of additional kinds of molluscicides, e.g. there are needs for highly active molluscicides of low mammalian toxicity that are relatively cheap, combined herbicide-molluscicide compounds, and products highly specific for snails. Other desirable attributes include good chemical stability, ease and safety of application, and low cost of application [WHO, 1965a]. Although it is unlikely that a single compound will be found to have all the desirable characteristics of the 'ideal molluscicide', it is important to combine as many merits as possible. There are presently several highly rated molluscicides, but each has some disadvantages, among which are biocidal activity, lack of ovicidal activity and high cost of production.

Laboratory screening for molluscicidal compounds may be done in two steps, *preliminary* and *definitive*. Preliminary screening can be either an empirical test or a fundamental investigation with a standard test. The latter, although desirable, is not always deemed expedient by chemical companies, who are primarily responsible. Certain compromises may be indicated to expedite this work, since standardized definitive tests are a sequel. The use of a non-host snail has been suggested for testing by companies in non-endemic areas where severe quarantine regulations are imposed. The cost of snail culture can be further minimized by using immature specimens that can be reared in 2 to 3 weeks in mass numbers on simple diets [ROWAN, 1958; RITCHIE[1]].

A standard method of testing against both amphibious and aquatic snails is a prerequisite for definitive laboratory screening. Such tests have been extensively evaluated and revised according to the experiences of a number of investigators (see annex), thus allowing comparison of results obtained by different workers and serving as a basis for a battery of tests for comprehensive laboratory evaluations. Representative species of host snails should be used in definitive screening tests.

1   RITCHIE, L. S.: in WHO unpublished document MOL/INF 15 (1964).

Comprehensive Laboratory Evaluations

Comprehensive laboratory evaluations of molluscicides may be classified under three headings: (1) characterization of molluscicidal activity; (2) effects of physico-chemical factors; and (3) toxico-pharmacological evaluations. A battery of tests is necessary to fulfil each of these categories. These tests are largely based on the WHO standardized test and some are still not developed. The sequence in which they are performed and the integration of field tests into the series is important, relative to cost-efficiency.

Characterization of Molluscicidal Activity

a) *Time-concentration relationships (T × C)*. Among the comprehensive tests used in evaluating molluscicides, time-concentration relationships should be given priority in order to provide information essential for effective planning of field-screening tests. Moreover, this evaluation affords basic information for other comprehensive evaluations. T × C tests were made first by HOFFMAN and ZAKHARY [1953], and developed by GILLET and BRUAUX [1961], PAULINI *et al.* [1961], and RITCHIE *et al.* [1964]. The shortest exposure time giving maximum efficiency varies for different molluscicides [GILLET and BRUAUX, 1961; BRUAUX and GILLET, 1961; RITCHIE, 1964]. Niclosamide and N-tritylmorpholine are highly active even with 1-hour exposures or less [GILLET and BRUAUX, 1961; EL TAWIL[2]; RITCHIE, 1964; RITCHIE *et al.*[3]; CROSSLAND[4]]. For the organo-tins and DNCHP, a 6-hour exposure approximates the shortest interval that will give maximum efficiencies. Even longer times may be required for copper compounds, organo-leads and NaPCP.

HAIRSTON[5] discussed the theoretical and practical importance of T × C tests, and recommended plotting concentrations for specific mortalities (LC_{50} and LC_{90}) against time on double logarithmic paper. His comment that studies on factors affecting the T × C relationships may be rewarding supported the earlier report of PAULINI [1956]. He observed that resistance to the toxic effects of $CuSO_4$ and NaPCP increased proportionately with concentration up to a certain point, beyond which the relationship was reversed.

2   EL TAWIL: in WHO unpublished document MOL/INF 14 (1963).
3   RITCHIE, L.S.; FOX, I.; BERRÍOS-DURÁN, L.A., and FRICK, L.P.: in WHO unpublished document MOL/INF 18 (1964).
4   CROSSLAND, N.O.: in WHO unpublished document MOL/INF 16 (1964).
5   HAIRSTON, N.G.: in WHO unpublished document MOL/INF 4 (1962).

Time of exposure for aquatic snails in static water is related to stability of the chemical. As the time of exposure increases, the concentration gradually decreases. Consequently, $T \times C$ is a continuously changing relationship. For flowing water, the same situation appears to prevail, but because of different circumstances. Surface water at the centre of a stream or channel moves faster than water at the margins or bottom, resulting in a progressive dilution and a reciprocal increase in contact time as the chemical is carried downstream; again the $T \times C$ is a changing relationship. Niclosamide has been reported to be equally effective with 1- and 24-hour exposures, but less efficient with 6 hours. Serving as a hypothetical case, such a molluscicide might kill all snails for a distance with a 1-hour application, then fall short of 100% mortality for a limited distance, and again kill all snails.

Although studies on $T \times C$ relationships may be rewarding, their real value depends on correlation with field evaluations. It is essential that these studies be made in both standing and flowing water, with benefit of chemical analysis, to provide concentrations and time of exposure. Corresponding evaluations for amphibious snails may not be feasible when applications are on moist soil, but should be possible in standing water.

b) Basic chemical stability of molluscicides. Niclosamide was storage-stable for 9 months under sub-tropical conditions [STRUFE and GÖNNERT, 1962], while Fox *et al.* [1966] reported loss of activity within 3 years. Experience with NaPCP, DNCHP and CuSO$_4$ indicates that they are sufficiently stable in storage.

In laboratory tests the concentration of NaPCP remained unchanged at 10 ppm for 72 days [DOBROVOLNY and HASKINS, 1953]. This marked stability was reflected in field tests in Egypt, but not in Brazil [WRIGHT *et al.*, 1958]. Studies were made on the basic stabilities of molluscicides by allowing LC$_{90}$ concentrations (24-hour exposures) to stand for increasing intervals before exposing snails [RITCHIE and BERRÍOS-DURÁN, 1969]. Onsets of decay in days were: NaPCP in excess of 32; DNCHP between 16 and 32; organo-tins and organo-leads after 8 days; CuSO$_4$ after 6 days; and niclosamide after 6 days. MEYLING *et al.* [1962] found 1 ppm of niclosamide undiminished (by analysis) after 13 days, but WEBBE [1961] reported reduction of this product after 24 h in standing water (field test).

Information is too limited to state categorically how stable a molluscicide should be. This will depend on other qualities of the chemical, type of habitat, toxicity hazards and the balance of nature.

c) Snail behaviourisms that protect from or enhance exposure. Such observations are commonly made in conjunction with other tests, but special studies may be indicated. Protective behaviourisms include crawling-out of water, quick contraction into the shell, and secretion of mucus. Distension of the body, and inability to contract deeply into the shell enhance exposure. It is essential to make these observations in field evaluations.

d) Residual potentials of molluscicides. BARBOSA *et al.* [1956] and BARBOSA [1961] reported a remarkable residual potential for copper carbonate. Five of 13 slow-flowing streams remained snail-free for one year after treatment, and mud collected from some of these streams after one year still contained enough copper to kill snails. Cuprous oxide (SCS), when placed on filter paper, persisted as a lethal residue for snails after three months with weekly changes of water [FRICK *et al.*, 1964]. FLOCH and DESCHIENS [1962a] also evaluated the residuals of SCS and other insoluble compounds with good results. Residual copper may have a biocidal spectrum that is very destructive to the balance of nature [SHIFF and GARNETT, 1961]. NaPCP and triphenyltin acetate with 5 and 8 g/m², respectively, in field-plot tests (Philippines) still killed *O. quadrasi* introduced after three weeks [WHO][6].

e) Prolonged concentrations. HOFFMAN and ZAKHARY [1953] recognized possible benefit from prolonged applications. Field-trials using $CuSO_4$ as a 'chemical barrier' were first conducted in the Sudan [SHARAF EL DIN and EL NAGAR, 1955], subsequently in Egypt [AYAD, 1961, 1962], in Kenya [TEESDALE *et al.*, 1961], and again in the Sudan [MALEK, 1962]. Laboratory studies by OLIVIER and HASKINS [1960] gave further impetus for evaluating prolonged applications. Although concentrations of 0.05 and 0.1 ppm of NaPCP did not kill snails after 7 to 8 days, oviposition was reduced, and eggs recovered at 24-hour intervals were all dead. YEO [1965] outlined a plan for prolonged applications that might make non-ovicidal molluscicides practicable. The feasibility of this plan has been tested by CROSSLAND *et al.*[7] and BOYCE *et al.* [1966].

RITCHIE *et al.* [1965] suppressed cercarial emergence *(S. mansoni)* with 0.05 ppm $CuSO_4$. The snails survived a month, but within that time emergence of cercariae had almost stopped. With 0.1 ppm $CuSO_4$, the snails were killed within a week, during which time the number of cercariae was reduced.

Further studies on prolonged or continuous application of molluscicides are indicated. The more stable compounds may be more practicable in this regard when the chemical must be carried by water for long distances. MALEK

6   WHO: Reports from Philippines-9 schistosomiasis control pilot project; in WHO unpublished document MOL/INF 16 (1964).
7   CROSSLAND, N.O.; BEESLEY, J.S.S., and MESMER, E.T.: in WHO unpublished document MOL/INF 20 (1965).

[1962] was of the opinion that NaPCP should prove cheaper than CuSO₄ in prolonged applications.

Prolonged exposure of snails to molluscicides could be greatly facilitated by the biocidal rubber formulation reported by CARDARELLI *et al.*[8]. In this case the molluscicidal agent incorporated was bis(tri-*n*-butyltin) oxide. Prolonged effective release against *Biomphalaria glabrata* was demonstrated by BERRÍOS-DURÁN and RITCHIE [1968], HOPF and GOLL[9], and DE SOUZA and PAULINI[10]. The latter also reported successful field trials.

f) Susceptibilities of different stages and sizes of the snails. In addition to mature snails and eggs for evaluating molluscicides, HOPF[11] and WEBBE and STURROCK [1964] reported using 'young' snails. Others have used a more complete stage-size array [RITCHIE *et al.*, 1963b, c, d; FRICK *et al.*, 1964a, b; FRICK and DE JIMENEZ, 1964]. Most of these studies have been made with *Biomphalaria* snails.

Some molluscicides are ineffective against snail eggs, including *N*-tritylmorpholine. The ovicidal compounds include niclosamide, NaPCP, DNCHP, organo-tins, Gramoxone and Reglone. CuSO₄ and tributyl-lead acetate are active against eggs, but less so than against hatched snails. GÖNNERT [1961] reviewed studies on niclosamide, and concluded that it is equally effective against eggs at all stages of incubation. RITCHIE *et al.* [1965] were in accord when exposures were for 24 h, but with 6-hour treatments, eggs incubated for 4 to 5 days were less susceptible than newly-laid eggs. With 24-hour exposures, all hatched snails were about equally as susceptible as eggs, while for 6-hour exposures, mature snails and adolescents (8–10 mm) were less susceptible. A review of literature by OLIVIER and HASKINS [1960] and OLIVIER *et al.* [1962] showed that NaPCP is similarly active against embryos and hatched snails, but as both increase in size they become a little less susceptible [OLIVIER and HASKINS, 1960; RITCHIE *et al.*, 1963d]. DNCHP was effective against embryos of all ages with 24-hour exposures, but with 6-hour exposures the older embryos were less susceptible. Although CuSO₄ is toxic for eggs [CAMEY and PAULINI, 1962; OLIVIER *et al.*, 1962] a review of the literature by the latter showed lack of agreement on whether they are as susceptible as hatched snails. Recent observations indicate that the eggs are less susceptible [BRUAUX and

8   CARDARELLI, N.F.; KELLER, R.F., and JACKSON, D.L.: Unpublished report to the B.F. Goodrich Co., Akron, Ohio, USA (1966).
9   HOPF, H.S. and GOLL, P.H.: in WHO unpublished document PD/MOL/69.4 (1969).
10   DE SOUZA, C.P. and PAULINI, E.: in WHO unpublished document PD/MOL/69.9 (1969).
11   HOPF, H.S.: in WHO unpublished document MOL/INF 4 (1962).

GILLET, 1961; JOBIN and UNRAU, 1967; RITCHIE *et al.*, unpublished; EL GINDY, 1968; NELSON, pers. comm.]. SCS was less effective against eggs than against hatched snails [FRICK *et al.*, 1964b; PAULINI *et al.*, 1963]. Organo-tin compounds were highly ovicidal at 0.1 ppm with 24-hour exposures [HOPF[12]; FRICK and DE JIMENEZ, 1964; WEBBE and STURROCK, 1964; CAMEY and PAULINI, 1964]. Gramoxone and Reglone (herbicides) are ovicidal at favourable levels [CAMEY *et al.*, 1966; WEBBE and STURROCK, 1964]. The latter two compounds were molluscicidal even after absorption by algae [PAULINI and CAMEY, 1968].

For eggs of oncomelanid snails, CHI and WINKLER [1962] found $CuSO_4$ effective at 10 ppm with prolonged exposures, NaPCP at 2 ppm after one week. Since these eggs are often laid above the water level on moist soil or objects [WAGNER and WONG, 1956; WAGNER and MOORE, 1956], ovicides are not very practicable. Since newly-hatched oncomelanid snails are aquatic, it might be more feasible to destroy them rather than the eggs [WILLIAMS *et al.*, 1957].

Hatched snails generally become less susceptible to molluscicides as they increase in age, but not always. Deviations appeared to be related to length of exposure and kind of chemical. Newly-hatched snails (1–24 h old) were more sensitive than older stages to NaPCP, $CuSO_4$, SCS and organo-tins. On the other hand, newly-hatched specimens were as resistant, or more so, than mature specimens against DNCHP. All hatched snails were equally susceptible to niclosamide with 24-hour exposures, while with 6-hour exposures the newly-hatched and juveniles were more susceptible than older specimens. The juvenile (3–5 mm) tends to be a susceptible stage, while the adolescent (8–10 mm) may be similar to either the juvenile or the mature snail. With some chemicals there may be a susceptibility gradient in correlation with increasing size. The LC_{50} for N-tritylmorpholine increases as *B. glabrata* grows from 3 to 20 mm in diameter [BOYCE *et al.*, 1967].

Chemical Degradation of Molluscicides Due to Physicochemical Factors

a) The effects of light. Ultraviolet light sources have been used for laboratory testing, because of ease of standardization and better reproducibility of results. However, variability is common in the quality of ultraviolet light from different lamps, so results should be validated by tests using sunlight [WHO, 1965a].

12   HOPF, H.S.: in WHO unpublished document MOL/INF 6 (1962).

Apparently CuSO$_4$ is not affected by light, while NaPCP has been reported repeatedly to be photosensitive [STRUFE and GÖNNERT, 1962]. These investigators found that light reduced niclosamide, but to a lesser degree than NaPCP. The photosensitivity of niclosamide was found to be affected by the amount of calcium and magnesium in the water. Sodium silicate had the same effect in high concentrations, but with low concentrations it had a stabilizing influence. The pH values from 5 to 9 did not affect photosensitivity of niclosamide. Other reports support the conclusion of GÖNNERT and STRUFE [1961] that niclosamide is relatively photostable [SHIFF, 1961; MEYLING et al., 1962; GILLET and BRUAUX, 1961; ABDALLA and NASR, 1961].

When LC$_{90}$ concentrations for 24-hour treatments were placed in intense sunlight for 4 h, there was no loss in activity for niclosamide, DNCHP and tri-n-butyltin acetate. On the other hand, NaPCP was reduced considerably after 1 h, NaPCP by 50% [RITCHIE et al., unpublished].

The seriousness of photosensitivity of molluscicides under field conditions has not been fully determined. The best evidence is provided by NaPCP. It showed marked stability in field trials in Egypt, where a concentration of 10 ppm was easily maintained in a canal 30 km long, and persisted for 6 weeks in adjoining drainage canals [WRIGHT et al., 1958]. In Brazil, higher concentrations were required and the results were erratic [DOBROVOLNY and BARBOSA, 1953]. MEYLING et al. [1959] reported that degradation of NaPCP was enhanced by hard water. These investigators and PITCHFORD [1961] were convinced that NaPCP cannot be used successfully in the Transvaal because of photosensitivity. HIATT et al., [1960] suggested that turbidity of the water in Egypt protected it from sunlight. Turbidity due to soil inactivates NaPCP, but this may not be conflicting, as 'cloudiness' of the water can be due to different kinds of matter. There are other protective factors against photodegradation, including depth of the water and shade due to plants. Therefore, it is essential to survey environmental conditions whenever a molluscicide is to be selected.

b) The effect of pH on molluscicides. HOPF et al. [1963] showed that copper compounds were more molluscicidal with acid pH values. GÖNNERT and STRUFE [1961] found that niclosamide was unaffected within a range of pH 5 to 9, while FOX et al. [1963b] noted detoxification beyond both limits of this range. MEYLING et al. [1959] found NaPCP unaffected by pH. On the other hand, DE SOUZA and PAULINI [1967] reported that niclosamide and pentachlorophenol showed higher toxicity for *B. glabrata* at pH 6, decreasing at pH 7 and 8. This was more pronounced with eggs than mature snails. The activity of organo-tins was unchanged within a range of 5 to 8.5 [FLOCH and

Deschiens, 1962b]. The hydrolysis of *N*-tritylmorpholine is rapid below pH 7 [Beynon *et al.*, 1967; Meyling *et al.*, 1966]. These results indicate that the effects of pH must be determined for each candidate molluscicide.

    c) Inactivation of molluscicides by physical and chemical adsorption. That $CuSO_4$ is adsorbed by mud has been reported repeatedly [Paulini, 1958]. At least 20 to 30 times more chemical is required in the field to equal laboratory mortalities. NaPCP is also inactivated by mud and even fine sand [Dobrovolny and Barbosa, 1953; Dobrovolny and Haskins, 1953; Pereira and Mendoça, 1954; Klock *et al.*, 1957]. In parallel tests, Strufe and Gönnert [1962] showed that niclosamide was adsorbed much less than NaPCP, but for both, adsorption was irreversible. Duhm *et al.* [1961] demonstrated adsorption and inactivation of niclosamide by plants by using a sample labelled with ^{14}C.

    Inactivation of molluscicides by adsorption and absorption is important and warrants clarification. As an empirical test, the extent of inactivation caused by mud may seem adequate, but it does not reveal the factors involved. The need for more effective testing is indicated.

    d) The effects of water hardness on molluscicides. Gönnert and Strufe [1962] reported that 0.5 ppm niclosamide in water containing different combinations and concentrations of minerals of water hardness (342 to 500 ppm at 30 °C) still killed nearly all of the snails after the mixture of molluscicide and minerals had stood 5, 10 and 15 days. NaPCP was nearly as stable, while $CuSO_4$ showed progressive inactivation. On the other hand, Meyling *et al.* [1962] reported that the activity of niclosamide (0.5 and 1.0 ppm) was reduced in naturally hard water (total hardness, 400 ppm $CaCO_3$).

    e) The effects of temperature on molluscicides. Chandler [1920] noted that temperature influenced the activity of $CuSO_4$, and Hoffman and Zakhary [1951] found that the LC_{50} values were 13 and 0.25 ppm at 14 and 26 °C, respectively. Kuntz [1957] reported that snails were remarkably more susceptible to DNCHP, NaPCP and $CuSO_4$ with higher temperatures. Only half as much DNCHP was required from June to September as compared with the cooler months [Kuntz and Wells, 1951]. In comparative tests, involving NaPCP and niclosamide, the latter was affected slightly less by temperature [Strufe and Gönnert, 1962; Gönnert and Strufe, 1962]. However, temperature had little effect unless it went as low as 11 to 13 °C. The greater activity induced by higher temperatures must be equated against other factors, e.g. complications with agricultural pursuits and less availability of labour during the warmer months [Kuntz, 1957].

    f) Bacterial degradation of molluscicides. Etges *et al.* [1965] isolated a Gram-negative coccobacillus from a snail aquarium that degraded molluscicides (probably genus *Pseudomonas*) [BELL *et al.*, 1966]. It derived total nitrogen, but not carbon, from niclosamide, *N*-tritylmorpholine, DNCHP and 2-tert.-butyl-4-6-dinitrophenol. The first three and especially niclosamide were reduced in activity after 5 to 7 days of bacterial action. Bacterial growth did not occur with NaPCP and 2–4-dinitro-6-phenylphenol. The authors concluded that bacterial degradation of molluscicides might account for significant loss of activity, especially in sluggish streams and standing water. Moreover, they noted the protective benefits of bacterial degradation against cumulations of pesticides. Subsequently, molluscicide-degrading bacteria were recovered repeatedly in field surveys of four Caribbean areas [ETGES *et al.*, 1969].

g) Absorption of molluscicides by living cells. Recently, it was reported that absorption of NaPCP and niclosamide by yeast cells accounted for considerable loss of these molluscicide [DE SOUZA and PAULINI, 1968]. The same has been found true for the organo-tin and organo-lead compounds[13]. The absorption of Gramoxone and Reglone by algae also occurs [PAULINI and CAMEY, 1965], but these compounds were still molluscicidal after absorption.

Field Evaluations

It is virtually impossible to duplicate in the laboratory the great variety of factors, and an even greater number of combinations thereof, that may affect molluscicides under field conditions. Consequently, field observations on the performance of a candidate molluscicide are indispensable as one phase of its evaluation. However, one must be aware of the limitations of field testing, because of variability and combinations of factors involved. Therefore, generalizations based on results obtained in the field should be made with reservation until there has been extensive replication of tests.

Before starting field evaluations on highly active molluscicides, the practical economic aspects of these endeavours must be considered. The number of compounds tested in a given period of time must be limited because the various stages of field evaluation require much time, the number of suitable testing sites is often limited, and seasonal factors (drought or rainfall) often ruin field tests with loss of both time and molluscicide. Therefore, it is justifiable to limit field evaluations to compounds that have: (1) cost-efficiency ratios equal to, or better than, NaPCP; (2) special, uncommon properties

13   PAULINI, E.: in Annual grant report to WHO, for the year 1968.

(residual or herbicidal effects, etc.); and (3) been formulated in new, unique ways, which promise greater efficiency.

In order to carry out field evaluations with a minimum waste of time, energy and material, it is advisable to distinguish three distinct and consecutive stages in the work: (1) field screening; (2) field trials; and (3) transmission control projects. These stages have points in common, but each has distinct objectives in addition to difference in magnitude. There are certain general requirements, some of which are self-evident, while others are inadequately fulfilled as pointed out by Paulini[14] who emphasized the need for: (1) better standardization of tests for aquatic snails; (2) more information on the environment; (3) different time-concentration relationships with at least two of the lower concentrations giving partial kills; (4) more replicate tests; and (5) use of reference molluscicides. To these may be added the need for more adequate sampling of the snails before and after treatment, with data from a comparable non-treated control [Hairston, 1965].

Regarding the environment, the following information should be reported in increasing detail with each stage of field testing [WHO, 1965b]:

(a) nature and size of water body, with rate of flow, if applicable;

(b) type and amount of vegetation;

(c) temperature, pH and turbidity of the water;

(d) characteristics of the bottom stratum;

(e) intensity of sunlight; amount of ultraviolet light if indicated;

(f) complete water analysis, whenever possible.

The desirability of a sequential plan for integrating laboratory and field evaluations has been recognized [WHO, 1965a]. The objectives are to designate an order for performing laboratory and field tests that will: (1) reduce the time required for final evaluation; (2) provide better defined cut-off points for candidate molluscicides that prove inadequate; and (3) avoid introducing time-consuming tests prematurely for chemicals that will ultimately be abandoned. The validity of such a plan is based on the premise that merits and demerits of a product are not of equal significance. A precise sequence is not possible, but each investigator should envisage a plan, based on his own insight. The following plan may serve as a useful model.

After laboratory screening, the first comprehensive evaluations should involve time-concentration relationships and basic chemical stability in working dilutions (LC_{90} values), and storage stability tests should be started. If indicated, field screening tests may follow and, if these are favourable, lab-

14   Paulini, E.: in WHO unpublished document MOL/INF 15 (1964).

oratory evaluations started on the stage-size array susceptibilities, prolonged low concentration tests against normal and infected snails, biocidal tests against other animals and crops, and mammalian toxicity tests to reveal any hazards in handling. In the meantime types of formulation must be developed and evaluated both in laboratory and field screening tests before 'field trials' are started. If the results of field trials are poorer than expected from prior testing, possible ill-effects of physico-chemical factors of the environment should be explored. A good example of this need is NaPCP, which gave superior results in Egypt, was moderately effective in Brazil and relatively ineffective in the Transvaal. Finally, after exhaustive preparation including repeated determinations of snail population densities, recording of data on environmental characteristics of the snail habitat, and observations on the status of the infection in the human and other possible hosts, 'transmission control' projects may be started. This should include the assistance of specialists in ecology, malacology, engineering and parasitology.

A brief outline of the objectives, principles, and techniques related to each stage of testing are given in the following paragraphs.

Field Screening

This may be carried out under somewhat artificial, controlled conditions, in order to: (1) compare the effectiveness of candidate molluscicides against various species of medically important snails; (2) examine the effects of molluscicides on other aquatic animals and plants; (3) test the effectiveness of various time-concentration regimes in type-habitats; and (4) evaluate molluscicidal formulations. The repeated use of the same test site is indicated, to afford better comparisons. The use of caged snails is acceptable in order to perform tests more frequently. Laboratory-reared snails may be preferable to those of natural populations, because of availability and uniformity in size. Proper control tests must be included to ensure that transplanting the snails does not weaken them. In field screening tests the LC_{90} values obtained in the laboratory should be used, and concentrations two and four times this amount. It is not suitable to determine LC_{99} and LC_{100} by extrapolation [WHO, 1965a].

Field screening tests on the amphibious oncomelanid snails, involve small plots either in dry irrigation ditches or swampy areas with or without conspicuous water [RITCHIE and MCMULLEN, 1961; PESIGAN and MASILUÑGAN, 1950; KOMIYA et al.[15]]. Small baskets filled with soil have also been used in the

15 KOMIYA, Y.; YASURAOKA, K., and HOSAKA, Y.: in WHO unpublished document MOL/INF 19 (1965).

Philippines. Field screening tests are currently being run in Japan and in the Philippines. Starting doses of 1, 5 and 10 g/m² are indicated.

When field tests are carried out against aquatic snails, it is necessary to consider the different conditions associated with two main types of habitat, namely stationary and flowing water.

Stationary water might include pools, ponds, lakes, reservoirs, inundated fields, marshes and combinations thereof. It is not always possible to find natural testing plots of suitable size in sufficient numbers. Generally, replicate tests in small plots provide results of greater significance than those obtained from one or a few pools. In Puerto Rico, BERRY *et al.* [1950] tested NaPCP and other halogenated hydrocarbon compounds in roadside ditches, drainage ditches, small ponds, rainwater pools, and discontinuous swampy areas, part of which served as controls. PAULINI[16] used watering pits on truck farms for testing molluscicides in serial dilution, and sub-divided drainage ditches by earthen dams into sections of 10 m. WEBBE [1961] tested niclosamide at varied concentrations in pools holding about 40 m³ of water. JOBIN and UNRAU [1967] tested chemicals in standing water in different parts of Puerto Rico with critical attention to ecological conditions.

If small natural pools are not available, artificial ones can be made by forcing drums with open ends into the substratum of suitable snail habitats, e.g. at the margins of lakes, reservoirs or marshes. These small circumscribed volumes of water make it possible to test three or more concentrations in two-fold increments, starting with the LC₉₀ value for 24-hour laboratory exposures as the lowest. A reference molluscicide should be tested in parallel, and there should be one or more untreated plots.

When the plots are small, exhaustive search for snails and egg masses can be made, returning them to the plot after counting. In the case of artificial pools or if the existing population is sparse, both snails and eggs can be introduced, and restricted in cages or fences if indicated. In larger pools any of the commonly used snail sampling methods, e.g. snails/man-hour, snails/dip, or snails/m², may be used to note long-term changes in snail population; however, pre- and post-treatment mortalities may be considered adequate for field screening tests.

The molluscicide is applied in proportion to the water volume, requiring average length, width and depth measurements before application. In case of deep mud at the bottom of the pool, depth of the mud should be included. The required molluscicide may be diluted with water and applied

---

16   PAULINI, E.: in WHO unpublished document MOL/INF 16 (1964).

over the surface of the entire plot with a sprinkling-can or a portable pressure sprayer.

On the day of the application, as much information as possible should be collected on air and water temperature, pH, light intensity during the day, identification and relative amounts of vegetation in the plots and the kind of animals present. Water samples can be taken to check the actual concentration of the chemical by analyses, if a method is available; periodic samples will reveal the rate of detoxification.

The reactions of the snails and other aquatic animals to the chemical should be observed. The mortality of the snails and eggs will be determined only 2 to 5 days after application. Some molluscicides like Bayluscide and Frescon act rapidly, whereas organo-metal compounds and Gramoxone, at low concentrations, may require several days to cause death. Concomitantly with the final snail collection, the nature and extent of the effect of the chemical on aquatic flora and fauna should be recorded. Any residual potential of a chemical may be revealed by introducing caged snails and egg masses periodically after the application.

The percentage mortalities obtained in field screening tests may be represented graphically on log-probit paper, including results for the reference molluscicide, and the data may be treated statistically as in laboratory tests.

Flowing water habitats should include small natural streams, and man-made canals or ditches that are representative and readily accessible. The amount of chemical available for the screening test will be a limiting factor as to size of stream or canal chosen. Flowing water has inherent advantages over standing water, since controls can be kept in the same water, upstream from the application point. Also, the same body of water can be used repeatedly for different time × concentration regimens, since the chemical is quickly carried away.

Only a few standardized field-screening tests against aquatic snails in flowing water have been described. CROSSLAND et al.[17] used a series of especially designed irrigation canals, and a similar series was developed for use in Egypt [WHO][18]. In Puerto Rico, BERRÍOS-DURÁN et al. [1968] used a cement-lined sector of a stream and a conjoined natural section. Also in Puerto Rico, JOBIN and UNRAU [1967] used streams in various parts of the island, giving critical attention to ecological conditions. They determined downstream effectiveness

17 CROSSLAND, N.O.; BEESLEY, J.S.S., and MESMER, E.T.: in WHO unpublished document MOL/INF 20 (1965).
18 WHO: WHO unpublished document MOL/INF 19, sections I and VIII (1965).

and determined the 'half-life' by bioassay in an artificial canal with recirculating pump.

Small natural streams or artificial canals or ditches are acceptable for field-screening tests if they are representative of natural snail habitats. The test must be small, because only small amounts of chemical may be available. To further reduce cost of testing, the sites should be readily accessible. The flow rate in the stream or canal should be determined by a triangular or rectangular weir, Parshall flume or by determining the dilution of a known amount of some chemical that has been added.

In selecting the distance between point of application and the location of caged snails, one must choose between two objectives: (1) to determine the effectiveness of various dosages (time × concentration) at a given distance downstream; (2) to determine the effectiveness of a given dosage at various distances downstream. For the first objective a relatively short distance is sufficient (200–500 m), while several kilometers may be needed for the second; indeed, a suitable long sector of a stream can serve both objectives. Factors influencing these distances will be considered in more detail below under 'dispersal patterns', one of which is velocity. For a velocity of 0.2 m/sec, stations might be conveniently placed at distances of 300, 1,000, and 3,000 m downstream, while for greater velocities proportionately greater distances need to be used.

Exposure to the chemical may be for a relatively short period of 2 to 8 h, or for 1 to 2 days and even longer with correspondingly lower concentrations. For the various intervals, the LC_{90} values obtained in the laboratory may be used initially and then increased, if needed. Application of the molluscicide in turbulent water or over a weir will assure quick mixing. Effectiveness can be determined on the basis of pre- and post-treatment mortalities, as corrected for mortalities among the controls. The data should reveal how fast the molluscicide activity is lost by downstream carriage. This will indicate the basic chemical stability and the effects of environmental factors such as sunlight, physico-chemical adsorption, and absorption by micro- and macro-flora. Loss of activity should be checked against chemical analyses, if possible, since activity of a molluscicide may be affected by a characteristic feature of flowing water. With downstream carriage, a dilution of the chemical occurs which modifies the shape of the curve, but does not change its area. Thus the concentration becomes increasingly lower, but the time of the exposure increases correspondingly.

The field screening tests should be followed by a decision on whether any further work should or should not be carried out on each candidate molluscicide.

Field Trials

These should be carried out under natural conditions, in order to: (1) test the effectiveness of promising molluscicides under a variety of natural conditions; (2) examine the effect of physical and chemical factors on performance; (3) investigate the distance that the molluscicide is effective downstream in flowing water; and (4) evaluate handling properties.

The field trials should be conducted in a variety of snail habitats and the results should be based primarily on natural populations, rather than caged snails. The dosages selected should be the lowest concentrations that gave complete kill in 'field screening' tests and, if necessary, followed by increased concentrations until the effective dosage is determined. When expected results are not obtained, an attempt should be made to determine what environmental or physico-chemical factors, or combinations thereof, may have been involved. Chemicals for field trials must be few in number, and proper choice depends on good 'field screening' tests and some comprehensive laboratory evaluations. It is essential to have field tests made in a number of endemic centres. That this is being accomplished is shown by the following reviews.

Field trials in Japan from 1947 to 1955 indicated about equal cost-efficiency ratios for NaPCP and DNCHP against the amphibious *Oncomelania nosophora*, when sprayed on moist soil of irrigation systems during the months of October and April. Also, it was demonstrated that repopulation control might be possible by applying low concentrations of DNCHP to irrigation water repeatedly during the summer against the aquatic juvenile stage [WILLIAMS *et al.*, 1957]. Subsequently, Japanese investigators [HOSAKA *et al.*, 1957] reported in favour of NaPCP over DNCHP on the basis of cost efficiency. More recently, calcium arsenic compounds [reported from China by SU, 1954], niclosamide and bromo-nitro-benzenes were reported effective against *O. nosophora*. Niclosamide was found to be more active than NaPCP, but the cost-efficiency factor was in favour of NaPCP [KOMIYA, 1961; KOMIYA *et al.*, 1962; KOMIYA *et al.*, 1964; IIJIMA *et al.*, 1964]. In comparison, 'field screening' tests in the Philippines indicate the same efficiency for niclosamide against *O. quadrasi*.

In Egypt, after initial field trials with NaPCP, $CuSO_4$ and DNCHP [KUNTZ and WELLS, 1951; WRIGHT *et al.*, 1958; VAN DER SCHALIE, 1958], preference went to NaPCP, although the effectiveness of DNCHP was impressive, and the low cost per unit of $CuSO_4$ has kept it among the current molluscicides of choice. More recently field tests have been carried out using niclosamide in comparison with NaPCP. Acrolein, a molluscicide-herbicide, was tested by UNRAU *et al.* [1965] and found to be active against snail hosts and aquatic weeds at 20 to 25 ppm. Resurgence of snails was delayed for 8 to 12 months and damage to crops was not deemed significant. Field tests with *N*-trityl-morpholine in the Egypt-49 project were strikingly effective in primary irrigation channels with prolonged application of 0.04 ppm. A critical comparison of niclosamide and NaPCP made by Dawood *et al.* [1966], indicated that cost-efficiency indices for these products were similar for main canals of irrigation systems. However, where water carriage of the molluscicide is not fully effective, requiring spray applications, the cost-efficiency index for niclosamide was more favourable. The handling hazard for NaPCP, with extra cost for added supervision, were factors that gave preference to niclosamide as the molluscicide of choice for the project areas and probably the entire Nile Delta.

In the Sudan, Malek [1962] field-tested copper sulphate, using a 'blanket' exposure of 30 ppm, followed with continuous applications of 0.125 ppm. The former was effective, but the canals were suitable habitats under the maintenance dose for snails placed in cages. However, Malek concluded that the principle of continuous application is probably sound. Acrolein was also tested in the Sudan by Ferguson *et al.* [1965] with a 98- to 99-percent mortality against *Bulinus* and *Biomphalaria* at 25 ppm with a downstream carriage of 1.6 km. No phytotoxicity occurred with furrow irrigation, but with flooding irrigation seedlings were damaged at 15 ppm.

In Rhodesia, Shiff [1961] reported a field trial with 1 ppm of niclosamide in impounded and flowing water. He concluded that this product represents a major step forward in snail control, as compared with NaPCP and copper sulphate. Although mildly biocidal, the resulting biological imbalance was restored to normal in about one month [Shiff and Garnett, 1961]. A successful field test with *N*-tritylmorpholine was reported by Shiff [1966]; 1 ppm for 15 min and 0.5 ppm for 1 to 2 h gave effective results against *Bulinus (Ph.) globosus* snails and similar sensitivities were obtained for *Biomphalaria pfeifferi* and *Lymnaea natalensis*. A second application after 14 to 21 days was recommended because of the non-ovicidal nature of the chemical. Snails in silt were protected. Many fish were killed but microfauna survived.

In Tanzania, Webbe [1961] tested niclosamide in ponds and concluded that the greater toxicity of this molluscicide against snail hosts of schistosomiasis and their eggs may permit great advances in snail control, with consequent impact on the incidence of infection. In natural flowing water Foster *et al.* [1960] also obtained good results with niclosamide. Using this molluscicide in irrigation systems, Crossland [1963] reported that treated areas were free of snails for 7 months with possible eradication in some sections. The drainage system, however, contained pockets of snails which accounted for dramatic resurgence of the population. CROSSLAND [1967] applied N-trityl-morpholine with a prolonged low concentration (0.025 ppm for 30 days) at the headwaters of a 5000-acre irrigation system in Tanzania and obtained good control against B. pfeifferi for 3 to 4 months.

In Kenya, TEESDALE et al. [1961] tentatively concluded that 0.25 ppm copper sulphate in continuous application was lethal for snails. With 0.125 ppm, results were intermediate but better than those reported by MALEK [1962]; PAULINI[19] related this difference to pH and alkalinity of the water.

In the Republic of the Congo, GILLET et al. [1961] tested niclosamide in irrigation systems at 0.5 to 1 ppm, killing all planorbids and lymnaeids for 7 km. It was considered to be more effective and more economical than NaPCP in a concentration of 5 to 20 ppm.

In the Transvaal, field tests with copper sulphate and NaPCP gave un-satisfactory results [MEYLING et al., 1959; PITCHFORD et al., 1960]. It was concluded that neither of these compounds could be effective in the Transvaal. The poor results with NaPCP were related to photo-instability.

In Brazil, WRIGHT et al. [1958] reported field tests with NaPCP, DNCHP, and copper sulphate. NaPCP was deemed most effective in relation to cost and availability. By repeated application of NaPCP, PARAENSE and PEREIRA [1957] eradicated B. glabrata from one stream by four applications over a period of four months, but this was recognized as possible in only a few localities; single applications were ineffective. BARBOSA [1961] evaluated copper carbonate in slow-flowing streams, using 30 g/m². Mortalities of 100% were reported in 11 of 13 streams and 5 streams were free of snails after 12 months. Mud taken from some streams after 12 months still showed residual activity. BARBOSA and ARRUDA[20] tested Molucid and obtained 100% mortalities with 1 ppm in both still and flowing water. These same authors[21] evaluated N-tritylmorpho-line in field trials, using a wettable powder and an emulsifiable liquid con-centrate in both still and flowing water. High mortalities with 0.5 ppm were obtained, especially with the emulsifiable liquid formulation. Repopulation occurred soon after treatments with N-tritylmorpholine. PAULINI[22] evaluated several of the newer molluscicides in static and flowing water. The emulsifiable liquid concentrate of N-tritylmorpholine gave a 99-percent kill in pools with

19   PAULINI, E.: in WHO unpublished document MOL/INF 15 (1964).
20   BARBOSA, F.S. and ARRUDA, F.: in WHO unpublished document MOL/INF 16 (1964).
21   BARBOSA, F.S. and ARRUDA, F.: in WHO unpublished document MOL/INF 14 (1964).
22   PAULINI, E.: in WHO unpublished document MOL/INF 16 (1964), and in WHO un-published document MOL/INF 20 (1965).

0.05 g/m², or 0.2 ppm. Double this application was necessary in flowing water for equal results. Copper dimethyl-dithiocarbamate at 1 g/m² killed 95% of snails in still water, while two applications of this amount were necessary for equal results in flowing water; it proved non-irritating to handlers, gave a good suspension, and did not affect plants; its lethal action was slow. Different methods of application with niclosamide were tried, including the use of water impoundments as the molluscicide reservoir, application on the basis of area rather than volume of water, and the use of a granule formulation. Paraquat and Réglone, which are molluscicide-herbicides, killed eggs and mature snails at 2 to 10 ppm. Vegetation was killed but heavy growth reduced the molluscicidal activity of the chemicals.

In Puerto Rico, NaPCP was chosen for extensive field tests, and applied either by power sprayer to still water, or by the drip method to flowing water. The application rates were 3 to 5 mg/l with 24-hour treatments for flowing water [KLOCK et al., 1957]. In addition to molluscicidal activity, information on dispersion patterns was obtained. Subsequently, NaPCP was put into operational use by the Department of Health. Field tests were also conducted with acrolein, which clearly established that this product is highly efficient as a molluscicide in irrigation canals with high velocity, but relatively unsatisfactory in small streams because of its volatile nature [FERGUSON et al., 1961]. Acrolein is now in regular use by the irrigation authorities for weed control. The most recent field study was a parallel testing of niclosamide, CuSO₄ and TFM; the latter has been used against lamprey eel in the Great Lakes (USA). In comparison with NaPCP as a reference, it was clearly established that niclosamide is superior. The eelicide, TFM, also proved useful in ponds where it is desirable to protect fish, since it is non-toxic for most species at concentrations needed to kill B. glabrata. The tests indicated that CuSO₄ was not found to be satisfactory for field use in Puerto Rico [JOBIN and UNRAU, 1967]. Niclosamide has been introduced into the regular schistosomiasis control programme in Puerto Rico with 15 mg/l for 1 h in flowing water and 0.3 to 1.0 mg/l in still water.

Control of Schistosomiasis Transmission by Molluscicides

This constitutes a long-term study with observations on: (1) reduction of new cases, particularly in children; (2) quantitative changes in existing infections; (3) changes in the snail population dynamics; (4) reduction in numbers of cercariae; (5) long-term effect on flora and fauna; (6) the possible reduction of trematode infections in domestic animals; and (7) operational costs. Presently there are no reported investigations that embrace all the above points, but reduction in transmission of schistosomiasis by molluscicides has been reported in several endemic areas.

In Japan, HUNTER *et al.* [1962] reported reduction of schistosomiasis in Nagatoishi-cho, Kyushu, following a decade of control effort by means of NaPCP, and finally by cementing irrigation channels. In 1948 the infection rate was 73%, and in 1960 2%; clinical manifestations had essentially ceased. Subsequently a general programme of control with NaPCP was carried out by the Japanese in their endemic centres with about 70 to 80% reduction of snails with each application [KOMIYA, 1961]. Personal communications indicate that schistosomiasis is currently of little concern in most endemic areas of Japan although prevalence rates are still high in a few isolated foci.

In Egypt, the results of transmission control efforts have been summarized by AYAD [1961]. In the Dakhla Oasis, sulphation eliminated *Bulinus* and the prevalence of infection has dropped from 65 to 3%; remaining cases are those coming from the Nile Valley. The effect of molluscicides on transmission throughout Egypt has not been reported, but snail infection rates dropped from 1.27 to 0.13% in the case of *Bulinus* snails and from 3.76 to 0.16% for *Biomphalaria*. Considerable effort has been given to snail control, primarily with copper sulphate, and new methods of application have been tried, including 'focal-radial' applications in relation to population centres, continuous application of low concentrations, and shore sulphation in main irrigation canals. Between 1954 and 1956, NaPCP was employed for control of *Bulinus (B.) truncatus* and *Biomphalaria alexandrina* in the Warraq El-Arab area near Cairo, Egypt [WRIGHT *et al.*, 1958]. The area comprised approximately 25 km² with a population of about 50,000. Three applications of 10 ppm of the chemical each year effectively controlled both snail hosts in the Sawahil Canal and its branches. Single yearly urine and stool examinations of primary schoolchildren within the area indicated a reduction of prevalence of infection although for various reasons an adequate sampling was not possible. In an experiment in which it was possible to evaluate results more carefully, FAROOQ *et al.* [1966] reported that molluscicides applied to two areas near Alexandria had a significant effect in reducing both incidence and prevalence of *Schistosoma haematobium* and *S. mansoni*. No decrease in either measure of endemicity was found in an adjacent area where molluscicides were not applied. Niclosamide and NaPCP were equally effective in interrupting transmission of *S. haematobium*, but niclosamide was more effective against *S. mansoni*, probably because of the difficulty encountered in applying NaPCP to drains, which are the primary habitats for the intermediate hosts of *S. mansoni*.

In Rhodesia, CLARKE *et al.* [1961], and CLARKE [1965] observed some reduction in transmission of *S. haematobium* after applying molluscicides over an area of approximately 20,000 km². The decrease in prevalence did not occur in places where there was constant migration of people, or where physical difficulties prevented efficient application of molluscicides. Moreover, there was a decline in liver fluke infection in cattle. The control programme included: (1) a 'blanket' application to all natural waters; (2) 'focal' treatment the second year where snails persisted; and (3) 'surveillance' thereafter. The snails were reduced to such a level that as few as five could be collected per man-day. As indicated by MCMULLEN [1963] this endeavour was unique, because it was based on watershed units, involved unusual co-operation between government and farmers, and also afforded marked control of fascioliasis.

In Venezuela, JOVE and MARSZEWSKI [1961] achieved marked reduction in prevalence of *S. mansoni* in children under 5 years of age through use of molluscicides (NaPCP, CuPCP and copper sulphate) in conjunction with other measures.

The Puerto Rico Department of Health has operated a mollusciciding programme since 1955, involving six watersheds, or 10% of the land area, and protecting 200,000 people. Annual surveys of first-grade school-children showed a decline in occurrence of schistosomiasis of from 10 to 30%; even to zero in three of the six areas. Prevalence in witness area showed decline during the long period of observation, but increased thereafter. One of the watersheds was Vieques Island where no first-grade child was found positive after 1962, and no new cases occurred in the general population [FERGUSON *et al.*, 1968]. Control measures included mollusciciding, drainage of snail habitat, biological control with *Marisa cornuarietis* and therapy.

Correlation between the Results of Laboratory and Field Evaluations

The role and relative value of laboratory versus field evaluations have not been clearly established. In general, the results have been compatible. Those obtained in the laboratory, using *Biomphalaria glabrata* have correlated well with results obtained in the field with other species of *Biomphalaria* and *Bulinus*. The toxicities obtained in the laboratory with niclosamide and *N*-tritylmorpholine were confirmed under field conditions. Differences encountered were often related to the problem of formulation or to differences in the susceptibility of field and laboratory snails. In contrast, copper sulphate and NaPCP under field conditions have not always performed as well as laboratory tests indicated they should. In the case of copper sulphate, 20 to 30 times as much was required in the field. While NaPCP performed well in the field in Egypt, it was less effective in other countries. Clarification of these inconsistencies and others have depended upon laboratory tests. In one instance, the performance of niclosamide in the field exceeded the results in laboratory tests [FOSTER *et al.*, 1960]; it is now apparent that this was due to use of distilled water in the laboratory. Thus, it is apparent that the aim in developing laboratory tests must be to provide results that are realistic in terms of field conditions. Furthermore, laboratory tests must be used to reveal causes for diverse results obtained in the field, as occurred with NaPCP in Egypt, Brazil and the Transvaal, where results ranged from marked success to near-failure, due to variations in ecological conditions of the snail habitat.

Summation of Properties of 'Available' and 'Candidate' Molluscicides

Currently Available Molluscicides

Satisfactory statements of advantages and disadvantages of molluscicides are difficult to make because general objectives, methods of use, formulation and conditions of habitat all affect the adequacy of a product. Also, commercial availability is important, e.g. it has proved difficult to provide a suitable, inexpensive, safe container for acrolein, an otherwise impressive molluscicide-herbicide. On the basis of effectiveness and completeness of evaluation, niclosamide, NaPCP, copper sulphate and *N*-tritylmorpholine may be classified as 'available' molluscicides (table I).

Niclosamide (Ethanolamine Salt of 5,2'-dichloro-4'-nitrosalicylicanilide)
The base compound is relatively insoluble, but the ethanolamine salt is effectively formulated as a wettable powder; recently, a liquid concentrate was developed. The wettable powder tends to clog equipment used in applying it. The compound acts quickly in low concentrations with about equal efficiencies for 1- and 24-hour exposures. The ppm $\times$ h values range from 2 to 7 and are about the same in field and laboratory tests. The LC_{90} concentrations for 24-hour exposures show a loss of activity after six days standing in the laboratory; degradation occurs sooner under field conditions. In streams with numerous impoundments, it may not be effective very far downstream. Storage-stability is satisfactory, but some deterioration does occur within two to three years. Its effectiveness is reduced slowly by sunlight, slightly by ad-

Table I. Advantages and disadvantages of selected molluscicides

Molluscicide	Advantages	Disadvantages
Niclosamide	Highly toxic to snails and eggs. Safe to handle and use. Probably the cheapest chemical per unit volume of water treated. Does not upset the biota as much as some compounds.	Difficult to formulate. In certain types of habitat available formulations do not disperse effectively. Equipment is clogged by sediment.
NaPCP	Kills both snails and their eggs. Excellent penetration downstream has been achieved. Widely used for other purposes and so not dependent on a molluscicide 'market'.	Irritating and potentially dangerous to the handler. Doses required relatively high compared with new molluscicides Activity may be reduced by bright sunlight.
Copper sulphate	Kills both snails and their eggs, but eggs are less susceptible. More active at a low pH. Somewhat less toxic to fish than other molluscicides. Safe to handle. (It may be possible to exploit insoluble copper compounds for use under some conditions.)	Absorbed by soil and organic material. Ineffective at a high pH. Corrosive to equipment. Of variable toxicity to snails under field conditions.
N-tritylmorpholine	Rapidly and highly molluscicidal. Low toxicity for other biota. Relatively safe toxicologically. Safe to handle and apply. Adequately stable. Good selection of formulations. Cost-efficiency on a *par*.	Does not kill snail eggs. Repeated or prolonged application required. Hydrolyses below pH 7.0.

sorption on mud and colloidal particles, and to a limited degree by high concentration of minerals of water hardness. The pH values found in the normal range of natural waters have no effect. The toxicity of niclosamide is low for mammals and it is not irritating. Its biocidal activity is inclusive, but restoration of the biota occurs rather soon. It is about equally effective against all stages and sizes of aquatic snails with 24-hour exposures, but for 6-h the ppm

$\times$ h value for mature and adolescent snails is about double that for other stages. Field tests in Tanzania, South Africa and Egypt have given excellent results. It is considered the molluscicide of choice for most habitats encountered in the Rhodesia snail control programme. It was declared molluscicide of choice in the Philippines [PESIGAN, 1967].

Sodium Pentachlorophenate (NaPCP)

This highly soluble molluscicide is formulated as flakes, pellets and briquettes. Its efficiency is low with 1-hour exposures, and with 6-hour exposures mature snails are relatively less susceptible than with 24-hour exposures. Newly-laid eggs are more susceptible than 4- to 5-day-old embryos, and newly-hatched and juvenile snails are more susceptible than adolescent and mature specimens. In flowing water, exposures of 8 to 10 h are effective with 50 to 80 ppm $\times$ h values. In non-flowing water, the concentration can be reduced, and on moist soil it is applied at the rate of 4 to 10 g/m². It is ovicidal against eggs of aquatic snails. The use of prolonged low concentrations holds promise as NaPCP is highly effective against newly-laid eggs; storage-stability is satisfactory; it is basically a stable compound, but is photosensitive. It is unaffected by the normal pH range of natural water, it is reduced by hard water, and is irreversibly adsorbed by mud. Careless handling can be dangerous, particularly in the flake formulation; the briquettes are safer and more practicable for flowing water. The biocidal spectrum is inclusive, but the biota is soon restored. NaPCP has been one of the most effective of all the molluscicides, when application is by water carriage in canal systems and watersheds where intense ultraviolet light is not a problem. In general, NaPCP has been a relatively reliable molluscicide in Japan, Egypt, Rhodesia and Venezuela.

Copper Sulphate (CuSO₄)

This stable, easy-to-handle compound is usually applied as a solution in aquatic habitats only. Its activity is rapid when relatively high concentrations are used, but its effectiveness is reduced in the presence of organic material, certain types of dissolved solids, and a high pH. Evidence of this variability is shown by the wide range of ppm $\times$ h values that have been reported to be effective, i.e. 48 to 300 ppm $\times$ h. CuSO₄ is ovicidal, but at higher concentrations than required for hatched snails. For reasons cited above, the compound is applied throughout the habitat at 30 ppm, rather than depending on water carriage. It has been used with continuous application at low concentrations ('chemical barrier'). CuSO₄ is a good molluscicide, but to obtain reliable results, its advantages and limitations under local conditions must be understood. Extensive use of this compound in control programmes is now confined to Egypt and Sudan.

N-tritylmorpholine

Commendable studies by the following investigators warrant the inclusion of this product as an 'available' molluscicide: BOYCE et al. [1967a, b]; CROSSLAND [1967]; CHAPMAN [1967]; BEYNON and THOMAS [1967]; BEYNON et al. [1967]; BEYNON and WRIGHT [1967]; BROWN et al. [1967]; MEYLING and MEYLING[23].

N-tritylmorpholine is presently the most active molluscicide against hatched snails. It is active at 0.1 to 0.5 ppm with 1-hour exposures, and at 0.01 to 0.05 ppm with 24-hour exposures. In these relationships it is not effective against snail eggs. There is evidence that longer exposures may prove toxic for the eggs, therefore, prolonged applications at low concentrations are recommended. Moreover, any eggs that develop and hatch will be killed. As snails grow in diameter, there is a progressive increase in the LC_{50}. Environmental factors, such as light, mud and plants, have not proven to be limiting factors in the efficacy of N-tritylmorpholine. However, it is rendered less active, due to hydrolysis, at pH values below 7.0. Toxicological studies indicate a good margin of safety, but a chlorinated solvent used in one formulation is believed to have been accountable for liver and kidney damage in rats. Admixture of 100 ppm in rat food for 90 days did not cause ill-effects. Small amounts of the active ingredient have been detected in rice plants. Snail control apparently will require repeated applications or prolonged treatments at low concentrations because of its non-ovicidal nature. Fish susceptibilities vary with species, but can be minimized by use of a granular formulation or use of prolonged low dosages. Formulations include emulsifiable concentrates, water dispersible powder and granules, spreading oils, and baits. Analytical determinations for field use have been developed. It has been priced to compete with other molluscicidal products.

Candidate Molluscicides

A number of chemicals with varied combinations of merits are designated as 'candidate' molluscicides. These are listed in table II along with 'available' products.

23 MEYLING, A. H. and MEYLING, J.: in WHO unpublished document PD/MOL 69.8 (1969).

Table II. Molluscicides and their properties[1]

Common and/or trade name	Physical form of technical material	Active ingredient	Solubility in water	Toxicity of technical material[2]				Stability of technical material affected by					Handling qualities		Formulations	Field dosage		Range of application
				snail LC₉₀, ppm × h	snail eggs LC₉₀	herbicidal activity	LD₅₀, rats, acute oral, mg/kg	ultraviolet light	mud, turbidity	pH	algae, plants	storage	safe	simple		aquatic snails (ppm × h)	amphibious snails on moist soil	
Acrolein[3] (Aqualin[4])	liquid		22% w/w 20°C	30–75	15–24	yes[5]	30–40	?	yes	yes	yes	yes	no	no	86% acrolein volatile liquid	75–100 ppm		flowing water where control of submerged weeds also necessary
Niclosamide[6] (Bayluscide)	crystalline solid	ethanolamine salt of 2',5-dichloro-4'-nitrosalicyl-anilide	230 ppm	5–8	2–4	no	5,000	yes[6]	nor-mal	opti-mum 6–8	no	no	yes	yes	wettable powder containing 70% active ingredient	4–8	0.2 g/m²	flowing and static water
Carbamates e.g., zinc dimethyl-dithio-carbamate	amorphous solid		65 ppm	50	50–100	no	1,400	?	no	?	no	no	yes	yes	(1) granules 50% + 50% CaCO₃ (2) micronized powder (90% active ingredient)	10 g/m³ 5[7]		where killing of fish is undesirable
Copper compounds (1) soluble e.g., copper sulfate	crystalline solid		32%	20–100	50–100	yes[8]	?	no	yes	yes	yes	no	yes	yes	crystals of CuSO₄·5H₂O	20–30[9]		static and flowing water
(2) insoluble e.g., cuprous oxide	amorphous solid		insoluble	7–100	50–100	no	2,000	no	yes	yes	yes	in part	yes	yes	powder	60[10]	–[11]	static water where killing of fish undesirable

Table II (Continued)

Common and/or trade name	Physical form of technical material	Active ingredient	Solubility in water	Toxicity of technical material[a]				Stability of technical material affected by					Handling qualities		Formulations	Field dosage		Range of application
				snail LC90, ppm × h	snail eggs LC90	herbicidal activity	LD50, rats, acute oral, mg/kg	ultraviolet light	mud, turbidity	pH	algae, plants	storage	safe	simple		aquatic snails (ppm × h)	amphibious snails on moist soil	
Dinitro-phenols[12] e.g., DNCHP (Dinex[4])	crystalline solid	2-cyclo-hexyl-4,6-dinitro-phenol	0.072%	30-60	20-40	yes	60	?	no	?	no	no	va-ries	no	40% wettable powder	30-55	0.1-5 g/m²	various
Paraquat[3] (Gramoxone)	crystalline solid	1,1'-dimethyl-4,4'-dipyri-dilium dichloride	highly soluble	60-100	6-10	yes	200	no	yes	no	yes	no	yes	yes	liquid: 2 lb. paraquat per UK gal (200 g/l)	5-10[7]		not yet defined
Organo-tin compounds e.g., tri-phenyltin acetate; tri-n-butyltin acetate	liquids and crystalline solids		varies from < 1 to about 50 ppm	1-10[13]	1-2	no[14]	150	yes	?	yes	no	no	yes	yes	20% wettable powder	7-14	—[13]	not defined
Diquat[3]	crystalline solid	1,1'-ethylene-2,2'-di-pyridilium dibromide	highly soluble	60-100	6-10	yes	200	no	yes	?	yes	no	yes	yes	liquid: 2 lb. diquat per UK gal (200 g/l)	5-10[7]		not defined
NaPCP	crystalline solid	sodium pentachloro-phenate	33%	20-80	3-30	no	40-250	yes	no	no	no	no	va-ries	yes	(1) flakes 75% (2) pellets 80% (3) briquettes 80%	50-80	0.4-10 g/m²	flowing and static water

Name	Physical form	Chemical name	Water solubility				Toxicity							Formulation	Dosage	Type of water
N-trityl-morpholine (Frescon)	crystalline solid	N-trityl-morpholine	insoluble	1–2	240	no	1,400	?	?	yes	no	no	yes	yes	(1) 16.5% w/v emulsifiable concentrate (2) granular bait	1–2 (0.2?) / 150 lb./acre	flowing and static water
Yurimin	solid	3,5-dibromo-4-hydroxy-4'-nitroazo benzene	low	15	4–5	no	168 (mice)	no	?	yes	?	?	yes	yes	powder granules	? / 5 gm/m²	flowing and static water
Diaphene	solid	3,5,4-tribromo-salicylanilide	low	3–8	3–8	?	?	yes	?	yes	?	?	yes	yes	liquid	?	flowing and static water
Fluorophene	solid	3,5-dibromo-3'-trifluoro-methyl-salicylanilide	low	12–25	12–25	?	?	yes	?	yes	?	?	yes	yes	liquid	?	flowing and static water
Nicotinanilides (Dowco-212-1, 215-2, 216-2)	solids	nicotinanilide	low	4–7	high	no	2,000 (mice)	no	?	?	?	?	yes	yes	not formulated	2 ppm static water	where killing of fish is undesirable
Phenyl-salicylanilide (PSA)	solid	2',5-dichloro-4'-nitro-3-phenyl-salicylanilide	low	0.3–1.2	10	?	164	?	?	?	?	?	?	?	liquid	2.4	flowing and static water

1 In order to present a summary of the properties of molluscicides for easy comparison, many details have been omitted. It would be impossible to include the entire range of results reported by different workers, the exact species of snails against which molluscicides were tested, the maturity of the snails, or the precise conditions of laboratory and field tests. Furthermore, properties listed under group headings such as 'organo-tins' and 'carbamates' are not necessarily applicable to all members of the group. Additional details on any subject can be provided upon request.

2 'Toxicity' to snails: the standard of comparison—ppm × h—is normally calculated on the basis of a 24-hour exposure. As appreciable variations in CT (concentration × time) values may occur during such a period, the figures given might prove unrealistic if applied to a short exposure of, say, 1–2 h.

3 Name recommended by the International Organization for Standardization (ISO).

4 Not available outside the USA.
5 For submerged weeds only.
6 Depending upon salt content of water.
7 Static water.
8 Algae only.
9 For 24 h or more.
10 5 ppm for 12 h.
11 Not effective against amphibious snails.
12 Not readily available commercially.
13 No figures obtainable for Oncomelania due to low activity against amphibious snails.
14 Phytotoxic to certain irrigated crops.

Acrolein

This product was developed recently as a herbicide to control aquatic vegetation in irrigation canals, and is applied to give a concentration × time value of 30 to 75 ppm × h. It is molluscicidal and kills snail eggs at herbicidal concentrations. It is a volatile material that is irritating to eyes and mucous membranes, but this serves as a warning, because harmful levels are well above the limits of mammalian tolerance. Effective metering devices have been developed, in order to give proper dosages and to protect personnel making the application. Experiments in Egypt showed that when the dosages are properly controlled the treated water can be used for irrigation. In fact, crop yields were greater in the experimental plots than controls. Acrolein may not be practical for snail control except in combination with control of immersed plants, but should be less expensive than separate snail and weed-control programmes. Field trials in Puerto Rico, Sudan, Tanzania and Egypt have shown effective control of weeds and snails in irrigation systems.

Organo-Tin Compounds

Several of these fungicidal compounds have proved to be highly molluscicidal. Bis (tri-*n*-butyltin) oxide, tri-*n*-butyltin acetate and tri-*n*-propyltin oxide are comparable in activity to Bayluscide. Deschiens and Floch [1968] included the oxide of tributyltin and triphenyltin chloride in their selection of the six most practical molluscicides. However, they are slower acting and not efficient with 1-hour exposures. Eggs and hatched snails are about equally susceptible. The newly-laid eggs and newly-hatched snails are especially sensitive. The organo-tins are basically stable and they are not seriously degraded by environmental factors. They are formulated as emulsifiable liquid concentrates or wettable powders. Field-screening tests in Tanzania and in Puerto Rico indicate that these compounds warrant further evaluations. From laboratory tests, it was concluded that they will not be effective against *O. nosophora*. They can be handled safely, but are more toxic for mammals than Bayluscide.

Dinitrophenols

Among these compounds, DNCHP (2-cyclohexyl-4,6-dinitrophenol) is the most active. This basically stable, relatively insoluble compound, has been formulated as a wettable powder and a 30-percent liquid concentrate can be prepared in xylene. It is uniformly and equally effective against all stages and sizes of aquatic snails with both 6- and 24-hour exposures. DNCHP is not vulnerable to environmental factors. It is applied at a rate of 1.0 to 5.0 g/m² against oncomelanid snails. Evidence of snail resistance after several years of use has been reported from Japan. It is relatively safe for animals and plants, and not dangerous to apply. Its cost-efficiency index is somewhat less favourable than for NaPCP. Compounds related to DNCHP are both molluscicidal and herbicidal and may warrant evaluation on this basis.

Paraquat and Réglone

These soluble compounds are effective both as molluscicides and herbicides. They are quaternized, dipiridyl derivatives prepared as liquid concentrates. The LC_{90} values against mature B. glabrata with 24-hour exposures are 4 to 6 ppm, while newly-laid eggs are decidedly more susceptible. These products are not affected by sunlight or pH, but are reduced by mud. They are rapidly absorbed by algae, but still retain their activity. Accordingly they may be called 'systemic molluscicides'. Neither paraquat nor Réglone kill fish. They are relatively toxic for mammals, but can be handled safely. The price of these products is comparatively high.

Insoluble Copper Compounds

Copper pentachlorophenate is relatively insoluble and has been distributed in the snail habitat by applying NaPCP and $CuSO_4$. A chemical reaction provides a fine suspension of CuPCP that gives a residual effect in non-flowing water. It has been used to control B. glabrata in Venezuela, and in Australia for control of fascioliasis.

Copper carbonate is a stable, relatively insoluble compound that is applied by spraying or dusting. It is most effective in standing or slow flowing water and moist soil. It is applied on the basis of area at the rate of 30 to $60 g/m^2$. Remarkably good results were obtained in Brazil with $30 g/m^2$. It has been the molluscicide of choice for many years in controlling the aquatic hosts of non-human schistosomes in lake habitats in the USA.

Cuprous oxide, in the form of stabilized 'chevreul salt' (SCS) is highly insoluble and has a good residual effect. It is slow acting and is more effective at 24- than at 6-hour exposures in laboratory tests. There is evidence indicating that: (1) the cupric ion is the active principle; (2) the residual effect is related to low solubility and possibly other characteristics; (3) the effect on snails is similar to that of other copper compounds; and (4) it kills some fish but not others at recommended concentrations. Studies on this compound have drawn attention to the limited knowledge that exists about the action of the cupric ion, even though a copper compound was used as the first molluscicide.

Carbamates

Interest in these compounds developed because it was reported that they had a prolonged effect, and did not kill fish. At least four (Rhodiacid, Cuprobam, Sevin and Zectran) have received limited tests; they produce a relaxation of the snail body. High concentrations are required and some species of fish were killed. Apparently they are not very promising as selective molluscicides. However, it is possible that these insecticidal compounds should be considered for combined control where schistosomiasis, mosquito-borne diseases and onchocerciasis (transmitted by *Simulium*) occur together.

Organo-Leads

Molluscicidal qualities of these compounds are being studied. At least five are known to be active below 1 ppm with 24-hour exposures. Triphenyl-lead acetate and tributyl-lead acetate are among the more active compounds. The latter may be more uniformly active against all sizes of hatched snails and with shorter exposures. Eggs are susceptible, but relatively less so than hatched snails. It has been suggested that organo-leads may be more practical than organo-tins, being more selective for snails than rice seedlings, less degraded by mud, and probably less expensive. Toxicity hazards require further study.

Yurimin (P-99)

Yurimin (3,5-dibromo-4-hydroxy-4'-nitrobenzene) in field tests was found to compare favourably with NaPCP on a cost-efficiency basis against *Oncomelania nosophora* [IIJIMA *et al.*, 1964]. In laboratory immersion tests, the results were also good [KOMIYA *et al.*)[24]. Against *B. glabrata*, it was several times more active than PCP. Newly hatched snails were particularly susceptible, and eggs were also more susceptible than mature snails [PAULINI and DE SOUZA, 1968]. It was not degraded by water hardness, its stability was unaffected by sunlight, giving it an advantage over NaPCP, but acid waters (pH 4.5 to 5.2) decreased its effectiveness somewhat [KOMIYA *et al.*][24]. The latter also reported that LC_{50} of Yurimin (active ingredient) for mice was 167.9 mg/kg and 10 times that figure for a 5-percent granular formulation. It was not toxic for plants but was piscicidal.

Diaphene and Fluorophene (Halogenated Salicylanilides)

Diaphene is a mixture of 5,4'-dibromosalicylanilide and the 3,5,4'-tri-

24   KOMIYA, Y.; YASURAOKA, K., and HOSAKA, Y.: in WHO unpublished document MOL/INF 66.22 (1966).

bromo derivative, the latter being the active substance, and fluorophene is 3,5-dibromo, 3-trifluoro-methyl salicylanilide [HOPF et al.][25]. Both products are bacteriocides and fungicides. Diaphene is more active, with LC_{50}/LC_{90} values of 0.05 and 0.1 ppm. Thus it should compete with niclosamide; moreover, it has the advantage of a liquid formulation. It is degraded by an acid pH (5.5), whereas fluorophene is more stable. Their sensitivity to other physico-chemical factors remain to be determined. These products warrant further comprehensive evaluations.

Nicotinanilides

For mature B. glabrata, the LC_{90} values were 0.18, 0.27 and 0.21 ppm for Dowco 212, 215 and 216, respectively. Corresponding figures for newly-hatched snails were higher and eggs were even less susceptible, especially those newly laid. These results were obtained with 24-hour exposures and up to 6-day recovery periods. In field trials, mature snails were all killed at 2 ppm, but some eggs survived. Of special importance, was the selective action of these compounds, with no mortalities among four species of fish, frogs and plants [DE SOUZA and PAULINI[26]]. Mice tolerated 2 g/kg. Similar results were obtained by FENWICK[27] for Dowco 212-1 in both laboratory and field trials. In the latter, it was effective against B. pfeifferi, Bulinus (B.) tropicus and Lymnaea natalensis, but not against two other snails. FENWICK[27] further reported that sunlight did not degrade Dowco 212 and it was effective in the field in spite of precipitation onto mud. Because of its 'selective' action, it warrants consideration as a 'candidate' molluscicide.

PSA (Phenylsalicylanilide)

The chemical formula for PSA has been given as 2',5-dichloro-4'-nitro-3-phenylsalicylanilide. The addition of the phenyl radical to the base compound used in preparing niclosamide introduced new molluscicidal qualities. PSA was found to be more efficient with 1-hour exposures than with 3-, 6- and 24-hour exposures on the basis of ppm × h values. It is more highly efficient against hatched B. glabrata, especially against newly-hatched specimens. Against eggs it is less efficient than niclosamide [RITCHIE and FOX, 1968]. This product warrants further comprehensive evaluations.

25   HOPF, H.S.; DUNCAN, J.; GOLL, P.H., and RICHARDSON, H.: in WHO unpublished document PD/MOL 69.3 (1969).
26   DE SOUZA, C.P. and PAULINI, E.: in WHO unpublished document PD/MOL 69.7 (1969).
27   FENWICK, A.: in WHO unpublished document PD/MOL 70.10 (1970).

A Critique on the Characteristics of Good Molluscicides

There is obvious need for a wide variety of molluscicides and for a diversity of formulations to meet the challenges resulting from variations in the nature of different snail species, differences in conditions of the habitat and limitations imposed by terrain, climate and human activity. Consequently, it is difficult to give a concise description of an ideal molluscicide. Rather, it should be emphasized that compounds with varied combinations of molluscicidal merits and versatility are needed. However, there are certain general characteristics that are desirable in a molluscicide: (1) it should have low toxicity for man, domesticated animals, crops, game, fish, and the natural biota should be quickly restored after its use; (2) it should be reasonably safe in the hands of trained, but relatively unsophisticated, people; (3) it should be active at very low concentrations since this reduces the cost of transportation and burden of carrying it to points of application; (4) it should be versatile in different time × concentration regimens; (5) it should be stable in storage and in the habitat after use; (6) it should kill not only the snails but also their eggs; (7) it should be usable with simple, durable equipment or none at all; (8) tests should be available to measure the concentrations used in the field; and (9) it should have a low cost so that it can be employed economically.

No practical molluscicide is likely to have all these characteristics, and it is quite possible for an excellent molluscicide to lack one or more of them.

Practical Aspects of Chemical Control of Intermediate Hosts

Introduction

Advances have been made in chemical control of snails during the past decade. More active molluscicides and improved formulations allow more realistic means of application; characteristics of the activity of molluscicides and their stability are better understood. Moreover, there is awareness that chemical control of snails can be enhanced through better understanding of changes in population densities and the periodicity of transmission, through exploiting controls imposed by nature itself, through combining chemical with biological control, and by increasing efficiency in water management and agricultural practices. Nevertheless, for each major control endeavour, continued ingenuity will be needed for proper selections of molluscicides and formulations thereof, and for selecting and implementing the best procedures for a variety of habitats. Alertness will always be needed to ensure that control efforts do not cause harm to humans, crops, domestic animals, or other biota of economic importance. Skilled and unskilled personnel participating in control must attain high proficiency and obtain evaluation data correctly and completely. Cost must be minimized by using simple, inexpensive, yet efficient methods of application.

Dispersal Patterns of Chemicals

Dispersal Patterns in Habitats

This important subject has not received adequate attention until recently; our present knowledge is based on a limited number of field observations. It is desirable that systematic investigation be carried out to increase our understanding of the various phenomena involved in the process of dispersal and disappearance of molluscicides from natural waters.

The application of a molluscicide aims at the uniform distribution of the chemical in the entire body of water in order to kill all the snails and possibly also their eggs. Since it is not practical, and sometimes impossible, to secure the thorough mixing of the chemical in natural bodies of water by mechanical means, reliance has to be placed upon the natural forces which work towards its uniform distribution. These natural forces in decreasing order of importance are:

  (i) wave action;
 (ii) turbulent flow;
(iii) molecular diffusion;
(iv) thermal or gravity currents.

Dispersion in Still Water

A molluscicide applied to standing water is usually distributed over the surface by means of a sprayer or sprinkling-can without causing much mixing except in the top few centimeters. Then the mollucicide diffuses into the lower layers and attains equilibrium, i.e. uniform concentration in all parts of the pool after a considerable time. The progressive changes in the concentration of the chemical in the top and bottom layers in relation to time are shown in figures 1 and 2. The reciprocal slopes in the two lines show that the concentration became uniform after one hour in water that was 20 cm deep and after 3 h in water 70 cm deep. This example applies to a product which is very dilute (less than 0.5% of strength) or to emulsions of any strength when their specific

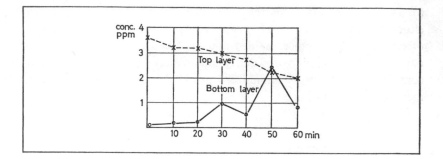

Fig. 1. Niclosamide applied to a shallow water. Depth = 20 cm.

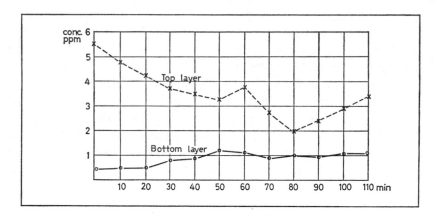

Fig. 2. Niclosamide applied to a deep pool. Depth = 70 cm.

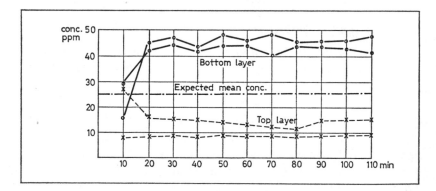

Fig. 3. Concentrated molluscicide applied to a deep pool. Depth = 70 cm.

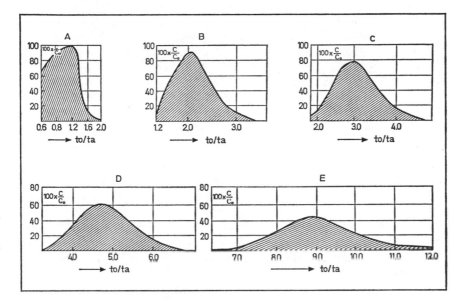

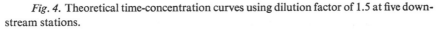

Fig. 4. Theoretical time-concentration curves using dilution factor of 1.5 at five downstream stations.

gravity is not different from that of the water. However, when a wettable powder or a water-soluble molluscicide at a concentration above 5% is used, the drops of the solution or suspension are not retained in the surface layer but fall to the bottom, forming a concentrated bottom layer (fig. 3). The tendency of this heavier bottom layer to disperse is much smaller than in the previous example. Stratification of the molluscicide was observed also by CROSS-LAND when treated water having a lower temperature (and consequently higher density) flowed into a reservoir containing water of higher temperature [CROSSLAND, 1963].

Dispersion in Flowing Water

If the molluscicide is added to a stream at a place of high turbulence, rapid and uniform distribution of the chemical in the water is assured. As long as the chemical is added at a rate which maintains a constant proportion to the volumetric rate of flow, the concentration of the chemical remains at a given level as can be observed in samples taken downstream, not too far from the application point. The chemical thus added forms a 'plug' moving downstream with the average velocity of the stream. During its travel, the

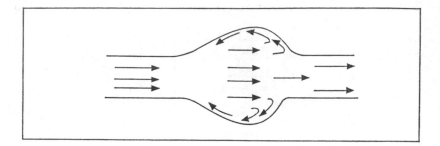

Fig. 5. Dilution effect caused by irregular margin of the stream.

'plug' expands both in the direction of and against the flow, with the result that the average concentration of the 'plug' becomes progressively less as the distance travelled increases. The changes which occur in the concentration of the chemical in relation to the time are best described graphically in the C × T curves (fig. 4).

These curves were taken in a hypothetical case, at increasing distances downstream from the application point. If no chemical was lost during its travel, the areas under the curves remain the same, although the shape of the curves changes. The changes are brought about by a number of factors, namely: (1) the diffusion coefficient of the chemical; (2) velocity of the flow; and (3) irregularities on the bottom, or along the margin of the stream (pools, vegetation, etc.). Without further details regarding each factor one can state that their cumulative effect results in continuous dilution of the molluscicide. The process of dilution caused by irregularities along the margin is represented in figure 5.

The degree of dilution of the molluscicide depends on the number and size of the irregularities (pockets, pools, static places) caused by aquatic vegetation, etc. [DOBROVOLNY and BARBOSA, 1953; KLOCK *et al.*, 1957]. The cumulative effect of these factors can be expressed in the form of a proportionality factor, and it is proposed to call this the 'dilution factor'. It should be emphasized that the dilution factor may show both great variation and high values (1.5 to 3.0 or more) in natural streams and in poorly maintained irrigation canals, while low values (near 1.1) with less variation in range may occur in irrigation canals free of vegetation and carrying large volumes of water.

KLOCK *et al.* [1957] observed that the distance of effective treatment downstream was related directly to the time used in applying the chemicals. Following this observation, it was found that the shape of the C × T curve

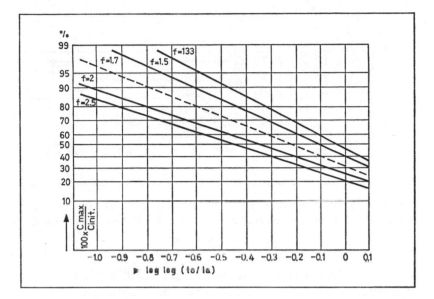

Fig.6. Maximum relative concentrations in function of relative time of travel for various dilution factors.

observed at a given point in a particular stream is dependent both on the duration of application and on the travel time of the chemical to reach the point of observation. The influence of these two factors can be reduced to only one by dividing the time of travel (t_o) by the time of application (t_a). The fraction t_o/t_a has been called 'relative time of travel'. In figure 6 typical C × T curves are shown with increasing relative time of travel at a given 'dilution factor' $(f = 1.5)$.

When in model experiments C × T curves have been plotted at various distances downstream and using different dilution factors, it was observed that the maximum concentration of the molluscicide showed dependence on both the dilution factor and relative time of travel. The relation is linear when the maximum concentration is plotted in probit versus the log of relative time of travel. It is stressed again that these relationships apply only to cases where no loss of molluscicide occurs.

The graphic widening of the C × T curve with increasing time of travel may be used with advantage for the damping of oscillations of the concentration caused either by variation of the rate of application, or by changes in the volumetric flow of the stream $(f = 1.3)$. In the example given in figure 7,

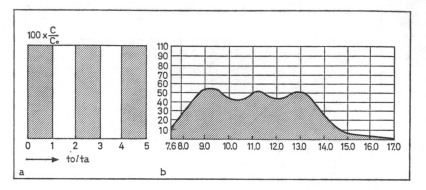

Fig. 7. Time-concentration pattern from intermittent application at two stations. *a* Application pattern at upstream station. *b* Observation at downstream station.

the variation between peaks and valleys was reduced from 100% at the point of application to 20% after a relative time of travel equal to 8.

In order to know the characteristics of a stream, or part of it, dependence has to be placed on field tests made with 'tracer' compounds. The tracer should be readily available, inexpensive, not harmful to the handler and to the aquatic life, should not be affected either by the composition of the water or by inorganic and organic matter present in the water and on the bottom of the stream; the quantitative assay of the tracer should be possible with a given accuracy, preferably in the field. Experiments in Brazil were done with NaCl solutions which were introduced into the water for only short periods (5 to 10 min) at a rate which gave 100 to 200 ppm of final concentration. Fluorescent dyes and radioactive tracers have also been used in water-movement studies in various parts of the world.

Once the principal characteristics of a stream are known, an experimental run with a molluscicide would show whether any significant loss of the latter occurs in the area under study. For this purpose a comparison can be made of the $C \times T$ curves obtained both by the tracer and the molluscicide. If the two curves can be superimposed, probably no loss occurred; if one curve lies below the other, loss of the chemical can be suspected. Using this technique, PAULINI found no appreciable loss of NaPCP and a small (20%) loss of niclosamide as compared with sodium chloride in an irrigation canal over a distance of 0.5 km. Under the same conditions copper sulphate suffered a 75-percent loss over the first 0.1 km, and only 2% of the copper applied passed the 0.5-km mark during the expected period of time (pH of water 6.5 to 7.0).

The characteristic behaviour of the chemical wave in flowing water may, in the near future, permit the calculation of the optimal rate of application and the estimation of the effective distance for a given molluscicide.

Choice of a Molluscicide

Qualities in Relation to Habitat and Species of Intermediate Host
As 'available' molluscicides increase in number and their characteristics become fully known, more than one may be used, even in a limited area, to provide maximum efficiency in varied habitats. One product might be dispersed at the headwaters of a stream, another applied to marginal swamps or pools along the stream and yet another used in ponds or reservoirs. The three products might be different formulations of the same chemical or entirely different chemicals. Wise and efficient use of a molluscicide is possible only when detailed information is available on the characteristics of its action and its stability under physico-chemical factors of the environment.

The effectiveness of a molluscicide must be known for each snail species in the varied habitats of each endemic area. Consequently, some testing in the laboratory and trials in the field are indicated before a product is selected for major control efforts.

Of special consideration are herbicides that are molluscicidal. In some endemic situations, particularly irrigation channels, a product serving these roles is desirable if it can be used without damage to crops. Moreover, the removal of aquatic plants makes the habitat less suitable for surviving snails, since vegetation serves for food, protection, and as a site for depositing eggs.

Formulations, According to Field Conditions
A widening of the range of available auxiliary surface-active agents (emulsifiers, spreaders, stickers, wetters, dispersants), naturally-occurring and synthetic fillers, stabilizers (e.g. anti-oxidants and water scavengers) and solvents, and the accumulation of considerable knowledge about their use have made possible considerable advances in the formulation of pesticides for agricultural purposes and for the control of insect hosts of disease. It is, therefore, generally possible, though not necessarily easy, to formulate active ingredients in such a way that the resulting formulations are stable and have an acceptable storage life in the tropics.

The physical properties of the active molluscicide tend to dictate the kind of formulation that can be made. It is generally not possible to formulate liquid active ingredients as water-dispersible powders with a high content of active ingredient, and it is virtually impossible to prepare liquid concentrates of active ingredients that are sparingly soluble in organic solvents.

In snail control the variety of conditions in which the molluscicide has to be applied is greater than in any other form of pest, disease, or weed control. A number of different formulations to meet these conditions is required.

Experience with insecticides has shown that biocidal performance can vary with different methods of application, and also with the particle size of the active material in water-dispersible powder formulations. This also occurs with molluscicides. For example, with N-tritylmorpholine the percentage kill of adult $B.$ $glabrata$ exposed for 24 h to 0.06 ppm suspensions of the toxicant, ground to different particle sizes, was as follows:

Particle size, μm	1–2	2–6	6–15	10–25
Percentage kill	100	70	40	0

Also, the performance of a toxicant may vary when different solvents and emulsifiers are used in preparing an emulsifiable liquid. Therefore, it is very necessary that all the known factors be taken into account and assessed during the development of any formulation for field use.

In addition to work on water-dispersible powders and emulsifiable oils, experimental work has been undertaken on granules (either floating or sinking), slow-release slabs, capsules, resin formulations, oil-bound solids, pastes, solutions with good spreading characteristics, electrolytically-released copper, baits, molluscicidal soaps, and micronized powders that can spread over the surface of the water and then slowly become dispersed throughout the water. This range of formulations has arisen in order to cope with particular circumstances encountered in field operations.

Granules can be applied from the air or thrown, mechanically or manually, from the bank of a stream or from a boat. In the floating form, they appear to be more successful with water-soluble than with water-insoluble compounds.

Oil-bound solids and pastes, as alternatives, do not seem to have any advantages over water-dispersible powders. Resin formulations, painted on wood or metal plates that can then be lowered into the infested water, depend on the random wandering of the snail for their efficacy and have not been successful in tank experiments.

High spreading solutions and floating micronized dusts appear to offer advantages under conditions similar to those in which floating granules can be used. The final choice would probably depend upon cost, which in turn would be influenced by the price of the auxiliary chemicals (emulsifiers, stabilizers) and the ease or difficulty of producing the formulation.

Although baits as residual molluscicides seem promising and the laboratory work encouraging, difficulties have arisen in the field which need to be studied in greater detail before a final decision about their potential value can be made. The difficulties are microbial decomposition of the bait, silting over with mud, and consumption by fish. The toxicity of some molluscicides to fish, however, is far less as a stomach than as a contact poison.

Molluscicidal soap, which permits the continuous application of low doses of molluscicide without any labour costs, constitutes a novel approach to the snail control problem. It might have some application in very limited areas.

The incorporation of water-soluble molluscicides in porous slabs from which the molluscicide would be leached by water movement, could be effective and economical in conditions in which the prolonged application of very low dosages provides effective snail control. It would seem that the solubility of the molluscicide in water is a limiting factor and that the technique described below for continuous low dosages would prove the more effective in use.

Recent field experiments on the distribution of small quantities of concentrated formulations added to water as single doses at regular intervals suggest that this method is adequate for snail control. If this is confirmed and snail control achieved, the concentrated molluscicide formulation could be encapsulated and the capsules placed in water at appropriate intervals. Alternatively, measured 'shots' could be applied by a syringe or suitable measure.

A biocidal rubber formulation, incorporating bis(tri-n-butyltin) oxide into elastomeric matrices, has afforded a slow, long-lasting release of this toxicant. The residual effect has persisted on surfaces in sea water, keeping them free of marine organisms for more than a year. The toxic hazard of the organo-tin for man is seemingly minimized in this formulation, but its molluscicidal activity lasted as long as 200 days in laboratory test. One field trial in still water was successful. Such prolonged activity also warrants considering control of schistosomiasis by destroying miracidia and cercariae. Extensive investigations of the possibilities of biocidal rubbers appear warranted, and field evaluations should be extended.

Few quantitative field observations have been made regarding the influence of formulation upon the dispersal of a molluscicide. A spreading oil formulation has been tested on a few occasions and has shown promise. Emulsifiable concentrates injected below the surface of the water at regular intervals gave a uniform distribution after 24 h in a small pond. Sparingly soluble, solid molluscicides may get lost in standing water when the bottom is muddy, but give complete solution and good distribution when applied to flowing water in the form of wettable powders of suitable particle size.

Safety in Handling Molluscicides

A molluscicide must be relatively safe for handling because the demands of the job sometimes result in taking undue chances, and warnings will not be meaningful to some labourers. Supervision of application must be increased for toxic molluscicides and the cost is correspondingly greater. For this reason, DAWOOD et al. [1965] down-graded NaPCP; however, BLAIR [1961] concluded that simple precautions should be adequate for its wide-scale use. Solid formulations of NaPCP tend to minimize its handling hazards and increase its efficiency, e.g. briquettes and a new preparation for slow release [RITCHIE et al., 1969]. Even a relatively dangerous compound, such as acrolein with combined herbicidal and molluscicidal activities, may warrant the expense of hiring individuals specially trained to handle it safely. The formulation of a molluscicide may account for increasing toxicity, e.g. in a liquid concentrate a chemical may be more readily absorbed through the skin and mucous membranes. However, these concentrates can be used safely in drip application into flowing water, particularly if the product can be applied without prior dilution and especially if the shipping container is of a suitable size and adaptable for drip application. The liquid concentrates may not be safe in spray applications.

Phyto- and Faunal-Toxicities of Molluscicides

Toxicities of molluscicides for man and his domestic animals are paramount in importance, primarily because applications to water used for drinking cannot always be avoided. At concentrations required to kill aquatic snails, none of the current molluscicides appear to be very dangerous, but there is always the possibility of excessive application at some critical point, particularly in standing water. In treating the multiple tributaries of natural streams, the use of unattended applications by drip systems or solid formulations would afford a saving in labour, but would constitute a hazard for the curious. Solid formulations would be safer because they can be better hidden in the streams. Since control efforts might well involve more than one molluscicide, the least toxic, though more expensive, could be selected for situations where the applications might be hazardous. Niclosamide is the least toxic of all currently available molluscicides [GÖNNERT, 1961; HECHT and GLOXHUBER, 1962], and N-tritylmorpholine is also relatively low in toxicity, while most others require precautions (see table II).

The danger of molluscicides for crops is critical in irrigation systems, but of little concern in natural waters. Nevertheless, even acrolein, an effective herbicide, was used in irrigation systems in Egypt and Sudan with negligible damage to furrow crops [UNRAU et al., 1965; FERGUSON et al., 1965]. Phenolic compounds are generally toxic in high concentrations, but NaPCP at 5 ppm with 6- to 8-hour exposures did not harm crops in Japan and the farmers asked for DNCHP in their rice fields, believing it stimulated growth and controlled insects [RITCHIE and McMULLEN, 1961]. GÖNNERT [1961] found NaPCP to be phytotoxic in concentrations required to kill snails; however, this has not been borne out in field usage. Molluscicides selected for use in each endemic area should be tested against local crops with the time-concentration relationship that is to be used.

Even though piscicidal activity of molluscicides is of no concern in many snail habitats, there are many places where the use of such a compound would be disastrous, because fish from ponds and streams are a major source of animal protein for some indigenous populations. Of the 'available' molluscicides, niclosamide and NaPCP are highly piscicidal while copper sulphate is somewhat less so. Paraquat is not lethal to fish at molluscicidal concentrations. DESCHIENS and his colleagues emphasize the non-piscicidal activity of cuprous oxide and cuprous chloride [DESCHIENS et al., 1964a, b; FLOCH et al., 1964]. However, these compounds have not yet been used successfully in the field. In determining piscicidal activity of molluscicides, the choice of fish for testing is important. Recently it has been shown that different species of fish vary in susceptibility to the same molluscicide and for different compounds one species of fish may be relatively susceptible to one and tolerant of another in molluscicidal concentrations [BERRÍOS-DURÁN et al.[28]]. Also, SHIFF et al. [1967] found that one species of Tilapia survived molluscicidal concentrations of N-tritylmorpholine while a second species succumbed. The granular formulation of this product proved less toxic for fish, and BOYCE et al. [1966] showed that the margin of safety for fish increased when N-tritylmorpholine was used in prolonged applications with lower concentrations. There is an enormous literature on toxicity of chemicals for fish that does not include molluscicidal evaluations. A few selected points may be helpful in determining piscicidal activities of molluscicides [WHO, 1965a]. The use of the guppy (Lebistes) for

28 BERRÍOS-DURÁN, L. A.; RITCHIE, L. S.; FRICK, L. P., and FOX, I.: in WHO unpublished document MOL/INF 18 (1964).

fish toxicity tests was discontinued in one laboratory, because it was generally more resistant than other species. In this case, the harlequin fish *(Rasbora)* was substituted because it was considered a better indicator for trout reactions. For different organo-phosphorous compounds against a single species of fish, the highest LC_{50} was about 100 times the lowest, and for Delnav the LC_{50} for gold-fish was over 900 times greater than for bluegills. Therefore, several different species are essential for determining the piscicidal actions of molluscicides; in selecting a non-piscicidal product for use in endemic foci of schistosomiasis it is essential to know the species of fish that needs to be protected. If edible fish are killed, it should be known whether it is safe to eat them. Fish killed by NaPCP in Japan and Africa were consumed without ill effects. Any information of this type should be reported.

The use of any pesticide imposes a responsibility for knowing the effect it has on ecological balances in nature. Even with non-piscicidal compounds, their action on flora and fauna may indirectly affect the fish population. A single investigation of this type in the molluscicidal literature [SHIFF and GARNETT, 1961] revealed that most organisms were re-established in biologically stable ponds within one month following the use of NaPCP and niclosamide. However, the effects of copper sulphate were longer-lasting and certain forms did not reappear within the period of observation.

Cost Efficiency Considerations

There are many inter-related factors that must be equated in cost/efficiency determinations, making it very difficult to arrive at valid conclusions. Examples of these factors include type of habitat, equipment needs, labour requirements, and the supervision necessary for application.

There are two approaches that may be taken in evaluating the cost/efficiency ratio of a molluscicide. One is to determine the cost in relation to the population protected, i.e. the *per capita* cost. This method may prove to be partially fallacious because a high-priced molluscicide used in a sparsely populated area might be costly on a *per capita* basis, while if used in a heavily populated area it would be reasonably economical. On the other hand, cost/efficiency can be calculated on the cost per unit of snail habitat that is controlled in relation to the population protected. In undertaking any schistosomiasis control programme, the cost and efficiency of chemical control should be compared with that of other measures. The expense of any such campaign cannot be viewed entirely from a monetary standpoint, but should be considered in the light of resulting benefits. Control of other communicable diseases, tuberculosis and malaria for instance, has been costly also.

Recently JOBIN [1968] developed a mathematical model for selecting a molluscicide for major control effort. It incorporates data on toxicity, stability under field conditions, stream characteristics, and costs of chemical and labour.

Essential Preliminary Information

Only fundamentals can be stated here, as some of the details are included elsewhere in this manual; basic references include HAIRSTON [1961]; HAIRSTON [1965]; WHO [1961, 1965b].

Taxonomic Identification

Identification of probable snail hosts is essential and infectability experiments should be made, since variations in snail susceptibility to infection supposedly occur not only for different species of host but also for geographically different strains of the same species [KUNTZ, 1955]. However, some of these findings require validation because the predatory activity of chaetogastrid worms against miracidia could have accounted for faulty results. Moreover, susceptibility to molluscicides varies for different species of snail host [SHIFF and WARD, 1966]. The identity of the snail in relation to infectability and reaction to molluscicides is essential to assure use of proper concentrations of chemicals and to avoid unnecessary applications. In planning major control efforts in new endemic areas, preliminary laboratory and field tests should be made.

Locating Snail Habitats

Locating all habitats may or may not be necessary, depending on whether an 'area' or 'blanket' application of the molluscicide is used in order to destroy all snails [CLARKE et al., 1961; FERGUSON, pers. comm.] or whether chemical control is to be limited to transmission foci ('focal-radial' control) [AYAD, 1961]. In both cases, detailed maps are necessary for recording the location of water bodies, occurrence of snail colonies and infected specimens, and other epidemiological information. Sampling of the snail population to determine density and frequency of infection must meet statistical requirements. Of primary concern is a random sampling coverage based on as many small samples as possible. The accuracy of a sampling method in the hands of each group of investigators should be determined by replicate collections in the same habitat at short intervals. One, if not more, 'control' areas that will not be treated with molluscicides should be selected and sampled at the same time as the area to be treated. The relative susceptibilities of infected and non-infected snails can be determined if sufficient infected snails occurred in pre-treatment collections. A total of 30 such obtained with proper sampling is sufficient [HAIRSTON, 1961].

Ecological Information

Knowledge relating to the habitats of the intermediate hosts of human schistosomes is accumulating rapidly, and its importance for more effective use of molluscicides must be assessed. In planning chemical control in new endemic areas, certain basic ecological information must be obtained, for it is important in the choice of the molluscicide. Moreover, to whatever extent is possible, new information should be sought. Areas of interest that may be explored are as follows: (1) physico-chemical characteristics of the environment; (2) biological agents or qualities; (3) natural history of the snail; (4) behaviouristic responses of snails to various ecological factors; (5) influences affecting propagation, causing mortalities and otherwise inducing changes in snail population density; and (6) conditions contributing to infection of the snail and transmission to humans. The following review of the above points is not intended to be complete, but rather to include examples.

Among physico-chemical factors, hydrological patterns and temperatures may limit snail activity and transmission to a relatively short part of the year. In other areas where these factors are more uniform, either because of meteorological conditions or the installation of irrigation systems, conditions are more favourable for transmission throughout the year. Even so, hydrological influences and temperature may adversely affect snails sporadically or periodically. Snails located in flowing water may be 'washed out' by floods, but this may be countered by dense vegetation. On the other hand, droughts may cause high mortalities in standing water. Interruption of irrigation water for short intervals has been observed to cause mass destruction of *Biomphalaria* in Puerto Rico, which probably was due to an increase in temperature. When there is an increase in temperature in the laboratory, due to an air-conditioning failure, mortalities among infected snails are much higher than among uninfected stocks. Related observations should be made for field situations. Seasonal or even sporadic occurrence of snail propagation and infection transmission must be exploited in timing chemical control. Moreover, this may vary for different types of habitat in the same area. Water qualities may also have a more direct bearing on chemical control, constituting a factor in the choice of molluscicides, e.g. greater efficiency on the part of

NaPCP in Africa as compared with results in Brazil was probably due to water qualities [WRIGHT et al., 1958; HIATT et al., 1960], and copper compounds are more effective in acid than in alkaline pH values [HOPF et al., 1963].

Among biological agents, guppies may be important in controlling transmission by consuming cercariae [PELLEGRINO et al., 1966]. Unfortunately, the guppies are killed by most of the current molluscicides. Consequently, the effectiveness of the guppy as an agent of control and its capacity to repopulate must be quantified and equated against the benefits of piscicidal molluscicides. Only limited exploration has been made of the occurrence of molluscicidal biota in snail habitats, and the importance of foods in relation to control is only generally known.

Although natural history studies on snails are time-consuming, biological factors such as growth, maturation, egg production, and the reproductive and life-span are basic for evaluating the influences of ecological factors. The marked capacity of Biomphalaria to survive exigencies of nature and artificial control measures is linked with an egg-to-egg cycle of one month and a peak laying capacity exceeding 100 eggs per snail per day [RITCHIE et al., 1963a, 1966]. That these potentials are suppressed at times by some unknown environmental factors is certain, and it is urgent that these factors be identified and evaluated; PAULINI and CAMEY [1964] reported that low temperature is one such factor.

Behaviouristic responses of snails to temperature, light, dryness or moisture, and to foods and plants in their environment will provide an understanding of some aspects of distribution within their habitat, and of movements that may occur daily, seasonally or in response to weather changes. This information may be useful in timing chemical control operations. For instance, dose rates of less than 100 g/m^2 of NaPCP, copper sulphate and dinitro-o-cyclohexylphenol were ineffective against aestivating hosts of S. mansoni in north-east Brazil. At 100 g/m^2 only NaPCP proved effective against aestivating and retracted Biomphalaria straminea on dry ground under a thick cover of grass. After the first rains, NaPCP and dinitro-o-cyclohexylphenol at rates as low as 25 g/m^2 destroyed all B. glabrata and B. straminea under grass and on wet ground [WRIGHT et al., 1958].

Characteristic snail behaviour resulting from exposure to the molluscicide must be observed, and this may be influenced by environmental factors.

Suppression of snail propagation may occur even when meteorological conditions are seemingly favourable. Eggs laid under laboratory conditions often fail to hatch after apparently normal development. Propagative failures occur in nature, even though eggs are being laid; the reasons for this are not known. Often, propagation ceases after a period of great increase in the snail population, but it is not known whether this is due to physico-chemical factors or a biological control linked with crowding. Factors suppressing propagation could be a very rewarding field of investigation in relation to chemical control. Causes of death must be varied and many, for the different stages and sizes of snails, but few are known. Investigations will be tedious, even difficult, yet they may reveal biological controls that can be exploited.

Factors affecting exposure of snails to miracidia under field conditions are essentially unknown. The first investigation of this kind in the laboratory was that of CHERNIN and DUNAVAN [1962] in which they demonstrated that the miracidia have considerable facility in locating and infecting snails in both vertical and horizontal spatial dispersion. PURNELL [1966] found that the mortality of miracidia of *S. mansoni* was uniformly low after maintenance for 2 h at temperatures of from 12 to 33 °C, but increased in a linear manner with temperature after maintenance for 6 h at the same temperature.

WEBBE [1966] studied the influence of water velocities on infection of snails exposed to different numbers of *S. mansoni* miracidia in a flowing water system. High infection rates were obtained at water velocities of between 0.5 and 1.5 feet per second; at exposures of about one miracidium per snail there was only a slight reduction in infection rates. WEBBE thought that water velocity may enhance the effective scanning capacity of miracidia, so that snail hosts may be located and infected under conditions of high water velocity and low miracidial density.

Predation of miracidia by a chaetogastrid worm that infests the head and foot of aquatic snails may afford some protection against schistosome infections in these hosts [MICHELSON, 1964].

Controls imposed against snail hosts and their infections by natural forces are indeed inadequate in themselves, but they should be known and understood in order to exploit them to whatever extent possible as a means of reducing the cost of chemical control.

Human Infection Rates

The rate of infection in the human population before and after control operations should be made in a standard way, using the same techniques throughout. The repeated examinations that are required over a period of years should be carried out in the same month of each year. The earliest possible evidence of interruption of transmission is provided by the pre-school-children (3–5 years). However, it is much more convenient to obtain stools and urines from school-children. The choice of one of these groups may be influenced by the method(s) used to determine infection, e.g. the efficiency of the intradermal test is greater with increasingly older age groups. Determining the relative efficiencies of the various methods for diagnosing schistosome infections has been exceedingly difficult. Attempts to evaluate and standardize certain of these by survey have been sponsored by WHO.

FAROOQ [1966] stressed the importance of recognizing transmission sites in planning the control of schistosomiasis. He recommended infection rates and egg-counts in children 5 years old as the means to this end. Control priorities could then be given to areas of high risk. In Egypt, exposure risks were found to relate to type of watercourse and water uses.

Training of Personnel

This is imperative before instituting control measures. All personnel, both skilled and unskilled, should receive broad training on the importance of schistosomiasis and other snail-borne diseases that may be present. They should understand the life cycle, particularly how infections are acquired, and the methods used for achieving control. Successful control depends largely on the efficiency of each participant in the programme and the co-ordination of the entire group working as a team. This alliance, or team work, will be achieved only when each member realizes the significance that his particular job bears in relation to the main objective, namely, the disappearance of snails serving as intermediate hosts of human and animal parasites.

Selection of Techniques and Equipment

Although the newer molluscicides are far more toxic to snails than older ones, and their applications are easier and more effective, the material and equipment must be used intelligently. As fewer labourers are needed, it is possible to train them more effectively to ensure that the molluscicides are properly applied and concentrations maintained at proper levels. An improperly trained staff will result in wastage of chemicals, inefficient coverage of the snail habitats, and poor evaluation.

Each type of habitat has formidable features, requiring varied procedures for calculating field dosages and making the applications. In the case of moist-dry habitats, vegetation sometimes must be cut, water may have to be carried, and the effort of application provided by man or machine. In flowing water, the energy for dispersal is provided by movement of the water. For standing water and swamps, merely finding the habitats may be a great burden; however, the static feature assures maximum exposure time. In the case of large bodies of water, applications will be limited to margins, and the determination of dosages is difficult. Swamps are probably the most troublesome, because of dense vegetation that lessens the assurance of complete coverage. Marginal swamps and disjunct pools along streams add to the difficulty of clearing snails from natural water-ways. In such habitats, intelligent use of filling or drainage may reduce propagation of snails and simplify application of the molluscicide. In irrigation systems, dispersal of the chemical is complicated by the large volumes of water that have to be treated and loss of chemical activity in seepage water that collects in drainage ditches. In natural streams, application is complicated by the multiplicity of head-waters and by determining how far downstream the chemical is effective.

The computing of water volumes is not as simple nor is it commonly accomplished with the accuracy implied in the methods described below, except in field trials. Major control efforts may have to rely more on the capacity of operators to estimate volumes, a skill they will acquire with experience. In flowing water, excesses of chemical will not be wasted but will extend the downstream carriage. Recently, PAULINI [1968a, b] described a weir that he states is simple and usable under a wide variety of field conditions. The calculation of the rate of flow and the quantity of molluscicides to be applied are simplified by means of two specially constructed graphs.

Chemical analyses for use in the field are an essential adjunct for determining downstream concentrations, but the benefit is related to the simplicity of the procedures. The very low concentrations required with some of the newer molluscicides complicate the matter of analysis, particularly for low concentrations in prolonged application.

Regarding equipment, the ideal situation is no equipment at all, and this might prove possible for flowing water. The shipping containers for liquid concentrates might serve as the dispenser, and solid formulations could be affixed inconspicuously in the streams. Nevertheless, equipment will be necessary for other habitats, but no effort should be spared in achieving simplicity in the equipment required; personnel should receive careful training in the use of the equipment chosen.

Strategy for Molluscicide Application

Natural Drainage Systems

Two general strategies for snail control are in current use, localized or 'focal' control, and watershed or 'area' control. The concept of localized control is valuable in very large watersheds where transmission occurs only in limited sites, usually near areas of heavy population density. On the other hand, watershed control is practised where the transmission is occurring throughout a relatively small watershed.

A control programme aimed at localized transmission foci requires detailed epidemiological study to locate the important foci. Once these have been located, the application of molluscicides is begun on a regular basis, including repeated applications whenever the snails reappear. Since snails will continue to re-infest the treated area from the surrounding untreated areas, molluscicid-ing must be continued indefinitely. Once the mollusciciding is stopped, the snail populations will build up again and transmission will resume.

Control of an entire watershed is initially more difficult than localized control, but it offers the possibility of eventual eradication of the snail. This means that the control programme can be reduced to surveillance after a num-ber of years. In watershed control, the habitats must be treated in a rigid sequence. First, the sources of all streams must be freed of snail populations; quite often these sources are muddy, seepage areas where chemicals have no effect, so the areas must be ditched and dried out.

After the stream sources are free of snails, the marginal swamps and small tributaries just below the swamp sources have to be treated individually. In some cases the flow will be very slow and the tributaries can be treated as if they were standing water bodies, applying the chemicals with sprayers or as pellets or briquettes. When the head-water tributaries are free, then the major streams can be treated. If these streams have fairly rapid flow, a drip system can be used to apply the chemical.

A great deal of thought must be given to strategies which will reduce the costs inherent in treating the multiple sources. One such strategy is the synch-ronized treatment of all tributaries in a given drainage area, as opposed to the usual treatment of one tributary at a time.

Consider figure 8 which is a problem drainage basin in Aibonito, Puerto Rico. If the usual simple method of molluscicide application is used on this system, it would require applications at points A through L (after ponds, intermittent streams, seepage areas, and upstream marshes are rid of snails) plus applications at points M through S where dilution drastically lowers the incoming molluscicide concentration. This makes a total of 20 application points. The amount of chemical used is proportional to the summation of discharges at each application point. Assuming each branch contributes 10 l/sec, this would total 120 l/sec for the 12 tributaries and 600 l/sec for the treatments below junctions, or 720 l/sec.

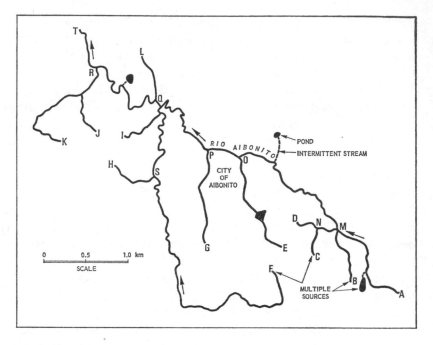

Fig. 8. Aibonito natural drainage system (Puerto Rico).

The alternative is a synchronized treatment based on the following approach. If the travel times for the water in each tributary and branch are measured by tracers, it is possible to prepare a time-table for molluscicide applications. This time-table can be arranged so that the chemical applied at point A will reach junction M at the same time that the molluscicide from point B arrives. Similarly, the chemical from points D and C should meet at junction N and then arrive at M with the doses from A and B, and so forth throughout the system. In this way, the concentration of molluscicide in the flow below each junction will not be diluted by entering tributaries, since all tributaries will be carrying the molluscicide.

If the entire system is treated in the synchronized manner, treatment will require application points only at A through L for a total of 12 points. Total discharge treated would be only 120 l/sec. Comparing costs for the two methods, labour is proportional to the number of applications, so the synchronized treatment will need only 12/20 or 60% of the labour for the simpler type of treatment. Chemical required for the synchronized treatment will be 120/720 or only 17% of the chemical required for the simpler treatment. It is obvious that synchronization of the treatment for this drainage basin would cut the total cost in half, if not more.

There are limitations to the use of synchronized treatment. If the lengths of tributaries are very long and the average flow velocities quite low, it is possible that the molluscicide wave will have decayed and be less than toxic before the outlet of the drainage system is reached. In this case, it is then necessary to sub-divide the major drainage system into smaller units and treat each unit separately. The size of a unit is a function of travel times/decay rate of the chemical and the C_0/C_t ratio used.

For example, if the travel time in figure 4 is about 100 h from A to T and the area is being treated with niclosamide at 15 mg/l with a 1-hour application (a is 50 h, C_0/C_t is 5), then the approximate concentration of the molluscicide will be 7.5 mg/l half-way through the system (T = 100 h). Under these conditions, the entire watershed can be treated as one unit since the C_t is 3.0 mg/l. But, if the travel time from A to T were 200 h, it would be necessary to divide the system into two or three units, perhaps one from A to Q, one from F to Q, and the other from Q to T.

In general terms, the longest travel time, T_{max}, on any stream in the unit, should be equal to or less than T_t, the time of effective treatment for each molluscicide application. Then

$T_t = K_2 \log C_0/C_t.$
If $T_{max} = T_t$, then,
$T_{max} = K_2 \log C_0/C_t,$
or
$T_{max} = 3.3 \text{ a} \log C_0/C_t.$
For the case above, a is 50 h and $\log C_0/C_t$ is log 5 or 0.7, so
$T_{max} = 3.3 \times 50 \times 0.7 = 116 \text{ h.}$

At the other extreme is the very small watershed with relatively high flow velocities. In this case the molluscicide might pass through the entire system with only slight decay. The waste of molluscicide is minimized by lowering the C_0/C_t ratio of the applied dosage.

Irrigation Systems

In irrigation systems, the application of chemicals is simpler than it is in natural drainage systems. The water originates from one large reservoir and is delivered through large accessible main canals. Again, the treatment must proceed from upstream to downstream, but in this case one upstream application will pass through the entire irrigation system along with the flow.

In some systems, night storage ponds will interrupt the treatment since the chemical will be detained in these structures. In this case it will be necessary to treat the pond as a standing water body.

Application of Chemicals to Large Water Bodies

Large lakes and rivers will require a special treatment outside the routine treatment programme. In most cases the volumes of water involved will prohibit a complete treatment and the localized control concept must be applied, limiting the mollusciciding to those portions of the lake or river which are most important in the transmission of schistosomiasis.

Large swamps present the same problem as large lakes, except that treatment may become much more difficult because of inaccessibility of the habitat. In many cases it will be cheaper to drain the swamp than to treat it with chemicals.

Re-treatment Schedules

Repopulation of habitats after chemical treatment is a common occurrence, due to snails which were temporarily out of the water during the treatment, or due to snails which were introduced from other habitats. In Puerto Rico, repeated exposures at intervals of two to four weeks for several months have been tried, particularly after the snail population has been reduced to distinct foci [FERGUSON and PALMER, 1961; FERGUSON et al., 1968]. In areas with pronounced seasonal changes, all of the treatments may be done during a few months of the year. In areas such as Puerto Rico, however, the molluscicide is applied throughout the year.

Basic Planning for Applying Molluscicides

The objective of mollusciciding is to reduce the snail population sufficiently to interrupt transmission of the infection. Experience has indicated that eradication of the snail is virtually impossible, thus necessitating a prolonged control programme. To limit cost, maximum efficiency must be achieved through knowledge of snail reproduction in each endemic area to ensure proper timing of mollusciciding, proper choice of molluscicides and formulations, judicious selection of equipment, and use of other methods of snail control where indicated, e.g. drainage of swamps. In relation to each of these points, the nature of the habitat is critical.

Basic planning should include a choice between 'focal-radial' and 'area' control, prolonged applications in comparison with repeated applications, and specific repopulation control measures, e.g. chemical barriers.

The equipment requirements for control programmes can be specified only after the molluscicide is selected and the major habitat types are known. The least possible amount of equipment should be used, in the simplest manner. In addition, the availability of spare parts and facilities for maintenance are factors of major importance in equipment selection. Available equipment is described below, as well as that currently in use.

Equipment for Applying Molluscicides

General Considerations

The objective of this section is to review the factors that bear on the selection and design of equipment for effective application of molluscicides, to describe suitable items of equipment that are available, and note their adaptability to various types of habitat. Although a wide range of commercial insecticide equipment can also be used for molluscicides, some specialized equipment is needed.

The wide variety of snail habitats is a primary factor in the selection and design of equipment for applying molluscicides. The main types of habitat include:

(1) soil areas alternating from dry to moist conditions;

(2) shallow swamps;

(3) still water bodies – natural and artificial; and

(4) flowing water – natural and artificial.

Formulations of molluscicides can sometimes reduce their toxicity hazards, but the main function of formulations is to provide the optimal opportunity for the molluscicide to come into contact with the snails. It follows that the equipment chosen should be compatible with this objective. The immediate equipment requirements, then, can usually be based on four conditions:

(1) the accuracy of placement required;

(2) the accuracy of dosage required;

(3) the capacity required, which should be based on the rate and time of application; and

(4) requirements imposed by the formulation (e.g. adequate provision for agitation, if suspensions are dispensed).

Having narrowed the field of choice to this extent, it is appropriate to consider conditions under which the equipment must be used.

Portability or mobility is a frequent requirement, which relates to the terrain and accessibility of points where applications must be made. Weights that can be carried will vary with the physique and practices, or customs, of the local people. These should be followed, as a guide, in choice of equipment that may be carried on the head, back and shoulders, or between people.

The capacity of available labourers for training and their skill in maintaining equipment are important in relation to types of equipment that can be used. With rising costs of labour everywhere in Africa [HIGGINS[29]] it is evident that relatively low-grade, unskilled labour will have to be used.

Hazards imposed by the way in which the equipment discharges the molluscicides and danger from the equipment *per se* constitute a vital matter. A chemical as toxic as NaPCP has been shown to be dangerous in spray or dusting application. Leakage from equipment carried on the back or shoulders may be dangerous with some chemicals. Equipment carried on the head, or shoulders and back must not have sharp projections or cutting edges. Any form of equipment employing air or gas under pressure at any stage of operation must be designed to give the user adequate protection in the event of failure. Pressurized containers should be provided with a mechanism to release the pressure before they can be opened. For all such equipment, tests at twice the working pressure should be made at designated intervals by means of a hydrostatic pressure test in which all air is excluded from the system. In relation to the physical comfort of labourers, equipment carried on the back must be properly supported and padded, and a shaped bracket on the back-rest should be provided to allow free circulation of air over the back. If equipment is carried between people in stretcher form, they must have a clear view of the ground. A light harness over the shoulders that is fitted to handles will free the hands. If supporting poles are borne on the shoulders adequate padding must be provided. In tropical areas, consideration should be given to protection against metal parts that become hot due to radiation of the sun.

That simplicity of design and operation of equipment is the keystone of success, is stressed by each of the above paragraphs. Even where skilled workers are available, complexity should be avoided if possible. The more items that can be taken apart or removed, the greater the likelihood that parts will be lost, in grass or muddy water. Worn or damaged items should be easily replaceable without excessive 'stripping down' or removal of parts. A simple design also enhances cleaning and reduces corrosion. Simplicity of operation is frequently a deciding factor in the success of any programme. The easier

29   HIGGINS, A. E. H.: in WHO unpublished document MOL/INF 22 (1966).

the task can be made, the more likely it is that personnel will co-operate. Field work at best is most arduous and often unpleasant, and labourers may not always be under constant supervision. Therefore, when evaluating equipment, particular consideration should always be given to the field personnel, and it should be tested under conditions simulating those where it must be used.

Cost of equipment should be considered at an early stage of a control programme. Too frequently the amount of money allocated to equipment is dictated by what remains when all other financial decisions have been made, rather than in relation to the programme as a whole, and especially to the molluscicide and possible formulations. It has been demonstrated that careful selection of equipment will result in savings in labour and materials, sometimes enough to actually pay for the equipment. When deciding on expenditures for equipment, three possibilities exist:

(1) expendable equipment can be chosen for single or short-term uses;

(2) equipment can be chosen with a moderate life and

(a) used thereafter for spare parts, or

(b) serviced periodically with replacement of worn or damaged parts; and

(3) equipment can be chosen on the basis of a specification for a definite period of life.

The last possibility is the most logical and satisfactory, but the required specifications do not always exist, nor are there agencies to test the equipment against specifications.

Kinds of Equipment

a) Dispensers for Flowing Water

Liquid feeders have been widely used because of their simplicity. Basically, they consist only of a reservoir and some device for regulating discharge (valve or orifice). The reservoir is normally portable, and may be a steel drum or wooden barrel with a capacity of as much as 200 l. With an open reservoir and valve, the rate of discharge decreases as the reservoir empties, requiring repeated adjustments of the valve. However, a constant head can be provided simply by inserting an open box with float valve between reservoir and orifice, or by inserting an air tube near the bottom of a closed drum. The rate of feed may be regulated by adjusting a valve setting, by using orifices of different sizes, or by adjusting the head acting on a fixed orifice. In order to standardize and thereby simplify the procedure, it is possible to select one of a series of orifices of graded sizes and then vary only the amount of chemical placed in the tank (fig. 9).

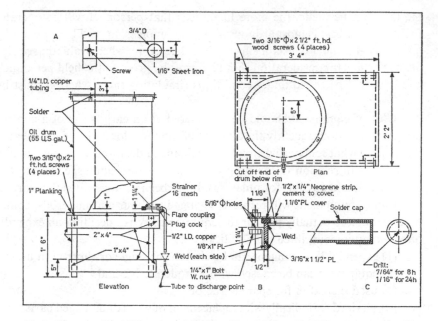

Fig.9. Constant-head Dispenser. Liquid orifice. Notes: (1) Adjust length of orifice tube to give desired flow. (2) Lumber to be Douglas fir or equivalent, nailed in addition to screws shown. A = Funnel support detail, B = cover and seal detail, C = orifice detail [from Snail Control in the Prevention of Bilharziasis. WHO Monogr. Ser. No. 50, p. 172].

If fluctuations in stream flow are of concern, there are liquid dispensers that automatically adjust the rate of application. An example is the device of GRAM and JOBIN [1965] that employs a Sutro weir as the flow-recording device, and a diaphragm-operated valve that regulates the pressure of feed solution behind a series of metering orifices.

The volume of flow that can be treated by a single gravity dispenser depends on the capacity of the reservoir and the amount that can be dissolved or satisfactorily suspended. A 200-litre tank will hold enough $CuSO_4$ or NaPCP for 80 l/sec. For greater flow rates, two or more reservoirs can be interconnected, while the greater potency of some molluscicides compensates.

b) Hand Sprayers

There are two types of hand sprayers. One operates by a plunger pump using either air or liquid to provide pressure, while the other is operated by a piston using only liquid (ram pump). The basic difference is the position of the liquid seal. The plunger type has a cup leather fastened to the end of the plunger shaft, while in the piston sprayer, a gasket is placed at the top of the cylinder through which a solid piston moves at the end of the plunger shaft.

c) Knapsack Sprayers

These comprise six principal types, distinguished by the method used to propel the liquid:

(1) sprayers with self-supplying syringe, and those of the slide-type pump operated by plunger or piston;

(2) sprayers with diaphragm pumps operated by hand lever;

(3) sprayers with plunger pumps operated by hand lever;

(4) compression sprayers into which air is pumped before use;

(5) pressure-retaining compression sprayers into which liquid is pumped against an initial pressure; and

(6) powered mist blowers.

Type 1 sprayers usually cost less than any of the others, and the slide-type pump in particular is one of the simplest and the easiest to use and maintain.

The powered mist-blower, type 6, included in the knapsack category is an entirely different item of equipment. It consists of a light-weight two-cycle motor running on a petrol-oil mixture for fuel. This drives a fan or blower producing a powerful air blast which is discharged from a nozzle held and directed by the hand. The spray liquid is introduced into the nozzle from a container via a feed pipe where it is sheared by the air velocity into small droplets which are then projected for distances of 25 feet (7.5 m) or more. The whole unit is built into a framework provided with carrying straps so that it can be used as a knapsack sprayer.

d) Spray Pumps

These consist of various types. The simplest is the stirrup pump, of value where only limited areas have to be covered. Larger manually-operated pumps are available and can be modified into wheelbarrow sprayers or into stretcher or pole-carried devices.

Power-operated pumps are either rotary, plunger or piston reciprocating types. They are heavier than manually-operated pumps, and vary in weight between 85 and 200 lb. (39 and 91 kg), according to capacity. In the rotary category, gear pumps, vane or roller-impeller pumps are the ones usually employed for spraying; all give pressures up to about 125 p.s.i. (8.9 kg/cm²), with rates of delivery in the medium range. For higher pressures and greater rates of delivery, multi-plunger or piston pumps are used.

e) Circulating Pump

A simple method of introducing liquid molluscicide into flowing water is by bleeding it into the suction line of a pump which circulates water from the stream. A pump which will deliver 100 to 200 l/sec against a head of 8 m, driven by a one-horse-power petrol engine, is adequate for practically any conceivable rate of application. Since the vacuum produced at the pump suction will vary somewhat from one situation to the next, a regulating valve and rotameter (or other flow meter) must be installed for adjustment of the feed rate, which normally will remain relatively constant.

f) Aircraft

In the light of current developments in dispersal of insecticides by aircraft, consideration might be given to their use for molluscicides [HIGGINS[30]]. Their use will be limited to large areas of water, such as swamps or lakes. However, consideration should be given first to the feasibility of draining even large swamps.

Equipment Currently in Use for Applying Molluscicides

HIGGINS[31] reported types of equipment presently in use for applying molluscicides in Africa. The principal types included liquid dispensers, powered compression-type knapsack sprayers, stirrup pumps, power-operated barrow sprayers, and trailer-type hydraulic sprayers.

A simple gravity-flow dispenser (open, calibrated 200-litre/drum) with only a stopcock to regulate discharge is deemed adequate for control programmes. For research purposes, the power-driven constant flow dispenser of CROSSLAND and ADAMS [1965] is in use. The sediment of wettable-powder formulations tends to clog the orifices of any kind of dispenser and a satisfactory agitator is not available. In Puerto Rico, the Gram dispenser is in use for both control programmes and research projects.

Compression type, powered knapsack sprayers of several makes are in use. The Hudson X-pert and the Galeazzi sprayers conform to WHO specifications, but the No. 21 Yorktown sprayer (D. B. Smith and Co., Inc., Utica, N. Y.) used in Rhodesia, is considerably cheaper. The stirrup pump ('Nesthill', UK) serves as an alternative to compression sprayers in Rhodesia. Wettable powders can be mixed by occasionally directing the nozzle into the bucket containing the molluscicide.

30   HIGGINS, A. E. H.: in unpublished documents WHO/VBC 50, WHO/MAL 639, or WHO/Fil 79 (1967).
31   HIGGINS, A. E. H.: in WHO unpublished document MOL/INF 22 (1966).

Power-driven hydraulic sprayers of varying sizes and types, either barrow or trailer mounted, which may also be operated from boats for dam spraying, play an important role. Suitable reservoirs of 25- to 200-litre/drums are readily available and good hydraulic agitation can be achieved through the by-pass return feature. In Puerto Rico, the Hudson X-pert and John Bean powered, positive displacement sprayers are mounted for two-man carrying. They function at 150 p.s.i. (10 kg/cm²) and deliver about 250 l/h (John Bean Div., FMC Corp., Lansing 4, Mich., USA).

Recently, investigators at the Egypt-49 project introduced the veterinarian drenching pistol (with long extension) for applying small measured amounts of molluscicidal liquid concentrates to standing or sluggish water; however, the pistol is tiring to operate. In lieu of this, HIGGINS [pers. comm.] has developed a knapsack, metered-dose applicator that ejects each dose for a distance of 25 to 30 feet (7.5 to 9.0 m).

A list of equipment is provided in table III, including that used up to the present time, and suggestions for additional equipment that might prove advantageous. Moreover, requirements for different types of habitat are given. Reference might also be made to WHO [1964] for more extensive descriptions and photographs of equipment.

Problems of Application Related to Kinds of Habitat
a) Dry-Moist Habitats
Oncomelania snails are commonly controlled in Japan by applying NaPCP to dry-moist soil of irrigation channels and rice fields in spring and autumn when irrigation is not in progress. The chemical is applied in solution (10–15%) at the rate of 0.4 to 10 g (active ingredient) per m². DNCHP is equally effective at lower concentrations, but the cost-efficiency index has been judged more favourable for NaPCP. When applications are made to dry soil, higher concentrations are necessary, up to five times more. The equipment used has been mainly stirrup pumps, knapsack sprayers and hand garden-sprinklers. Cutting or burning of dense vegetation is necessary for effective application.

b) Shallow Inundated Areas
Such habitats include swamps, seepages, shallow pools, paddies, etc. The vegetation is dense and the water, which may not be permanent, is shallow and still. CuSO₄, NaPCP and niclosamide have been used primarily, and the equipment includes the stirrup pump or a high-pressure power pump that discharges sprays or jets 40 feet (12 m) into the swamps. Power sprayers providing pressures of 100 to 400 p.s.i. (7 to 28 kg/cm²) are desirable. Tractors

Table III. Summary of equipment used for molluscicide application and of other equipment worthy of trial

Used up to the present	Additional equipment suggested

Habitat (1): dry-moist soil areas

Watering ean	WHO compression sprayer as used in Malaria
Stirrup pump	Eradication Programme
Knapsack sprayer	Powered knapsack mist-blower
Knapsack duster	Tractor-mounted ground or row-crop sprayer
Powered high-pressure pump	Granule applicator
Portable pumps	Pellet applicator
(a) manually operated	
(b) powered	

Habitat (2): shallow inundated areas

Stirrup pump	Knapsack sprayer
Powered high-pressure pump	Knapsack metered dose applicator
	Portable pumps
	(a) manually operated
	(b) powered
	Tractor-mounted ground or row-crop sprayer
	Granule applicator
	Pellet applicator
	Aircraft application

Habitat (3): still water of various extents, depths and configurations

Stirrup pump	Knapsack sprayer
Powered high-pressure pump	Knapsack metered-dose applicator
Portable pumps	Granule applicator
(a) manually operated	Pellet applicator
(b) powered	Porous container
Briquette and burlap or hessian bag	Aircraft application
Dry feeder	

Habitat (4): flowing water of various extents, depths and configurations

Solution dispensers of various types	Dispensers for solid materials
Briquette and plaster of Paris balls	Metering displacement pump
Burlap or hessian bag	Porous container
Canisters holding bags or	
canisters of molluscicide	

equipped to perform in swampy places might be used to power mounted rotary or displacement sprayers and carry reservoirs for the molluscicide.

c) Still Water of Varying Extents and Depths

This type of habitat includes wells, ponds, lakes and reservoirs. The entire smaller bodies of water require treatment, while it is feasible to treat only the margins of the larger bodies. The molluscicides, formulations and equipment used are the same as for shallow inundated areas, except that boats serve well to carry the equipment and make applications to the larger accumulations of water. However, there is no specific method or item of equipment that is outstandingly good. For smaller amounts of static water, jet discharges from knapsack sprayers or the newly-introduced knapsack metered-dose applicator might be adequate. Granules, briquettes and porous containers may warrant trials. Porous containers may hold either solids or liquids that diffuse into the water at controlled rates from special ceramic containers, such as are used for applying hypochlorite to wells in public health work, or at uncontrolled rates as in case of $CuSO_4$ in burlap or hessian bags.

d) Flowing Water

Natural watercourses and man-made channels, or canals, make up this category. Flowing water serves to disperse chemicals in the channel, but lateral stagnant areas due to great width of streams or marginal vegetation, conjoined swamps and impoundments must be treated as standing water. Even extensive sections of the stream or canal must sometimes be treated as swamps, because of dense vegetation and intermittent flow, e.g. irrigation drains.

Artificial channels and natural streams differ in several respects that bear on mollusciciding. The volume of flow increases in streams, due to tributaries and ground water, while in channels used for irrigation, there is a decrease as water is discharged into laterals. The resulting dilution of the chemical in streams must be dealt with by applying an excess at repeated treatment points and by synchronizing applications in tributaries so that the chemical applied in them will admix in the main stream. Another advantage in irrigation channels is existing gates or other hydraulic means of measuring volume of flow, while less accurate computations must be used in streams unless weirs are installed. Vegetation is generally heavier in streams, since artificial canals must be cleaned periodically to maintain their carrying capacity.

Annex

Definitive laboratory screening—standard methods

---

1. Snail source	*Immersion test – aquatic and amphibious snails* Aquatic snails: laboratory-reared snails, and/or uninfected local host snails. Details to be given in reports. Amphibious snails: as for plate test.	*Plate test – amphibious snails only* Active, freshly collected (24–48 h) field snails.
2. Standard strain	Use of the same strains of snails in all laboratories would be the ideal but is probably not feasible; the strain might cease to be standard in the different conditions of culture and might preclude successful use of a specific molluscicide in certain endemic areas where snails of high susceptibility occur. Each collaborating laboratory should therefore use its own strain and differences in existing strains should be confirmed.	
3. Nature of container	The containers and the composition of the materials used in the containers have various advantages and disadvantages, depending on the compound being tested. Each laboratory should experimentally evaluate the possible effects of the containers, and report the type(s) used. For amphibious snails, as for plate test but with dish 3 cm in depth.	15 cm × 1 cm Petri dish, of glass or disposable plastic.
4. Container size (ml) 5. Volume/snail (ml)	Not less than one-litre vessels should be used in which 10 snails are exposed at 100 ml/snail.	
6. Bottom covering		One sheet of fine-grained filter paper.

Annex (continued)

7. Number of containers	Three containers at each concentration with 10 snails each are deemed a test minimum. The use of 5 snails per test with four containers at each concentration is an acceptable alternative.	(a) Two when a single concentration is used. (b) One for each concentration if three or more concentrations are used.
8. Number of snails	30 snails should be exposed to each of at least three concentrations which lie between the levels giving 5- and 95-percent mortality.	10 per container, placed in the centre of the paper.
9. Snail age	Aquatic snails should be young-mature and relatively uniform in age and size. Daily or weekly use of control tests with a reference molluscicide would detect unfavourable changes in susceptibility with increased age. Amphibious snails as for plate test.	Mature snails, uniform in size.
10. Cover	Should snails show a tendency to crawl out of the test solution, this must be prevented by covering the top of the beaker just above the water level. Glass is recommended. Should the water level be too far below the top of the beaker, it should be raised by the addition to the beaker of glass beads. If other methods are used to prevent snails from leaving the test solution, these should be fully described and, if possible, evaluated by comparison with the recommended procedure at the LC_{50}.	The Petri dish cover.
11. Water	Dechlorinated tap-water. Aerated standard reference water (10% hardness) should be used to assay the influences imposed by local water.	Dechlorinated tap-water.

Annex (continued)

12. Chemical concentration	A 10-fold dilution (solution, suspension, emulsion, etc.) series of 0.1, 1.0 and 10 ppm appears to be in general use and, in some cases, a twofold series is further used after the critical range is determined.	(a) 100 ppm for single concentrations; (b) 10, 100, and 1000 ppm for multiple concentrations and a twofold series can be used after the critical range is determined. If not soluble in water, use a volatile solvent if possible. If insoluble, use finely divided material to get a suitable distribution.
13. Preparation of solutions	Some laboratories use serial dilutions, others dilutions prepared by micropipette.	As in immersion test
14. Volume used		2 ml evenly distributed on filter paper
15. Aeration	Aeration is not necessary during the exposure or recovery periods.	
16. Pre-exposure handling		Allow solvent to evaporate
17. Wetting of impregnated paper		3 ml of water at time snails are added
18. Light	Laboratory lighting with normal diurnal light changes. Experimental evaluation of the effects of laboratory lighting is indicated as this may affect the result.	As in immersion test
19. Mixing	Mixing during test not considered necessary.	
20. Temperature	This factor is important and should always be kept constant (recommended temperature is 25 ± 1 °C).	26–28 °C

Annex (continued)

21. Period of exposure	Exposures of 24 h are thought adequate and a matter of convenience. Other exposure intervals may be used for comprehensive evaluation and in experiments with operculated amphibious snails.	4 days
22. Observations during exposure	Behaviour that may be protective is important, but specific testing is indicated as a part of comprehensive evaluation.	First day: Observe three times, note reactions, centre snails, add water as required to keep paper well moistened but leave no free water. Second day: Observe once, note reactions, centre snails, and add water as required. Third day: As on previous day. Fourth day: Note reactions and prepare for final examination.
23. Washing	For aquatic snails, 3 changes of standard water. For amphibious snails, as for plate test but place snails in a clean Petri dish.	In small strainer. Place washed snails in respective Petri dish lid, add water to cover.
24. Recovery period	The recovery period should be varied according to the action of specific chemicals. The possibility of a carry-over of the chemical on the snail into the recovery water should be borne in mind.	
25. Criterion of death	Death criterion for aquatic snails: by examination (discoloration, heart rate, activity of muscle, etc.) and/or crushing. For amphibious snails, as for plate test.	Crush all snails showing no activity.

Annex (continued)

26. Food during test	Feeding is not necessary during exposure or recovery period as snails are able to survive some days without apparent ill-effects.	As in immersion test
27. Snail controls	Two containers with 10 snails each are a minimum requirement.	5 containers, 10 snails in each
28. Molluscicide control	Trials using a reference compound should be repeated regularly.	Determine LC_{50} with NaPCP at concentrations of 20, 50, and 100 ppm, 2 containers for each concentration, once per month.
29. Determination of LC values	LC_{50} and LC_{90} values should be computed, particularly when the standard test is used in comprehensive evaluations. The use of the probit analysis method appears to be replacing the LITCHFIELD and WILCOXON statistical method[1].	As in immersion test
30. pH	pH of test solution should be measured at the beginning of exposure.	
31. Removal of dead snails	Dead snails should be removed to prevent fouling the recovery water.	

1 LITCHFIELD, J. T. and WILCOXON, F.: J. Pharmacol. exp. Ther., *96:* 99 (1949).

References

ABDALLA, A. and NASR, T. S.: J. Egypt. med. Ass. *44:* 160 (1961).

AYAD, N.: Bull. Wld Hlth Org. *25:* 712 (1961).

AYAD, N.: The rôle of molluscicides in combating bilharziasis; in WOLSTENHOLME and O'CONNOR Bilharziasis, p. 339 (Churchill, London 1962).

BARBOSA, F. S.: Bull. Wld Hlth Org. *25:* 710 (1961).

BARBOSA, F. S.; FILHO, J. C.; MORAES, J. G. DE, and CARNEIRO, E.: Publ. avuls. Inst. Magalhaes *5:* 7 (1956).

BELL, E. J.; ETGES, F. J., and JENNELLE, L. J.: Amer. J. trop. Med. Hyg. *15:* 539 (1966).

BERRÍOS-DURÁN, L. A. and RITCHIE, L. S.: Bull. Wld Hlth Org. *39:* 310 (1968).

BERRÍOS-DURÁN, L. A.; RITCHIE, L. S., and WESSEL, H. B.: Bull. Wld Hlth Org. *39:* 316 (1968).

BERRY, E. G.; NOLAN, M. O., and OLIVER-GONZALES, J.: Publ. Hlth Rep., Wash. *65:* 939 (1950).

BEYNON, K. I. and THOMAS, G. R.: Bull. Wld Hlth Org. *37:* 47 (1967).

BEYNON, K. I. and WRIGHT, A. N.: Bull. Wld Hlth Org. *37:* 65 (1967).

BEYNON, K. I.; CROSSLAND, N. O., and WRIGHT, A. N.: Bull. Wld Hlth Org. *37:* 53 (1967).

BLAIR, D. M.: Bull. Wld Hlth Org. *25:* 597 (1961).

BOYCE, C. B. C.; CROSSLAND, N. O., and SHIFF, C. J.: Nature, Lond. *210:* 1140 (1966).

BOYCE, C. B. C.; TIEZE-DAGEVOS, J. W., and LARMAN, V. N.: Bull. Wld Hlth Org. *37:* 13 (1967a).

BOYCE, C. B. C.; TYSSUL JONES, T. W., and VAN TONGEREN, W. A.: Bull. Wld Hlth Org. *37:* 1 (1967b).

BROWN, V. K.; STEVENSON, D. E., and WALKER, A. I. T.: Bull. Wld Hlth Org. *37:* 73 (1967).

BRUAUX, P. and GILLET, J.: Bull. Wld Hlth Org. *25:* 519 (1961).

CAMEY, T. and PAULINI, E.: Rev. brasil. Biol. *22:* 47 (1962).

CAMEY, T. and PAULINI, E.: Rev. brasil. Malar. *16:* 487 (1964).

CAMEY, T.; PAULINI, E., and DE SOUZA, C. P.: Rev. brasil. Malar. *18:* 235 (1966).

CHANDLER, A. C.: J. agric. Res. *20:* 193 (1920).

CHAPMAN, T.: Bull. Wld Hlth Org. *37:* 43 (1967).

CHERNIN, E. and DUNAVAN, C. A.: Amer. J. trop. Med. Hyg. *11:* 455 (1962).

CHI, L. W. and WINKLER, L. R.: Amer. J. trop. Med. Hyg. *11:* 851 (1962).

CLARKE, V. DE V.: The relationship between acquired resistance and transmission of Schistosoma Weinland, 1858, in man, and its influences on the prevalence of *S. capense* (Harley, 1864) and *S. mansoni* Sambon, 1907, in Southern Rhodesia; (Dissertation for the degree of Doctor of Philosophy) Rhodes University, Salisbury, Southern Rhodesia (1965).

CLARKE, V. DE V.; SHIFF, C. J., and BLAIR, D. M.: Bull. Wld Hlth Org. *25:* 549 (1961).

CROSSLAND, N. O.: Bull. Wld Hlth Org. *29:* 515 (1963).

CROSSLAND, N. O.: Bull. Wld Hlth Org. *37:* 23 (1967).

CROSSLAND, N. O. and ADAMS, W. M.: Bull. Wld Hlth Org. *32:* 144 (1965).

DAWOOD, I. K.; DAZO, B. C., and FAROOQ, M.: Bull. Wld Hlth Org. *35:* 357 (1966).

DAWOOD, I. K.; FAROOQ, M.; UNRAU, G. O.; MIGUEL, L. C., and DAZO, B. C.: Bull. Wld Hlth Org. *32:* 261 (1965).

DESCHIENS, R. and FLOCH, H.: Bull. Soc. Path. exot. *57:* 292 (1964a).

DESCHIENS, R. and FLOCH, H. A.: Bull. Soc. Path. exot. *61:* 640 (1968).

DESCHIENS, R.; FLOCH, H., and FLOCH, T.: Bull. Soc. Path. exot. *57:* 377 (1964b).

DE SOUZA, C. P. and PAULINI, E.: Rev. brasil. Malar. *19:* 413 (1967).

DE SOUZA, C. P. and PAULINI, E.: Rev. brasil. Malar. *20:* 155 (1968).

DOBROVOLNY, C. G. and BARBOSA, F. S.: Publ. avuls. Inst. Magalhaes *2:* 121 (1953).

DOBROVOLNY, C. G. and HASKINS, W. T.: Science *117:* 501 (1953).

DUHM, B.; MAUL, W.; MEDENWALD, H.; PATZSCHKE, K., and WEGNER, L.: Z. Naturforsch. *16B:* 509 (1961).

EL GINDY, H. I.: J. Egypt. med. Ass. *51:* 977 (1968).

ETGES, F. J.; BELL, E. J., and GILBERTSON, D. E.: Amer. J. trop. Med. Hyg. *14:* 846 (1965).

ETGES, F.J.; BELL, E.J., and IVINS, B.E.: Amer. J. trop. Med. Hyg. *18:* 472 (1969).

FAROOQ, M.: Amer. J. Epidem. *83:* 603 (1966).

FAROOQ, M.; HAIRSTON, N.G., and SAMAAN, S.A.: Bull. Wld Hlth Org. *35:* 369 (1966).

FERGUSON, F.F. and PALMER, J.R.: Bull. Wld Hlth Org. *25:* 721 (1961).

FERGUSON, F.F.; DAWOOD, I.K., and BLONDEAU, R.: Bull. Wld Hlth Org. *32:* 243 (1965).

FERGUSON, F.F.; PALMER, J.R., and JOBIN, W.R.: Amer. J. trop. Med. Hyg. *17:* 858 (1968).

FERGUSON, F.F.; RICHARDS, C.S., and PALMER, J.R.: Publ. Hlth Rep., Wash. *76:* 461 (1961).

FLOCH, H. and DESCHIENS, R.: Bull. Soc. Path. exot. *55:* 300 (1962a).

FLOCH, H. and DESCHIENS, R.: Bull. Soc. Path. exot. *55:* 816 (1962b).

FLOCH, H.; DESCHIENS, R., and LE CORROLLER, Y.: Bull. Soc. Path. exot. *57:* 124 (1964).

FOSTER, R.; TEESDALE, C., and POULTON, G.F.: Bull. Wld Hlth Org. *22:* 543 (1960).

FOX, I.; RITCHIE, L.S., and FRICK, L.P.: Exp. Parasit. *13:* 167 (1963b).

FOX, I.; BERRÍOS-DURÁN, L.A.; FRICK, L.P., and RITCHIE, L.S.: J. Parasit. *49:* 648 (1963a).

FOX, I.; RIVERA, G.A.; RITCHIE, L.S., and FRICK, L.P.: Bull. Wld Hlth Org. *34:* 307 (1966).

FRICK, L.P. and DE JIMENEZ, W.Q.: Bull. Wld Hlth Org. *31:* 429 (1964).

FRICK, L.P.; RITCHIE, L.S.; BERRÍOS-DURÁN, L.A., and FOX, I.: Bull. Wld Hlth Org. *30:* 292 (1964a).

FRICK, L.P.; RITCHIE, L.S.; FOX, I., and JIMENEZ, W.: Bull. Wld Hlth Org. *30:* 295 (1964b).

GILLET, J. and BRUAUX, P.: Bull. Wld Hlth Org. *25:* 509 (1961).

GILLET, J.; BRUAUX, P.; NANNAN, P., and LUKALL, G.: Ann. Soc. belge Méd. trop. *41:* 35 (1961).

GÖNNERT, R.: Bull. Wld Hlth Org. *25:* 483 (1961).

GÖNNERT, R. and STRUFE, R.: Z. Tropenmed. Parasit. *12:* 220 (1961).

GÖNNERT, R. and STRUFE, R.: Comparative investigations of some molluscicides; in WOLSTENHOLME and O'CONNOR Bilharziasis. Ciba Foundation Symposium, p.326 (Churchill, London 1962).

GRAM, A.L. and JOBIN, W.R.: Bull. Wld Hlth Org. *32:* 237 (1965).

HAIRSTON, N.G.: Bull. Wld Hlth Org. *25:* 731 (1961).

HAIRSTON, N.G.: Bull. Wld Hlth Org. *32:* 289 (1965).

HECHT, G. and GLOXHUBER, C.: Z. Tropenmed. Parasit. *13:* 1 (1962).

HIATT, C.W.; HASKINS, W.T., and OLIVIER, L.: Amer. J. trop. Med. Hyg. *9:* 527 (1960).

HOFFMAN, D.O. and ZAKHARY, R.: Science *114:* 521 (1951).

HOFFMAN, D.O. and ZAKHARY, R.: Amer. J. trop. Med. Hyg. *2:* 332 (1953).

HOPF, H.S.; DUNCAN, J., and WOOD, A.B.: Bull. Wld Hlth Org. *29:* 128 (1963).

HOSAKA, Y.; IIJIMA, T., and SASAKI, T.: Igaku to Seibutsugaku (Med. Biol., Tokyo) *44:* 134 (1957).

HUNTER, G.W., III; OKABE, K.; BURKE, J.C., and WILLIAMS, J.E.: Ann. trop. Med. Parasit. *56:* 302 (1962).

IIJIMA, T.; ITO, Y., and SAKAMOTO, K.: Jap. J. Parasit. *13:* 70 (1964).

JOBIN, W.R.: Publ. Hlth Rep., Wash. *83:* 594 (1968).

JOBIN, W.R. and UNRAU, G.O.: Publ. Hlth Rep., Wash. *82:* 63 (1967).

JOVE, J.A. and MARSZEWSKI, P.: Rev. venez. Sanid. *26:* 615 (1961).

KLOCK, J.W.; GERHARDT, C.E.; ILDEFONSO, V., and MATEO SERRANO, J.: Bull. Wld Hlth Org. *16:* 1189 (1957).

KOMIYA, Y.: Bull. Wld Hlth Org. *25:* 573 (1961).

KOMIYA, Y.; YASURAOKA, K., and HOSAKA, Y.: Jap. J. med. Sci. Biol. *15:* 119 (1962).

KOMIYA, Y. et al.: Jap. J. Parasit. *13:* 65 (1964).

KUNTZ, R. E.: Amer. J. trop. Med. Hyg. *4:* 383 (1955).

KUNTZ, R. E.: Amer. J. trop. Med. Hyg. *6:* 940 (1957).

KUNTZ, R. E. and WELLS, W. H.: Amer. J. trop. Med. Hyg. *31:* 784 (1951).

MALEK, E. A.: Bull. Wld Hlth Org. *27:* 41 (1962).

McMULLEN, D. B.: Amer. J. trop. Med. Hyg. *1:* 671 (1952).

McMULLEN, D. B.: Amer. J. trop. Med. Hyg. *12:* 288 (1963).

McMULLEN, D. B. and HARRY, H. W.: Bull. Wld Hlth Org. *18:* 1037 (1958).

McMULLEN, D. B.; HUBENDICK, B.; PESIGAN, T. P., and BIERSTEIN, P.: J. Philipp. med. Ass
    30: 615 (1954).

MEYLING, A. H.; MEYLING, J., and PITCHFORD, R. J.: Bull. Wld Hlth Org. *35:* 733 (1966).

MEYLING, A. H.; SCHUTTE, C. H. J., and PITCHFORD, R. J.: Bull. Wld Hlth Org. *27:* 95 (1962)

MEYLING, A. H.; MEYLING, J.; SCHUTTE, C. H. J., and PITCHFORD, R. J.: Trans. roy. Soc.
    trop. Med. Hyg. *53:* 475 (1959).

MICHELSON, E. H.: J. Parasit. *50:* 441 (1964).

MIYAGAWA, Y.: Iji-Shimbun (Med. News) *890:* 1; *891:* 5 (1913).

NARABAYASHI, H.: Chugai Iji Shimpo (Int. med. J.) *855:* 1381 (1915).

OLIVIER, L. and HASKINS, W. T.: Amer. J. trop. Med. Hyg. *9:* 199 (1960).

OLIVIER, L.; HASKINS, W. T., and GURIAN, J.: Bull. Wld Hlth Org. *27:* 87 (1962).

PARAENSE, W. L. and PEREIRA, O.: Rev. Serv. Saúde públ., Rio de J. *9:* 179 (1957).

PAULINI, E.: Rev. brasil. Malar. *8:* 545 (1956).

PAULINI, E.: Bull. Wld Hlth Org. *18:* 975 (1958).

PAULINI, E.: Rev. brasil. Malar. *20:* 139 (1968a).

PAULINI, E.: Rev. brasil. Malar. *20:* 225 (1968b).

PAULINI, E. and CAMEY, T.: Rev. brasil. Malar. *16:* 499 (1964).

PAULINI, E. and CAMEY, T.: Rev. brasil. Malar. *17:* 349 (1965).

PAULINI, E. and DE SOUZA, C. P.: Rev. brasil. Malar. *20:* 147 (1968).

PAULINI, E.; CAMEY, T., and PEREIRA, J. P.: Rev. brasil. Malar. *15:* 41 (1963).

PAULINI, E.; CHAIA, G., and DE FREITAS, J. R.: Bull. Wld Hlth Org. *25:* 706 (1961).

PELLEGRINO, J.; MARIA, M. DE, and MOURA, M. F. DE: Amer. J. trop. Med. Hyg. *15:* 337
    (1966).

PEREIRA, O. and MENDONÇA, F.: Rev. Serv. Saúde públ., Rio de J. *6:* 425 (1954).

PESIGAN, T. P.: J. Philipp. med. Ass. *43:* 861 (1967).

PESIGAN, T. P. and MASILUÑGAN, V. A.: J. Philipp. med. Ass. *26:* 17 (1950).

PITCHFORD, R. J.: Bull. Wld Hlth Org. *25:* 559 (1961).

PITCHFORD, R. J.; MEYLING, A. H.; BRUMMER, J. J.; DU TOIT, J. F., and VORSTER, S. V.: Cent.
    afr. J. Med. *6:* 97 (1960).

PURNELL, R. E.: Ann. trop. Med. Parasit. *60:* 182 (1966).

RITCHIE, L. S.: Comprehensive evaluations of candidate molluscicides; in CORRADETTI Pro-
    ceedings of the First International Congress of Parasitology, Rome, vol. 2, p. 728
    (Pergamon Press, Oxford/Tamburini, Milano 1964).

RITCHIE, L. S. and BERRÍOS-DURÁN, L. A.: Bull. Wld Hlth Org. *40:* 471 (1969).

RITCHIE, L. S. and FOX, I.: Bull. Wld Hlth Org. *39:* 312 (1968).

RITCHIE, L. S.; BERRÍOS-DURÁN, L. A., and DEWEESE, R.: Amer. J. trop. Med. Hyg. *12:* 264
    (1963a).

RITCHIE, L. S. and McMULLEN, D. B.: Milit. Med. *126:* 733 (1961).

RITCHIE, L. S.; BERRÍOS-DURÁN, L.A., and SIERRA, R.: J. Parasit. *51*: suppl. 2, No. 54 (1965).

RITCHIE, L. S.; BERRÍOS-DURÁN, L.A., and SIERRA, R.: Bull. Wld Hlth Org. *40*: 474 (1969).

RITCHIE, L. S.; HERNANDEZ, A., and ROSA-AMADOR, R.: Amer. J. trop. Med. Hyg. *15*: 614 (1966).

RITCHIE, L. S.; BERRÍOS-DURÁN, L.A.; FRICK, L.P., and FOX, I.: Bull. Wld Hlth Org. *29*: 281 (1963b).

RITCHIE, L. S.; BERRÍOS-DURÁN, L.A.; FRICK, L.P., and FOX, I.: Bull. Wld Hlth Org. *31*: 147 (1964).

RITCHIE, L. S.; FOX, I.; FRICK, L.P., and BERRÍOS-DURÁN, L.A.: Bull. Wld Hlth Org. *29*: 545 (1963c).

RITCHIE, L. S.; FRICK, L.P.; BERRÍOS-DURÁN, L.A., and FOX, I.: Bull. Wld Hlth Org. *29*: 421 (1963d).

ROWAN, W.B.: J. Parasit. *44*: 247 (1958).

SCHALIE, H. VAN DER: Bull. Wld Hlth Org. *19*: 263 (1958).

SHARAF EL DIN, H. and EL NAGAR, H.: J. trop. Med. Hyg. *58*: 260 (1955).

SHIFF, C.J.: Bull. Wld Hlth Org. *25*: 533 (1961).

SHIFF, C.J.: Bull. Wld Hlth Org. *35*: 203 (1966).

SHIFF, C.J. and GARNETT, B.: Bull. Wld Hlth Org. *25*: 543 (1961).

SHIFF, C.J. and WARD, D.: Bull. Wld Hlth Org. *34*: 147 (1966).

SHIFF, C.J.; CROSSLAND, N.O., and MILLAR, D.R.: Bull. Wld Hlth Org. *36*: 500 (1967).

STRUFE, R. and GÖNNERT, R.: Pflanzenschutz-Nachrichten 'Bayer' *15*: 50 (1962).

SU, T.L.: Chin. J. publ. Hlth *2*: 81 (1954).

TEESDALE, C.; HADMAN, D.F., and NGURIATHI, J.N.: Bull. Wld Hlth Org. *25*: 563 (1961).

UNRAU, G.O.; FAROOQ, M.; DAWOOD, I.K.; MIGUEL, L.C., and DAZO, B.C.: Bull. Wld Hlth Org. *32*: 249 (1965).

WAGNER, E.D. and MOORE, B.: Amer. J. trop. Med. Hyg. *5*: 553 (1956).

WAGNER, E.D. and WONG, L.W.: Amer. J. trop. Med. Hyg. *5*: 544 (1956).

WEBBE, G.: Bull. Wld Hlth Org. *25*: 525 (1961).

WEBBE, G.: Ann. trop. Med. Parasit. *60*: 85 (1966).

WEBBE, G. and STURROCK, R.F.: Ann. trop. Med. Parasit. *58*: 234 (1964).

WHO Expert Committee on Bilharziasis: Wld Hlth Org. techn. Rep. Ser. *214* (1961).

WHO: Equipment for Vector Control (World Health Organization, Geneva 1964).

WHO: Bull. Wld. Hlth Org. *33*: 567 (1965a).

WHO: Snail Control in the Prevention of Bilharziasis; 4. Chemical Control. World Health Organization: Monogr. Ser. No. 50 (Geneva 1965b).

WILLIAMS, J.E.; OTORI, Y.; MOON, A.P.; FRICK, L.P., and RITCHIE, L.S.: Amer. J. trop. Med. Hyg. *6*: 304 (1957).

WRIGHT, W.H.; DOBROVOLNY, C.G., and BERRY, E.G.: Bull. Wld Hlth Org. *18*: 963 (1958).

YEO, D.: Bull. Wld Hlth Org. *33*: 144 (1965).

Chapter 11

Epidemiology and Control of Schistosomiasis, pp. 533–591
(Karger, Basel and University Park Press, Baltimore 1973)

Biological and Environmental Control of Snails

D. B. McMullen

with the collaboration of Z. Buzo, E. Chernin and F. F. Ferguson

Introduction

Available evidence presented in previous chapters indicates that snail control is the most effective single measure for the control of schistosomiasis. The chemical control of the intermediate hosts has been discussed on pages 458 to 532 and this chapter will be devoted to biological and environmental snail control measures. In introducing a discussion of these methods it must be understood that *control* is not equated with the *eradication* of snails. The latter will be attained only in very localized and special situations. Also, it should be made clear that these measures are not presented in an effort to supersede those discussed elsewhere in this volume. In fact, it is now generally accepted that the goal of schistosomiasis abatement in many foci will require an intelligently selected combination of control measures.

If the biological and/or environmental control of snails is to be used effectively, it is essential to know a great deal about the ecology of the habitats. For this reason considerable attention will be given to describing in general terms snail habitats in natural, irrigation and other man-made environments. It cannot be assumed that public health engineers are fully familiar with the technical aspects of snail control measures required in natural and man-made habitats. Accordingly, engineering design and construction methods are given in a general and somewhat non-technical way so that public health engineers, biologists and epidemiologists can gain some understanding of the engineering methods of snail control.

Nature and Scope

The biological control of intermediate host populations is brought about by stresses produced by other organisms. Environmental control involves physical changes which make the habitats untenable or less suitable for the snails. The factors that affect both types of control measures usually are interrelated, e. g. a change in the environment may increase snail deaths from disease, or competitors may reduce the snails' food supply or bring about physical changes inimical to the snail colonies. The factors which limit snail populations include: (1) diseases; (2) predators; (3) competitors; (4) types of available egg-laying surfaces; (5) foods; (6) plant associations; (7) water body substrates; (8) photic responses; (9) water evaporation rate; (10) water temperature; (11) relative humidity; (12) climate; (13) water body level changes; (14) water chemical quality; (15) water turbidity; (16) water pollution; (17) large water bodies related to surface distribution; (18) wave action; (19) water depth; (20) water pressure; and (21) water velocity.

Environmental control of snails, although currently in limited use in anti-schistosomiasis campaigns, has a notable antecedent in the successful control of malaria in some situations by eliminating or modifying the habitats of the larvae of various vector mosquitoes. Less is known about the biological control of snails but available information will be discussed later.

As in the case of chemical control of snails (pp. 458 to 532), the biological control of snails and environmental control of their habitats have not always lived up to expectations. The reasons for this are similar to those cited as the difficulties encountered in the use of molluscicides: (1) the ecological diversity and extent of the habitats; and (2) the habits of the species and strains of the snail intermediate hosts that live in them. The degree of success of a snail control programme depends on the extent to which these have been considered and assessed as factors affecting the objective. The difficulties encountered and the methods to be used in overcoming them will be discussed in this chapter.

Biological Control

The literature contains numerous incidental observations on the harmful effects of various predators, parasites and competitors on the intermediate hosts of the human schistosomes. The elimination of aquatic plants by biological agents can also have a marked indirect effect on snail populations. A list of the organisms affecting the snails directly or indirectly would include species of bacteria, fungi, protozoa, helminths, annelids, arthropods, molluscs, amphibia, fish and birds [MICHELSON, 1957]. Few of these organisms have been evaluated as snail-controlling agents in the laboratory or field.

Limnogeton fieberi (Belostomatidae, Hemiptera), a 4- to 5-cm long aquatic bug living in the Nile Delta was proved by VOELKER [1966] to be an obligatory snail eater. Neither in the field nor under laboratory conditions were these bugs seen to attack other animals (fish, amphibia, arthropods). In a quantitative assessment of the food devoured by 28 *Limnogeton* from the first day of life to the final moulting (43 to 51 days), 3,547 snails were killed, i.e. a daily average of 2.7 snails per bug. It is probable that this insect plays an important role in reducing the bulinid snail population in Egyptian waters.

Observations on the biological control of one of the intermediate hosts of a human schistosome have been most extensive and over the longest period of time in Puerto Rico and a neighbouring island. An ampullarid snail, *Marisa cornuarietis*, was accidentally introduced into Puerto Rican waters about 1950. Field and laboratory observations showed that the introduced snail affected *Biomphalaria glabrata* in at least two ways: (1) as a competing, voracious feeder; and (2) egg masses and young of the intermediate host were ingested [OLIVER-GONZÁLEZ et al., 1956; CHERNIN et al., 1956]. The judicious use of chemical control and the introduction of *Marisa* into *B. glabrata* habitats in Vieques Island has practically eliminated the latter snail and there is evidence that the transmission of schistosomiasis has ceased. *Marisa* is now used routinely by the Department of Health in Puerto Rico as a control measure in combination with mollusciciding, the cleaning of small stream channels and some land drainage [FERGUSON et al., 1968; RUIZ-TIBÉN et al., 1969].

Some time after the introduction of *Marisa* into Puerto Rico another exogenous snail, *Tarebia granifera mauiensis*, appeared in a few habitats and spread rapidly into many watersheds. There is evidence that this snail can also displace *B. glabrata* and it is thought to have been responsible for the gradual decline of incidence in 6- to 10-year-old children in the formerly highly endemic Caguas Valley [FERGUSON et al., 1968].

Neither of the snail species has become a nuisance or a pest in Puerto Rico. *Tarebia* is one of the snail intermediate hosts for the human lung fluke, *Paragonimus westermani*. Its introduction into new areas, therefore, cannot be considered lightly. *Marisa* is not known to serve as an intermediate host for any important parasites and all attempts to infect this snail with trematodes affecting man and domestic animals have failed. It is possible that this snail could affect certain crops grown in water. All possible dangers should be considered and carefully controlled experiments should be conducted before introducing any biological agents into new areas. The introduction of *Marisa* or *Tarebia* into endemic areas is no exception.

Following observations made by ANDRADE [1959, 1969], a series of laboratory experiments conducted by PAULINYI and PAULINI [1970] showed that a *Pomacea* sp. (Ampullariidae) occurring in Brazil in the area of Belo Horizonte is an efficient competitor and predator of *Biomphalaria glabrata*. This *Pomacea* sp. has been referred to as *P. haustrum* by ANDRADE [1969] and as *P. australis* by FERGUSON [1968].

Environmental Control of the Habitats

Knowledge of the ecological requirements of snails is needed to achieve the habitat modifications necessary to render a locality unacceptable to them. Where detailed knowledge concerning specific ecological requirements of snails is available, it is possible that small changes may be enough to make the habitat unsuitable, but where such information is not available, the measures taken will probably have to be more crude and fundamental. Most of the methods of environmental control which are employed involve relatively drastic changes in the habitat. Although not complete, present knowledge of snail ecology is sufficient to guide the design of such control measures [WHO, 1957].

The types of snail habitats and transmission sites for schistosomiasis are variable. In general, however, most endemic areas can be placed in one of two categories. The first of these includes endemic foci which are located in low-lying areas where often there is an abundance of water. The extent of such areas, the lush vegetation, and difficult terrain often make the use of molluscicides impracticable. Much of the information on the methods most suitable for the elimination or control of the intermediate hosts in such areas has come from a pilot control project at Palo, Leyte, Philippines, and from Japan [PESIGAN et al., 1958; HAIRSTON and SANTOS, 1961]. In these countries it has been shown that engineering and improved agricultural methods can be used in such foci to eliminate many colonies and reduce the total snail population by more than 95%. Stool examinations made before, and two years after, control was started show a reduction in prevalence in all groups below 15 years of age and in the 'under five years' age group, the reduction was

77% [PESIGAN and HAIRSTON, 1961]. At the same time, it has been possible to obtain greatly increased crop yields in the Philippines and to reclaim waste land. Snail colonies remaining after engineering control can be attacked successfully with molluscicides.

The second broad category includes foci that occur in arid and semi-arid areas where the provision of a water supply and its equitable distribution, with reference to space, time and people, is an ever-present problem. It has been reported repeatedly that the irrigation of arid lands, or the conversion from basin and partial irrigation to perennial irrigation, results in an increase in the prevalence and intensity of schistosomiasis [WHO, 1959]. This is because the same factors which make an endemic area more satisfactory for man usually also make it more suitable for the molluscan intermediate hosts. Some areas once quite inhospitable for man and snails now have dense populations of both, and millions of cases of schistosomiasis. There is some evidence that well-designed and constructed irrigation and drainage systems, properly prepared land, good water management, careful maintenance of the canals, and improved agricultural practices in a few areas in Iraq, Kenya, Ghana, and Puerto Rico have, at least temporarily, prevented the usual extension of schistosomiasis into irrigation schemes. The basic principles that must be used to achieve this are discussed on pages 558 to 583.

The problem is further complicated by the fact that many of the medically important snail species have a wide tolerance for most of the physical and biological variables in their habitats, and it is therefore seldom possible under field conditions to alter one of these factors sufficiently to effect control. Thus the optimum temperature range for many species varies between 18 and 28 °C, while the lower and upper lethal temperatures are about 0 and 40 °C. Although most species prefer a habitat with considerable sun exposure, there is experimental evidence to show that some can breed in total darkness provided that food is available. The pH range tolerance is also fairly wide; although the optimum for any particular species usually lies between 6 and 8, the lethal limits are normally beyond any practical range of artificially imposed variation. Water movement, in the sense of velocity of flow, turbulence or wave action, is a factor which is known to affect many species adversely, but limiting values for any of these effects are difficult to determine and they never apply uniformly to a whole habitat because no natural habitat is completely uniform. Even in places where the environment as a whole is unsuited to snail development, there are often small foci where water movement is restricted and snails are able to breed. Factors such as salinity, the presence of toxic ions and pollution all merit further investigation. Some species are very sensitive to small traces of salinity, while other species appear to tolerate much greater concentrations. There is no doubt that limited amounts of organic pollution are beneficial to snails, and such pollution should be prevented wherever possible. The benefit which snails derive from sewage pollution is probably both direct and indirect, for some species are able to feed directly upon faecal material, while at the same time the increased organic content of the water will encourage the growth of algae which form an important natural food for the snails. Places are often found which appear to be excellent snail breeding sites and yet no snails are present. Detailed studies of such places usually have failed to demonstrate the reasons for this habitat selectivity [PESIGAN et al., 1958].

The most devastating change which can be brought about in an aquatic habitat is, of course, the removal of water. If this can be done permanently and without affecting agricultural or other requirements, it is obviously the best method of destroying breeding sites of aquatic snails. If, however, withdrawal of water can only be effected for short periods, as is often the case in irrigation systems, the ability of the snails to withstand desiccation will be the most important factor in the efficacy of the method. Many of the aquatic intermediate hosts of fluke diseases have remarkable powers of aestivation which enable them to survive the dry season in their natural habitats. Some species survive for six months or more without water. There is evidence from laboratory breeding experiments and field observations that such periods of desiccation are necessary for the survival of certain species [WEBBE, 1962]. Unpublished data collected by the same author indicate that the emergence of Schistosoma haematobium cercariae can begin from recently-aestivating Physopsis nasutus productus as early as six days after the return of water to the habitat. In Brazil, however, observations on S. mansoni infections in Biomphalaria glabrata show that snails with mature or reasonably well-developed stages die during the aestivation period as a result of the stress produced by the infection and the adverse conditions. Snails with very young infections often survive, the parasites continue their development and may produce cercariae within two to three weeks after normal aquatic life is resumed [OLIVIER and BARBOSA, 1955]. In any case, of course, no transmission takes place in the absence of water. It is evident, therefore, that in some areas periods of drying of the habitats affects transmission.

Where drainage is not possible, alternative methods such as weed clearance, straightening of banks, deepening of marginal areas and prevention of sewage pollution tend to reduce the number of snail habitats. In artificial habitats water management is an effective measure, for rapid fluctuations in water level and flow rate have a disturbing influence on snails. Irrigation systems and reservoirs should be designed so that such operations can be performed without difficulty and aquatic weeds controlled more effectively. These approaches to environmental control are also of great value in mollusciciding campaigns, because they reduce the number and extent of foci to be treated and make application of the chemicals much simpler and more efficient, with a consequent reduction in cost.

If the costs of installation and maintenance are reasonable, the environmental control of snails should be considered. Only rarely do ecological factors act singly and usually there is a synergistic effect among a number of conditions, and these acting together can make a habitat suitable or unsuitable. Thus, it may not be necessary to alter any one factor greatly if several can be changed slightly at the same time. It is important to remember that the intermediate hosts do not occupy the whole habitat but exist only in suitable microhabitats within the larger environment. Control measures, therefore, should be aimed at eliminating features which create the microhabitat. One of the most effective ways of achieving this is by the destruction of the aquatic vegetation, since this removes a great deal of the substratum on which the normal algal food of the snails occurs and on which the aquatic snails commonly lay their eggs. It also removes a potential source of dissolved oxygen in habitats which tend to be deficient in this respect, and the protection the snails may get from the effects of water movement. The removal of aquatic vegetation does not always change the habitat sufficiently to control the snails. Indeed, in some situations this can result in more snails, more human contact with the site and more transmission.

Environmental control is likely to be more permanent in its effects than chemical methods. However, the cost of making permanent habitat alterations and the difficulty of obtaining the co-operation of the local people may preclude the immediate adoption of such measures in some situations. In cases where complete drainage is proposed for a natural habitat which also serves as a source of water for people, it will be necessary to provide an alternative water supply. If there is no human contact with the water in the first instance, it is unlikely that such a habitat is an important source of infection, and drainage is probably not justified unless the snails present are serving as a reservoir population for actual transmission sites. In many circumstances, for example in rice-growing areas and fish-ponds, some of the more drastic environmental changes might destroy the possibility of using the habitat for its intended purpose. Careful consideration must be given to each case; if the locality to be treated is one in which habitat modification is practicable, and if the cost of the necessary work is not likely to be much greater than that of repeated molluscicide treatment, then environmental control methods should be adopted. This approach should be given particular attention where there is a possibility that the repeated application of molluscicides without selective activity might destroy freshwater fish, thereby depriving the human population of this source of protein. Whatever methods are used, eradication of the snail host is desirable because there is, as yet, insufficient information on safe minimum population densities, and even a small residual population can rapidly re-infest a large area if control measures are relaxed.

Advantages and Limitations

With this introduction to the biological and environmental control of snails, it is possible to outline the principal advantages and limitations of these measures. Details supporting the points made will be found in later in this chapter.

Biological Control of Snails

The observations made on the effect of two species of snails on *B. glabrata* populations and the decline in prevalence of *S. mansoni* in Puerto Rico and Vieques make this the most extensively studied and most successful example of biological control of schistosome intermediate hosts. As has been stated previously, this method of control is used as an adjunct to several other measures. It is not at all certain that the use of these snails is universally applicable in other endemic areas, in other types of habitats, and against other species of intermediate hosts. All that can be said at present is that this approach as a widely used control measure has not been sufficiently studied.

There is some evidence that the 'shellcracker' fish, *Lepomis microlophus*, may be of some value in the control of snails in ponds. Other methods of biological control are receiving some attention but their value is even less well established than those mentioned above. It is obvious that a great deal more laboratory and field research is required to obtain quantitative data on the effectiveness of these and other biological agents in the control of the schistosome intermediate hosts before they can be considered for general use. Until this type of information is available, it is impractical to summarize the advantages and limitations of biological control measures.

Environmental Control of Snails

Advantages

(1) Local labour and materials can often be used.

(2) Under certain conditions, agricultural production is increased through utilization of waste land.

(3) Improved irrigation and agricultural methods generally reduce the number of snails and increase crop yields.

(4) Such a programme usually assists in the control of filth-borne and arthropod-transmitted diseases.

(5) Such measures reduce the area in which it is necessary to use chemicals on residual colonies.

(6) Environmental control usually has a more lasting effect than does the application of molluscicides.

Limitations

(1) The control programme generally requires a degree of co-operation between various public service agencies and the local inhabitants, which may not be easy to attain because of conflicting interests and ignorance of the problem.

(2) In most endemic areas, economic and educational levels are not advanced to the stage where local inhabitants are capable of employing modern agricultural practices and economical water use as a means of snail control.

(3) Cost may prove to be prohibitive since it usually involves heavy capital expenditure, careful planning, and close integration with other engineering activities.

(4) Environmental control, although often referred to as 'permanent', always involves periodic expenditure for maintenance which must be considered in cost accounting.

(5) Such control measures employed in some high rainfall or heavily irrigated areas will not eliminate all snail colonies, and molluscicides also will have to be used (see pp. 458 to 532).

(6) Since water is essential for economic development in arid areas, there is always the danger that its introduction or storage will not only encourage snail habitats but will also lead to concentration of human populations, hence increasing schistosomiasis transmission. Water for man and domestic animals must often come from storage reservoirs and irrigation canals, which frequently harbour snail hosts.

(7) In dry areas environmental control measures usually result in fewer indirect benefits than in wet areas. However, proper water management and drainage in irrigation schemes helps to prevent waterlogging and salt accumulation, which cause loss of fertility.

Measures Applicable to Natural Habitats

Although schistosomiasis is predominantly associated with irrigated areas in Egypt, Lebanon, Iraq, China (Mainland) and Japan, natural waters commonly provide the snails with suitable habitats and serve as transmission sites in the other endemic areas. Streams in the latter provide many of the major foci of infection particularly where ox-bow lakes, shallows, meanders, growth of water plants, or pooling in the dry season have led to reduction in the rate of flow, and to other conditions favourable to the establishment of permanent or semi-permanent breeding colonies of the intermediate hosts. Overflow during seasons of flood and seepage lead to the formation of marshes, swamps and pools which provide additional habitats for the snails. Human interference in the form of dam and culvert construction, of establishment of fords and crossings, and of pollution with excrement, often renders the environmental conditions still more favourable to the host snails.

These situations need equal attention with those developing as a result of irrigation. When villages are situated near such streams or marshes, all the conditions necessary for the transmission of the disease from man to snail and snail to man are present. In these circumstances, it is no less necessary to undertake measures for the reduction and eventual elimination of the snail habitats than under the artificial conditions created by irrigation systems.

Experience has shown that natural snail habitats are so varied that no single method can be devised which can be used for effectively eliminating or reducing all of them. Each snail colony requires individual investigation before the best approach can be selected. In general, however, the more radical the changes initially produced, the less maintenance is subsequently required. Radical environmental change, therefore, if it is found practicable, is apt to be the cheapest control measure in the long run.

Unfortunately, the initial cost of such measures is often high. This would be an almost intolerable economic burden if these measures resulted only in the reduction of the prevalence of schistosomiasis and the funds were all appropriated from the public health budget. Fortunately, the measures needed for snail control often serve other equally useful purposes; thus several environmental control measures applicable to snails may have a profound influence on the control of malaria vectors and pest mosquitoes. Moreover, such measures frequently coincide with those needed for modern agricultural practice. Water conservation and disposal, land reclamation and the proper management of fields and farms require, in many respects, the same kind of treatment of flowing and standing water and waterlogged soil as does snail control when carried out by radical measures. The agricultural benefits which result, therefore, may be great enough to offset completely, or at least in part, the cost of measures which would otherwise be prohibitively expensive. In any event the cost of radical environmental changes must be evaluated in the light of direct and indirect benefits, as well as in regard to the possibility of employing less expensive methods of control. It is only after a careful study of all factors concerned that a rational decision can be made.

Watersheds

In dealing with natural snail habitats, surveys and control measures should be planned on watershed units, starting from the upper reaches of the area and working down systematically. In this way, areas over which control measures have been instituted would be relatively safe from snail infestation from higher areas. Where, however, the endemic area is located in the lower regions of a very extensive watershed, control measures would have to be confined to part of the watershed. The chemical treatment of strategic points above the controlled area or the use of mechanical barriers may be of some value but re-infestation from the upper reaches can be expected in a relatively short time.

A thorough survey and study of the characteristics of the watershed should precede any attempt to initiate control measures. It is essential to determine the area of the watershed and its geological and topographical features, and to obtain information and data on rainfall, stream flow and land-use practices. Aerial maps and observations from low-flying aircraft or helicopters would enable the engineer to gain a useful general impression of the watershed.

From topographical maps and hydrological data the engineer will be able to determine the existing water-carrying capacities of the streams and gullies, and the extent of flooded areas. Consideration can then be given to methods for improving the general drainage pattern in order to eliminate or reduce snail habitats. These methods may involve river training, channel-ization, cut-offs, removal of obstructions in the channels, prevention or re-duction of flooding, etc. Such methods are especially applicable where the density of the human population is high but the cost would be prohibitive in most rural areas.

Capacities for which drainage channels should be designed are deter-mined from records of rainfall intensities and frequencies. In some endemic areas it has been found sufficient to design structures for average annual intensities. Where the drainage affects agricultural or settled land, or roads and irrigation, then the design may have to be based on 5- to 10-year fre-quencies.

Experience has shown that where rainfall and stream-flow records are not available, as is the case in many endemic areas, it is safer to base the designs of control works on field observations, estimated capacities of existing water-ways, culverts and bridges, and on information gathered from local inhabi-tants rather than on empirical formulae that may not apply to the local conditions.

Streams

Flowing waters differ widely in their characteristics, and therefore in their suitability as snail habitats. In natural streams the intermediate hosts are usually associated with a mud bottom which is rich in organic matter. Clean sand, stones and deep semi-liquid mud usually do not provide favourable conditions for these snails. It has been found convenient to place streams in three different categories, in relation to their suitability for the intermediate hosts. After these categories have been discussed, the basic ecological factors in these habitats will be considered.

Large Perennial Streams (Rivers)

The main body of any large perennial stream is frequently unsuitable as a snail habitat. The generally rapid flow often accelerated to a raging torrent during the flood season, the relative freedom from pollution, the fact that there is often a heavy silt load and the water is therefore highly turbid, the absence of aquatic vegetation, and the fact that the bed generally consists of stones, sand or alluvial clay with little or no admixture of organic matter, all tend to render it unsuitable as a snail habitat. However, a few scattered colonies may occur in protected and often inaccessible sites along the margins.

The Tigris and the Euphrates and their major tributaries are examples of this type of stream.

The cardinal factor, however, is the rate of flow. In gentler, slower and shallower rivers, conditions suitable for the snails may be found at many points along the course. Some rivers which are, in the main, unsuitable for snails, present limited stretches where the molluscs can establish themselves. These include the reaches where the current is gentle and pools, lagoons and marshy bays with aquatic vegetation occur along the banks; the Nile is an example. Moreover, many such rivers play an important role in disseminating the snails by transporting them to downstream sites.

Small Perennial Streams

It is in the small perennial streams that favourable conditions for the establishment of permanent breeding colonies of the molluscan intermediate hosts are more commonly found. These streams are more frequently infested by reason of their gentler flow, less marked changes of level, clearer water, and the more frequent occurrence of algae and aquatic vegetation which provide food and shelter for the snails.

Meandering, sluggish streams of this type in endemic areas as, for example, in the Philippines and in Brazil, are often clogged with aquatic vegetation and permanently harbour dense populations of snails. In other endemic areas, such as parts of Puerto Rico, high rainfall and varied topography are responsible for the occurrence of small, permanent streams of variable slope and flow characteristics. In such streams the snails are absent from the high gradient stretches in which rapid flow makes conditions unfavourable to their establishment, but are often present in abundance where the gradient is low, the current is gentle and the margins irregular. Such low-gradient reaches are usually associated with alluvial deposits, both on the lowland plains and in the upland valleys. Even in the steep reaches, however, snails may occur in disjunct pools, seepages and small tributaries, although they may be absent from the main stream.

In many endemic areas small snail-infected perennial streams may be found in upland regions, as relatively small tributaries of larger rivers. If such colonies exist and are allowed to remain, they tend to reduce the effectiveness of snail control measures in the lower portions of the watershed.

Intermittent Streams

These streams often serve as important transmission sites, especially when they stop flowing and the river bed is dotted with disconnected pools.

The rapid increase in the number of snails in the pools and the drought which compels the human population to use these same pools, leads to the establishment of ideal conditions for the transmission of infection. Where the pools dry up completely, the period of transmission is shortened but snails may survive by aestivation through being buried in the mud or protected by accumulations of dead vegetation.

Fundamental Ecological Factors

In the study of flowing waters from the point of view of schistosomiasis control, certain ecological factors are of cardinal importance. Some consideration of their nature and effect will therefore not be out of place at this juncture in the discussion.

The intermediate hosts differ to some extent in their capacity to maintain themselves in swiftly flowing water, the deciding factor being their ability to cling to a surface. When the current velocity is such that the snails are unable to relax their hold in the slightest degree without being swept away, they are unable to move or feed, and can therefore no longer maintain themselves in the given situation.

Little is known about the relationship between current velocity and snail ecology, but laboratory experiments show that a flow of 33 cm/sec causes immobilization and 65 cm/sec causes dislodgement of *B. glabrata* attached to a smooth surface [JOBIN and IPPEN, 1964]. The velocities causing these effects under natural conditions will vary with the nature of the substratum. Snails can cling more easily to a firm rough surface, such as that of concrete or stone, than to a firm smooth surface, such as that of the glass which has been used in some laboratory experiments, or to a loose and shifting surface, such as the silt beds and earth banks of many streams. Snails with conical shells, such as the oncomelanids and bulinids, show a slightly greater resistance to the dislodging effect of swiftly flowing water than snails with flat discoidal shells, such as the planorbids.

Higher rates of flow can be withstood in streams where the current is intermittent; the longer the intervening periods of stagnation, the higher the rate of flow which can be borne. Moreover, more rapid flow is tolerated when the water is clear than when it is silt-laden.

From the point of view of snail control it is desirable to establish, wherever possible, such minimal average, marginal and bottom velocities as will discourage the multiplication of the snails.

Factors that affect the velocity of flow and its measurement will be found later in this chapter.

Floods

Floods are usually harmful to snail populations because of rapid flows and, in some cases, a marked drop in temperature which is sufficient to interrupt breeding. Moreover, the presence of a heavy silt burden reduces the penetration of light; hence the algae and other aquatic plants, which provide the snails with food, are affected.

The seasonal occurrence of floods has some effect on the fluctuation of snail populations, since it not only dislodges or destroys many individuals but also interferes with, or temporarily prevents, breeding. Some individuals in sheltered spots usually succeed in surviving the floods and play an important role in subsequently repopulating the stream.

It must not be overlooked that flooding may lead to the creation of additional snail habitats outside the bed of the stream. Overflow may follow if floods in tributaries occur simultaneously instead of in succession, or at times when the main stream is itself in maximum flood. The resulting swamps and marshes may remain long enough to provide a large number of additional habitats. Snails to colonize these habitats are often transported to them by the flood waters.

Before embarking on any flood control schemes, it is desirable to have data respecting frequency and peak discharges. In some streams floods occur regularly and can be predicted with accuracy; in others they show unpredictable irregularity.

For small streams flood control is best carried out by enlarging and improving the channel; sometimes the raising of the stream banks by levees may prove practicable.

Aquatic Vegetation

Water plants form a desirable, but not an essential, feature of the habitat of the aquatic snail hosts. Bulinids appear to be slightly more dependent than planorbids upon the occurrence of aquatic vegetation, but both types of snails can subsist in its absence provided other food material is available.

Plants apparently favourable to the aquatic snails include, among many others, *Nympheaceae*, *Potamogeton*, *Pistia*, *Ceratophyllum* and *Myriophyllum*. Broad-leaved plants provide suitable surfaces for the deposition of eggs and for the growth of unicellular green algae which form a favourite snail food. There is no doubt that the micro-flora and fauna on the leaves of these plants are more important to the snails as a source of food than are the plants themselves.

Water plants also provide the snails with shelter and protection from intense sunlight and from the mechanical effects of fast current. In habitats exposed to bright sunlight, planorbids and bulinids are generally found sheltering on the underside of the leaves, where the temperature may be two or three degrees lower than in more exposed situations. Oxygen tension may also be higher, especially on the underside of leaves such as those of water-lilies which have no cuticle. The underside of leaves therefore forms a favourite microhabitat. In some cases, the translocation of oxygen to the roots of water plants provides water snails with a microhabitat having a high oxygen tension near the bottom.

The amphibious *Oncomelania* spp. are usually found in habitats with emergent vegetation or vegetation growing closely along the bank near the water's edge. Such plants shade the habitat, and their transpiration cools the air and makes the habitat more favourable to snails emerging from the water. Decaying vegetation from water plants assists in the formation of a suitable substratum and provides additional food for the snails.

Pollution

Pollution by decaying organic matter is a common phenomenon in streams but is markedly more pronounced in the vicinity of human habitations, owing to the casting of animal rubbish (bones, skins, fragments of meat, carcasses, etc.) and plant rubbish (vegetable parings and discards, waste fruit, etc.) into the water. Such pollution, if not enough to upset the biological oxygen demand seriously, is definitely favourable to the occurrence of snails that transmit schistosomiasis and appears to provide them with a rich source of additional food.

A moderate degree of pollution with human excrement is favourable to the establishment of large populations of snail hosts. It is not known, in most cases, whether this favourable effect is due to faeces or to urine, since the effects of these two types of excrement cannot normally be differentiated, but there is some evidence to show that the pollution of streams by urine alone has a favourable effect on the snail populations. A moderate degree of pollution with animal excrement also appears to be sometimes favourable.

Other Forms of Human Interference

In many sections of Africa south of the Sahara, the construction of dams for the purpose of soil conservation and water storage has led to the formation of favourable new habitats for aquatic snails.

For *Oncomelania* spp., the same result may occur, but the change in water-flow is usually on a much smaller scale. The repeated temporary damming of the small streams in order to catch fish, the presence of water-buffalo wallows, and the use of small dams to divert water to the rice-fields, are examples. These and similar diversions force the water away from any defined channel, soften the stream bed, make the flow more sluggish, and encourage the growth of semi-aquatic grasses and other plants which further impede the water flow. This vicious circle produces ideal habitats for *Oncomelania*.

Microhabitats

Reference has already been made to the existence of microhabitats in which the snails can survive and breed in streams in which the general conditions are unsuitable for their establishment. This is an important matter, since failure to detect microhabitats or to consider their possible formation may vitiate the effect of control measures.

Conclusion

It will thus be clear that, in devising environmental control measures directed against the intermediate hosts of the schistosomes in natural streams, particular attention should be paid to increasing the velocity of flow of the water, to the straightening of banks and elimination of pockets and pools, to the clearance of aquatic vegetation, to the avoidance of pollution and to the elimination of microhabitats. The success of the measures taken will depend to a large degree upon the extent to which these aims are achieved. The nature of the substratum will not generally be susceptible to alteration but will provide some guide as to the possible presence of snails during the preliminary investigations.

Reduction and Control of Snail Habitats in Streams and Non-Flowing Waters

Stream Channelization

Marshy margins, seepages and small tributaries of streams in many regions provide important breeding sites for host snails. Streams with these characteristics are always costly and difficult to treat with molluscicides. The vegetation-choked margins and the seepages along the banks tend to keep the chemical introduced upstream from penetrating many snail-infested areas.

Unless they are treated separately, each tributary is a potential pocket from which surviving snails may emerge to repopulate the treated portions. As the chemical flows downstream, additional water tends to reduce the concentration to impotency. For these reasons stream channelization, not only to improve the flow characteristics but also to facilitate effective application of molluscicides, is often necessary to eliminate or reduce snail breeding sites. After channelization, any remaining snail colonies can usually be eliminated by mollusciciding.

Stream channelization has been used to control *O. quadrasi* in Leyte, Philippines [PESIGAN *et al.*, 1958; HAIRSTON and SANTOS, 1961]. The following evidence indicates that it can be effective against aquatic intermediate hosts. In 1950 a section of the Latanier River extending for some distance above the Père Laval School at Ste Croix, through Port Louis, Mauritius, to the sea was channelized with concrete and rubble to prevent the breeding of mosquitoes. Before this was done, the stream served as a habitat for the local intermediate host of *S. haematobium*. A survey of the school-children showed that 63% had schistosomiasis. In 1959 snails were found in parts of the stream above the channelized section but were not present where the mosquito breeding sites had been eliminated by channelization. Seven years after the initial survey of the school-children, and after only partial habitat elimination in the watershed, it was found that only 25% were infected. The absence of protected nooks and relatively frequent flash flooding were factors that prevented the establishment of snail colonies in the channelized reach of the stream. These observations indicate that, in order to be completely effective, snail control measures must extend throughout the infested portion of the watershed [McMULLEN *et al.*, 1962].

Although stream regulation is a specialized field of civil engineering, the problems encountered in the channelization of streams as a snail control measure are not particularly difficult [KING, 1954]. It is, of course, desirable that engineers entrusted with stream channelization should have adequate training, experience, facilities for field investigations and access to experimental data and reports on similar works in various parts of the world. Literature on this subject is mainly found under the heading of 'river regulation'.

Field investigations consist of topographical, hydrographical and geological surveys. Topographical surveys are necessary for the determination of the physical features of the watershed such as its size, shape, drainage pattern, slope, vegetation cover, land use, tendency to erosion and any other special features. Hydrographical surveys furnish information on stream flow and facilitate the correct interpretation of rainfall data. The geological survey reveals the general land formation, soil types, and the presence of suitable materials that can be used for carrying out corrective measures.

Until recently most of our knowledge on stream-training methods was based mainly on field observations. Advances in the field of hydraulics have made possible the study of the behaviour of streams under controlled laboratory conditions. The critical application of both field and laboratory observations in the design and operation of training projects is necessary to ensure their effectiveness and to keep construction costs down to a reasonable level.

In the design of stream training projects, it is necessary to select cross-sections and grades that limit the maximum tractive forces to the value that will not cause scouring of the bottom and sides of the channel. Due to considerable variation in the resistance to erosion of the stream channel, it is not easy to determine this limit with any degree of accuracy. However, observations after the completion of the work will disclose local weakness and then remedial measures may be taken.

The capacity of the stream to transport the estimated quantity of sediment is another factor which must not be overlooked. Again, due to wide fluctuations in discharge stages and sediment load, only an approximate solution is possible. The maximum quantity of sediment is usually carried by a stream at its maximum flow and the hydraulic design should be based on this value. A rough estimate of the quantity of sediment transported over a given period may be made from the flow-duration characteristics of the stream and the density of sediment at various stages of discharge. For snail control work, stream regulation generally involves improvement of grade and stabilization, channel contraction and bank protection works. The stream bed should form a continuous gradient without depressions. At no point along its length should it be possible for water to accumulate so that snails can develop in residual pools if the stream dries out. Limited dredging may be carried out by manual labour or by use of heavy equipment including bulldozers and dragline excavators.

Grade correction and stabilization require the use of training walls and dykes to direct flow so as to establish favourable channels which will prevent scour and erosion. Concrete sills, mainly at scoured bends, may also be necessary. Choice of channel contraction methods depends largely on the need for re-alignment and the suitability of local materials. In some cases the use of concrete, steel-sheet piling or timber has proved effective. In other cases, wire baskets filled with stones have been satisfactorily employed. Bamboo or timber cribs and fascine mattresses may also be used. In Mauritius, masonry walls with cement joints have proved economical and durable. When stone or rock is not available, concrete blocks made from rather weak mixes may be used for bank protection works. In India the use of soil cement blocks has proved satisfactory; the blocks are made from a mixture of sandy soil and 5% Portland cement. Stabilized soil blocks may also be used for short-term protection. Small streams may be enclosed in corrugated metal or concrete piping, which also reduces human access to the water and exposure to schistosomiasis. Adequate training works may also be provided by rock fills or the planting of various trees, such as willows, and the grassing of the banks.

In stream-training work special measures are usually required at bridge, culvert and causeway sites to prevent scouring of the bank and to ensure the stability of the foundations. From the engineering point of view, scouring is especially dangerous where a roadway parallels a stream. Protection of the slope against stream erosion by the use of flexible mats, retaining walls of metal or concrete, timber or steel-sheet piling may be necessary. Such localities are also dangerous from the point of view of schistosomiasis transmission, since human access is easy and snail colonies may develop in the slack water on the convex side of bends.

Problems Where Streams Pass Villages

From the viewpoint of transmission of schistosomiasis three types of problems arise where snail-infested streams pass villages in endemic areas, namely: contact, pollution and blockage. Under these circumstances, it is desirable and perhaps possible to limit human access. However, methods of preventing human contact with the infested water will not be successful unless alternative sources of safe domestic water are provided.

Bathing pools, separate from any other bodies of water, preferably cement-lined and filled with clean chlorinated water, may justify the expense of their establishment by saving the cost of treating infected children. In hot climates children bathe frequently and, unless provided with safe bathing places, they will naturally use the infested streams.

Although rarely possible, it is desirable that villages should be sited as far away as possible from infested streams; a minimum distance of 500 m has been recommended. Where a new settlement is planned this may be done, but in other cases it may be easier to alter the channel of the stream so that it is directed away from human habitations. An alternative method of limiting human access is to flank the stream through the village, and for a distance of

500 m on either side, by high walls or fences. Perhaps the best method of access limitation, where engineering and budgetary considerations permit, is to enclose the stream completely within the same limits in a long culvert or underground channel.

Provision of latrines and of adequate waste-disposal facilities are obviously essential measures, but if they are to be effective the people must be induced to use them. This implies that an adequate and permanent sanitation service exists in the local health administration. It is the duty of local sanitarians to participate, together with public health officers and visiting nurses, in educating the people in health matters and in improved hygienic practices.

Discharges from public fountains and wells, and effluent from public lavatories and sewage-treatment plants must be disposed of properly, in order to prevent the creation of snail habitats. Effective snail control in such cases may require concrete filling, subsoil drainage or absorption trenches. Where, due to the presence of large quantities of water or to topographical features, it is necessary to effect drainage by open channels, provision should be made for periodic treatment with molluscicides.

Where limitation of access as described above cannot be practised, it is important to ensure that nothing is dumped in the stream which may cause blockage which, in turn, will lead to obstruction of flow and ponding, and thereby provide favourable snail habitats.

Seepages

Seepages along the margins of streams may give rise to pools or even to swamps and marshes in which the intermediate hosts find favourable conditions for breeding. In the Philippine Islands *Oncomelania* is able to maintain colonies on patches of ground kept moist by small perennial seepage flows. It is therefore important to eliminate seepages wherever possible.

Where a stream is flanked by low-lying, level ground, a considerable area of this may be affected by seepage. In such cases it is necessary to lower the water table on either side of the stream by the construction of drainage ditches or by the installation of a subsurface drainage system such as French drains or perforated pipes laid in trenches filled with broken bricks or stones.

On slopes near the source of the stream and, more rarely, on lower and more level ground further down the course of the stream, seepage from springs may constitute a serious problem. Drainage in such cases will involve the construction of interception ditches by which the water can be conducted into the main stream channel without the formation of pools or marshes. It is obvious that the drainage ditches must themselves conform to the principles laid down for the prevention of the formation of snail habitats.

The principal source of seepage along the course of many streams is the permeability of the levees or dykes constructed to confine the additional discharge during times of flood and prevent overflow. Seepage may decrease with the passage of time if the waters of the stream carry a heavy load of silt, since the fine particles tend to fill the voids in the levee; for this, however, it is generally necessary to take some steps to reduce its permeability. Prevention or reduction may be accomplished during construction of the levee by the use of less permeable material, such as clay mixed with sand or gravel and well puddled or rammed. The same effect may be achieved by lining the levees on the water side with an impermeable layer of well-tamped clay, clay mixed with sand or gravel, or concrete. In swiftly flowing streams it may be necessary to protect the puddled material from erosion by a layer of coarser material.

Plastic film, butyl sheeting and asphalt-coated fabrics can be used also to reduce the permeability of levees. These materials are less subject to blowouts than is clay. The liner should be anchored in a trench, well below the bed of the stream, brought up over the embankment, anchored in the top of the embankment, and covered with at least two feet of fine-textured earth topped with gravel or other non-erosive material.

Marshes and Swamps

Flood plains and low-lying marshy ground bordering rivers and streams or fringing shallow lakes are not uncommon in some endemic areas. In some cases the stream loses its defined channel and spreads out to become a swamp. Another type of marsh or swamp is that which forms in a shallow depression surrounding a spring. All of these are commonly colonized by the snails. Drainage, filling, ponding, or pumping may either eliminate the breeding sites or reduce them to a point where it is practicable to apply molluscicides.

The planning of drainage schemes must be preceded by thorough investigations of the hydrological factors, topographical features, and the soil properties of the area involved. This must be followed by the selection of the methods of construction and the types of equipment that will be needed. The drainage channels should be located in such a way as to facilitate farming operations and provide easy access to the various sub-divisions. The over-all planning and budgeting for such a scheme should include the location of building sites, roads, safe water supplies and waste disposal. Provision must also be made for the maintenance of the drainage system.

In marshes of limited extent, engineering operations are relatively simple, and most of the work may be carried out by local labour with hand-operated equipment. As the water drains away, the initial trenches can be deepened to the desired level. Then, after a short period of drying and consolidation of the soil, light excavators may be used to dig wider and deeper drainage channels. In the reclamation areas in Holland, a snow-plough type of ditcher has been used successfully to excavate shallow drains.

Light trenching machines for use in relatively soft ground are now available. One type weights less than 1,000 kg, digs a trench 12 inches (30.5 cm) wide by 30 inches (76.28 cm) deep, can excavate over 100 feet (30 m) per hour, has tracks that spread the weight to 518 lb/ft^2 (2,526 kg/m^2), is only 3 feet (approximately 0.92 m) wide, 3 feet (0.92 m) high and 7 feet (2.15 m) long, with a bulldozing blade 3 feet (0.92 m) by 18 inches (46 cm), and can be easily transported on a trailer. The total price, including the trailer, is approximately $3,000 in the USA.

Drainage channels must be kept free from aquatic growth and may have to be treated periodically with molluscicides, since the snails which formerly inhabited the marsh probably will now be confined to them. Drainage channels are less likely to support breeding populations of molluscan hosts if the drainage flow (which usually is relatively small) is concentrated in lined inverts laid with a uniform gradient. This discourages the growth of rooted water plants at the bottom and makes cleaning an easy matter.

Vertical drainage wells dug into a porous substratum have also been successful in draining some isolated marshes.

For marshes of limited extent, where drainage involves relatively small quantities of water, subsoil drainage may be used to advantage. Investigations in many areas have shown that the income from the cultivation of such low-lying areas is considerable and would pay for the cost of drainage in a few years. The engineering aspects of subsoil drainage are treated in some detail on pages 110–112 of the WHO publication *Snail Control in the Prevention of Bilharziasis* [WHO, 1965].

In any drainage scheme where the land is to be used for cultivation, filling and grading are essential for good crop yields and help to eliminate snail breeding sites. While this appears to be self-evident, there are many areas where it has not been done. The material used for filling can be obtained from the levelling of higher areas, earth removed from the drainage channels or ponds, and suitable types of refuse. In coastal areas where sand is available, this can be used as fill; if covered with a foot of soil it can be used for crop production.

In places where drainage and filling are not practicable, or are only partially effective, periodic pumping from wells or channels may be a satisfactory method of drying up marshes. Where pumping is required daily or every few days, pumping stations should be established. If electric power is not available, diesel engines should be used. Where pumping is not required frequently, a truck-mounted pumping unit driven by a petrol engine could be used to cover several water-collection points.

In some localities, marshes have been eliminated by constructing ponds and using the earth excavated as fill. This has somewhat the same effect as drainage channels, in that it allows cultivation of more land and confines the snails to limited habitats where supplemental measures can be applied. This has been used successfully in Australia and the USA to control the snail intermediate host of *Fasciola hepatica*, a trematode causing serious loss among domestic animals. It has also been effectively used in the marshy-margined, slow-flowing streams in Leyte to control *Oncomelania quadrasi*. By this method the amphibious intermediate host is eliminated from the drained marsh, and the ecological conditions in the ponds do not provide a suitable habitat for it. Unfortunately, these ponds often serve as excellent habitats for the aquatic intermediate hosts of *S. mansoni* and *S. haematobium;* even so, such ponds tend to limit the number of breeding sites and make fertile soil available for cultivation.

Drainage and reclamation of extensive marshy areas are highly specialized and relatively expensive operations, requiring the use of a wide range of excavating and earth-moving equipment. In addition, pumps may be required to obtain satisfactory drainage after the channels have been constructed. For these reasons, large-scale drainage schemes ordinarily are impractical as a disease-control measure alone, and must be a part of a land reclamation and utilization programme to be economically feasible. Fortunately, the long-term value of such reclaimed land is often far greater than the cost of the drainage works.

Lakes and Ponds

The association of the amphibious snails with lakes has never been reported. Lakes differ in their suitability as habitats for the aquatic intermediate hosts, but are often potentially or actually favourable to their establishment. No lake in an endemic area can be considered free from these snails until it has been thoroughly investigated along the whole length of its shore-line, since favourable habitats may be restricted to very limited areas. Snail control in large permanent lakes need be carried out only along stretches of the shore with which there is human contact and in adjacent areas from which snails and cercariae may be brought by the current.

Where host snails occur in lakes they are usually established in the shallows along the shore-line. Only one species, *Biomphalaria choanomphala*, an intermediate host for *S. mansoni,* has been reported from deep water in Lake Victoria. Where shallow water species are involved in transmission, the habitat may be rendered less suitable by the deepening and straightening of the margins and by clearance of all aquatic vegetation. In natural lakes much of the clearance of aquatic vegetation must be done by dredges or drags, operated either from shore or from a boat. This was carried out successfully on long stretches of shore-line on Lake Kivu, Congo (Kinshasa) [GILLET *et al.,* 1960].

In lakes and ponds with marked seasonal changes in water level, such work can be done most effectively with graders or bulldozers when the water is low. Provision should be made for roads along, or close to, the edge of the lake to provide access for weed control and mollusciciding operations. Where the presence of swamps or dense forests make treatment from the shore difficult or impracticable, weed control and mollusciciding operations may have to be carried out from boats or barges. In this connexion, however, it has been observed that in Ghana and Rhodesia snails do not thrive where vegetation along the margins of impounded waters is very dense. Such dense vegetation also limits human contact and transmission. Ultimate control can generally only be achieved by the subsequent application of molluscicides.

In arid, tropical or subtropical endemic areas many of the smaller lakes are not permanent or sharply differentiated from marshes. Excessive evaporation under the intensely hot summer sun and, in certain areas, very low relative humidity, together with great variation in inflow of water due to fluctuation in precipitation, lead to great and rapid changes of level. Thus, a body of water which in one year or at one season may be deep and extensive, and justify the name of lake, may in another year or at another season be shallow, with emergent vegetation everywhere, and be justly regarded as a marsh. Such fluctuations of water level are not necessarily inimical to the snails since they take place slowly enough for the molluscs to adapt themselves to the changing conditions. Such marsh-lakes which frequently harbour abundant snail colonies can generally only be dealt with as part of a major land reclamation programme.

In addition to lakes, ponds in endemic areas almost invariably offer favourable conditions for bulinid and planorbid snails and therefore require particular attention. Moreover, they are often important foci of infection, since people are tempted to use them for domestic and recreation purposes and as watering points for domestic animals.

Filling-in is the most satisfactory method of control in such cases, but rarely practicable. Fencing such ponds to limit human access has been tried with success in some areas. Resort may be had to treatment with molluscicides. It is obvious that provision of alternative, safe supplies of water for human needs is essential wherever a pond which has played an important role in the life of the local community is thus brought under control.

Soil Erosion

Soil erosion in endemic areas may result in the creation of suitable snail habitats by blocking water courses and drains, by increasing flood flows and in other ways interfering with the natural drainage of the area. Methods that have been developed recently to control soil erosion, such as improved land-use practices, not only result in considerable economic benefits but also contribute to snail control.

The provision of soil erosion control works has become important enough to require the services of specialists in the field of soils, agriculture and engineering. Where such a programme is under way, the reduction or elimination of snail habitats will be relatively easy. In regions where such is not the case, however, the engineer may have to fall back on his own resources and carry out such works as controlled drainage, filling, slope stabilization, grassing and afforestation.

Measures Applicable to Irrigation Schemes

The considerable increase in the prevalence of schistosomiasis which has followed the establishment of irrigation schemes in most endemic areas of Africa and Asia has been viewed with serious concern by national and international agencies concerned with public health and land development. Attempts have been made to study a number of such schemes in order to ascertain the characteristics which tend to limit the creation of snail habitats and which facilitate snail control measures. These characteristics will be discussed in the following sections in the hope that they will receive the consideration of authorities engaged in the planning of new irrigation schemes and in the improvement of existing ones.

The Planning of Irrigation Schemes

The successful development and utilization of an irrigation scheme are so intimately related to community interest and activities that the planning should be on a broad basis. Consideration should be given to the available land and water resources, climate, crops, people, health aspects and the effect of other water-use development such as hydro-electric power, water supply, flood control, navigation, fish and wildlife, and recreation.

The detailed planning of the scheme should be based on thorough investigations of topographical features of the proposed area, soil properties, climate and hydrological factors, crops and their water requirements. It should also take into account the prevalence of human and animal diseases, vital statistics and available scientific data applicable to irrigation schemes, organization, engineering services, operation, management, and economic and marketing factors. In many schemes engineering design and construction are concerned only with the dam and main canal, leaving the distribution system in the hands of the cultivators. Inadequate preparation of the fields and faulty distribution lead to unnecessary waste of water and soil, and result in low productivity. Often complex and antiquated land tenure laws and water rights further hinder the efficient distribution of water.

Water resources are limited and their development requires huge capital investment. It is therefore all the more necessary that their planning be based on sound economic considerations. Cost estimates should include recurrent as well as capital expenditure. Under recurrent expenditure full provision should be made for regular maintenance and for any special measures required for snail control, such as the cost of barriers and of treatment with molluscicides.

In some areas where snail control has been carried out for a period of several years by molluscicides alone, it has been possible to determine the annual cost of the chemical and the labour required for application. It has been found that such a programme may cost up to $1.20 per irrigated hectare annually. It is believed that costs of this magnitude should be considered in the planning and design of irrigation systems, especially since corrective measures can be used to reduce this figure.

The Gezira scheme in Sudan and the Miwani scheme in Kenya may be cited as examples of well-planned and well-managed irrigation projects in areas in which schistosomiasis is endemic. In the first area, reasonable snail control has been achieved by the use of molluscicides and screens at an annual cost of less than one dollar *per capita* of population. In the Miwani scheme, effective control of irrigation water and efficient farming practices have apparently prevented the establishment of transmission sites in the area.

In other schemes where the planning and management are of a lower standard, snail control methods would be inefficient from the viewpoints of both cost and effectiveness. Moreover, such schemes are characterized by wasteful use of water, poor agricultural practices, low crop yields, inadequate maintenance and management, and poor health and, as a consequence, these communities cannot afford the cost of snail control. It is important that demonstration control projects be started in such areas as an educational activity.

Some of the more important considerations in the design and operation of the components of an irrigation scheme are presented below.

Storage

The selection of reservoir sites should be preceded by surveys of the prevalence of human schistosomes and their intermediate hosts. Storage reservoirs usually provide suitable habitats for some species of aquatic intermediate hosts, and if these are present in the watershed they may invade the reservoir.

In other cases snails do not adapt themselves readily to the reservoir environment but may be able to migrate through it to suitable habitats in the irrigation system below the dam. Thus, *Bulinus* and *Biomphalaria* are both present in the upper reaches of the Blue Nile; but, while the former is found in both the reservoir and the irrigation system, the latter is found only in the irrigation system [Malek, 1958]. In Japan and the Philippine Islands the intermediate hosts of *S. japonicum* have not been found in reservoirs, although ecological conditions along the margins of the reservoirs seem favourable for the establishment of snail colonies.

Where evaporation losses are high, additional water has to be stored to meet the requirements of the irrigation project. This additional storage increases the length of the shore-line and consequently the extent of snail breeding sites. Evaporation losses from the Sennar Reservoir in Sudan are estimated at 135,000,000 m³ per year, representing one-fifth of the water diverted for irrigation. If losses of this order can be reduced, the marginal area which is suitable for the establishment of host snails may be similarly diminished. The application of a monomolecular film of hexadecanol may reduce evaporation losses appreciably [LAURITZEN, 1963]. Experiments by the United States Bureau of Reclamation and the Commonwealth Scientific Industrial Research Organization of Australia have demonstrated that evaporation losses can be reduced by the application of hexadecanol at moderate cost. The success of such application depends on wind velocity, and is very marked in areas where this seldom exceeds 15 km per hour.

Where alternative sites are available, preference should be given to areas either where snails are not present or where control measures are relatively easy. It is also sometimes possible to select areas which are relatively sheltered from strong winds and thus reduce evaporation losses. However, because of freedom from wave action, sheltered areas tend to provide more suitable snail habitats than do exposed areas, and this drawback may offset the advantages of reduced evaporation losses.

It is standard practice to clear reservoir sites before inundation, and the extent of such clearing depends on the utilization to be made of the water. For irrigation purposes it is not usual to carry out as thorough a clearing as for water supply schemes, but sufficient clearing must be done to prevent damage to regulators and spillway gates from floating debris and driftwood. In addition, work should also be carried out for the purpose of facilitating snail control. In shallow areas, edges of reservoirs and vegetation usually provide suitable snail habitats, which may necessitate a number of control measures. The shore-line may be shortened and steepened by the construction of dykes or by deepening and filling. Shallow pockets especially may be deepened, graded, filled or connected with the main body of water so that they do not become isolated pools when the water level drops.

Where appreciable seepage under the dam or around the abutments occurs, it must be either stopped or drained away. In some cases such seepages, particularly during the first few months after construction, are important enough to warrant corrective measures from considerations of water loss alone. In small reservoirs, clay and plastic linings may be used. In earth dams such as have been built in Ghana and Togo, seepage and overflow around and over the spillways and their channels provide suitable snail habitats, which may be eliminated by channelization and subsoil drainage. Often paving of the spillway channel with concrete or stone would facilitate snail control.

Water-level fluctuation as a means of mosquito control has been practised with considerable success for some time. There may be instances where such a procedure would be effective and practicable for the control of aquatic snails in small reservoirs. It is possible that certain species of snails would not survive long periods of desiccation on exposed marginal areas under conditions such as are prevalent in Africa, eastern Mediterranean countries and Brazil. For water-level fluctuation fairly large outlet gates are required. Such gates will also permit lowering of the water level just before rainy seasons, and thus assist in getting rid of deposited silt, enable a grader to trim the shoreline, facilitate removal of weeds and carry out any other maintenance work.

The provision of water take-off pumps and valves would considerably reduce the need for human contact with infested water in reservoirs. Fencing of small reservoirs as a means of preventing contact with, and pollution of, snail-infested water should also be considered.

Where human access to a reservoir is unavoidable, jetties might be erected so that people will not come into contact with snail-infested water near the shore, since the cercariae may be expected to be more frequent there.

Where excessive silting takes place, dams have to be constructed to store additional water, thus again creating potential snail habitats. By the institution of soil conservation practices in the watershed silting may be checked, and for the same extent of surface area greater volumes of water become available.

Diversion

Location, design and construction of diversion works play an important part in the efficient operation of irrigation schemes and the reduction of the number of snails introduced into the distribution system. The type of structure used depends on whether diversion involves an impounded reservoir, a weir, or a pumping station.

For a diversion from a reservoir, intakes should be located some distance from the shore or the dam. They should be well submerged, and should be provided with galvanized screens having three meshes to the centimetre and protected by coarser screens.

Where diversion is from a low weir the chances of snails passing into the distribution system are greatly increased. It is advisable, therefore, to provide baffles as well as fine screens similar to those mentioned above. Investigations in the Gezira area have shown that about 70% of snails carried by the current are transported on trash at, or near, the surface of the water, and that no snails have been observed to be carried below a depth of 50 cm [ABDER RAHMAN and SHARAF ED DIN, 1961]. This finding may be used as a guide in the design of baffles and screens in snail control work, taking into consideration the characteristics of the canal and of the flow, such as velocity and turbulence, which may affect the vertical distribution of the water-borne snails.

The canal intake structures should be located at right angles to the flow of the river. Provision should then be made, by means of baffle walls and a gate through the weir and close to the intake, to induce either a continuous or an intermittent flow in front of the intake in order to keep it free from sediment. The bottom of the intake should be a few feet above the stream bed, in order to prevent the entry of bed-load sediment. Racks should be provided to keep out trash and to protect the fine screens. The works should be located on a straight stretch of the river or near the end of an outer concave bank, where the flow and bed-load are deflected away from the bank. Some river-training works may be necessary for stability and for the control of bed-load deposition.

Where water is diverted by pumping, care should be exercised in locating the suction pipe well away from the river bank and providing a strainer of three meshes to the centimetre. Snails have been reported to pass through centrifugal pumps unharmed, and have established thriving colonies in the distribution channels [PITCHFORD, 1953]. Snails have also been found in concrete pump-wells and tanks.

The design of diversion structures should provide for the quantity of water required to meet the expected consumption, the irrigation losses and the conveyance losses under conditions of partial blockage of the trash-racks and screens.

Where silt traps are provided, the installation of baffles and screens is greatly facilitated. It is often more economical to prevent silt from entering canals than to remove it periodically or to provide for its transportation in suspension directly to the fields.

Distribution

The dam and the main canal of an irrigation scheme are usually well designed and constructed. It is in the distribution and field channels where evidence of inadequate and incompetent planning, design, construction and operation is often found. The intermediate hosts are commonly found and much of the schistosomiasis transmission takes place in this part of the scheme. This is particularly true of distribution systems that are poorly designed and inefficiently operated. In the following paragraphs some of the features which will facilitate snail control in a well-conceived and well-operated irrigation scheme will be contrasted with practices that hinder it.

In general, where the layout and construction of the distribution and field channels are left in the hands of the farmers, or where the responsibility of the irrigation authority ends with the diversion of the water into the lateral canals, the snails are numerous and difficult to control. In some schemes the fields are irrigated only during the day. Many of these provide for the augmentation of the day-time flow by storing the night flow in reservoirs (night storage dams) or in long lateral canals. These provide exceptionally good snail habitats which are difficult to control, especially in the reservoirs.

Excessive seepage, with the formation of waterlogged areas, and overflows into natural drainage channels and gullies are common in poor distribution systems. These also lead to the creation of snail habitats which are very difficult to treat effectively with molluscicides.

In some endemic areas the distribution systems are designed and operated on a continuous flow basis. This tends to reduce seepage by preventing cracking which may follow the turning off of water when rotation is practised. Continuous flow also reduces the danger of overflow. While both features facilitate snail control operations with molluscicides, continuous flow usually provides ideal conditions for the snails within the distribution system. On the other hand, in schemes where rotation is used, the intermittent absence of water often affects the snails adversely. If the periods when the water is off are sufficiently long and the system is provided with efficient shut-off gates and the channels are adequately maintained so that they drain and dry out quickly, snail populations will be greatly reduced. In any event, it is essential to have complete control of the water in the distribution system to get effective snail control. Effective water management in the distribution system benefits agriculture and schistosomiasis control by preventing: (1) loss of water; (2) reduced delivery to irrigated areas; (3) waterlogging of adjacent lands which may be rendered useless; (4) damage to roads, bridges and other structures; (5) an increase required in the capacity of drainage works; and (6) creation of snail habitats.

Canal Linings

As far as snail control is concerned, the lining of canals does not necessarily prevent the establishment of snail colonies. Snails do not occur in the lined canals in Mauritius, but observations in Tunisia and elsewhere have shown that concrete flumes and concrete-lined canals can sometimes provide suitable habitats for snails. However, the relatively high velocities which are possible in lined canals, and the relative absence of aquatic vegetation, not only make them less attractive as snail habitats than earth canals but also facilitate rapid drainage and drying. Moreover, lining reduces seepage to low-lying areas which may otherwise become potential breeding sites. Finally, the application of molluscicides, where advisable, is more effective and less costly in lined canals than in earth canals. Other advantages of the lining of canals, and some of the engineering aspects are treated in the following paragraphs.

Excessive seepage losses from irrigation canals can be reduced by the use of various types of lining. However, it is first necessary to establish the economic benefits to be derived from such a step and to carry out field investigations to ascertain the most suitable type of lining to be used. In some cases it may only be necessary to line sections of the canal that run through the more permeable soils or unstable foundations. In other cases lining may be carried out in stages as water requirements increase.

In the design and construction of hard-surface linings such as concrete and bitumen, the preparation of the sub-grade is most essential in order to provide sufficient support for the lining and to avoid cracks caused by settlement. The principal types of canal linings are Portland cement concrete, bituminous concrete, bituminous membrane, plastic membrane, asbestos cement lining and clay lining. Brick may be available in some areas.

The Portland cement concrete linings are usually 5 to 10 cm thick and are not reinforced. Transverse joints are provided at intervals of 2 to 3 m. Pre-cast concrete slabs and block sections have also been used successfuly. Bituminous concrete linings are usually 5 to 7.5 cm thick and are placed on soil which has been treated with some chemical to prevent weed growth. The mixture contains 5 to 10% by weight of bitumen. It is placed as a hot mix and packed by rolling. After compaction, a sealing coat is usually applied.

In buried membrane linings, excavation of the canal section is extended by about 30 cm and the sides are given a two-in-one slope (two horizontal to one vertical). Before application of the hot bitumen, the sides and bottom of the canal are sprinkled with water and a hot spray at a pressure of 3.5 kg/cm² is applied at the rate of 8 l/m². Three coats are usually necessary to produce a thickness of 6 to 8 mm. The bitumen is then covered promptly with 15 cm of earth, and then another 15 cm of gravel are added to bring the cross-sections of the canal to the desired dimensions. In the USA a 50–60 penetration catalytically-blown asphaltic cement is used. In order for such linings to be serviceable, a special grade of asphalt must be used.

The use of asbestos cement sheets for canal linings has given satisfactory results in Rhodesia and in Bulgaria. In Rhodesia, prefabricated corrugated asbestos cement sheets with relatively flat corrugations have been used. Sheets are rolled into a parabolic shape and are specially cast to accommodate curves in the canal. The sheets are bolted, and no joint filler is used. In each case, preparation of the sub-grade is important. In Bulgaria, half-round asbestos cement sections varying in diameter from 30 to 110 cm and in thickness from 5 to 12 mm, have been used successfully.

Other buried linings, such as plastic films and butyl sheets, may be employed. Installation of these materials requires a limited amount of equipment, and a better water barrier can be assured where inexperienced help must be used.

The choice of any particular type of lining depends on local conditions, initial cost and maintenance. These factors can only be evaluated for any particular locality by adequate investigations. For example, observations have shown that where canal velocities are low and excessive silting takes place, silt removal from lined canals may be more expensive than the removal of both silt and weeds from an unlined canal. There is also the likelihood of damage to the soft linings by livestock and equipment. Research in this field of irrigation is still under way in various parts of the world and especially in the USA. While the various types of linings have their particular fields of application, for snail control the most suitable type is concrete.

Closed Conduits

The use of closed conduits for the conveyance of water in distribution systems is rather limited due to the higher cost as compared with that of open conduits. In some cases, as in California for instance, the low cost of making concrete pipe and the high crop returns from well-managed farms render the use of closed conduits well justified on economic grounds. The Miwani Sugar Estates in Kenya, mentioned earlier, use closed conduits to deliver water from the pump station on the river to the field canals. This practice, and the irrigation cycle used, appear to prevent snail breeding on these estates.

In endemic areas, the use of pipes for the carrying of moderate discharges requiring pipe sizes of up to 1.5 m in diameter may be justified on the grounds of irrigation considerations alone and, at the same time, may bring about the elimination of important snail breeding sites. In some countries much larger conduits have been used but for conditions in eastern Mediterranean countries and Africa the sizes should be limited in accordance with facilities for precasting concrete pipes in field factories and transporting them to the sites.

Pipes for use in irrigation schemes can be readily manufactured in field factories by moderately skilled labour at reasonable cost which, depending on local conditions, may be no higher than for concrete lining of canals.

The use of pipes results in a number of benefits which may more than offset the capital outlay. For instance, water losses due to seepage, evaporation and transpiration by weeds are either greatly reduced or entirely eliminated. This saving of water would allow additional land to be irrigated. On account of the adoption of relatively high velocities, silting is practically prevented. The use of pipes greatly facilitates water control, reduces maintenance, makes more land available for cultivation and facilitates transport and farming operations. In endemic areas, considerable savings in labour and molluscicides would result from the use of pipes as against open canals, since no snail control work would be required. Of all snail control measures, the use of closed conduits is the most effective.

Regulation

Effective regulation of water flow in an irrigation scheme is necessary to ensure adequate supplies to the fields: to reduce fluctuations in demand and hence the need for large canals in the distribution system; to prevent damage to canals and structures from overflow; to reduce water losses; and to enable sectors to be isolated for maintenance and repairs. This latter facilitates periodic drying-out of the habitats and is necessary for the efficient application of molluscicides.

Control structures comprise gates at the main intake and distribution system, balancing reservoirs, large-capacity holding canals, fixed overflow spillways, spillways provided with gates, automatic water-level regulators, gates for isolating various sections of the canals, and various types of meters or other water-measuring devices. The most commonly used type of gate in irrigation schemes is the vertical slide gate of various designs, depending on size. The radial gate has now largely superseded the slide gate where a large regulator is required. In some cases gates are used for metering the water deliveries. Elsewhere, specially constructed propeller-type or blade-type meter-measuring devices are used, such as the Dethridge meter used extensively in Australia. More recently, various types of automatic water-level regulators have been used. These consist essentially of radial gates operated by floats, and are used for either upstream or downstream regulation in an irrigation canal.

Provision for isolating areas of an irrigation scheme, regulation of water flow, and measurement of discharge are of special importance in snail control; for this purpose an adequate supply of gates is necessary.

Silting

Silting in irrigation canals reduces velocities and encourages the growth of aquatic weeds, and these conditions in turn contribute to making suitable snail habitats. Observations have shown that snails thrive much better in field channels where silting is excessive than in main canals where it is usually moderate. In endemic areas therefore, the prevention of, or reduction in, the deposition of silt in canals is of benefit not only to the functioning of an irrigation scheme but also to a snail control programme.

The costs of silt removal from distribution systems are quite considerable. In the Gezira scheme in Sudan, in a canal system supplying about 400,000 hectares, the cost amounts to 250,000 Sudanese pounds (US $700,000) a year. In Mozambique, the cost of silt removal from concrete-lined canals is also considerable, and greater than that of removal of silt from earth canals. In Egypt also, silt removal from canals is very costly and as the number of irrigation canals increases it is becoming more difficult to keep up with their desilting. In Iraq, considerable quantities of silt are removed annually from canals and heaped up on the sides. After a number of years the ridges grow to such heights that it becomes cheaper to excavate a new canal than to continue removing the silt in the old canals. Silt removal from irrigation canals also creates the problem of disposal of the silt, especially where this consists mainly of fine sand without any fertilizing value. Another problem created by silting is the difficulty of maintaining the various regulating structures in working order.

The design of distribution systems should provide for most of the sediment that enters the main canal to be kept in suspension and to be carried through to the fields. This can only be done by the adoption of relatively steep grades, which reduce the area that can be brought under irrigation. However, such reduction in the irrigable area is often offset by the savings in the annual cost of silt removal.

Fluctuations in the discharge of irrigation canals, and variations in the quantity and size of silt introduced at the river-diversion site, make some silting unavoidable. In certain cases it may be far cheaper to reduce the quantity of silt entering a canal by the provision of silt traps than to provide steep grades to maintain it in suspension. The shutting-off of the supply to the irrigation area during periods of high silt-load, such as occur in flood time, also decreases the amount of silt entering the distribution system.

Further aspects of silting are discussed below.

Velocities

The effect of water velocities on the establishment of snail colonies in irrigation canals depends on a number of factors. In earth canals aquatic vegetation provides adequate shelter and anchorage for snails even though the average velocity may be of the order of 0.6 m/sec.

Until recently no investigation had been made of the variation of flow in different parts of the cross-sectional area of streams and channels, with particular reference to the peripheral conditions favouring the establishment of snail colonies. The following facts have now been established in respect of irrigation canals running through silty loam rich in clay and having a width of up to 4 m and a depth of up to 1.2 m [DE AROAZ, 1962]:

(1) Water velocities along the periphery of the cross-section have a mean value of 0.40 of the velocity on the water surface at the centre line and may vary only within 12% of the mean value from the water edge to the centre point on the bottom.

(2) The discharge in cubic metres per second is expressed by the following formula:

$$Q = 0.549 \, WHV_0,$$

where

W is the width of the channel at the water surface in metres,

H is the water depth at the centre line in metres,

V_0 is the water velocity in metres per second, measured on the surface at the centre line.

(3) The mean water velocity, as determined by dividing the rate of flow by the area of the cross-section, is 0.729 of the velocity on the water surface at the centre line.

(4) The water velocity at a point on the centre line at a depth from the water surface equal to 0.755 of the total depth at the centre, has the same value as the mean velocity of the water flowing throughout the channel.

Figures 1, 2 and 3 [DE AROAZ, 1962] illustrate the lines of equal velocity in different types of channels.

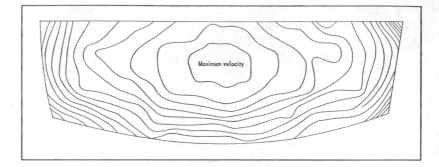

Fig. 1. Lines of equal velocity in a regular channel.

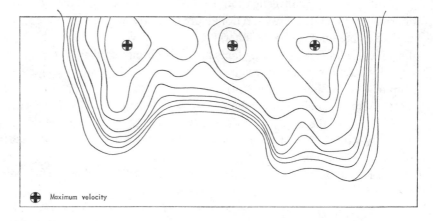

Fig. 2. Lines of equal velocity in an irregular channel (adapted from KING, 1954).

While it is important to appreciate that the velocities in irrigation canals are not, in general, high enough to prevent snail breeding, they are nevertheless an essential factor in determining the suitability of habitat. Evidence indicates that there is a range of critical velocities for each species of snail above which anchorage is difficult or impossible but it must be remembered that such velocities are only effective if they reach the microhabitat. Wherever practicable, therefore, irrigation systems should be designed so that water velocities in canals are as high as the nature of the soil and configuration of the ground would permit without causing erosion. Some of the more important factors influencing choice of velocities will be considered in the following paragraphs.

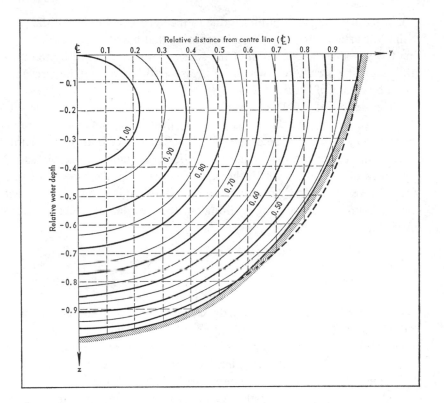

Fig. 3. Lines of equal velocity in a typical earth canal.

Determination of optimum velocities in an irrigation scheme depends not only on the topographical features of the area and the properties of its soil, but also on the operating conditions of the distribution system. Velocities in earth canals should be high enough to prevent silting without causing at the same time serious scouring of the bottom and sides of the canal.

Although many attempts have been made to evaluate the various factors that determine the range of optimum velocities under a given set of conditions, it is still necessary for engineers to rely largely on their own observations and assessment of local conditions. Both silting and scouring may be expected over a period of several years, but the choice of proper velocities should result in stable canals where silting during floods would be counteracted by limited scouring during periods of normal clear-water flows.

Observations show that in irrigation schemes silting is a far more serious problem than scouring. Whereas silting is likely to increase with the age of the canals, scouring tends to diminish due to the ageing and lining of the canals with silt. Furthermore, any possible scouring that may take place during the first few years of the operation of the scheme may be checked by the use of grade-reducing structures, whereas excessive silting cannot be prevented, except by means of silt traps.

The design of stable irrigation canals should be based on the latest concepts of the regime theory to guard against silting and on the tractive forces theory to prevent excessive scouring. The use of both these methods requires the determination of the properties and quantities of silt and the properties of the soil in which the canal is excavated. As a result of many years of research and field observations, the factors that determine whether a canal will suffer from scouring or silting have been evaluated with some degree of reliability.

Weed Control

Weeds in irrigation canals and drains provide suitable habitats for snails, and where they hamper the application of molluscicides their removal becomes necessary. In addition, they reduce the carrying capacities of the distribution system, use up considerable quantities of water and thus reduce the amount available to crops. The control of weeds is therefore important, not only for snail control but also for the proper functioning of an irrigation scheme. A reduction of one-third to one-half of the carrying capacity of an earth canal in from three to five years is not unusual.

Weed control is a problem even in concrete-lined canals, although not to the same extent as in unlined canals. Submerged weeds grow in the deposited silt or through construction joints and cracks, while bank weeds reach down to the water level, shedding their seeds which are transported through the distribution system to cultivated fields. Further, their branches and leaves provide anchorages for the establishment of snail colonies.

Biological control of weeds in irrigation schemes is being investigated. At present both mechanical and chemical methods are widely used. The selection of method or a combination of methods depends on local conditions, the size and characteristics of the irrigation area, types of weeds and relative costs. Mechanical methods comprise dredging, pulling out by specially designed scrapers, burning, chaining, cutting, mowing and grazing. Chemical methods comprise the use of selective herbicides such as 2,4-D, TCA, Dalapon and CMV for bank weeds, and aromatic solvents for aquatic weeds. The effectiveness of chemical control depends largely on the choice of herbicide, which is governed by the type of weed, and on the method, timing and frequency of application.

As far as snail control work is concerned, weed removal is an important factor. With mechanical methods, snail habitats are either destroyed or seriously disturbed. However, such disturbance may also facilitate the movement of snails by floating them down irrigation canals to new areas.

The number of selected herbicides is being continually extended and some of them are lethal to host snails (pp. 488, 489). Such a double effect may result in substantial savings in areas where snail control has been established and molluscicides are used.

Weed control operations are facilitated by the provision of places for the application of herbicides, and roads for the use of mechanical equipment. In certain circumstances, provision should be made for the use of boats, both for herbicide application and for cutting of weeds. In some areas flat-bottomed boats, paddle-propelled and fitted with cutting knives, have been found practicable for this purpose. The cut weeds float downstream and are collected at convenient stations.

A comprehensive account of methods is given in Manual No. 36 of the Food and Agriculture Organization, entitled *Methods of Weed Control*.

Water Supply

Where water supply to villages for domestic purposes, washing, recreation and gardens has to be obtained from irrigation canals, adequate provision should be made for appropriate take off structures, protected with strainers. The water may flow by gravity to the village in a pipe to feed a ground reservoir, from which it may be pumped to elevated tanks. If gravity flow is not possible, then a pump must be installed close to the canal to feed elevated tanks in the village.

Snail breeding in such cases may take place in concrete channels, washing troughs, valve chambers and reservoirs. Effective snail control would involve surveillance, covering of the various concrete structures and filters, and the provision of a storage period of 48 h to ensure that any cercariae that may have gained access to the water supply would perish before the water is used. It should be remembered that it has been demonstrated repeatedly that viable cercariae can pass through sand filters. As a matter of general preventive medical practice, wherever possible water supplies should be chlorinated.

A chlorine residual of 1.0 ppm for 30 min will kill schistosome cercariae. Lower residuals are also effective for this purpose after more prolonged exposure.

Land Preparation for Irrigation

The levelling, grading, sub-division and layout of irrigation field ditches are very important operations requiring design and technical skill and equipment, and they are generally best handled by a constituted authority or some other organization prepared to do this type of work. When entrusted to individual farmers such work cannot, as a rule, be properly executed, and the result will be uneven water application, water waste, formation of stagnant pools, reduced crop yields and creation of numerous potential snail habitats.

Furthermore, the works of a more or less permanent nature in efficient irrigation require some field preparation before every irrigation season, and maintenance of ditches and border-strip dykes. This work is greatly facilitated by the use of light mechanical equipment that can be operated by a tractor. A good example of an irrigation scheme where field preparation is efficiently practised is the Gezira scheme in the Sudan.

For sprinkler irrigation, the need for land preparation is considerably reduced. Although this type of irrigation has not been used to any extent in areas where schistosomiasis is endemic, its employment would lead to reduction in the number of snail habitats and hence in the number of snails. Since field channels are not necessary and excess water is avoided, two important factors in the creation of breeding sites for snails are eliminated.

This method of irrigation has been more widely used in the past 15 years, mainly owing to the increased availability of lightweight pipes and easily operated pumping units. The method can be applied, without causing soil erosion, to areas of limited extent which are too steep or irregular for surface irrigation, and fairly uniform application of water is possible where the design is satisfactory and reasonable care is exercised. In one irrigation scheme in Rhodesia sugar cane yields were 15% higher in sprinkler-irrigated than in gravity-irrigated fields.

Some of the limiting factors of this method of irrigation are: wind interference; clogging of channels or pipe perforations by debris; the difficulty of ensuring a constant supply of water; and the need for power. Moreover, this method involves high investment cost and skilled technicians.

The general layout of any type of farm distribution system is governed by topographical features, soil texture, methods of water application, infiltration rates, size of irrigation stream, condition of soil, and types of crops. Some of these factors vary during any one irrigation period, and the layout can only provide for average conditions. The detailed layout of the farm distribution system should take into account the supply to the various fields, the location of control structures, roads and drainage, and agricultural practice such as seeding, tillage and harvesting.

While there are variations in detail, a general pattern of distribution is discernible in many irrigation schemes. The main supply canal to the farms is located on the highest ground and is usually large and short so as to provide some balancing storage. Water flows into the various fields in more or less permanent earth ditches, having grades of about 1 to 5 per thousand, and velocities of about 0.610 m/sec. These are located along the field boundaries. Temporary ditches are then used for conveying the water from the edge of the field to individual furrows or border checks. Lining of some permanent farm ditches may be advisable to reduce seepage, silting and weed growth. Materials for this purpose have been discussed on pages 564 to 566. Various special control structures and devices are necessary for efficient use and even application of water. These may be either permanent, temporary or portable, depending on local conditions, available funds, methods of cleaning the canals, and expected changes in farming practices. Flumes and inverted siphons and culverts are required to cross gullies and roads, railways, streams and other canals. Division boxes and turn-outs and gates to control and guide the water, are required. Drop-structures are used to prevent scouring when the grade is too steep. Check-weirs are used to raise the water surface to feed some laterals.

Flow-measuring devices are most important in preventing unnecessary waste and collections of excess water. Typical examples of such devices are the Parshall flume, weirs, calibrated gates, orifices and gauges, and Dethridge meters. In the layout of the farm distribution channels, adequate provision should be made for drainage to handle excess irrigation water as well as surface run-off from rainfall.

Topographical features and types of crops usually determine the size and shape of fields and their preparation for irrigation. The more common methods of irrigation requiring specific land preparation are border strips, basins, furrows and corrugations.

Border strips consist of fields level in the transverse direction and having a uniform slope not exceeding 1% in the longitudinal direction, varying in width from 6 to 15 m and in length from 60 to about 400 m, depending on soil types, land slope and depth of irrigation. The fields are divided by low ridges up to 15 to 20 cm high running down the slope. These prevent the sheet of water from spreading beyond the desirable width. The total infiltration may be much higher at the top of the field if, due to improper design or grading, the water is allowed to remain there much longer than on the bottom portion of the field. This method of irrigation is efficient from the viewpoint of water use, time and labour required. It is used mainly for close-growing crops, hay and pastures.

Basically, the design, which involves the relationship between the intake rate, the size of stream, and area of the strip, should be such that the water will flow into the strip during the period of time required for the desired amount to enter the soil. The total volume applied must equal the desired depth of application multiplied by the area. The longitudinal slope is relatively important, but must not be so steep as to cause erosion. It should be flattened at the bottom end of the strip to provide some storage, which will improve the uniformity of application along the strip. Some allowance for less than 100% uniformity in application must be made.

Basin irrigation is sometimes practised where land slopes are rather flat and infiltration is slow. Low dykes are built around the field and water is turned in and allowed to soak into the soil. The size and shape of basin are determined by topography, the nature of soil and the source of water available. Where these factors are taken into account, this method of irrigation can be efficient.

Furrow irrigation is most common for row crops, orchards, vineyards, cotton, corn and potatoes. In this method water flows in furrows between rows of plants and infiltrates to the roots. The land slope, soil texture, length of furrows and the depth of water application and the size of irrigation streams are important factors in controlling even application and preventing soil erosion.

Where transplanting of crops is practised, or where soil moisture is insufficient for germination in the case of sown crops, furrows are formed after sowing. The spacing of furrows depends on the distance between rows of crops or fruit trees. In some cases two rows of crops are planted between furrows.

For rather steep land slopes, close-growing crops and soils with low infiltration capacity, small furrows called corrugations are used. Corrugations are only a few inches deep and are spaced from 18 to 36 inches (45.72 to 91.44 cm) apart. In areas where there are significant intervals between the use of the furrows, and water is not allowed to stand, the snails usually do not find suitable habitats.

Application of Irrigation Water

This phase of irrigation practice affects not only crop yield and soil and water utilization but also the extent and cost of snail control measures that may be necessary. Yields are adversely affected by considerable variations in the depth of water application and by the loss of soil fertility through leaching and erosion. Observations have shown that young and inexperienced farmers can profit a great deal from demonstration and extension courses in this phase of irrigation.

Where flood irrigation is practised the rate at which water is applied is governed by the texture of the soil, land slope, and width of strips. Control of the size of irrigation streams can be achieved by using pipes or siphons to convey the water from the supply ditch on to the fields.

In furrow irrigation the practice of using earth dams in the supply ditch and the cutting of openings through the side of the ditch result in loss of good soil, poor water control and silting of the furrows. These can be overcome by using siphons and spiles to divert and control the water on to the furrows.

In sprinkler irrigation, the control of application is relatively simple, and over-irrigation is not likely. Rates of application can vary from 0.1 to 1.0 inches (0.254 to 2.54 cm) per hour, depending on the absorption capacity of the soil. The design and layout should provide for limiting the variations in the depth of application within a reasonable range, in order to avoid excessive irrigation in one part and insufficient water in another part of the field. Where necessary or desirable, irrigation at low application can be carried out at night without involving any labour.

There are a number of commercial types or sprinkler systems operating at pressures as low as 15 lb/in^2 (1.0546 kg/cm^2), and embracing a variety of sprinklers and perforated pipes. The choice of design will depend on local conditions, source of water and other factors.

Where the capacities of delivery canals are not sufficient to meet the irrigation requirements during daytime, the deficiency is made up by storing the night flow of the delivery canal in special storage reservoirs, usually referred to as night storage dams. This practice presents serious problems in the control of schistosomiasis. In endemic areas most of the dams and canals that are used for storage become snail hatcheries and transmission sites. If, in spite of this, such storage is used in an irrigation scheme, provision must be made for control measures.

In cases where the length of the delivery canal is not great, an enlargement of the canal to supply the full irrigation requirements during daytime hours may be cheaper than the provision of a large number of night storage dams. In the Gezira scheme, night storage is provided by surcharging the minor canals by 9 to 18 inches (22.86 to 45.72 cm). There is some evidence that this practice encourages the establishment of snail colonies. Where the delivery canal is rather long, or where the quantity of water diverted must be continuous, then storage in a small number of large reservoirs may be cheaper than storage in a large number of small reservoirs.

Drainage

Importance
Lack of drainage in irrigation schemes results in the formation of stagnant pools, wet areas and seepages which are often good snail habitats. It is therefore important that in irrigation schemes in endemic areas adequate drainage be provided if snail control is to be successful. In addition to facilitating snail control work, adequate drainage has important beneficial effects on the productivity of an irrigation scheme. There are instances of irrigation schemes that have failed to achieve the expected productivity because of lack of adequate drainage. In some places salt accumulation and waterlogging have become so serious within only a few years of the introduction of irrigation that valuable lands have been rendered useless. The reclamation of such lands may be feasible, but at considerable cost.

Planning
In the planning of irrigation schemes, funds for the construction of irrigation canals are more easily allocated than are funds needed for drainage. The function of canals is readily understood, but that of drainage is often considered to be of minor importance. Planners and engineers are sometimes under governmental pressure to provide for the maximum areas to be irrigated for a given grant, and to give little consideration to the long-term benefits of such developments. In addition to the economic losses resulting from the creation of habitats for intermediate hosts of parasites, both in humans and animals, lack of adequate drainage adversely affects crop yields and seriously hampers such farm operations as tillage, land preparation, harvest, maintenance of roads and control of water.

In planning irrigation schemes it is essential to provide for adequate drainage at the outset, even though under certain conditions the implementation of this part of the development may be carried out in stages as the need arises. For example, drainage for the removal of surface run-off from rains and from excess irrigation should be provided at the outset, whereas drainage required for conditions brought about as a result of several years of irrigation practice may be provided later.

Design

The design of drainage schemes is far more difficult than the design of irrigation schemes. There are such factors as rainfall intensities and frequencies, the quantity of excess irrigation water, the length of time crops can be subjected to flooding without affecting their yield, the soil properties that control the rate of movement of water, the nature of the ground surface as it affects the movement of water overland and, in some areas, provision for the leaching-out of salt accumulations. It must be pointed out, however, that even the approximate determination of the above factors requires a great deal of investigation and long periods of observation and often the engineer has to fall back on his experience and judgement. Nevertheless, steady progress is being made in the various aspects of drainage design, and it is now possible to attempt such design with some confidence. Some of the more important factors will be considered in the following paragraphs.

In some countries high rainfall intensities impose a heavy load on the size of drainage to be provided; for example, the drainage system of the Kpong irrigation experimental station in Ghana has been designed for a storm intensity of seven inches (17.78 cm) per hour, and a considerable network of surface drains has been provided. While this is by no means typical of irrigation schemes in endemic areas, it illustrates the importance of providing for the drainage of surface run-off resulting from rainfall. A fairly reliable estimate of the volume of run-off, and the frequency of its occurrence, may be made from an examination and analysis of rainfall data and stream-flows. Of particular interest in irrigated areas is the limiting time during which crops may be inundated without suffering any damage, and this determines the rate at which water should be removed.

Other sources of water are excess irrigation, overflows, and seepage from dams and canals. All these vary considerably from place to place, but an estimate of their magnitude is necessary for the design of a drainage system. Some authorities state that the minimum quantity to be allowed is one-tenth of the irrigation application and that as much again should be allowed for leaching applications. This, of course, depends on soil texture and quality of the irrigation water. Others recommend a drainage coefficient of between ¼ and ½ inch (6.35 and 12.70 mm) every 24 hours.

Having estimated the quantity of water to be drained in a given time, the layout and sizes of surface and tile drains can be determined. In many irrigation schemes drainage is effected by large open channels. Their design should take into consideration the reduction in carrying capacity which results from poor maintenance, scouring, silting, and growth of weeds. The capacities of the drains provided at Kpong, Ghana, for example, have been reduced by the tendency of the very fine- textured soil to cake and form clods.

Owing to considerable fluctuations in the quantity of water carried and the prolonged periods of very small flows, open drains provide important breeding sites for snails. Wherever possible, such open drains should be provided with subsoil drains so that during small flows they may be completely dried out.

The problem of control by the application of molluscicides becomes even more difficult when there is not sufficient flow to carry molluscicides through the entire length of the drains. The large amount of vegetation often present also tends to prevent dispersion near the margins. In such cases molluscicides may have to be sprayed over the drains, and may necessitate weed removal or destruction.

The design of drainage channels is usually based on Manning's formula, using a coefficient of roughness of 0.025 to 0.040, and taking into consideration all the other factors discussed on pages 91–92 and 94–101 in *Snail Control in the Prevention of Bilharziasis* [WHO, 1965].

Underground drainage is used to a limited extent in the drainage of irrigated areas where schistosomiasis is endemic. It is much more widely used in the USA, and a great deal of investigation and data are now available to facilitate the design and construction of subsoil drains.

Where water quantities are small it may be cheaper to use pipe drains than open drains, as maintenance of open drains is not only costly but often neglected.

In subsoil drainage, the depth and spacing of pipes depends on the texture of the soil and the desired level of the water table. Existing data are only empirical, and field observations have to be used as guides. For example, if the water table must not rise to a level higher than 4 ft (1.219 m) below the ground surface, open drains may have to be 8–10 ft (2.433 to 3.048 m) deep, and subsoil drains 6–8 ft (1.829 to 2.438 m) deep; in both cases, the depth depends on the spacing of the drains and also on whether saline ground waters have to be kept low.

The following basic information is required for the design of a subsoil drainage scheme:

(1) Soil permeability, which may be determined by field measurements of the hydraulic conductivity of the soil as, for example, by means of the auger-hole, or piezometer methods.

(2) Drainage requirements which depend on expected run-offs from rains and irrigation applications.

(3) The determination of soil properties. It has been suggested that borings need not extend to depths greater than 10 ft (3.05 m) for tile drains, and 15 ft (4.57 m) for open drains. This, of course, depends on the soil profile stratification. If highly permeable strata are present within depths of 25 ft (7.62 m) or more, they will have an important effect on the drainability of the soil.

(4) It is essential that a very accurate topographical survey be prepared to enable the layout of the main drains and the laterals to be determined.

Costs

The cost of tile drainage is surprisingly low compared with the value of the land reclaimed and the benefits in terms of increased crop yields resulting from keeping the water table within the desired distance of the root zone. In the current reclamation work in the Nile Delta, the cost of subsoil drainage, using 4- and 6-inch (10- and 15-cm) diameter concrete subsoil pipes, is about $28 per hectare. This represents about one-tenth of the market value of the land reclaimed. However, this cost is completely offset by the saving in land which would otherwise be required if open drains were used. In addition, there would be hardly any maintenance costs involved as compared with open drains.

Larger pipes may very well be used to replace some of the existing open drains and thus eliminate potential snail breeding sites at no additional expense. An example of such use is the Qala drain in Beira Province, Egypt.

Special Structures

Special structures required for the proper functioning of an irrigation system and for the control of host snails should be made part of the irrigation scheme during the planning stage. Such structures comprise mechanical snail traps, molluscicide-dispenser sites, crossings over or under siphons, flumes, drop structures, chutes, culverts, bridges, division boxes, turn-outs, checks and waste-ways. Provision should also be made for the protection of the distribution system by means of lateral spillways, drainage inlets and drainage of natural water courses over or under the irrigation canals. It is also desirable from the viewpoint of efficient operation to provide bridges to facilitate traffic movement and the transport of cleaning and maintenance equipment. For the application of molluscicides it is desirable to establish staff gauges in canals to indicate discharges at various depths.

Maintenance and Management

Observations in many parts of Africa, Asia and the USA show that many irrigation schemes suffer from lack of adequate maintenance and efficient management. In some cases this is largely due to failure on the part of the responsible authorities or the individual farmers to make adequate provision for trained staff and recurrent maintenance expense. In other cases it is due to lack of efficient organization with adequate powers to control the irrigation works and distribution of water. In some countries complicated water and property rights based on long traditions and customs prevent the development of efficient irrigation; as a consequence, the expected benefits from such developments are not realized and, in areas where schistosomiasis is endemic, measures to check its spread are either very difficult or impracticable.

In order to reduce the extent and cost of maintenance and to ensure efficient management, irrigation schemes should be designed and constructed to as high a standard as possible. Adequate provision should be made for facilities, equipment, materials and staff to carry out regular repairs and maintenance. Where this has been done, the extent and cost of maintenance are considerably reduced. The bulk of maintenance work is in the distribution canals and drains, and involves silt removal, weed-clearing and repairs to banks. Of smaller magnitude but of equal importance is the maintenance of control works, such as head-gates, delivery gates, bridges, culverts, screens, meters, and so on. Regular inspection and prompt repair and maintenance of this part of the irrigation system will pay in terms of increased yields, of reduction of snail populations and in the improved well-being of the people and promotion of good health. These objectives are further promoted by close collaboration between irrigation and public health authorities.

The importance of management in the successful operation of an irrigation scheme is perhaps best exemplified by the Gezira scheme in Sudan. There it has been demonstrated that by planning and co-ordinating the interests and contributions of the various departments such as agriculture, irrigation, public works, public health, education and rural councils, a well-balanced development has been made possible. Land and water resources are used to best advantage, and a high degree of snail control has been achieved by the provision of mechanical barriers, the application of molluscicide, and adequate surveillance for focal treatment of snail habitats.

Irrigation requirements in the Gezira area are carefully assessed for each zone, compiled and passed on to the engineers at the Sennar dam, and the correct discharge is allowed down the main canal. In the Murrumbidgee irrigation scheme in Australia, water requirements are made known to the field supervisors on 48 hours' notice, and this also facilitates the allotment of water to the various users.

Training of field supervisors in extension service courses would help in the general adoption of scientific methods in irrigation practice. FAO training should precede the commissioning of any irrigation scheme in order to enable the farmers to adopt the proper methods and practices. In some countries metering of irrigation water has proved an effective means of reducing losses. In such cases the farmers pay a fixed amount for the right to have water on their land, and another amount based on the total volume of water used. It has been pointed out that payment for water may result in smaller quantities being used for irrigation than are required for maximum crop yield. However, taking the over-all view, it would seem that for best use of water resources some form of metering and payment for water used is necessary.

Organizations or agencies responsible for the operation of an irrigation system can do this successfully only if granted adequate administrative powers by the Government. The Gezira Board is a good example of an agency with such powers. Under such conditions protection and promotion of public health become important functions in an irrigation scheme. In Iraq, the Irrigation and Embankments Law of 1923 empowers irrigation engineers with control of distribution. However, difficulty is caused by inherited water rights which are often based on quantities disproportionate to the areas served. Under the 1923 law, engineers can fix dimensions of channels, limit pump capacity and, if necessary, requisition labour for maintenance. The law provides for the imposition of fines upon conviction by a District Magistrate. Under this law provision is also made to regulate the building and maintenance of flood embankments.

Improvement of Existing Irrigation Systems

Opportunities for major improvements in the basic features of existing irrigation schemes with the objects of increasing their efficiency and facilitating snail control are in general rather limited. However, such opportunities should be explored and attempts should be made to carry out whatever modifications or improvements seem practicable both physically and financially. Before corrective measures can be considered surveys should be conducted to locate both actual and potential snail breeding areas.

In most existing schemes there is room for improvement and intensification of the maintenance of the canals, drains, structures and regulators. Regular clearing, weeding and desilting of the canals and restoration of their original cross-sections are not only necessary to maintain full supply to the farms, but are also justified on economic grounds when the useful life of the scheme is taken into consideration.

Some reduction in the number of snail habitats along the shores of storage reservoirs can be effected by the methods outlined on pages 560 to 562.

As the silt-carrying capacities of existing canals cannot be increased, attempts should be made to reduce the amount of silt entering the system by the installation of sand traps and desilting basins at the head of the main canal.

Improvement in the distribution system may involve relocation of limited sections of the canals, provision of structures for canal crossings, of flumes, of concrete or masonry lining of unstable sections, and measures to reduce excessive seepage. Snail habitats at regulator bays and watering places may be reduced or eliminated by the revetment of the canal banks and by the provision of concrete aprons.

Main head gates may need either repair and adjustment or complete renewal. Often due to lack of adequate maintenance, corrosion of the gates and lifting gear is severe, and their operation becomes either difficult or unsatisfactory.

The installation of screens at the head of the main canals would prevent most of the drifting snails from being carried into the distribution system. It must be remembered, however, that the installation of screens simply minimizes the introduction of snails from upstream. If the canals below the screens are suitable as habitats, the breeding capacity of a few snails can soon populate them unless other control measures are used.

The overtopping of canal banks may be prevented by the construction of overflow spillways at selected sites.

The need for drainage is usually obvious in most irrigation schemes. Unsatisfactory agricultural practices and lack of maintenance result in gradual reduction in the carrying capacities of the drains. Additional drainage may be required to take away seepage from irrigation canals, and for this purpose tile drains may be used to advantage, as the quantities of water are usually small. In some cases pumping may be necessary, and where this is done the water may be returned to the distribution system and used for irrigation. Drainage may also be required where the ground water table has risen too close to the surface after long periods of irrigation.

In some schemes supply canals terminate in dead-ends which are usually enlarged to form pools for watering purposes. These should be drained completely or provided with gates that will facilitate their periodic drying and thus prevent the establishment of snail colonies.

Good management of existing irrigation schemes can greatly increase their economic benefits and also facilitate snail control. Vigorous and enlightened efforts should be made to train farmers to discard inefficient practices such as night storage in canals for daytime irrigation, and to adopt practices in the selection of crops and methods of cultivation and irrigation that will result in higher productivity. Observations have shown that water management is one of the most important factors in sound agricultural production, and that it has the added advantage of checking the establishment of snail colonies. A great deal can be achieved by proper organization and by training of staff to ensure that water is well used and that the amount of excess is kept down to a minimum.

Improvements in engineering structures, and in the operation and management of existing irrigation schemes make snail control practicable from the viewpoints of both effectiveness and cost. Additional details will be found in the following section.

Agricultural Practice

Soil Properties and Water Requirements

An accurate knowledge of the properties of the soil and the water requirements of the crops to be irrigated is necessary for the success of an irrigation scheme. Soil properties under given climatic conditions will largely determine the kinds of crops that may be grown and methods of field preparation and water application, and these in turn will determine the extent of snail control work which will be necessary.

The determination of soil properties such as depth, composition, structure and texture enable the planner to leave out areas of poor soil which may be used for engineering works such as canals, control structures, roads, housing, etc. Where water is limited, only the best areas are considered for bringing under irrigation. Composition of soil determines its potential fertility, capacity to promote crop growth and fertilizer requirements. Structure and texture determine the properties of the soil as they affect tilth, water movement and retention, extent of root zone, field capacity and wilting-point.

The water-holding capacities of soils depend on their texture, condition and the presence of organic matter. Coarse soils hold less water than fine soils; the following values are given as a rough guide:

Type of soil	Depth of available water per foot depth of soil	
	in	mm
Sandy soil	¼	6.35
Sandy loam	¾	19.05
Fine sandy loam	1¼	31.75
Silt and clay loams	2½–3	63.5–76.2

Methods have been developed for estimating water requirements for various crops [WHO, 1965]. To determine the total volume of water which must be diverted into the irrigation area, the expected losses in the distribution system and in the conveyance of water must be added to the water requirements of the crop. The next step is the preparation of the fields and the drawing up of a schedule of irrigation. The amount and frequency will depend on local conditions, soil properties and seasonal rainfall. In general, irrigation in any one unit will be started when the moisture available is halfway between the wilting-point and the field capacity, and will be completed before soil moisture drops to a quarter of this value.

Once the total water requirements for optimum yield have been determined, it is possible to control and regulate irrigation heads rather precisely. This prevents the unnecessary waste of water and limits the creation of snail habitats. At the same time it improves land use and crop yields, and facilitates snail control measures directed against persistent colonies.

Crop Selection

In areas where schistosomiasis is endemic, selection of crops, rotation and farming practices can play an important part in a control programme. If preference is given in the selection of crops to varieties not requiring a large amount of water, control or elimination of snail habitats is greatly facilitated. Thus, in Egypt, the prevalence of schistosomiasis is less in areas where wheat and barley are grown than where rice is grown. Crop rotation makes possible irrigation practices that could prevent snail breeding, especially of the amphibious species. For example, in areas where *Oncomelania* is prevalent such crop rotations can be used to control or even eradicate them [PESIGAN *et al.*, 1958]. For the control of aquatic snails, crop rotation is only effective where the distribution system is so designed that channels supplying un-cropped fields may also be dried out. The sequence in which crops are grown affects tillage, seeding, weed control equipment, fertility, erosion, cultural practices and profitable land use.

Farming practices may be scheduled with some regard to seasonal fluctuations in snail breeding so that the water may be turned off at suitable intervals to interrupt this activity. Major breeding periods may occur one or more times a year, but the pattern must be known before planting, irrigation and harvesting operations can be used to obtain the control of snail popu-lations.

The practice of planting or sowing rice in rows simplifies weed control and increases yield. The attendant cultivation tends to eliminate *Oncomelania* snails in the fields, as has been demonstrated in Leyte and Japan [PESIGAN *et al.*, 1958].

Because of the high water requirements and methods of cultivation, rice-growing is a major problem in any snail control programme. It is therefore essential that attempts be made to cultivate varieties requiring relatively less water. One type developed in Egypt in a five-year programme by the Food and Agriculture Organization of the United Nations (FAO) and now called NAHDA, gave the lowest reduction in yield when subjected to reduced water applications. As a result of this work the growing of this variety increased from 38% of the total production in 1955 to 85% in 1957. While the extent to which reduced water application may facilitate snail control operations is not clearly known, it may be safe to expect that it will be of some benefit.

Further research in Egypt led to the selection of varieties, methods of cultivation and application of fertilizers that resulted in an increase in yields from 3.67 tons of rice per hectare in 1953 to 5.61 tons per hectare in 1957. Rice in Egypt is irrigated for four days at intervals of four days. When the period of irrigation was changed to six days with a 12-day interval, the yield of the NAHDA variety was reduced by 14.8% whereas for other varieties the reduction in yield rose to 25%. This loss in yield should, however, be considered in relation to the benefits that may result from the effect of such practices on snail control.

Results of experiments in Japan show that under certain conditions water application for rice-growing can be reduced by as much as 50% without affecting yield. The method recommended is as follows: water is applied to maintain the soil moisture at about 75% of field capacity from the period of transplanting to the beginning of heading; then the application is increased sufficiently to maintain a depth of water in the paddy field of 2.3 cm for 30 days; finally the application is cut back so as to maintain the moisture content at 75% of field capacity until just before harvesting. A reduction in the water application can prove an effective means of preventing snail breeding in rice fields, drains and canals, if it is consistent with good rice culture.

Of course, in the final analysis the effectiveness of any of these experimental results as snail control measures depends on their acceptance and use by the entire farming community.

Measures Applicable to Other Man-Made Habitats

General

Engineering operations associated with the construction of public works, utilities, industrial activities and mines often involve excavations, fills and hydraulic structures which may provide additional breeding places for host snails. Such places include roadside ditches, borrow-pits, quarries, gullies, obstructed drainage channels, bridges, culverts, causeways. Even the laying of a water supply pipe may create potential breeding sites. In one case the excavation of the trench on each side of a bridge and excavation for pipe supports caused surface erosion, and leakage from an air valve and pipe joints supplied the necessary water for snail colonies to be established.

All these potential snail breeding sites result from careless engineering practices, and their elimination can be effected by the responsible government agencies.

The importance of such habitats in the transmission of schistosomiasis has been amply demonstrated by careful investigations in Iraq, Iran and elsewhere. They provide suitable breeding areas for host snails, they attract human pollution, and provide opportunities for human contact with infested water.

The elimination of these snail habitats by engineering methods does not involve a great deal of work or expense. Where water bodies cannot be eliminated by these methods, snail control may be effected by treatment with a molluscicide.

Borrow-Pits

Borrow-pits in and near villages often serve as a place for the disposal of all kinds of wastes and debris. They often serve also as transmission sites for schistosomiasis. Borrow-pits no longer used for mining clay or storing water may be eliminated by filling, grading and drainage. Where such methods are not practicable the pits may be dried out by periodic pumping during the snail breeding season. Fencing of the pits may prove an effective means of preventing human contact. Where borrow-pits are used as water reservoirs, fencing and the provision of a satisfactory means of drawing water, such as a pump, are necessary to prevent transmission.

In recent years evidence has accumulated which indicates that sewage stabilization ponds are effective in solving disposal problems in many situations. It appears that they would be very practical in many areas endemic for schistosomiasis but there has been some question whether the eggs and miracidia of the parasite and the snails could survive in such ponds. Laboratory experiments indicate that the eggs and miracidia are killed in the stabilization pond environment, if the facility has been constructed and operated properly. Preliminary experiments show that snails can survive in raw sewage for long periods of time but they do not lay eggs. In certain concentrations of diluted sewage, eggs are laid by the snails but they fail to hatch [KAWATA, 1965]. It is possible that village borrow-pits could be fenced and modified in some situations and be used as sewage stabilization ponds. Whether this is used or more sophisticated stabilization ponds are constructed, it will be necessary to conduct studies under field conditions, in order to verify the laboratory work cited above.

Stream Crossings

In endemic areas, stream crossings present important transmission sites, whether the crossing is a ford or a bridge. They are of special importance when located near centres of population or schools. Methods of control here should be aimed at prevention of snail breeding and of human contact with the water.

At fords the provision of a foot-bridge and fenced approaches would go a long way towards reducing human contact with the stream. By fencing also the critical reaches of streams, transmission was greatly reduced in one area in South Africa. In this case it was necessary to provide safe water for drinking and bathing.

Causeways often create snail breeding pools either above or below the crossing. They also serve as washing and bathing sites for nearby villagers. Pools upstream of the causeway may be drained by the provision of pipes of sufficient size to take the normal flow of the stream and thus prevent water from flowing over the causeway. Pools downstream of the causeway may be eliminated by the construction of concrete or masonry aprons.

Where culverts are used for stream crossing, scouring is difficult to prevent, and pools are often formed either above or below the crossing. Sometimes the inverts are either too high or too low, and to eliminate the pools the culvert may have to be reconstructed so that the invert lies at the normal stream grade. Where the culverts are too high, it may be more convenient and cheaper to lay pipes at the correct level to take the normal or low flows. Where the culvert is placed too low, it is necessary to raise it or to fill the portion below the channel grade with concrete or grouted masonry, and provide additional waterway. Unless steps are taken to eliminate such habitats, other methods of control must be considered.

At bridge sites scouring of the banks and stream bed creates pools in which host snails may breed. As such sites are much frequented by nearby villagers the opportunities for transmission are considerable. In such cases, control measures would have to provide for alternative sources of water supply for domestic and recreational purposes.

Miscellaneous

Important snail habitats are sometimes created by the blockage of water courses or roadside ditches by dumping soil from excavations, by silt and flood debris, by weeds and by caving-in of the banks. In some areas abandoned rice-fields and unkept ponds provide suitable breeding sites. In a snail control programme, provision should be made for applying measures in such situations; regular inspection and maintenance and the use of molluscicides should be considered.

References

ABDER RAHMAN, K. and SHARAF ED DIN: Bull Wld Hlth Org. *25:* 699 (1961).

ANDRADE, R. M. DE: Rev. brasil. Malar. *11:* 653 (1959).

ANDRADE, R. M. DE: Rev. brasil. Malar. *21:* 59 (1969).

ARAOZ, J. DE: Bull. Wld Hlth Org. *27:* 99 (1962).

CHERNIN, E.; MICHELSON, E. H., and AUGUSTINE, D. L.: Amer. J. trop. Med. Hyg. *9:* 297, 308 (1956).

FERGUSON, F. F.: Hyacinth Contr. J. *7:* 7 (1968).

FERGUSON, F. F.; PALMER, J. R., and JOBIN, W. R.: Amer. J. trop. Med. Hyg. *17:* 858 (1968).

GILLET, J.; BRUAUX, P., and WOLFS, J.: Ann. Soc. belge Méd. trop. *40:* 643 (1960).

HAIRSTON, N. G. and SANTOS, B. C.: Bull. Wld Hlth Org. *25:* 603 (1961).

JOBIN, W. R. and IPPEN, A. T.: Science *145:* 1324 (1964).

KAWATA, K.: The effects of sewage stabilization ponds on the ova and miracidia of *Schistosoma mansoni;* thesis, The John's Hopkins University School of Hygiene (1965).

KING, H. W.: Handbook of Hydraulics, pp. 9–1, 9–2 (McGraw-Hill, New York 1954).

LAURITZEN, C. W.: in HODGE Aridity and man, p. 266 (Amer. Ass. Adv. Sci., Committee on Desert and Arid Zones Research, Washington 1963).

MALEK, E. A.: Bull. Wld Hlth Org. *18:* 691 (1958).

MCMULLEN, D. B.; BUZO, Z.J.; RAINEY, M. B., and FRANCOTTE, J.: Bull. Wld Hlth Org. *27:* 25 (1962).

MICHELSON, E. H.: Parasitology *47:* 413 (1957).

OLIVER-GONZÁLES, J.; BAUMAN, P. M., and BENENSON, A. S.: Amer. J. trop. Med. Hyg. *5:* 290 (1956).

OLIVIER, L. and BARBOSA, F. S.: Publ. Avuls. Inst. Magalhaes *4:* 79 (1955).

PAULINYI, H. and PAULINI, E.: Laboratory observations on the control of *Biomphalaria glabrata* by *Pomacea* sp. (Ampullariidae). OAU Symposium on Schistosomiasis, Addis Ababa 1970. Document CS/13/I (1970).

PESIGAN, T. P. and HAIRSTON, N. G.: Bull. Wld Hlth Org. *25:* 479 (1961).

PESIGAN, T. P.; FAROOQ, M.; HAIRSTON, N. G.; JAUREGUI, J.J.; GARCIA, E. G.; SANTOS, A.T.; SANTOS, B. C., and BESA, A. A.: Bull. Wld Hlth Org. *18:* 481; *19:* 223 (1958).

PITCHFORD, R.J.: Publ. Hlth, Johannesburg *17:* 325 (1953).

RUIZ-TIBÉN, E.; PALMER, J. R., and FERGUSON, F. F.: Bull. Wld Hlth Org. *41:* 329 (1969).

VOELKER, J.: Z. Tropenmed. Parasit. *17:* 155 (1966).

WEBBE, G.: Bull. Wld Hlth Org. *27:* 59 (1962).

WHO: Study Group on the Ecology of Intermediate Snail Hosts of Bilharziasis. Report, Paris 1956. Wld Hlth Org. techn. Rep. Ser. 120 (1957).

WHO: WHO Chron. *13:* 19 (1959).

WHO: Snail Control on the Prevention of Bilharziasis, Geneva. Wld Hlth Org. Monogr. Ser. No. 50 (1965).

Chapter 12

Epidemiology and Control of Schistosomiasis, pp. 592–608
(Karger, Basel and University Park Press, Baltimore 1973)

Chemotherapy in Control

A. DAVIS

Introduction

Despite intensive chemotherapeutic research over many years, encouraged and assisted by WHO, schistosomicidal drugs, potentially useful in control, have remained depressingly few in number. There is no doubt that the perfect drug would be an immense help in both control and eventual eradication, but as yet the ultimate criteria of absolute efficacy combined with non-toxicity to the human host have not been achieved.

Theoretically the use of mass chemotherapy in control possesses outstanding advantages. The effective treatment and cure of all infected people, by eliminating the excretion of eggs, blocks an essential stage in the life cycle of the parasite. Drug therapy relieves the symptoms of schistosomal infections, can be expected to improve the general health of an infected population and wins the confidence of those sick people who have been cured. There is evidence that treatment can lead to the reversal of pathological lesions in the acute or sub-acute stage, and can halt the progression of such lesions in the chronic stage. Regular chemotherapy in highly endemic areas may retard the development of the chronic insidious sequelae of schistosomal infections.

The importance to a community of the younger age groups, possessing as they do the future productive capacity and its attendant economic potential, cannot be over-emphasised. Yet in endemic areas schistosomiasis is one of the most important diseases of childhood and young adult life, those times of maximum physiological growth and activity. Usually showing the highest prevalence rates, the younger age groups contribute a major proportion of infection potential to the transmission cycle, and it is these age groups which derive maximum benefit from treatment.

Whilst the serious sequelae of infection with either *Schistosoma japonicum* or *S. mansoni* have been recognized for decades, the recent demonstrations, by intravenous urography, of radiological abnormalities in a high proportion of children and adolescents with *S. haematobium* infection but otherwise clinically normal, have negated the view that infection with this parasite is essentially benign.

The justification for the treatment of the individual is plain, but several technical and pharmacological factors have retarded the use of chemotherapeutic drugs in control. Due to the inefficiency of many methods of egg isolation from excreta, a proportion of low density infections will escape detection during screening programmes. Time-consuming multiple examinations may be needed to detect all infected cases within a community. The same criticism can be applied to serological methods which, although useful as a primary screening procedure, are neither sufficiently sensitive nor specific.

Mass treatment campaigns must contend with the imperfect efficacy of the available drugs, few of which will give 100% cure in the field, their toxicity, actual or potential, with consequent failure to complete treatment, and the difficulties of monitoring large numbers of people. Failure to achieve adequate population coverage will leave a residue of infected cases to maintain a transmission cycle.

The failure of certain schistosomicides to affect the larval stages of the parasites may lead to pre-infections, i.e. infection acquired immediately prior to chemotherapy, becoming manifest after drug treatment. Continued exposure to infected water may result in re-infection after chemotherapy, while the presence of reservoir hosts in *S. japonicum* and possibly in *S. mansoni* infections, all compound the difficulties of control by chemotherapy alone.

The biological characteristics of different endemic zones may indicate an alternative method of control; measures suitable for an isolated focus of infection, such as an oasis or island, can scarcely be expected to be applicable to a diffuse inland area with multiple pockets of infection. Chemotherapy as a tool in control must be considered in relation to these variables and not as an absolute method *per se*.

Pre-control data on the epidemiology, clinical patterns of infection, incidence and prevalence of complications, morbidity and/or mortality are essential. Methods of population survey, screening programmes and their techniques, operational protocols, etc., must be planned and discussed exhaustively bearing all possible adverse factors in mind before starting treatment. The services of a professional statistician will be a necessity.

An approach to chemotherapeutic control, or even mass chemotherapy, based on laudable though vague criteria, such as a general desire to improve population health can only be regarded as misguided. The highest scientific standards in planning and approach should be followed, for only then will the results be of value in the detection of operational mistakes and a reliable guide to future policy.

Available Drugs

Antimonial Compounds

Although organic trivalent antimonial compounds have been used as the cornerstone of individual treatment of schistosomiasis since the introduction of tartar emetic by CHRISTOPHERSON in 1917 [CHRISTOPHERSON and NEWLOVE, 1919], knowledge of their pharmacological properties has been slow to accumulate. In recent years the use of improved and sensitive methods of detection such as radioactive labelled antimony in humans and neutron-activation analysis in rodents, have clarified many debatable points on the absorption, distribution, excretion and mode of action of antimony.

Although effective and successful in the treatment of the individual patient with schistosomiasis, antimony fell far short of perfection due to its toxicity, and because therapeutic courses required prolonged intravenous or intramuscular administration. Attempts to diminish toxicity yet retain therapeutic effectiveness led to the use of a variety of treatment regimes depending essentially on a lengthening of the time between individual injections. Schedules involving the intravenous administration of antimony sodium tartrate or tartar emetic once, twice, or thrice weekly became popular, but extensive Egyptian experience with these regimes showed a wide range of cure rates, side-effects and patient absenteeism. Short-term intensive antimonial treatment was generally abandoned because of high toxicity rates.

The three antimonials most frequently used are antimony sodium tartrate (AST), which has generally replaced the original tartar emetic (antimony potassium tartrate); sodium antimonyl gluconate; and stibocaptate (antimony sodium dimercaptosuccinate). The first two drugs are given by intravenous injection whilst the dimercaptosuccinate has the advantage of intramuscular administration.

Table I. A comparison of the effects of three antimonial drugs in the treatment of *S. haematobium* infections in East Africa

Drug	Sodium antimonyl gluconate	Stibocaptate	Antimony sodium tartrate
Trivalent antimony content, %	36	25–26	39.3
Dilution in water, %	5.4	10	6
Total dose of trivalent antimony for adult (58 kg) given over 15 days[1], mg	527	530	530
Number of patients treated	60	50	50
Number of patients completing treatment	58 (97%)	24 (48%)	15 (30%)
Number of patients with side-effects	30 (50%)	47 (94%)	48 (96%)
Cumulative number of failures at three months after a complete course	14/58 (24%)	1/24 (4%)	0/15 (0%)
Cumulative number of failures at one year after a complete course	20/58 (34%)	4/24 (17%)	1/15 (7%)
Cumulative number of failures at one year after an incomplete course	2/2 (100%)	5/26 (19%)	8/35 (23%)

1 The antimony content of the daily dose of each drug was similar.

Comparative Trial of Antimony Sodium Tartrate, Sodium Antimonyl Gluconate and Stibocaptate

The results of a comparative trial of these compounds against *S. haematobium* in Tanzania [DAVIS, 1968] are summarized in table I.

General experience indicates that similar findings would result from antimony treatment of *S. mansoni* and *S. japonicum* infections, but absolute failure rates would be higher.

The outstanding feature of the trial was toxicity. Despite the near ideal conditions with careful and continuous medical supervision of hospitalized patients, more than half of those given stibocaptate and AST discontinued the course of treatment either on their own initiative or that of the physician. Under the special circumstances of the trial good cure rates were achieved, even among those whose treatment was terminated prematurely, but comparable results would not be expected in the field. Infections with either *S. mansoni* or *S. japonicum* would present similar or more pronounced problems.

Other relevant conclusions from the trial were:

(1) There was little therapeutic difference between intravenous antimony sodium tartrate and intramuscular stibocaptate (antimony sodium dimer-

captosuccinate) when given at equimetallic dose over the same period of time. Both drugs, if given in adequate doses, will cure the majority of cases of *S. haematobium* infection in East Africa. Sodium antimonyl gluconate was less effective at equivalent dosage but this was offset by the fact that tolerance was greatly superior.

(2) As the total antimony content of the therapeutic courses dropped below 400 mg, failure rates increased inversely.

(3) The prospect of complete parasitological cure was inversely proportional to the pretreatment egg output as noted in other trials [JORDAN, 1965].

(4) The major proportion of therapeutic failures (80–90%) became manifest in the first three months after treatment and only a small proportion, 1 or 2 in 10, showed an initial late relapse between three and six months after treatment. Nearly all failures should be detected in the first six months after therapy.

(5) If the cases becoming urine-positive initially at nine months or one year after treatment were regarded as true re-infections, which appeared justifiable in the light of the over-all therapeutic results, then the number of re-infections occurring in adults in one year after curative treatment in a highly endemic area was small and much less than hitherto considered likely. Re-infection rates in children in East African endemic zones, given stibocaptate, have been shown to be of the order of 1 in 4 during the first two years after treatment [JORDAN, 1968].

(6) Even in those adults who were not parasitologically cured, egg output was reduced markedly throughout the year of follow up, and similar observations have been made in children [JORDAN, 1968].

(7) Follow-up studies supported the concept that passage of black eggs, if unaccompanied by microscopically viable or hatching eggs, did not necessarily denote impending relapse, and the presence of such eggs alone after chemotherapy was compatible with parasitological cure. The long-term prognosis in cases passing only black eggs in early follow up did not differ to a significant extent from those cases in which no eggs were found.

Toxic Effects of Antimony in Man

All antimony compounds may produce undesirable side-effects, particularly antimony sodium tartrate and stibocaptate.

Care is essential during intravenous injection to avoid perivenous leak and subsequent painful local inflammation. An intravenous injection should be abandoned if vomiting, cough, severe substernal pain or syncope occur. Intramuscular injections require the selection of a deep site, and local pain may follow.

A variety of symptoms and reactions may occur during treatment, usually, but not inevitably, in the later stages parallel with accumulation of the metal.

Gastro-intestinal symptoms are frequently prominent and much distress may be experienced by patients from anorexia, nausea and vomiting.

Liver function tests may show changes indicative of hepatocellular disturbance.

There may be complaints of general weakness, and arthralgia and myalgia are common.

Substernal discomfort or pain and the well-known electrocardiographic changes of T wave inversion and QT lengthening are indicative of cardiotoxicity. Changes in serial electrocardiograms may occur in as many as 40 to 80% of treated patients. Two further cardiovascular syndromes are fortunately rare: one involves the myocardium with the development of a cardiac arrhythmia, and death may ensue; the other is a shock-like state with some of the characteristics of anaphylaxis.

Various types of skin rash may be associated with antimonial treatment: urticaria, herpes simplex, a fine desquamation of the skin; severe exfoliative dermatitis is rare. Herpes zoster may arise after treatment.

Use of the Antimonials in Mass Chemotherapy

The combination of the difficulty of administration and toxicity render the antimonials unsuitable for mass chemotherapy in situations where medical supervision is not available. Stibocaptate is the most easily handled preparation and, provided it is not given in daily doses, is likely to achieve greater population coverage than the intravenous preparations (see *suppressive management*, p. 607).

The cumulative disadvantages make it inherently unlikely that the antimony compounds will be used extensively in attempts at chemotherapeutic control.

Non-Antimonial Compounds

Thioxanthones

Lucanthone hydrochloride
The properties of this drug were reviewed in 1958 [BLAIR, 1958]. The hydrochloride, 1–2(diethylaminoethylamino)-4-methylthioxanthone hydro-

chloride, is a bright yellow, almost odourless crystalline powder, soluble in both warm water and warm alcohol, and is formulated in different strengths as plain uncoated or enteric sugar-coated tablets. It is effective given orally.

Early clinical trials were conducted with a variety of dose regimes and, predictably, the therapeutic results were also variable. A fairly high cure rate can be expected in *S. haematobium* infections after a total dose of 100 mg/kg. The impression is that *S. mansoni* is rather less susceptible than the urinary form of the parasite but this has not been subjected to formal trial and statistical confirmation. Initial trials against *S. japonicum* [PESIGAN *et al.*, 1951] gave such poor results that they have not been repeated.

Although the efficiency of a total dose of 100 mg/kg is agreed, the occurrence of side-effects often negates attempts to achieve this dose level. It is usual to give a total dose of 60 to 75 mg/kg over three to six days. Even at this level toxic effects may cause the time of administration to be extended, and various regimes lasting from three to 20 days at this total dose level have been described.

Toxicity. Short-term courses produce side-effects in a high proportion of treated patients. Gastro-intestinal symptoms are frequent and often lead to failure to complete the course. Anorexia, nausea, vomiting which can be severe and distressing, loose stools or diarrhoea sometimes accompanied by intestinal colic, may be encountered in various combinations.

Vertigo, insomnia and general weakness can occur. Very occasionally states of mental confusion, excitement or mania arise and are an indication for the cessation of treatment, and sedation.

The urine becomes yellow during treatment and a yellow non-icteric staining of the palms and soles, disappearing after completion of the course, may be seen.

Tolerance to lucanthone apparently varies in different regions. Caucasians tend to be less tolerant of the drug than others.

Many attempts have been made to diminish the frequency and severity of the side-effects while retaining the schistosomicidal action of the drug. The use of simultaneous belladonna alkaloids or sedatives, the preparation of different salts, the formulation of slow-release resinates or enteric-coated preparations have, however, all been unsuccessful. Recent trials of lucanthone tablets coated with cellulose acetate phthalate gave disappointing therapeutic results in both *S. mansoni* and *S haematobium* infections although side-effects were not troublesome.

Use in mass chemotherapy. The advent of new schistosomicides, the high frequency of unwanted side-effects of treatment and the relatively poor therapeutic effect have all led to diminished use of lucanthone for short-term curative courses. Because of its ease of administration, it retains a place in the mass treatment of children whose tolerance is superior to that of adults. Its suppressive use in low doses over longer time periods seems distinctly more promising than its short-term curative use.

Hycanthone

1-{[2-(Diethylamino) ethyl] amino}-4-(hydroxymethyl)-thioxanthen-9-one.

Suspicions existed for some time that the therapeutic action of lucanthone was due to one of its many metabolites. The discovery that a mould *Aspergillus sclerotiorum* could convert lucanthone biologically into a mixture of new substances led to the eventual separation and identification of a hydroxymethyl derivative named hycanthone [ROSI *et al.*, 1965]. Treatment of experimental infections confirmed that the schistosomicidal activity of hycanthone was greater than that of lucanthone itself and it was thought that the compound was the active metabolite of lucanthone.

Given in human schistosomiasis as hycanthone methanesulphonate, its outstanding advantage was that the total dose could be administered as one intramuscular injection. The drug was presented as an orange-yellow powder base in vials, and was made up to a 10-percent solution with sterile water. The usual dose was 3.0 mg of base per kg of body weight.

Initial clinical trials soon demonstrated its curative efficacy against both *S. haematobium* and *S. mansoni*. Despite varying modes of therapeutic assessment the majority of investigators reported high cure rates of from 65 to 95% against both parasites. Since the early enthusiastic reports, there have been indications that cure rates in *S. mansoni* infections may be distinctly lower than those obtained against *S. haematobium*. Field trials involving large numbers of patients are now under way and a balanced judgement of the therapeutic effect should be available in the near future. In all the trials conducted with quantitative methods of assessment, reduction of egg output in patients not parasitologically cured was of a very high order and usually greater than 90% of pretreatment output.

Toxicity. In the conduct of clinical trials to date, considerable attention has been paid to the side-effects of hycanthone.

Vomiting was a common complaint and affected more than 50% in some series. It rarely lasted for more than a day and seemed to be much less distressing than that induced by lucanthone. A variety of other symptoms have been noted including anorexia, nausea, abdominal pain, diarrhoea, headache and vertigo, most of which have not been of serious consequence. Minimal and transient electrocardiographic changes of doubtful significance have been observed. Pain at the site of injection which can be associated with induration or abcess formation have been recorded. It is essential to employ a deep intramuscular injection to avoid local complications and the preferred site is the gluteus minimus muscle high up under the iliac crest.

Although general side-effects are mild, there have been reports of post-treatment jaundice. Serum transaminase levels frequently show a transient rise after hycanthone. Of more disturbing import is the knowledge of a few deaths after treatment in which hepatic necrosis was confirmed. While faulty case selection was occasionally contributory, a precipitating role of hycanthone could not be excluded. The incidence of such events is extremely low and it appears that the risk of acute hepatotoxicity associated with hycanthone at established dose levels is no more than that accepted with some other drugs used in routine practice. However the hazard cannot be ignored since mass treatment of schistosomiasis will be undertaken in areas, many of which have less than adequate medical facilities, and where the population may have been subjected to a variety of liver diseases.

Adherence to both absolute and relative contraindications to the use of the drug is essential and emphasis should be placed on the monitoring of reactions in patients subjected to retreatment. Vomiting following hycanthone treatment should not be treated with phenothiazines which may themselves cause a sensitivity-type cholestasis on rare occasions.

It is important to appreciate that none of the available schistosomicides are free from the potential of side effects at accepted therapeutic doses.

Acquired resistance to hycanthone in one particular strain of *S. mansoni* in an experimental rodent model has been noted recently [ROGERS and BUEDING, 1971] but similar investigations using other strains have not reproduced the finding. The relevance of this observation to man is not clear. Epidemiological surveillance of patients treated with the drug on more than one occasion, though often difficult, is desirable.

The possibility of mutagenesis, raised by experiments conducted with a limited number of test systems [HARTMAN *et al.*, 1971], has not been confirmed by further extensive investigations, as yet unpublished. Authoritative clarification of this issue is expected shortly. Information on the mutagenic and carcinogenic potential of other schistosomicides is insufficient to allow relative evaluation.

Use in mass chemotherapy

Since the total dose of hycanthone can be given as a single intramuscular injection, the potentialities for population coverage in endemic areas are great. Therapeutic efficacy is high against both *S. haematobium* and *S. mansoni*.

The extended use of hycanthone, under medical supervision, continues and is likely to increase in the future.

Niridazole (Nitrothiazolylimidazolidinone)

Chemically a nitrothiazol, 1-(5-nitro-2-thiazolyl)-2-imidazolidinone, niridazole is a yellow crystalline powder, practically insoluble in water or most organic solvents, and is formulated as tablets for clinical use.

Detailed experimental studies in animals showed it was an effective schistosomicide against all three common schistosomes of man and without significant pharmacodynamic effects. As it was known that chemically similar substances, the nitrofurane derivatives, could induce sterility in rodents, special studies were made on the effect of niridazole on spermatogenesis, fertility and teratogenesis. The results indicated an inhibition of spermatogenesis in various species after high doses, but the effect was short lived and reversible after cessation of treatment. No statistically significant teratogenicity was demonstrated in rats, mice or rabbits. Slight inhibition of fetal growth was seen but this finding may occur with other drugs. It was considered that the dosage used in clinical practice would not produce sterility or embryopathy, and this supposition has been confirmed by the data accumulated in the last few years of extensive clinical use.

The drug is active when given by mouth and maximum blood concentrations are attained in 6 h. Experimentally, absorption was increased if the daily dose was given in two divided amounts than if given as a single portion. Within the body, metabolism is complete and the metabolites are excreted slowly, though completely, in the urine and faeces. After absorption and passage through the liver where metabolism occurs, most of the drug exists in the form of inactive metabolites bound to plasma albumin. The active fraction of the compound is the small amount of circulating non-metabolized drug which is concentrated in the germinal cells of the schistosomes and in their eggs.

Niridazole has been used widely for the treatment of *S. haematobium* and *S. mansoni* infections, and to a lesser extent against *S. japonicum*. A total dose of 175 mg/kg of body weight will cure a high proportion of *S. haematobium* infections, ranging from 75 to 95% depending on sampling variables. Cure rates in children infected with *S. mansoni*, and probably also in adults infected with this parasite, are lower at this dosage, although success rates equivalent to those obtained in the treatment of *S. haematobium* infections have been claimed. Infections due to *S. japonicum* do not respond so well.

The total dose may be given as 25 mg/kg/day for 7 days, or as 35 mg/kg/day for 5 days. Increasing the daily dose above 35 mg/kg is not recommended. Whilst there is clinical evidence that division of the daily dose into two portions, one given at least 6 h after the first, gives superior therapeutic results, this may be impracticable in the treatment of large numbers. In at least one large trial, side-effects were more prominent after twice-daily dosage and fewer patients completed treatment than after a single dose per day.

Toxicity

Although many minor side-effects have been reported, tolerance in general is good. Anorexia, nausea, vomiting, abdominal pain, diarrhoea, headache and vertigo have all been noted. Occasionally skin rashes are seen. Excretion of metabolites produces a brownish discoloration of the urine and patients should be warned of this symptom. An increase in heart rate may occur, and serial electrocardiography may reveal flattened T waves which are of little clinical significance.

The major side-effects, which fortunately occur only rarely, involve the central nervous system. Hyperexcitability, mania, depression, hallucinations, confusional states or generalized epileptiform attacks have been described. While serial electro-encephalographs may show changes during treatment, there is poor correlation between the type of abnormal tracing and the subsequent onset of neuro-psychiatric symptoms. Usually the acute episodes subside within 48 h of withholding the drug, but a normal mental state may not be resumed for some three weeks after treatment. Adults exhibit such symptoms more frequently than do children, and the incidence is greater during the treatment of *S. japonicum* and *S. mansoni* infections than in those due to *S. haematobium*.

The pathogenesis of the mental changes is thought to be associated with high levels of the active non-metabolized fraction of the drug in the peripheral blood, resulting from by-pass of the liver through portal-systemic vascular communications found in long-standing cases of *S. japonicum* or *S. mansoni* infections with portal hypertension. This factor, rather than the state of liver cell function, predisposes to the occurrence of mental symptoms during treatment. Neuro-psychiatric changes occur less frequently in cases of *S. mansoni* infection when this is in a relatively early stage and is mainly confined to the bowel. That this is not the sole explanation is demonstrated by the occurrence of mental changes in the treatment of infections due to *S. haematobium* where no double infection with *S. mansoni* has been shown. Such occurrences have been termed idiosyncratic. The evidence that concurrent administration of antihistamines or sedatives reduces the frequency of neuro-psychiatric symptoms during niridazole treatment is unconvincing.

Contra-indications

If the use of niridazole is contemplated for mass chemotherapy, due attention must be given to the exclusion of cases known to carry high risk factors predisposing to neuro-psychiatric change.

The drug should not be given to any patient with a previous history of mental disease or any form of epilepsy. Poor liver function forbids its use and niridazole is absolutely contra-indicated when portal-systemic vascular communications are present. Patients with hepatosplenomegaly and/or ascites due to *S. japonicum* or *S. mansoni* infections should not be given niridazole in the field.

Anaemic patients tolerate the drug well, but the coexistence of schistosomiasis and severe heart disease, or a poor general condition, is a bar to its use. Pregnant women have been treated with no subsequent complications of the pregnancy or fetal damage, but treatment in the first four months of pregnancy should be avoided on general grounds.

Use in Mass Chemotherapy

The drug has probably been used for mass treatment more frequently than other non-antimonials, and many regard it as the current drug of choice for *S. haematobium* infections in children. Ease of administration, a relatively short course of treatment, high therapeutic efficiency against *S. haematobium*, and the infrequent occurrence of major side-effects have contributed to its popularity. Examples of its mass use in children can be found in reported trials from Tanzania, and in Iran it has been used on a large scale in all age groups.

There is less experience in the mass treatment of *S. japonicum* and *S. mansoni* infections due to fear of major side-effects and the necessity for a preliminary screening to exclude unsuitable cases.

Other Drugs

Metrifonate (0,0-dimethyl 2,2,2-trichloro-1-hydroxyethyl phosphonate)
Although this organophosphorous compound is ineffective against *S.*

mansoni, both in experimental models and in man [KATZ *et al.*, 1968], it has curative properties in infections due to *S. haematobium* and certain intestinal helminths.

When first used in clinical practice, the therapeutic results were rather variable. More recent trials [FORSYTH and RASHID, 1967a, b; DAVIS and BAILEY, 1969] have explored the effect of intermittent dosage given at intervals of 14 days or one month, to a maximum of three doses. A proportion of low density infections were cured after only one or two treatments, the optimum individual dose being 7.5 mg/kg of body weight. Cure rates to six months were about 75% in *S. haematobium* infections and the number of relapses was small. The mode of action of the drug is as yet unknown.

Toxicity

Tolerance has been good and only mild symptoms of abdominal pain, nausea or diarrhoea have been noted. Vomiting, or complaints of general weakness are occasionally reported.

After each dose of drug, both inhibition and recovery of plasma cholinesterase activity was faster than that of erythrocyte cholinesterase activity. While normal levels of the plasma enzyme were regained four weeks after the last dose of a three treatment course, the recovery of erythrocyte cholinesterase activity was much slower and pretreatment levels may not be achieved for 8–14 weeks. At established dosage, the compound appeared to be safe and well tolerated despite its inhibitory effect on blood cholinesterases [PLEŠTINA *et al.*, 1972]. No correlation between the degree of cholinesterase inhibition and the incidence or severity of side-effects has been demonstrated.

The combined use of pralidoxime, which may be given as the iodide, chloride or methanesulfonate, and atropine is effective in the treatment of poisoning caused by some organophosphorus compounds. The treatment of *S. haematobium* infections with metrifonate has been so devoid of major clinical incidents that little if any experience of these remedies is available. Nevertheless, the fact of their utility should be noted.

Use in Mass Chemotherapy

The drug must still be regarded as under trial. No information is available of its effect when used in populations previously subjected to organophosphorus insecticides, as in malaria control. The possibility of its use as a cheap, relatively non-toxic, orally-administered effective compound against *S. haematobium* is promising and further investigations are now being conducted.

Tris (p-Aminophenyl) Carbonium Pamoate (TAC Pamoate)

Following the demonstration of the schistosomicidal effect of this compound against *S. japonicum* and *S. mansoni* in mice and monkeys, clinical trials with the oral preparation pararosaniline pamoate were undertaken. Large scale field trials in the Philippines showed that the drug was effective in the treatment of *S. japonicum* infections, giving a cure rate of 72% at six months on the optimum dosage schedule [PESIGAN *et al.*, 1967]. The drug was acceptable to patients although transient and varied side-effects were seen in about one third. Although sebaceous and mammary gland tumours were observed in experimental rats after pararosaniline pamoate, there was no suggestion of a human carcinogenetic effect. However, the long course of treatment necessary to achieve cure, which may occupy 52 treatment days, makes it unlikely that this drug will be utilized in mass campaigns.

Dehydroemetine

The synthesis of dehydroemetine and the demonstration of antischistosomal activity [GELFAND *et al.*, 1962; SALEM, 1965] produced hopes that the drug would be less toxic than the natural alkaloid. Subsequent trials with parenteral dehydroemetine or an oral slow-release compound gave only moderate cure rates in *S. haematobium* and *S. mansoni* infections, and it is doubtful whether these compounds will be used in large scale treatment.

Use of Drugs in Control Programmes

Terminology

Variation in descriptions of drug administration may cause confusion unless a standardized nomenclature is adopted. Since chemotherapy may come into much wider use in control programmes, the use of generally agreed and understood terms is desirable.

Mass Drug Administration

One source of confusion lies in the use of the term *mass drug administration*. In the field of malaria, mass chemoprophylaxis or mass chemosuppression, if supervised strictly in a co-operative population, can be used as a control measure by the distribution of drugs to every member of the community, whether infected or uninfected. In schistosomiasis control, some modification of this procedure is necessary because of the greater expense and toxicity of the drugs available. Thus, in this context mass drug administration involves the distribution of the drug to those members of a community who are shown to be infected by preliminary parasitological screening. While it is unnecessary to treat individuals negative on screening, a proportion of those who are incubating infections will escape treatment during this procedure, and some follow-up mechanism is essential to detect and deal with such cases.

It may be appropriate to select a sub-group within a community, such as children under the age of 16 years, to whom mass treatment is given. This may be termed mass treatment or mass drug administration specific to an age group. It is usually justifiable only if it has been shown by previous quantitative epidemiological studies that the specific age group is reponsible for the major proportion of transmission.

As perfection is rarely attainable, it can be asserted that mass drug administration has been applied if it has covered at least 90% of the known number of positive infections.

Individual Drug Administration

The distribution of drugs to individuals is not classified as a major control measure in schistosomiasis. There are, however, occasions on which it may be utilized as an adjunct to other methods of control. For example, where an area of transmission is composed of multiple small foci of infected water bodies with a dispersed human population, and control by molluscicides is envisaged, those infected individuals shown by epidemiological studies to have frequent water-contact behaviour patterns could be given chemotherapy as a supportive measure to the main system of control.

When drugs are given to individuals, certain descriptions are commonly applied to the different methods of drug administration. Thus, drugs may be given *on demand*, *by persuasion* or *compulsorily*. The first term refers to the treatment of patients who report a history of illness. Drug administration by persuasion covers those situations where a specific campaign has been mounted against schistosomiasis, and a considerable propaganda element attempts to persuade people to receive treatment. The third term refers to those situations where treatment of any infection discovered is compulsory by law.

The Reasons for Drug Administration

Drugs may be given in schistosomiasis for several purposes. The principal ones are the radical cure of an infection to which the term *radical treatment* may be applied; and the palliative treatment of an infection to minimize ill effects by the reduction of egg deposition. This latter procedure may be termed *suppressive management* and it implies the periodic administration of sub-curative doses of a schistosomicide to produce a reduction of egg laying by the separation, sterilization or even death of a proportion of the body's population of worms. Although radical cure is not the primary aim, it may be achieved, as a bonus, in a certain number of low density infections. When drugs are used in this fashion, clinical symptoms commonly diminish in intensity or disappear, and the side-effects associated with the normal therapeutic use of the drug, are minimized.

Suppressive management was introduced originally and successfully by the periodic administration of stibocaptate in attempts to reduce the egg output of infected groups of patients, and hence to diminish transmission. Since that time many other schistosomicides have been used similarly.

It is not yet possible to use drugs to stop the maturation of an immature infection, and the prevention of cercarial penetration by repellant skin preparations or by other means has received little attention. These purposes are covered by the term *drug prophylaxis* or *chemoprophylaxis*, leaving the word *prophylaxis* to its proper meaning, the prevention of disease by whatsoever means.

Extent of Employment of Chemotherapy in Past and Present Control Programmes

Mention has been made of this subject on pages 388 to 421, and the drugs previously employed have been noted. With the exception of Brazil, Egypt, Iran, Venezuela, and possibly Rhodesia, chemotherapy has not played an important role in schistosomiasis control. Elsewhere, drugs have been used in a desultory manner and probably have had little effect either in reducing clinical manifestations or in promoting control.

For some years tartar emetic has been the standard treatment in Egypt, and wide population coverage has been attained by special teams. The relative efficacy of chemotherapy, in comparison with other control methods has been difficult to assess, but there is reason to believe that in Egypt extensive drug treatment has contributed to a reduction in the clinical severity of the disease.

The refining and quantifying of methods of assessing the curative properties of the new and potent drugs which are appearing, can be expected to stimulate the use of mass chemotherapy in control. There is already evidence that increasing interest is shown in its potentialities. The role of chemotherapy, either alone or in combination with molluscicides, will become increasingly well-defined only if adequate population coverage with drugs can be achieved.

References

BLAIR, D. M.: Bull. Wld Hlth Org. *18:* 989 (1958).

CHRISTOPHERSON, J. B. and NEWLOVE, J. R.: J. trop. Med. Hyg. *22:* 129 (1919).

DAVIS, A.: Bull. Wld Hlth Org. *38:* 197 (1968).

DAVIS, A. and BAILEY, D. R.: Bull. Wld Hlth Org. *41:* 209 (1969).

FORSYTH, D. M. and RASHID, C.: Lancet *i:* 130 (1967a).

FORSYTH, D. M. and RASHID, C.: Lancet *ii:* 909 (1967b).

GELFAND, M.; REID, E. T., and SIMPSON, B. E.: Trans. roy. Soc. trop. Med. Hyg. *56:* 77 (1962).

HARTMAN. P. E.; LEVINE, K.; HARTMAN, Z., and BERGER, H.: Science, *172*, 1058 (1971).

JORDAN, P.: Bull. Wld Hlth Org. *33:* 553 (1965).

JORDAN, P.: Trans. roy. Soc. trop. Med. Hyg. *62:* 413 (1968).

KATZ, N.; PELLEGRINO, J., and PEREIRA, J. P.: Rev. Soc. bras. Med. trop. *2:* 237 (1968).

PESIGAN, T. P.; BANZON, T. C.; SANTOS, A. T.; NOSEÑAS, J., and ZABALA, R. G.: Bull. Wld Hlth Org. *36:* 263 (1967).

PESIGAN, T.P.; PANGILINAN, M. V.; SANIEL, V. F.; GARCIA, E. G.; BANZON, T. C., and PUTONG, P. B.: J. Philipp. med. Ass. *27:* 242 (1951).

PLEŠTINA, R.; DAVIS, A., and BAILEY, D. R.: Bull. Wld Hlth Org. *in press* (1972).

ROGERS, S. H. and BUEDING, E.: Science, *172*, 1057 (1971).

ROSI, D.; PERUZZOTTI, G.; DENNIS, E. W.; BERBERIAN, D. A.; FREELE, H., and ARCHER, S.: Nature, Lond. *208:* 1005 (1965).

SALEM, H. H.: Trans. roy. Soc. trop. Med. Hyg. *59:* 307 (1965).

Chapter 13

Epidemiology and Control of Schistosomiasis, pp. 609–619
(Karger, Basel and University Park Press, Baltimore 1973)

Evaluation of Control Programmes

L. J. OLIVIER

Introduction

Evaluation must be an integral part of a control programme since it is the only objective means for judging the programme's success. It also forms the basis for improving and reorienting the programme.

The essential elements that must be evaluated are: (1) progress toward achievement of the goal; (2) cost; and (3) public acceptance. The first two can be evaluated objectively while the third must be measured with less precision and reliability.

Evaluation of the Efficacy of the Programme

The objectives of a control programme are discussed on pages 430 to 437, and measures that can be used for control are dealt with on pages 458 to 608.

The goal toward which control measures are directed is the reduction of human schistosome infection and mitigation of the disease and disability resulting from the infection. Therefore, evaluation of the efficacy of the control programme must be made in terms of its impact on human schistosome infection. No other measure can replace it. However, under some conditions other measures can supplement it, as will be seen.

In principle one evaluates the efficacy of a control programme by collecting meaningful data on the disease, the infection in man, and on other chosen parameters, before any control work is done. The control programme is then instituted and from time to time thereafter the same parameters are measured by exactly the same methods and procedures. In this way strictly comparable, consecutive records are obtained which can reveal, reliably and quantitatively, changes brought about by the control measures employed. Usually the measurements used to determine the efficacy of a control programme must be made separately and for the sole purpose of evaluation. Data collected in the pre-control studies will provide the basis for evaluation but usually cannot, themselves, be used for purposes of evaluation.

Various methods used to judge the efficacy of schistosomiasis control work can be divided into two groups: (1) those that measure the effects of control on human infection and disease; and (2) those that provide indirect evidence of control.

Measurement of Efficacy in Terms of Human Infection and Disease

General

Evaluation of efficacy involves measurement of the impact of control on the disease or the infection in man. The institution of control measures should result in a detectable change in (1) the prevalence of infection, (2) the intensity of infection, and (3) the severity of the symptoms of the disease. Therefore, study of any of these three changes should reveal the efficacy of a control programme. Each of the following procedures is designed to detect change in one of these three conditions.

Evaluation by Study of the Over-All Prevalence of Infection

It is conceivable that the efficacy of a control programme could be judged by changes observed in the over-all prevalence of infection in the population of the control area. A significant decline in transmission of infection should eventually result in a decline in prevalence. Therefore, the prevalence in the whole population, if the population is not too large, or of a carefully selected sample of the population, could be determined before control is begun, to be followed by measurements of prevalence in the same population as the programme progresses. The population sample would have to be standardized according to the proportions of sex, age, economic status and occupation, as well as other variables that could bias the results.

Aside from the sampling procedures, the method is relatively simple to execute. A standardized, non-quantitative method for urine or stool examinations would be used.

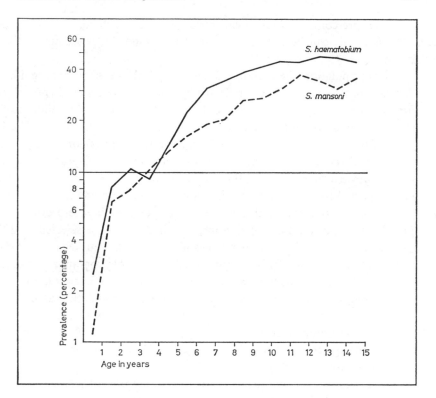

Fig. 1. Fig. 1. Prevalence of *S. haematobium* and *S. mansoni* infection in the project area. Age specific rates by single year in age group 0–14, 1962–1963.

This procedure is relatively insensitive to small changes which might result from control, and would probably require at least five years to produce meaningful data. Other procedures are more sensitive and therefore more useful and economical.

Evaluation by Study of Age-Prevalence in Children

This procedure is based on the fact that the prevalence in children increases rapidly from year to year, usually reaching a maximum by the age of 12 or 14. Moreover, children usually release eggs more consistently than do adults, and children are usually more available and more amenable for study. A characteristic age-prevalence curve for children is shown in figure 1.

The pre-control studies will have provided such an age-prevalence curve and this can be used as an aid in designing the procedure outlined below.

In a population of children, interruption of transmission or a significant decrease in transmission will be reflected by a progressive decline in prevalence for each age group as time passes. Thus, if the 11-year-old children of a selected population of adequate size have a prevalence of 62% while the 13-year-olds have a prevalence of 90% and transmission is completely interrupted for two years, it might then be expected that the 13-year-olds would have a prevalence closer to 62 than to 90%, the prevalence they could have been expected to have had transmission not been interrupted.

In order to detect and measure such a change in age-prevalence, a population, or a series of populations, of children must be selected, and the prevalence of infection in them measured by a standardized and tested technique. Then, annually or biennially as the control programme proceeds, the age-prevalence measurement in the children of the same population must be repeated, using exactly the same techniques. The population used should be stable and should spend all its time in the area to be controlled.

Two age groups can be used if the population is not large enough to provide one age group of sufficiently large size. A series of three or more age groups can also be employed.

A recommended method for conducting an age-prevalence study follows:

Before control begins, all children in a selected age group, such as the 6- to 10-group, in a series of selected schools or villages, are checked for infection using a standardized technique for stool or urine examination. The technique can be selected from among those described on pages 622 to 634. It need not be quantitative since in each case judgement will be made only as to whether eggs are detected or not. Obviously the sensitivity of the technique must not vary significantly from child to child or from year to year. This provides the base-line prevalence information. Then, at yearly intervals, a strictly comparable sample from the same school(s), village(s), or other unit is examined in exactly the same way. Care must be taken that the 'before' and 'after' samples are really comparable as to age and sex, and that no changes have occurred in the ethnic, religions or other social compositions of the sample. Moreover, the technique of stool or urine examination must be exactly the same for all the samples. If, as is usually the case, school-children are used, changes in the boundaries of school districts should be excluded as possible explanations for any differences observed in infection prevalence.

The infection prevalence should be recorded according to age and sex, and the data from each sampled group, such as the children from a given school, should be recorded separately.

The amount of data required before satisfactory conclusions can be drawn is estimated from preliminary results. The requirements are those imposed by the statistical test to be used in any comparisons that are contemplated. Except for very elaborate data, chi-square (χ^2) methods will be used and, in nearly all cases, the simple 2×2 table will suffice. For this test to be valid, the lowest average number may not be less than 10 (see pages 719 to 723).

This procedure is more sensitive than the study of over-all age-prevalence. Nevertheless, a modest though important change in transmission of infection might not be revealed by this procedure within three or more years.

Evaluation by Study of Change of Intensity of Infection

It has been shown that the rapid rise in prevalence of egg passers among young children of an endemic area is accompanied by a rise in the number of eggs per unit of urine or faeces. Thus, not only do more and more children acquire enough worms so that eggs are released in detectable numbers, but the children acquire progressively heavier worm burdens and so release more eggs per unit of time.

It has also been observed that the proportional rise in egg output by children is considerably greater than the proportional rise in prevalence. For example, in an Egyptian village when children aged 4 and 5 years were compared, the *S. haematobium* prevalence increased in the one-year interval from 27.3 to 33.3%, while the over-all average egg-counts increased from 8.8 to 60.0 eggs per 10 ml of urine. In the same children, while the prevalence of *S. mansoni* rose from 14.6 to 20.0%, the over-all mean egg-count rose from 0.35 to 6.3 eggs per 100 mg of faeces.

Since the egg-count can be expected to change more rapidly than prevalence and since egg-counts detect not only the presence or absence of infection but also its intensity, the method can be used as a sensitive and rapid way to detect change in transmission intensity. Whereas the prevalence in children should change significantly following substantial reduction or interruption of transmission, a modest reduction in transmission might not result in enough change to be readily revealed in reduced prevalence. Yet egg-counts on the same children might show a significant decrease as a result of the decreased transmission, and for that reason, the egg-counting method recommends itself for evaluating control.

Study of the age-prevalence curve in an area to be placed under control will reveal the age groups in which prevalence rises most rapidly. Egg-counts on children of those age groups can then be carried out to find the age groups in which the egg-count is rising most rapidly. These groups are the most sensitive indicators of change in transmission intensity.

The plan for the evaluation of transmission by egg-counting should proceed on the following basis:

If, for example, the 6-year age group is the group in which the egg-count rises most rapidly and transmission continues without substantial changes, children who are in this age group will in one year's time have an egg output similar to that of children in the 7-year age group. The aim of an evaluation study in that population would then be to collect the following data before control is begun:

(1) Egg output in an index population of children aged 6 last birthday.

(2) Egg output in an index population of children aged 7 last birthday.

(3) After the control programme has been in effect for one year, determine the average egg output of children in the population under study aged 7 last birthday and compare the data obtained with the predicted data for that age group.

If transmission had continued uninterrupted, the average egg output would be that expected of children aged 7 last birthday (see 2 above). If transmission was completely interrupted, the average egg-count would be near that for children aged 6 (see 1 above). Partial interruption of transmission would result in an intermediate average egg-count. It is conceivable that a change in transmission might be detected by this method in one year's time. In order to collect a greater amount of information in a small population of children, two or more age intervals as indices might be used instead of just one. Moreover, the comparisons should be continued for the duration of the control programme.

Egg output should, of course, be determined by a consistent, reliable, and quantitative technique which must not vary from year to year. Emphasis should be placed on reliability and consistency rather than on sensitivity of the method. Quantitative techniques are described on pages 622 to 634.

Evaluation by Study of the Clinical Gradient

The clinical gradient is a device for measuring the severity of the disease and is useful in judging the importance of the schistosomiasis problem (pp. 354 to 387 and 700 to 703). It can also be used for evaluating the efficacy of a control programme.

If transmission is reduced or interrupted there should eventually be a reduction in the severity of infection and so a reduction in the symptoms of the disease.

The classification of infected persons into four groups, with reference to apparent symptoms of the disease (pp. 700 to 703), is based largely on non-objective findings by a physician who makes his observations in local health centres or improvised examination posts. Although the judgements are largely subjective, care in selection of the samples and in grading may make it possible to make comparisons of disease severity before and after long-term snail control efforts.

The procedure for evaluation of control using the clinical gradient is to determine the clinical gradient in one or more population groups using carefully standardized criteria for the measurement of severity of symptoms and then, after an interval of time during which the control programme has been in effect, determining the clinical gradient in the same population groups. Since the clinical gradient can be expected to change relatively slowly even if transmission is completely interrupted, the first reassessment of the gradient should probably be done two years after the control programme is started.

Objectivity in determining such a clinical gradient is extraordinarily hard to attain. Repetition of the gradient by the same physicians would assure greater consistency of judgement as to severity of symptoms. Careful description of symptoms and their degrees of severity would also tend to make the data more reliable. A sheet used in one endemic area for collection of data relative to the clinical gradient is presented on pages 742 to 743.

Although demonstration of a change in clinical gradient resulting from a control programme is difficult and expensive, it is a highly important measurement to make since reduction in severity of the disease is the paramount objective of control work.

Evaluation by Objective Study of Damage to Infected Persons

Objective measurement of damage due to schistosomiasis could provide a sounder basis than the clinical gradient for judgement as to the efficacy of a control programme. If one or more clearly recognizable and measurable pathological conditions known to be closely associated with schistosome infection could be studied before and after a control programme was put into effect, one would have objective clinical evidence of the effect of the programme. Moreover, studies using such objective criteria could be the basis for comparing results from one area to another and from one country to another.

Selection and use of such objective criteria involve numerous pitfalls but the potential usefulness of the method justifies attempts at their use. In each case it would be necessary to develop a quantitative measure of damage which would not depend upon the judgement of the physician or technician making the measurement.

The following are objective criteria which might be developed:

S. haematobium infections

1. Haematuria measured quantitatively.
2. Bladder biopsy with objective measure of damage.
3. Bladder X-ray with quantitative measure of calcification.
4. Intravenous pyelogram to measure damage quantitatively.

S. mansoni and *S. japonicum* infections

1. Quantitative measure of haemoglobin in faeces.
2. Rectal biopsy with quantitative measure of damage.
3. Liver biopsy with quantitative measure of damage.

Evaluation of Efficacy Using Indirect Evidence

General

Although the true measure of the efficacy of a control programme must be in terms of human infection, indirect evidence of progress toward the control objective may be of some value especially if the evidence can be obtained more rapidly.

Evaluation by Study of Snail Populations

If snail control is a major part of the control programme, direct evidence of the value of control can be supplemented with indirect evidence in the form of snail population changes resulting from control. A snail control programme should quickly cause a drastic reduction in snail populations in most of the area under control. Presumably this should reduce transmission of infection to man, though the degree of snail population reduction necessary to cause a significant decline in transmission is not known. The estimation of snail population density is a difficult task and requires a high degree of skill and judgement. Therefore, it cannot be delegated to unsophisticated and unsupervised persons.

In general, to judge whether a snail control effort has been effective, and to measure quantitatively just how effective it has been, it is only necessary to compare measures of population density before and after control is attempted. In other words a series of collections are made which determine how many snails can be obtained under carefully standardized conditions. Then, after the attempt at control, a determination of how many snails can be collected using exactly the same method in the same places, is made. If the collections are done quantitatively and with statistical validity, the two operations can be compared and the effect of the control measures can be determined. It should be pointed out that the two measures referred to above need not be measures of the total snail population present at the time the collections are made. They need only give a reliable indication of a change in population density. Since the measures deal with less than the whole snail population, they can ignore some part of it, such as the eggs and very small snails, with the result that the labour of collecting may be greatly reduced and brought within practical limits. The technique, nevertheless, must account for a consistent proportion of the snails present, and it should be remembered that if data can be obtained, they will serve to indicate repopulation rates and the time of the next molluscicide application. Since snail control measures can reduce snail populations to a relatively low level, the evaluation collections must be intensive and relatively extensive so that even a small population can be detected.

It is necessary to test a collecting technique to determine whether it actually does obtain a consistent sample of the snails present. This can be done by comparing repeated collections in the same area, using suitable statistical tests. Thus, repeated quadrat samples on moist habitats can be evaluated, and repeated samples made with sieves or other collecting devices in aquatic habitats can be compared in a similar way.

It is obvious that population estimates can be no more accurate than the sampling technique on which they are based. It is necessary, therefore, to make every effort to discover the accuracy and constancy of the sample itself. This is distinct from the problem of 'sampling error' which is taken up in a later section. A sample may be inaccurate in a number of ways.

The simplest and most acceptable error is in missing a constant proportion of the snails present. Quadrat samples of amphibious snails of the genus *Oncomelania* have been shown to miss many snails shorter than 2.5 mm.

This often amounts to about half of the snails present, as determined by a more exhaustive technique. Inasmuch as the error is reasonably constant, it can be tolerated for many kinds of studies.

A less acceptable kind of error might occur when the efficiency of the sampling technique varies from time to time or from place to place. For example, a shallow dip-net, used in aquatic habitats, was found to yield counts that varied greatly in the same location from day to day. Closer study revealed that the difference was due to changes in water level and not to any appreciable change in the number of snails present or to the collecting techniques used. Variations can also be due to differences in skill of the collectors, and small variations in collecting equipment. All such variations must be carefully avoided.

Since snail populations vary greatly where there are seasonal climatic changes, the collections to be compared should always be made at the same season of the year and, to the greatest extent possible, when the conditions of the habitat are the same as those prevailing when the original index collections were made. If collections are made throughout the year their interpretation must take into account expected seasonal population changes.

Evaluation by Study of Infections in Snails

It is conceivable that one might, through control efforts, succeed in substantially reducing, or even eliminating, transmission of infection to man without eliminating the snails capable of transmitting infection. In such a situation schistosome infections in the remaining snails could provide a measure of reduction of transmission. Provided that significant numbers of snails more than 4 to 6 weeks old could be collected, the prevalence of schistosome infection in them could be determined and, through repeated collections in index habitats, change in the prevalence of their infections could be detected. A method for examination of snails for infection is presented in on pages 662 to 664.

In practice, study of snail infections is not a very sound method of studying transmission to man since the relationship between snail infection prevalence and human infections is not well understood nor are the factors that regulate the release of cercariae from snails and their chances of finding a human host. Snail infections may be very infrequent even in areas of very high endemicity. Consequently, a change in the prevalence of infections in the snails would be very hard to interpret in terms of transmission dynamics.

Other Possible Supplementary Methods for Evaluation

Immersion of white mice or other small rodents in suspected transmission sites has been used to detect cercariae. This has been a useful research tool, but it is impractical and of little use for evaluation of control.

In a few areas where human schistosomiasis is endemic, other trematodes parasitize snails of the same habitats as those used by the schistosomiasis snails. This is the case in Rhodesia where the snails transmitting cattle liver fluke infection occupy the same habitats as those transmitting human schistosomiasis. The prevalence of liver fluke in cattle was drastically reduced in some places where schistosomiasis control with molluscicides was attempted. The decline in liver fluke infection as judged by decline in the numbers of infected cattle livers was a rapid indicator of snail control and liver fluke control. Its significance in terms of control of human schistosome infection is not clear though study might show a strong correlation between liver fluke control and schistosomiasis control.

Theoretically, routine human morbidity and mortality data should reflect a change in the prevalence of severe schistosomiasis. However, such data are of little or no value in most endemic zones for evaluation of the efficacy of a control programme since they are not standardized and are highly variable in their consistency and reliability.

Chapter 14

Epidemiology and Control of Schistosomiasis, pp. 620–748
(Karger, Basel and University Park Press, Baltimore 1973)

Techniques, Statistical Methods and Recording Forms

A. Techniques
L. J. OLIVIER

B. Statistical Methods
K. UEMURA

C. Recording Forms
L. J. OLIVIER and K. UEMURA

A. Techniques
L. J. OLIVIER

Techniques for Studying Schistosomes in Various Developmental Stages

Introduction

A technique is defined here as a laboratory or field method for collecting a specific kind of information or for performing a specific function. A technique may involve the collection of information concerning one variable such as skin sensitivity to an antigen, the collection of information on one stage in the life-cycle such as the output of eggs in faeces, making a measurement such as finding the diameters of snails or making a calculation such as the volume of water passing a certain point.

Techniques are distinguished here from procedures which are defined as processes for arriving at a relatively more complex body of information usually by employing a series of techniques. Thus, evaluation of control is a procedure requiring use of a series of techniques including population sampling, a faecal or urine examination and statistical analysis. A procedure usually permits a choice of techniques which may be selected according to the preferences of the worker and the conditions under which the work is to be done. Therefore, a person determining prevalence of schistosome infection may choose to employ a direct smear technique for faecal examination instead of a concentration method. Either may be adequate if properly standardized and carried out with care and consistency.

Since the adoption of procedures related to schistosomiasis and its control permits choice of techniques, the presentation of techniques is omitted in other parts of this volume; instead, a series of recommended techniques is presented here. Where only one technique is presented for collection of a certain kind of information it is because that technique is considered clearly better than any other. When more than one technique is presented the relative advantages or disadvantages are usually indicated. Other techniques than those listed here exist and may be quite suitable. New ones may be developed that will eventually supplant some of those presented here. Skilful and knowledgeable choice of techniques can greatly increase the usefulness of a procedure but the choice must always be followed by careful standardization of the technique, meticulous training of all technicians involved, and care to ensure that the technique does not vary significantly from person to person, from time to time and from place to place. It is important that a technique should have reproducibility, acceptability, reasonable simplicity, reliability and consistency. Sensitivity may have to be reduced below the optimum to achieve these qualities.

There has always been a remarkable divergence of findings by workers in different endemic areas and in different laboratories. Some of these differences are doubtless due to variations in technique. If standardized techniques could be adopted for collection of some of the data on schistosomiasis and its control, not only would variations in results be reduced but direct and meaningful comparisons between areas, strains and procedures would be made possible. It is unreasonable to advocate the adoption of one or another 'standard' technique, but it is appropriate to make certain stipulations with respect to choice.

First, workers should choose their techniques carefully, having clearly in mind the expected uses of the data to be collected. Second, they should take steps to ensure that the selected techniques will be used without significant variation throughout the course of the programme. If a technique is changed, even in a seemingly minor way, the data obtained by that technique may be useless for comparison with data obtained earlier. Third, all technicians using a technique should be trained to use it in a demonstrably consistent and uniform way. This can be done by training them in one place and testing them for proficiency. Again, using faecal examination as an example, a suspension with a known egg-count can be used to test whether the technicians are equally competent to find and count the eggs. Fourth, the technicians should be retested frequently, without prior warning, to determine whether they are maintaining their skill and accuracy. Fifth, when possible it would be useful to compare the more important quantitative techniques adopted for a programme with other techniques used for the same purpose by others. For example, it would be valuable, if a standard direct smear technique is adopted for stool examination, to compare it for accuracy, efficiency and cost with another standard method in general use. This would provide a correction factor that could permit comparison of data obtained by different methods.

Diagnostic Methods

Diagnostic methods are used: (1) to establish the existence of an endemic focus by detecting infected individuals; (2) to determine the prevalence or severity of infection for the purpose of assessing the problem in an area; (3) to collect data useful for evaluation of a control programme; and (4) to collect evidence from infected individuals as to the course of the infection and the effect of therapy.

Selection of a diagnostic method is made on the basis of its suitability for the purpose for which it is to be used, and on the basis of other factors such as the human, material and financial resources available and the conditions under which the work must be done. However, no matter how skilfully the choice is made, the most crucial factor will be the skill and consistency with which the work is performed.

Detection of Eggs in Urine or Faeces

Whatever the purpose for which urine or faeces are examined, the technique used must be precise and reproducible even if some sensitivity in detecting light infections must be sacrificed to achieve these ends.

There are two aspects of excretal examination that must be controlled:

(1) The time, place and manner of collection of the samples must aim to provide that the largest and most reproducible phase of egg output be sampled. There is little freedom of choice for stool collecting in the field but care must be taken to ensure that faecal specimens are not shared, substituted, contaminated with soil or mixed with other faeces. However, the sampling time for urine can be chosen to advantage.

(2) It is necessary to examine a measured portion of the sample exhaustively for eggs. A consequence of this is that any precise technique used in a prevalence survey may also be used for egg-counts.

For most survey and evaluation purposes, examination of the urine and stool for schistosome eggs will be depended upon to provide the data on infections. As measurement of egg output provides the only practicable estimate of infection intensity, egg-counts are being increasingly emphasized.

There is an imperative need for a generally accepted standard technique for determining egg excretion. This technique should be both sensitive and accurate. Dilution techniques are relatively insensitive, and sedimentation techniques are of variable and often unknown accuracy. In recent years, filtration methods have supplanted the older procedures since they permit the use of large samples and provide lasting preparations.

Detection of Eggs in Urine

The techniques for examination of urine are relatively simple but they tend to be deficient in that they are not of proved accuracy and reproducibility. The technique using sedimentation in a urine glass is prone to error when the sediment is withdrawn. Resuspension of a centrifuged sample for removal to a slide is also prone to error. It is necessary, therefore, to standardize any chosen method carefully and test it for its inherent inaccuracies.

The sampling time should be standardized, preferably between 12 noon and 2 p.m. since in one area at least, the maximal egg output and reproducibility come at that time. Exercise prior to urination has no significant effect on the egg-count and there is no advantage in selecting only the terminal portion of the urine passed at one time.

Schistosoma mansoni eggs are occasionally found in the urine, as are *S. haematobium* eggs in the faeces.

a) Collection of urine specimens. In essence, one collects the whole contents of the bladder of the person to be examined and then either preserves the whole specimen or pours off a measured portion for preservation and examination. If the whole specimen is retained the collecting bottles must be large and the volume of preservative added will depend on the volume of urine collected. If only a portion of the specimen is retained for subsequent examination the whole specimen is agitated briskly and then a measured portion is delivered into the sample bottle, following which preservative is added. The required amount of preservative is a formalin solution of 5% or a 1:2,000 solution of merthiolate; the sample should not be less than 50 ml.

The method of urine collection used in Rhodesia is presented to illustrate how urine specimens can be collected effectively.

Two stout wooden boxes with carrying handles are built so that each holds 240 wide-mouth bottles with plastic screw caps; the bottles are identical and hold 110 ml. These bottles, which are numbered serially, are the sample containers.

One hundred somewhat larger (140 ml) bottles are used to collect the pre-sample urine specimens. These bottles are not labelled.

About 500 ml of a solution of methiolate (0.4%) and sodium citrate (4.0%) are carried separately in a dark, glass-stoppered bottle. This solution is made fresh for each survey. The citrate is necessary where there is substantial haematuria. An automatic, self-filling 1-ml syringe is used to deliver this solution.

When the specimens are to be collected the people are divided into groups of 20. Normally the collecting procedure starts in the middle of the morning since the objective is to collect specimens passed between 10 a.m. and 2 p.m.

Each member of the group is given one of the larger bottles and asked to pass urine into it. When the specimens are brought in, a record is made of the time the specimens from the group were produced and the specimens are then discarded. Exactly one hour later, each member of the group is given one of the smaller, labelled bottles and asked to empty his bladder into it. In that way, one-hour urine samples are obtained. These specimens are logged into the records as they are delivered and preservative-citrate is added to each before the bottle is capped. The samples are then ready to be transported to the laboratory.

b) Simple sedimentation. For rapid surveys of prevalence when precision and quantitative information are not desired, one may use a simple sedimentation method.

Materials
(1) Sedimentation flask, conical, 200 to 300 ml capacity.
(2) Pipette, long enough to reach the bottom of the flask.
(3) Glass microscope slides, 50 mm × 70 mm.
(4) Cover-glasses.

Procedure
(1) The urine to be examined is placed in the conical flask (at least 50 ml, and 200 to 300 ml may be used).
(2) Sediment for 20 to 30 min.
(3) With pipette, transfer the sediment to a slide in one or two drops.
(4) Examine until an egg is found or until all the sediment has been searched.

Alternatively, a portion of the thoroughly mixed sample may be poured into a centrifuge tube and spun at 800 to 1,000 rpm for 2 min, after which the sediment can be examined as described above.

Quantitative information can be obtained if all the eggs in the sediment are counted. However, since the method requires the transfer of urine and sediment, eggs may be lost. If the method is used quantitatively, its reliability and sensitivity should be determined experimentally using suspensions with known egg densities.

If centrifugation is used, quantitative information may be obtained as follows: agitate the urine vigorously and transfer 10 ml to a graduated centrifuge tube; centrifuge at moderate speed for 2 min; remove the supernatant urine down to the 0.2-ml level with a Pasteur pipette and agitate the remainder to resuspend the deposit; remove 60 mm^3 to a slide, cover with a cover slip and count the eggs, which are those present in 3 ml of the original urine.

c) Filtration. Schistosome eggs can be recovered successfully from urine by drawing all or part of a urine sample through a filter paper with suction. The eggs lodge on the surface of the paper where they can be killed, stained, and preserved for future examination. The technique can be applied either in the field or in a laboratory, the materials and method depending upon which is chosen.

The essential requirements for the technique are:

(1) A filter holder which is a perforated disc that will hold a small filter paper disc as suction is applied to it.

(2) Filter paper, Whatman No. 1, No. 541 or equivalent.

(3) Suction apparatus.

(4) Ninhydrin solution, saturated, aqueous. Ninhydrin should be kept as the solid in a dark bottle in a cupboard. The solution is made up twice weekly and kept also in a dark bottle, preferably in a drawer or cupboard. Very old stock solid to be found in some laboratories should be avoided in favour of that of known delivery date. Ninhydrin solution in pressure cans for chromatography has also been used successfully.

(5) Glass slides 50 mm × 75 mm.

(6) Glass cover slips or Perspex cover sheets.

Field filtration: A kit for field urine filtration has been devised [BRADLEY, 1965] which uses for the filter holder a Tenite 'field monitor' (fig. 2) with a perforated plastic disc and sampling tubes. Filter papers 37 mm in diameter are used. Suction is provided by a hypodermic syringe having a capacity equal to the volume of urine to be filtered through one paper.

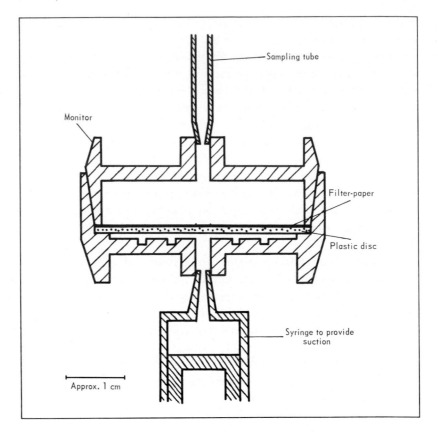

Fig. 1. Longitudinal section of urine filtration apparatus. Urine flow is from top to bottom of diagram [BRADLEY, 1965].

The field monitors, manufactured to carry precision cellulose-ester filters, are of two parts (as shown in fig. 1) which fit together to hold the filter paper supported by one of the perforated plastic discs. Each part has a Luer socket into which both the sampling tubes and syringes fit. The monitors are made of transparent plastic and are not easily broken. Plastic plugs are provided to close the sockets when not in use. Since the monitors replace the usual urine-carrying bottles, sufficient are taken into the field to allow one for each sample that day.

The monitors can be assembled in advance. In the field each person urinates into a wide-mouth jar. The sample is shaken vigorously and the sampling tube of a monitor inserted well into it after a syringe has been fixed

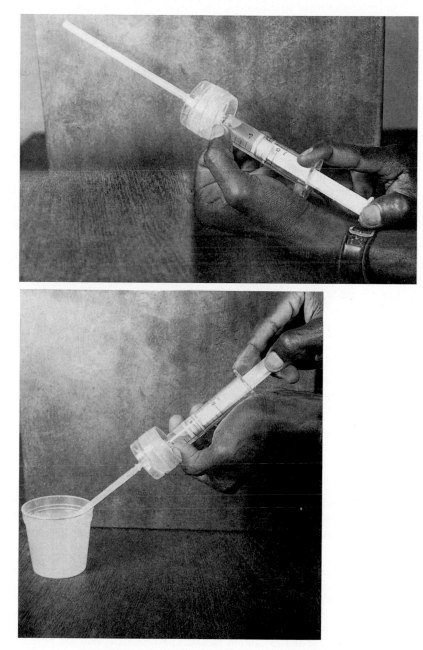

Fig. 2. Urine filtration apparatus. In field use the apparatus is kept vertical [BRADLEY, 1965].

to the filter end (fig. 2A). The plunger is withdrawn to the 5 ml mark, the whole apparatus removed from the urine and inverted (fig. 2B), and the urine filtered completely by suction from the syringe. The filtrate is discarded after the syringe has been detached from the monitor, whose lower end is then plugged. The sampling tube is then detached. The whole field procedure can be completed in a few seconds.

On return to the laboratory or camp, the dirtier samples and those containing blood may be washed with a dilute solution of Teepol detergent in saline, sucking with the syringe. The eggs are then killed by gentle heat or by formol. A few drops of saturated ninhydrin in saline, prepared less than a week previously, are added to the paper and the monitors are gently heated until dry. A temperature between 37 and 90°C is needed, and anything from a bacteriological incubator to a biscuit tin over a fire may be used.[1] The papers are then removed from the monitors which are reloaded for use the next day. The papers may be varnished with a drop of dilute Nobecutane, to attach the eggs to the paper, and stored. The cost of the kits is low and if many examinations are made, the cost can fall to US $0.02 per sample.

Laboratory filtration: Urine samples brought to the laboratory can be filtered with one of several filter holders and suction methods. The holder may be made of perforated Perspex (Lucite). The Millipore (Pyrex) filter holder (XX 10.047.00) is very suitable, taking 47-mm diameter papers.

Suction can be provided by a mechanical vacuum pump or by a water jet vacuum pump.

The filter paper should be held to the surface of the holder with a heavy brass ring, slightly smaller than the paper, which also prevents spillage of the sample over the edge of the paper.

Filtration is accomplished as follows:

With the paper and ring in place, apply suction to the holder. Mix the urine sample thoroughly and deliver a measured volume into the space formed by the ring. Usually a 10-ml portion will suffice if 47-mm paper is used. The

---

1   The ninhydrin reaction may be adversely affected by various factors. Formol saline and merthiolate-formalin solutions have a satisfactory pH for most purposes, provided the eggs are washed. Ninhydrin solutions must be freshly prepared every few days. It has often been inadequately realized that there are three stages of the ninhydrin reaction in eggs: (1) the egg needs to be dead to allow good penetration; (2) penetration by ninhydrin is a diffusion process requiring time and an aqueous medium; heat facilitates this; and (3) coloration requires heat and drying. It is likely that several failures to stain the eggs have resulted from over-rapid drying in the oven.

walls of the ring and the filter paper can then be rinsed with saline or water. If merthiolate was the preservative, a detergent (Teepol) may be added to the wash solution to lyse the red blood cells.

The filter paper is removed from the filter and wetted thoroughly with ninhydrin solution. In a closed dish it is then warmed or allowed to stand at room temperature overnight. The paper is then dried with heat (50 °C) in an uncovered dish.

Papers prepared by either of the above methods are dampened and viewed under a low-power monocular or dissecting microscope. For qualitative results each paper is scanned systematically until an egg is found or until all the paper has been examined.

Filtration is the method of choice for quantitative urine studies. The procedure is as follows:

Pour a known volume (usually 10 ml) of well-mixed urine through a filter paper with suction applied. Process the filter paper as described above and count all the eggs on the paper. The number obtained, divided by 10, will give the number of eggs per ml of urine in the sample.

Detection of Eggs in Faeces

Sensitivity is a problem in the precise examination of faeces for schistosome eggs since, whereas 10 ml of urine taken near midday contain about 2.5% of the daily *S. haematobium* output, 1 g of stool contains about 1.0% of the *S. mansoni* egg output.

Numerous techniques have been used for detection of schistosome eggs in faeces and a number of workers have compared techniques. However, techniques have rarely been tested for reliability, consistency or sensitivity with faecal material containing known numbers of schistosome eggs.

Several techniques will be described here. These and others are described in texts and in references to microbiological techniques. BAILENGER [1965] presents descriptions of numerous techniques for recovery of schistosome eggs from faeces. Whatever the technique or variant employed, it should be checked for consistency of results; it must be compared with another method, using heavily infected faeces, and the quantity of stool actually used should be recorded.

a) Collection and preservation of faeces. The most important consideration in the collection of faecal samples is that each be accurately identified, are fresh when examined or preserved, and are uncontaminated by water, soil or other substances which may contain organisms or their eggs.

The size of the sample, i.e. the amount requested from the individuals to be examined, need not be more than 5 to 10 g (a mass about as big as a thumb). If suitable containers are available (paper or plastic cartons of 200 ml capacity or larger) it is often more satisfactory to request the whole stool. The chief advantage in this arrangement is that it permits defaecation directly into the container and a proper sample for examination may then be selected.

When preservation is resorted to, the preferred preservative under usual circumstances is 10% formalin (commercial formaldehyde diluted with 9 parts water). Approximately 1 g (1 ml) of faeces is transferred to a vial or wide-mouth bottle of about 10 ml capacity or larger, and enough preservative is added, with stirring, to bring the faeces to a fluid-pasty consistency. Additional preservative is then added to half-fill the vial which, after being stoppered and vigorously shaken, is then nearly filled with preservative, stoppered and labelled.

Alternatively, the bottles or vials can be half-filled with formalin before they are taken to the field, and the faeces added and mixed when collected. The edges of an adhesive label, cut to a length slightly less than that of the vial's circumference and at a width equal to the depth of a 1-ml quantity contained in the vial, can be used to obtain accurate measurement of the faecal sample. The label is placed with its lower margin at the meniscus of a 4-ml quantity of the preservative-diluent. Adding faeces to bring the meniscus to the label's upper margin will give a 1-ml sample of faeces, measured by displacement.

b) Methods for Faecal Examination

1. Direct Smear Technique

Materials

(1) Wooden or bamboo applicator, toothpick or other type of disposable small shaft for transferring and stirring milligram amounts of faeces.

(2) Glass microscope slide, 25 mm × 75 mm.

(3) Glass or plastic cover-glass, 22 mm × 22 mm.

(4) Physiological salt solution (0.85% sodium chloride).

Procedure

(1) Place one drop of saline on the centre of a slide.

(2) With an applicator, take at random a 2-mg sample of faeces (1 mg of faeces is about 1 mm^3; it is better to take a correctly-sized sample and use all of it than to take a great excess and attempt to use only 2 mg of it).

(3) Stir the sample into the saline, making an even suspension without spreading the saline.

(4) Drag to the edge of the suspension and remove all gross elements such as fibres, seeds, sand, etc.

(5) Cover with 22 mm × 22 mm cover-glass.

(6) If the preparation is satisfactory in all respects, examine it; if not, discard it. No time should be wasted on a preparation that can only yield doubtful results if negative. A satisfactory smear is one that is of uniform density and contains a maximum of observable faecal elements without obscuring any object within the size-range of those being sought. The smear must not tilt the cover-glass nor contain large air bubbles.

(7) Examine the entire preparation systematically, in successive adjacent swaths, with low power (about 100 ×) of the microscope. Questionable objects may require inspection under higher magnification but, in properly-prepared smears, schistosome and other helminth eggs can be accurately identified and counted under low power.

The method is roughly quantitative though relatively insensitive. For quantitative measurement, count the schistosome eggs observed in the smear and record as 'eggs per smear'.

2. Direct Smear; Kato Procedure

Materials

(1) Wooden applicator or equivalent for transferring faeces.

(2) Glass microscope slides; 25 mm × 75 mm.

(3) Cellophane[2], *wettable*, 40 to 50 μm thickness cut in pieces about 22 mm × 30 mm.

(4) Glycerin-malachite green solution, aqueous (100 ml pure glycerin, 100 ml water, 1 ml of 3% aqueous malachite green).

Procedure

(1) Soak the cellophane pieces in the glycerin-malachite green solution.

(2) Transfer 40 to 50 mg of faeces to a slide (a 4-mm cube of faeces weighs about 60 mg). This amount can be secured accurately by the use of a simple tube with a plunger that will accept and release the correct amount of faeces [LAYRISSE *et al.*, 1969]. If the faeces are fibrous, 1 or 2 g of faeces may be put on a flat surface and a square of stainless wire cloth pressed down on them. The faeces to be used can then be scraped from the upper surface of the wire cloth (105-mesh steel bolting cloth).

(3) Cover the faecal sample with cellophane and press with a soft rubber stopper (No. 5) to spread in an even layer. Note: To judge the proper thickness of the layer of faeces requires experience. It is not necessary to spread the

2   DuPont No. 124 PD.

faeces to all areas of the cellophane cover; it is merely spread to about the circumference of an area equal to the width of the cellophane.

(4) Allow the smear to stand for one hour at room temperature or 20 to 30 min in a dry incubator at about 40 °C. This dries and clears the faeces, while the eggs retain their normal appearance. Note: If the film is over-dried, gas bubbles form, the eggs become distorted (especially hookworm eggs), and a dark air-cell may form around the eggs making them difficult to see.

(5) Examine the entire film under low magnification; experienced microscopists can readily detect and identify the larger helminth eggs under scanning lens (50 ×) magnification. Higher magnification can be used when needed.

This technique was developed in Japan for *Ascaris* surveys and its application for schistosome egg detection was described by MARTIN and BEAVER [1968]. It is a very simple, cheap, and accurate technique. As for sensitivity, it compares favourably with the gravity sedimentation method and the filtration method. It may be as sensitive as ether separation, since there is no egg loss in the procedure. If the amount of faeces is measured and all eggs on the smear are counted, the procedure is quantitative. This method is achieving increased acceptance.

3. Concentration by Sedimentation

Faeces normally contain a great variety of materials, most of which are either lighter or denser, smaller or larger than the eggs and larvae of worm parasites. The purpose in using a concentration method is to separate as completely as possible the parasite objects from elements of the faeces. In general, this is accomplished somewhat imperfectly, of course, by making a watery suspension which permits sorting of the elements, by screening which removes the larger objects, by sedimentation which removes the light elements in the supernatant fluid, and by flotation which separates the parasite stages from some of the mass of other elements. Several of the established concentration methods incorporate all three of these principles, usually in the order listed. An important requirement for efficiency of any concentration method is thorough mixing of the faeces in a diluent.

Gravity sedimentation is one of the most efficient methods for concentrating schistosome eggs. Because the eggs of schistosomes are relatively large and heavy they are effectively concentrated by this method. It involves simple procedures which can be carried out with inexpensive and readily available materials and equipment. For general surveys, the following technique is satisfactory:

Materials

(1) Diluent consisting of an aqueous solution of either 0.5% glycerol or 0.85% sodium chloride.

(2) Conical sedimentation flask, 50 to 200 ml (conical glass containers of any type will serve; several types manufactured for serving beverages are satisfactory).

(3) Wire or nylon gauze.

(4) Paper cup of about 50 ml capacity, or small beaker or sturdy 60-ml medicine or measuring glass.

(5) Wood applicator, toothpick or bamboo splinter.

(6) Pipette of suitable size for the sedimentation flask used.

(7) Slide and cover-glass.

Procedure

(1) In a paper cup or other small container (see 4 above), mix 1 cm³ of faeces in 1 or 2 ml of diluent.

(2) Dilute to capacity of the mixing container with the diluent and strain the suspension through gauze into the conical flask. Additional diluent can be used to rinse the gauze.

(3) Add diluent to fill the flask. Sediment for 20 to 30 min (neither more nor less) and decant.

(4) Resuspend the sediment in just enough diluent to make the suspension 2 cm deep, and allow to sediment for 10 min.

(5) Remove sediment from the bottom layer with a long pipette (a Pasteur pipette is very good for this), transfer two drops to a slide, add cover-glass and systematically examine the preparation. If considerable sediment remains, a second two-drop preparation should be similarly examined. For quantitative results all the sediment must be examined and all eggs in it counted. The results may be presented as eggs per cm³ or eggs per gram of faeces.

4. Ether Separation [RITCHIE, 1948]

To a measured volume (usually 5 ml) of a stool suspension of known faecal content in a 15-ml centrifuge tube add 4 ml of ether, stopper, and shake vigorously for 30 sec. Remove stopper and centrifuge for 2 min at about 2,000 rpm. Loosen the plug under the ether, decant the supernatant and examine the deposit in the bottom of the tube for eggs under the 10 × objective of a microscope. If quantitative information is needed, examine all the sediment and count all the eggs seen. The result is usually presented as eggs per gram of faeces.

5. Filtration

Schistosome eggs in faeces can be collected on filter paper by the technique of BELL [1963]. The urine filtration technique described previously was patterned on this. Reference should be made to page 625, c for additional information.

Materials
(1) Funnel.
(2) 0.5-mm mesh nylon gauze.
(3) Filter-paper holder attached to suction pump. A 7-cm diameter holder can be made of Perspex (Lucite). An alternative is to use the lowest part of a tripartite Hartley three-piece Buchner funnel and fix a perforated Perspex sheet to it, the usual porcelain disc having too few holes. Suction can be provided as noted under the description for urine filtration.
(4) Fresh saturated aqueous ninhydrin.
(5) Petri dishes.
(6) Incubator (between 37 and 60 °C).
(7) Whatman 541 filter paper or equivalent; 70-mm diameter.
(8) 2-ml pipette.
(9) Forceps.
(10) Microscope.
(11) Cover slip with grid.

Procedure
The stool suspension is shaken vigorously. A 1- or 2-ml sample is sucked through a 7-cm 541 filter paper after passing it through an 0.5-mm mesh gauze to remove large faecal debris. The deposit on the filter is well washed with water. The filter paper is laid on several drops of freshly made saturated ninhydrin solution and heated at 37 to 50 °C for several hours in a covered Petri dish. The cover is then removed so that the paper dries and is left to heat at about 50 °C overnight. The papers are cut in half, and placed on a large drop of water on a 50 mm × 75 mm slide. A cover slip with a grid is put over it, air bubbles being avoided. Eggs are counted under the low power of a microscope. After subsequent drying, the eggs may be fixed to the paper by immersion in a very dilute solution of Nobecutane in ethyl acetate.

In this way 100 or 200 mg of stool can be examined and egg-counts from that volume can be made. Theoretically using the faecal suspension described on page 630, § 3, the method will detect as few as 10 eggs per gram of faeces.

6. Dilution
Dilution techniques, as used by SCOTT [1937] and KLOETZEL [1963] can be used for egg-counting but they are relatively less sensitive than the filtration technique unless multiple counts are made.

7. Egg Hatching

Because the miracidia are negatively geotropic, the best method for concentrating those that hatch is to have a small surface area as compared to the volume of water in which hatching takes place. This result is obtained by fitting a 250- or 500-ml Erlenmeyer flask, with a conically-bored rubber stopper holding a vertical glass tube about 10 cm long. The bottom of the rubber stopper is cut off so as to preserve a smooth contour from the wall of the flask to the bottom of the glass tube. The water level is brought up to about 2 cm of the tube above the stopper. Miracidia collect towards the top of the water in the glass tube and can be observed by the naked eye or with the aid of a hand lens. When counts of miracidia are to be made, the water in the collecting tube is pipetted into shell vials which are observed under a dissecting microscope [INGALLS et al., 1949]. For other methods see HUNTER et al. [1946a, b]; PESIGAN and YOGORE [1947].

Immunodiagnosis

Of the immunological tests now available the most promising for screening purposes are the intradermal test, the slide flocculation test, and the fluorescent antibody test. They are of relatively little use for evaluation of control since the serological reactions persist for a time after the schistosome infection is lost. However, it is possible that longitudinal study of the serological reactions of young children might be used to measure incidence of infections in the very young as an index of transmission intensity.

It should be added that the correct evaluation of the results of these tests is a matter of considerable complexity and one requiring experience in the field. It is therefore strongly advisable, if immunological reactions are to be employed in assessing the results of control programmes, that the services of a suitable specialist should be enlisted.

Many kinds of antigen have been used and different tests employed. Improvements in preparation of the antigen and in execution of the tests have greatly increased their value. Nevertheless, it must be remembered that in judging the value of immunological techniques, the evidence obtained is indirect. Moreover, a false positive reaction may occur in response to substances antigenically related to schistosomes.

a) Transport, preservation and use of serum specimens. Most of the serological tests for schistosomiasis cannot be performed in the field because of the difficult conditions and the lack of adequate and specialized laboratory facilities. However, the serum required can be transported to laboratories for testing.

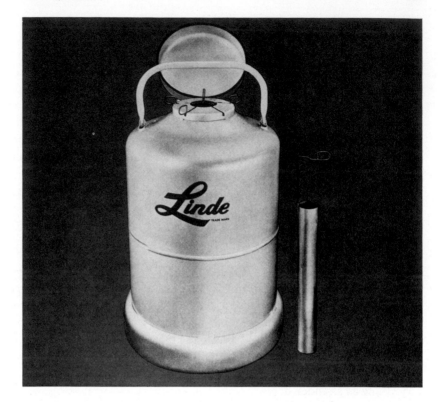

Fig. 3. The LR-10-5 liquid nitrogen refrigerator-transporter.

The problems of serum collection and transport in rural tropical field activities are well known and include risks of specimen contamination and of antibody decay. To provide adequate transport conditions for sera drawn in remote rural areas by vacutainer technique, the Linde liquid nitrogen transport refrigerator, previously used in the animal husbandry programme for preservation of bull sperm for artificial insemination, was adapted to serum transport by WHO. Figures 3 and 4 picture the model LR-10-5 refrigerator-transporter and give specifications. This equipment was adjusted to accommodate, in each of the three racks of its canisters, a total of 50 to 60 5-ml serum ampoules. A similar but larger model, the LR-10-6 transport refrigerator, with a capacity of 252 ampoules for 1-ml, 210 for 2-ml and some 90 ampoules for 5-ml serum is currently in use. The ampoules are stored in five or six canisters in the LR-10-6, each canister containing five insertable racks which hold the ampoules at a constant temperature close to $-196\,^{\circ}\text{C}$.

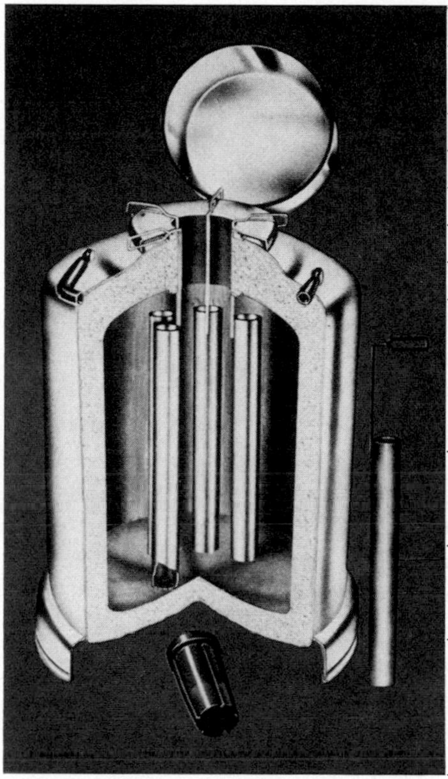

Specifications	
Rated liquid nitrogen capacity	9.9 litres
Height	44 cm
Outside diameter	26 cm
Entrance tube diameter	3.75 cm
Weight full	14 kg
Weight empty	5 kg

5 canister capacity	1032 ml
	90 ampoules (1.2 ml
	    racked and tubed)
	120 ampoules
	    (1.2 ml without tubes)

Canister size
    height
    outside diameter
	27.5 cm
	3.125 cm

Storage temperature	−320 °F. (−196 °C) below the liquid nitrogen level

Liquid nitrogen consumption rate (maximum)	0.40 litres per day
	    (without canisters)
	
	0.55 litres per day
	    (with canisters)

Fig. 4. Cross-section of the liquid nitrogen refrigerator-transporter showing canisters in place etc. and giving technical specifications. The LR-10-5 refrigerator-transporter and the slightly larger model LR-10-6 of a similar construction are designed for shipping and storage of biological specimens safely and economically. Originally designed for the preservation and shipment of bull semen in animal husbandry programmes this equipment has been adapted as described in this article to the use of rapid serum sample freezing at −196 °C and long distance transport to a base laboratory from the field. The liquid nitrogen refrigerator-transporter is an efficiently insulated double-walled container. Use of aluminium as its major construction material gives it high structural strength as well as light-weight design. It has a carrying handle and small size which assures portability.

The insulation of the LR-10-6 keeps the liquid nitrogen consumption extremely low, − 0.55 l per day.

Present experience shows that the LR-10-6 can actually be filled with liquid nitrogen in Europe and shipped by air to, say, Lagos (Nigeria) for subsequent road transport to the sampling points in the field, retaining sufficient capacity to be utilized and returned by road and by air to an overseas reference laboratory, still holding liquid nitrogen and freezing capacity after more than 21 days. This allows for the operations to be successfully carried out and for a *frozen base-line* for antibody determination to be obtained. Accurate base reference laboratory evaluation of test performance in a field laboratory has thus become more practical and certain, and proper studies can be undertaken of the influence of the time-temperature complex on antibody decay under more primitive conditions.

So far the freezing, transport and handling of sera by the method outlined has been found to be practical, efficient, safe and economical. Serologically inert, freeze-resistant, plastic tubes with an air-tight seal of Teflon-lined aluminium foil are more practical than glass ampoules. This avoids the use of blowlamps since no sealing is required.

The liquid nitrogen refrigerator transporter is without danger of explosion and is accepted by public carriers for air shipment (IATA). The air freight cost is reasonable, e.g., US $40 and US $45 between Lagos (Nigeria) and Copenhagen (Denmark). The total cost of liquid nitrogen needed for six shipments over the mentioned distances does not exceed US $35. The purchase cost of an LR-10-6 refrigerator transporter is US $200 to US $300.

b) Skin test (intradermal test). Persons infected with schistosomiasis may show specific cutaneous sensitivity at an early stage of the infection. Usually, the sensitization becomes evident in four to eight weeks after infection. It persists for years after the infection is lost.

The skin test is relatively inexpensive to administer, though the antigen is fairly expensive. It provides immediate results since the reaction is read within 15 min after the antigen is injected. Since great variation in sensitivity and specificity can occur due to the nature of the antigen, age and sex of the person tested and the site of the infection, it is necessary to standardize both the antigen and the procedure for the test.

The test is not very sensitive in detecting infection in children under 5 years of age, females are less reactive than males, marked differences in reactivity occur among different ethnic groups and the back is more sensitive than the arms. There are a number of false-positive reactions: cross-reactions occurring with other schistosomes, including bird schistosomes, and in persons with clonorchiasis and paragonimiasis. *S. mansoni* antigen should not be used in a *S. japonicum* area since the reactions are relatively poor.

For epidemiological surveys the intradermal test offers a means for getting information on the prevalence of infection. Not only are the results obtained immediately but blood-letting is avoided.

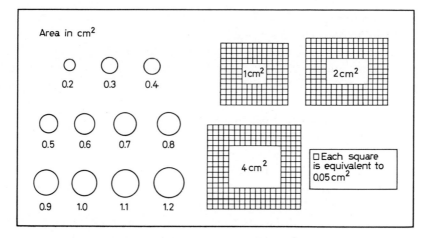

Area in cm²

0.2   0.3   0.4

1cm²   2cm²

0.5   0.6   0.7   0.8

4 cm²   □ Each square is equivalent to 0.05 cm²

0.9   1.0   1.1   1.2

Fig 5 Stencil for measuring area of skin tests.

The skin-test antigen: The World Health Organization has been instrumental in the preparation of a reference skin-test antigen which is an acid-soluble protein fraction of *S. mansoni* adults adjusted to 0.03 mg N/ml (Melcher's antigen). This should be used as a reference for any antigen employed in the skin test. It would be desirable to use only antigen prepared according to the method used for the reference antigen and calibrated against it. Techniques for preparation of antigen are presented in KAGAN and PELLEGRINO [1961].

Materials

(1) Antigen: the reference skin-test antigen is a sterile adult-worm acid-soluble protein fraction of *S. mansoni* or *S. japonicum* adjusted to 0.03 mg N/ml. Merthiolate has been substituted for phenol in the Coca's solution.

(2) Control: the control solution is composed of sodium bicarbonate buffer and 1:5,000 merthiolate.

(3) Hypodermic syringes: if possible, 0.25-ml tuberculin syringes should be used; however, 1-ml tuberculin syringes graduated in 0.1-ml amounts can be employed.

(4) Needles: sterile 27-gauge 0.4-mm steel disposable needles, or platinum skin-test needles with a short bevel are recommended.

(5) Alcohol lamp.

(6) Cellulose template for measuring the area of the weal (fig. 5).

(7) Small pad of paper.

(8) Ball-point pens.

(9) Watch.

(10) Alcohol and cotton wool.

Techniques for Handling Groups of Individuals for Skin Testing

For maximum efficiency a team of at least three individuals should be used; a clerk, an individual to inject the solutions, and an individual to read the test.

The clerk calls in the patient, writes his name, age, sex, etc., on a piece of paper (preferably 12 cm × 17 cm), gives him a number which is written on the paper and on the patient's arm.

The patient presents himself for skin testing, hands the paper to the doctor and is injected with the antigen and the control solution. The time of the last injection is recorded on the paper.

The paper is handed to the third member of the team who immediately adds 15 min which designates the time when the patient will be recalled and the test read. The patient is asked to wait and the slips of paper are arranged so that the patients will be recalled on time.

With this system, 50 to 60 patients per hour can be tested with ease. Where there is a language barrier and pronunciation of names is difficult, having the number on the patient and on the paper is very helpful and avoids errors in correlating *vitae* data and tests.

Techniques of the Test

After the site on the skin has been swabbed with alcohol, *exactly* 0.05 ml of the antigen and of the control solution are injected intradermally, with care and precision. In case of spillage or subcutaneous injection, a new site is selected and the injection is repeated. Women are tested above the neckline when the back is used; boys and men are asked to remove their shirts.

At 15 min and in good light, the edge of each area of *induration* is carefully outlined with a ball-point pen. Erythema around the weals is ignored. The paper (with patient's name, etc.) is slightly moistened with alcohol and the tracing transferred by pressing the paper over the inked areas.

Measurement of Reactions

When the tests have been completed, the area of each weal as indicated by the ink tracing is measured with the template and recorded.

On celluloid or thick cellophane a series of circles is drawn, so as to range from 0.2 to 1.2 cm² in area (difference of 0.1 cm² between two successive circles). At the side of these circles, three rectangles are drawn, with areas of 1.0, 2.0 and 4.0 cm². These rectangles are surrounded by a series of small squares, each corresponding to 0.05 cm². In order to determine the area of the weal, one places the celluloid on the transfer and reads off the area as follows:

(1) If the weal is rounded and does not exceed 1.2 cm², the area is determined by finding the circle on the celluloid whole area that is nearest the area of the transfer.

(2) If the weal is very irregular and its area is more than 1.2 cm², one of the rectangles is placed on the transfer, so as to remain within the outline of the latter. The small squares between the outline of the transfer and the rectangle are counted, their area is calculated (two are equivalent to 0.1 cm²) and is then added to the known area of the central rectangle.

An example of the celluloid template used to read the areas of the weals is given in figure 5.

The following classification of skin reactions has been adopted in Brazil.

Negative tests: weals with an area of 0.9 cm² or smaller.

Doubtful tests: weals with an area of 1.0 to 1.1 cm².

Positive tests: weals with an area of 1.2 cm² or over.

Probably the second group should also be considered positive.

c) Complement-fixation test. There is general agreement that the complement-fixation test is highly sensitive and specific using either cercaria or adult worm antigen. It becomes positive before the worms mature and eggs are produced. However, it remains positive for a long time after infection has ended.

The C-F test is reliable when performed under optimum conditions but it requires complex techniques that severely limit its usefulness.

The test is described and analysed in KAGAN and PELLEGRINO [1961] and in WHO [1967].

d) Fluorescent antibody test. The fluorescent antibody technique for the serodiagnosis of schistosomiasis in humans appears to be reasonably sensitive and specific. A modification has now been developed by which dried blood smears on filter paper may be used. In this way, drops of blood from finger pricks can be obtained in endemic areas, smeared on filter paper, dried, mailed to a central laboratory, extracted and used in the fluorescent antibody test. To obviate the necessity of maintaining a fresh supply of cercariae in the central diagnostic laboratory, a method has been developed whereby preserved cercariae can be used for the test without loss of reactivity. This technique is well suited to epidemiological investigations of human schistosomiasis since:

(1) collections of specimens may usually be obtained in endemic areas, even from infants, as only a few drops of blood are required;

(2) blood may be collected by puncture of finger, toe or heel with a minimum of apparatus;

(3) collection may be made by relatively untrained personnel without regard to sterility of the specimens; and

(4) dried blood smears may be placed in an envelope and mailed to a central laboratory where the tests can be performed with standardized reagents by adequately trained laboratory personnel.

Standards for the performance and interpretation of the test have been prepared and are available in published form [SADUN et al., 1960].

e) Slide flocculation test. The main advantages of this test are its reliability, relative simplicity, and economy. All the serologically reactive antibody for the test can be removed without any dilution by simple absorption with a calculated volume of washed, packed and essentially dry antigen-cholesterol-lecithin complex, thus permitting the standardization of antisera in terms of amounts of antibody nitrogen. As with all other schistosome serological tests, the slide flocculation test gives false positives with *Trichinella spiralis* antisera. A major drawback is the need for fresh serum. However, if serum is readily available, this may be the test of choice.

Standards for the performance and interpretation of results of the test have been prepared and are available in published form [ANDERSON, 1960]. The relationship of antibody and antigen to titre in this test has also been standardized [ANDERSON, 1961].

Detection of Cercariae in Natural Habitats

In order to study the factors that influence the success of cercariae in locating and successfully penetrating the human host, it is necessary to be able to collect free cercariae from the water of natural habitats and study their population dynamics in detail. It is essential to know when the cercariae are released into the habitat by the snails, how they are distributed in the habitat, what the factors are that speed their death or favour their survival, and many other such details that can only be learned by measuring their density from time to time by a precise method.

Until recently very few attempts had been made to collect schistosome cercariae from natural water. There have been many observations on the prevalence of infected snails in natural habitats but this is of limited value in study of transmission, since the factors causing release of the cercariae from

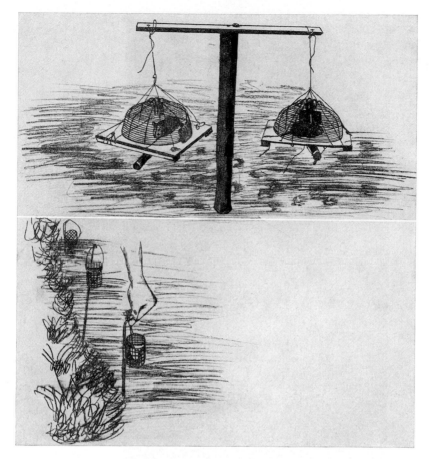

a

b

Fig. 6a and *b*.

snails are poorly understood and the presence of infected snails is not evidence
that there will be cercariae in the surrounding water.

Cercariae may be collected from the water either by exposing test animals
to the water and counting the worms that eventually develop in the animal, or
by processing the water in a way which will concentrate the cercariae and
permit their enumeration and study. Although the techniques described
below for collecting cercariae are not completely satisfactory, they are effective
enough to justify use in the basic epidemiological studies that precede control
operations.

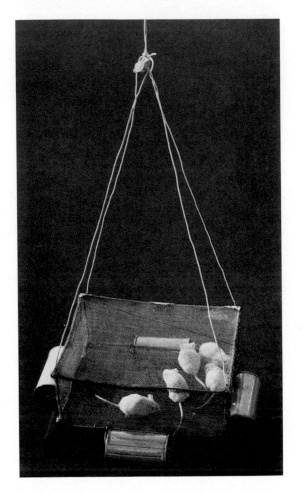

Fig.6c.

Exposure of Rodents

Small rodents, usually laboratory mice, have been used to test suspected transmission foci and to study the distribution of cercariae and their population dynamics.

The rodents are immersed in natural waters in wide-mesh wire cages or other restraining devices for a certain length of time, then removed, suitably labelled with all relevant data, and held until any schistosomes have matured. At autopsy, all schistosomes are removed, sexed, counted and identified.

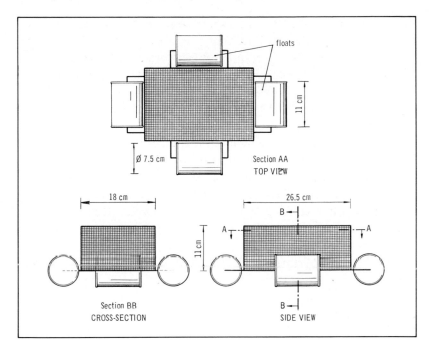

floats

11 cm

Ø 7.5 cm

Section AA
TOP VIEW

18 cm

26.5 cm

B

A

11 cm

A

Section BB
CROSS-SECTION

B

SIDE VIEW

Fig. 6d. Detailed drawing of the floating wire cage [Dazo, 1965].

The recommended procedure is as follows:

In each habitat to be studied mice should be exposed in one or more sets of five by fastening them to a device which, when placed at the surface of the water, will hold the mice partially submerged. The exposure time should be from 30 to 60 min. Longer exposure is undesirable since it risks death of mice through chilling. Exposure devices are pictured in figure 6a, b, c and d.

After exposure the mice should be held for a sufficient time to ensure not only development of adult worms but deposition of eggs since the latter may be necessary for recognition of species. Six weeks will be sufficient for *S. mansoni* and *S. japonicum*. *S. haematobium* cercariae have not been detected in natural habitats though attempts were made in South Africa. Should the method be tried in a *S. haematobium* habitat the rodents should be held for 12 to 15 weeks since the worms develop more slowly.

The rodents should be examined for adult worms by a perfusion method since perfusion is rapid and can be depended upon to expel all, or nearly all, the worms. The method which has had the most thorough evaluation is that developed at the National Institutes of Health in Bethesda on the basis of the method of YOLLES *et al.* [1947]. Typical eggs can be obtained by teasing the liver or the wall of the intestine. Under some circumstances, it may be useful to digest a portion of the liver or intestine in order to recover eggs.

The method has certain advantages. Infectivity of the cercariae is proved. Identification of the schistosomes is facilitated since schistosome adults, and especially the eggs can be recognized. Rodents can be used in any sort of habitat regardless of the condition of the water.

On the other hand the method has some disadvantages. The relation between the number of adult worms recovered and the number of cercariae present in the water at the time of exposure is not known. The method has been unsuccessful with *S. haematobium.* Large numbers of animals must be provided and housed for long periods. The desired information is obtained only after a very long delay.

Collection of Cercariae for Visual Examination by Concentration Methods

The cercaria population of a body of water can be measured if the cercariae in samples of the water can be concentrated and counted. This can be done by collecting the cercariae on filters or by centrifugation. Cercariae of non-human schistosomes will cause difficulties in some instances.

a) Filtration

Membrane Filtration

A device using a Millipore filter has been used to detect cercariae of *S. japonicum* in the Philippines. Water was dipped or skimmed from the habitat and poured through the membrane, and cercariae were detected successfully. The method has not been used elsewhere and its usefulness has not yet been evaluated adequately.

Paper Filtration

Cercariae can be collected with some success by forcing water containing cercariae through filter paper which will retain them.

In practice a portable filter holder and a suction device are used to draw the water through the filter. Such a filtration device [ROWAN, 1965] is shown in figure 7. A sheet of S and S No. 404 filter paper is held on a perforated plate fused into a large plastic funnel which is in turn fastened to a 20-litre bottle; suction applied to the bottle draws the water through the funnel. The suction is provided by a bicycle pump, modified for suction instead of pressure. All joints are sealed with elastic rubber compound. The filtered water is collected in the plastic bottle which is drained by means of a stoppered hole in its bottom.

Mechanical vacuum filtration can be done using a filtration chamber of

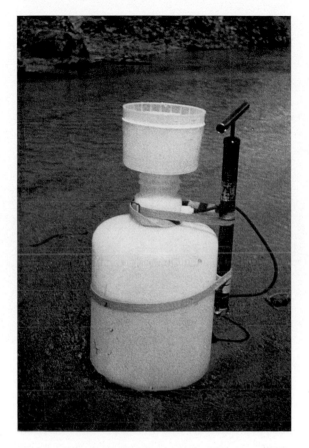

Fig. 7. Vacuum paper filtration apparatus [ROWAN, 1965].

stainless steel 33 cm in diameter with a plastic sieve plate mounted internally on which is placed the S and S No. 404 filter paper (24 cm in diameter) (fig. 8). The filter funnel is connected by plastic tubing to the intake port of a pump (Micro Mite Orion Mfg. Co., La Mirada, Calif.) driven by a 3.2 kg, 2-cycle, ¾-h.p. Ohlsson and Rice gasoline motor. A cut-off valve on the discharge port of the pump and shortout lever for the motor give finger-tip control to the filtering process.

If the water is not turbid, large volumes of water can be passed through the filter, and filtration is rapid. If the water is clear a 24-cm diameter paper will filter up to 100 l in 5 min.

At completion of filtration, the still-moist filter paper is placed over

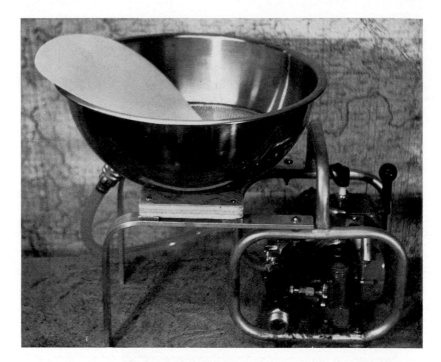

Fig.8. Apparatus for mechanical vacuum filtration [ROWAN].

several millilitres of 0.5% aqueous ninhydrin reagent in a flat pan and then heated rapidly to dryness without scorching the paper. The cercariae are stained blue and contrast with the white paper. The cercariae can be recognized by their shape, if not seriously distorted, and can be counted under low magnification by reflected light. For counting, the paper may be left dry or moistened with glycerin or xylene saturated with $NaHCO_3$. In laboratory trials 64% of test lots of cercariae were recovered from clear water, though some were distorted beyond recognition.

When the water is turbid the filter tends to clog rapidly. Prior flocculation of the water with filter alum is said to remove the turbidity but leaves the cercariae so that they can be filtered out. Nevertheless, in laboratory trials, the yield of cercariae from flocculated water was reduced.

It is important that the filtration process be brisk. Cercariae held to the paper by the current of water for more than a few minutes lose their tails and become difficult or impossible to recognize. Once the water sample has passed through, the paper must be transferred to ninhydrin and dried rapidly. Otherwise, further tail-loss will occur. Done correctly, brevifurcate cercariae are unmistakenly preserved for counting at a later date. The papers are mailable and can be stored for a year or more before counting, if kept dry.

When 100-litre samples were used under favourable conditions, cercariae were detected when no infected snails could be found upstream from the sample site, suggesting that the method may be very sensitive under some conditions.

Losses of cercariae through injury by the filtration process, as a result of turbidity, and by flocculation would need to be evaluated locally.

b) Centrifugation. Schistosome cercariae are heavier than water and can be concentrated by simple centrifugation. Recently, attempts have been made to concentrate cercariae from large volumes of water by continuous-flow centrifugation. Hand- and electrically-operated centrifuges have been modified for continuous flow, and preliminary trials have indicated that the method may be useful for study of cercaria populations in the field.

BARRETT and ELLISON [1965] have consistently recovered about 32% of the cercariae in 1-litre water samples introduced into a standard centrifuge adapted for continuous-flow operation. OLIVIER [1966] has modified an International Clinical Centrifuge by installing an inverted plastic funnel with four delivery tubes on the centrifuge 'spider'. Cercariae are collected in four small centrifuge tube shields (for 15-ml tubes). Flow time is up to 0.6 l/min. Rotation speeds of 600 to 1,000 rpm produced essentially equal recoveries of cercariae. The cercariae are poured, alive, from the tubes into Petri dishes to be stained with nile-blue hydrochloride and counted. Laboratory trials with clear water indicate that the instrument will recover from 60 to 90% of the cercariae in the water. The effect of turbidity has not been tested in the field but laboratory trials produced highly variable results depending on the nature of the turbidity. BUTLER *et al.* [1967] have reported successful recovery of cercariae with a shielded hand centrifuge and have tested the instrument in the field.

Conclusion

Progress made so far in development of methods for the recovery of cercariae from natural habitats is encouraging. Those engaged in the study of the epidemiology of schistosomiasis should consider using one or more of the methods outlined above. None is considered optimal for the job to be done, however. The Millipore system is not considered practical largely because the filter membranes are very expensive but also because the method has not yet been tested adequately. Mouse exposure is also of limited value due to its expense, the need to house many animals and the delay before the information is obtained.

Centrifugation offers promise of usefulness and should be given attention because of its potential.

The best method available at this time is paper filtration.

Detection of Worms in Laboratory Animals

In almost all work which requires the study of infections in laboratory animals, the number of worms in each animal must be determined with accuracy. Total worm counts of *S. mansoni* and *S. japonicum* from small laboratory animals can be made rapidly and efficiently by perfusing the liver and the portal systems. Although there has been much less experience with *S. haematobium*, the same procedure would probably be successful since the worms tend to inhabit the portal system of small laboratory animals.

Larger animals can also be perfused, though the technique is somewhat more laborious since blood vessels have to be tied off and larger volumes of perfusate have to be examined.

Perfusion is so simple, rapid, and efficient that it should be used for all routine examinations for adult worms. Dissection of the host's tissues and visual examination of the organs and tissues are not only more tedious but have not been shown to be more efficient in detecting worms.

Technique for Small Animals

a) NIH perfusion technique. A very rapid and highly standardized perfusion technique has been evolved at the NIH [DUVALL and DEWITT, 1967] for examination of laboratory mice. With minor modification, it is also useful for hamsters.

The animal is killed with sodium pentobarbital to cause the worms to move to the liver. The animal is prepared for perfusion by stripping the skin anteriorly and posteriorly from an incision in the belly area. The abdominal and pleural cavities are then opened to expose the viscera and large vessels (fig. 9). The portal vein is then opened, and citrated or heparinized saline solution is injected into the left heart under intermittent pressure from an automatic pipetting machine through a 20-gauge hypodermic needle on the end of a length of flexible rubber tubing. This washes all the portal system,

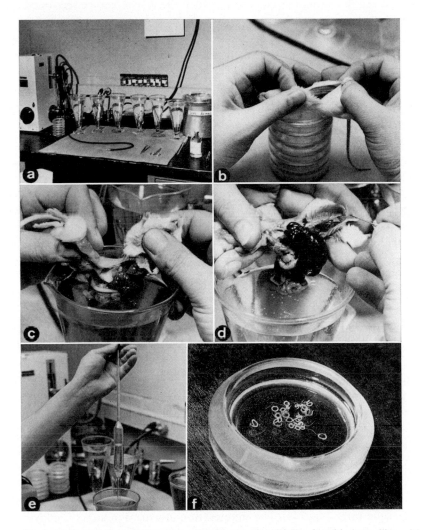

Fig. 9. (a) Complete perfusion apparatus for six mice. (b) Tearing skin by pulling with fingers prevents hair in perfusate. (c) Washing viscera in sedimentation glass. (A large beaker may be used for washing before perfusion and its contents discarded.) (d) Position of the animal during perfusion. Resting fingers on the rim of the glass allows better needle control. The liver lies over the severed portal vein and deflects the flow of perfusate directly into the glass. (e) Transferring the worms by an altered volumetric pipette. (f) Shallow counting dish containing schistosomes [DUVALL and DeWITT 1967].

including the vessels of the liver, since some of the fluid is forced through the hepatic artery into the liver. The perfusion fluid, with its content of worms, is collected in a urinalysis cone from which the worms can be recovered after they have settled.

An experienced operator requires about 3 min to perfuse a mouse and count the worms. The method recovers, consistently, over 98% of *S. mansoni*.

b) Suction technique. Another widely used technique is that of RADKE *et al*. [1961]. The method was designed for rapid collection of large numbers of worms for preparation of antigen. Its efficiency in detecting worms and its capacity to detect very small worms have not been measured.

c) Recovery of worms by dissection. If perfusion is not used, it is necessary to examine the liver and the vessels of the viscera for worms. Usually, the liver is pressed between slides to visualize the worms and the mesenteries are passed over a lighted glass plate on the stage of a dissecting microscope. Presumably all the large worms are seen by this method but the procedure is slow and worm recovery is difficult. Small worms are missed. Moreover, it is almost impossible to standardize the method.

Technique for Larger Animals

Perfusion of larger laboratory animals is practical and probably efficient though its accuracy has not been evaluated. It is necessary to tie off some of the larger vessels before perfusion to prevent gross leakage of the perfusion fluid into areas outside the portal system. Perfusion should be followed by examination of the viscera and liver for missed worms unless it can be shown that this is not necessary.

Detection of Worms at Autopsy

A standard operating protocol for schistosomiasis *post mortem* studies is given in form 4 (p. 744). The enumeration of worms in human cadavers has posed many problems. For *S. mansoni* and *S. japonicum*, portal mesenteric perfusion of cadavers for worms can be performed with apparently reliable results though it is slow, as will be seen below. Enumeration of *S. haematobium* in cadavers can only be done by laborious search involving press preparations and examination of tissues and blood vessels with transmitted light under low magnification.

Perfusion of Portal and Mesenteric Veins of Cadavers for S. mansoni

The method described here was developed by CHEEVER [1968]. Perfusion of the lungs has not, as yet, proved satisfactory and perfusion of other organs has not been attempted, hence the description will be limited to perfusion of the portal-mesenteric system. The time that elapses between death and perfusion is not critical.

1. Removal of Organs

(a) The organs are removed *en bloc*, the intestine being left attached to the mesentery.

(b) The thoracic viscera are then separated from the abdominal viscera as follows:

(1) The aorta is opened and cut.

(2) The oesophagus is dissected free of the diaphragm and is clamped or ligated to avoid spillage of fluid.

(3) The pericardium is removed and the inferior vena cava ligated, clamped and cut just above the diaphragm.

(4) The prosector can then proceed with dissection of the heart, lungs and neck organs while the perfusion is being carried out.

2. Perfusion of the Liver

(a) The organs are placed on an autopsy dissecting table (about 60 cm × 60 cm with sides approximately 1.5 cm high) which has a central drain used for collection of fluid.

(b) The rectum is ligated or clamped.

(c) A cannula is placed in the abdominal vena cava above the renal veins.

(d) A liver biopsy (2 cm × 1 cm) can be taken for histological study.

(e) The portal vein is opened and perfusion begun. Tap water can be used with line pressure serving as the pump, but further histological study would presumably be prejudiced. Alternatively, a water pump can be used with saline as the perfusion medium. A pump delivering 2 to 4 l/min at a pressure (at the pump) of 10 pounds per square inch (approximately 0.7 kg/cm^2) has proved satisfactory. The liver is perfused with a total of 10 l of fluid and is massaged during perfusion to ensure irrigation of all areas. No data have been sought regarding worms possibly not removed from the liver.

3. Perfusion of Mesenteric Veins

(a) Perfusion via the mesenteric arteries is the logical means of recovering worms in the mesenteric veins; however, perfusion of the arteries resulted in massive accumulation of fluid in the stomach and intestine (presumably due to rupture of autolysed capillaries) and poor flow of fluid from the mesenteric veins. Even when good flow is obtained from the mesenteric veins, some (and presumably most) worms present in the intestinal submucosa remain there, perfusion evidently being through only a portion of the veins. In addition, arterial perfusion results in massive submucosal oedema, complicating morphological evaluation of the intestine.

(b) Retrograde perfusion: Because of the inadequacy of arterial perfusion, mesenteric veins are perfused in a retrograde fashion, the cannula being introduced in the portal and larger mesenteric veins and the worms collected from the small mesenteric veins near the mesenteric insertion into the bowel.

(1) The bowel is removed from the mesentery, cutting as closely to the bowel wall as possible. Large and small intestine may be removed separately if differential perfusion is desired.

(2) The cannula is introduced into the mesenteric vein branches. (The main portal vein could be perfused but this would require fairly rapid flow, and the spleen, pancreas and stomach would be perfused unless proper precautions were taken.) Mesenteric veins are then perfused individually, roughly six branches being involved in the case of the superior mesenteric vein and only one for the inferior. The periphery of the mesentery is massaged to help expel worms and clots at this stage, and the vein opened afterwards to ensure the absence of clots.

The inferior mesenteric vein can be found at the junction of the splenic and superior mesenteric veins, sometimes joining one and sometimes the other. It may also be identified as it passes beneath the intestine at the ligament of Treitz. Its structure (one long main branch with numerous short branches to the intestine) makes it difficult to perfuse the entire length of the vein from the proximal end, hence, after initial perfusion, it is opened for a distance of 10 cm, perfused a second time and this procedure repeated a third or fourth time if possible. Good flow from perirectal vessels is thus obtained.

4. Examination of the Intestine

Following removal of the intestine from the mesentery, the intestine is placed in water and massaged to remove worms in the serosal veins which might otherwise be lost in subsequent handling. The intestine is then opened and washed, and biopsies for compression preparations and tissue for fixation removed. The worms cannot be seen through the mucosa, hence the mucosa and submucosa must be separated. This is done with scissors and is greatly facilitated by injecting water into the submucosa with a needle connected to the perfusion pump. Worms may be freed in the fluid that seeps out during dissection, therefore this work is carried out on the same table used for perfusion, and the fluid collected and examined. The mucosa is then examined by compression between the glass stage of a dissecting microscope and a glass plate. The serosal and mucosal surfaces of the bowel wall are also examined by the same method.

5. Collection and Counting of Worms

(a) The fluid is carried from the dissecting table to collection flasks by tubing; large-mouth 10-litre plastic flasks are convenient, small-mouthed flasks are difficult to clean. The supernatant fluid remaining after sedimentation is poured through a screen (about 0.7-mm aperture to catch floating worms) and then discarded. The last few litres of fluid and sediment are placed in 1-litre conical flasks and eventually the sediment transferred to ordinary conical urine sedimentation glasses, water being added at each step to haemolyse blood cells and dilute fine debris. The sediment is then transferred to Petri dishes and the worms counted, using a dissecting microscope.

Presumably the sedimentation procedures might be circumvented by placing a suitable cloth or other filter at the end of the collecting tube.

Clots do not interfere with the perfusions. When present in the sediment, they are pressed between glass slides to ensure that no worms are present in them.

6. Sites of Worm Recovery

Few worms are recovered from the liver, except when one sex greatly exceeds the other in number or when infections are massive. Most of the worms are recovered by retrograde perfusion (see 3b above). The proportion of the total worm recovery found in the other parts of the procedure is highly variable from one cadaver to another.

No part of the procedure can be omitted with assurance that an important percentage of worms has not been missed. Recovery is judged to be reasonably complete. As evidence for the efficiency of the method, it has been noted that in no case have viable eggs been demonstrated in the liver or in compression preparations of the intestine if no worm pair has been found. However, it is conceded that some worms may be missed.

7. Time Involved

All of the above procedures could be performed by a competent technician, hence theoretically only supervisory professional time is required.

(a) Perfusion: 20 min.

(b) Sedimentation and counting: 80 min (during which time compression preparations can be read, etc.); longer if numerous worms are present.

(c) Separation of intestinal mucosa and submucosa: 5 h (special technical competence not required).

(d) Examination of intestine for worms: 90 min (fluid and tissues).

Detection of Eggs in Tissues

The detection of eggs in tissues is useful in the study of the general pathology of the disease. Their enumeration is necessary in the study of the intensity of tissue damage and the relation of worm burden to pathology.

Press Preparations

Eggs can be detected simply by pressing bits of tissue between glass slides or plates and passing the preparation under a microscope. The method is slow, insensitive and not quantitative, but it detects eggs in all stages of development and permits easy distinction between living and dead eggs. Examination of the tissue is easier if the specimens are small and if they have been soaked in water for 5 to 10 min before compression.

For the pathologist wearing rubber gloves, it is convenient to have paired slides already prepared with attached pieces of adhesive tape. The slides may then be easily approximated and fastened together after a tissue specimen is placed between them.

The procedure at autopsy is as follows:

Two tissue fragments the size of a grain of rice are taken from the rectum, sigmoid, transverse colon, caecum, terminal ileum, mid-ileum, mid-jejunum and proximal jejunum, using biopsy forceps. Examination of two specimens is based on convenience, since both can be examined on the same slide. The use of more specimens would lessen error in individual cases.

Digestion

Digestion of portions of tissue for detection and enumeration of eggs is a rapid, quantitative and sensitive technique. It is preferred over press preparations. Formalin-fixed tissues cannot be used for digestion.

Alkali (potassium hydroxide) digestion techniques are most suitable, since they are more easily performed than enzymatic digestion and yield a clearer field for examination, allowing quantitation of small numbers of eggs with less effort. Distinction between living and dead eggs is difficult but rough estimates can be made.

Liver Digestion

Eggs of *S. mansoni* are distributed at random in the liver except in cases of pipe-stem fibrosis. Probably the eggs are also randomly distributed in cases of *S. japonicum* infection. One volume of liver is placed in 10 volumes of 4 to 5% potassium hydroxide solution, ordinarily 1 g of liver is sufficient. The liver is cut into pieces no greater than 0.5 cm in their smallest dimension before it is added to the hydroxide. The suspension is then left at room temperature for 12 to 24 h and is shaken occasionally. This allows deep penetration of the hydroxide. The suspension is then incubated at 45 °C for 6 h or 37 °C for 12 h. (In tests with mouse liver, egg-counts were reduced by digestion longer than 24 h at 37 °C; however, following the normal digestion time, eggs could be left in the hydroxide at room temperature or in the refrigerator for several days without significant loss of eggs.)

Eggs are best counted in 1-ml portions transferred to a Sedgwick-Rafter chamber (available from A.H. Thomas, Philadelphia, Pa., USA), a slide which holds 1 ml of liquid. One gram of liver per 10 ml of digestion fluid usually results in liquid sufficiently clear for accurate counts. Opaque fluid is usually due to the presence of fat and can be corrected by further dilution, if numerous eggs are present, or by centrifugation.

Three samples are usually counted for each tissue specimen. The counts are expressed as eggs per gram of liver. If very few eggs are present, the suspension may be centrifuged and the whole sediment examined.

Empty egg shells will be missed in the microscopic examination if the light is not reduced.

Alternatively, egg-counts can be made from smaller portions of the digest using ordinary slides and large cover-glasses with a proportionate loss of sensitivity and, possibly, of accuracy.

Lung Digestion

Lung tissue is digested by the same method as that used for liver but lung is harder to digest and must be minced before digestion if prolonged incubation, with possible loss of eggs, is to be avoided.

Other Tissues

Other tissues can also be digested. They should be minced before digestion and the duration of the digestion period would vary depending on the nature and density of the tissue.

Peptic digestion is usually not practical since the resulting suspension is very cloudy and difficult to examine.

Techniques for Studying Snails and Habitats to Plan Control Measures

Methods of Studying Snails

The snails transmitting schistosome infections are studied for two reasons; to gather basic information concerning the epidemiology of the disease, and to measure the effects of snail control measures. For the first purpose, a malacologist is usually employed and he may use a variety of techniques for snail study, not all of which will be dealt with here since space does not permit. For the second purpose, one uses a small number of standardized, quantitative methods directed toward measurement of snail populations as they change under pressure of control measures. These methods can be used by any well-trained technician.

Snail Measurement

Measurement of the size of the intermediate hosts is a necessary aid to the judgement of snail age and to the study of snail growth.

a) Amphibious snails (hosts of S.japonicum). The best single measurement for *Oncomelania* spp. is the greatest dimension, from the tip of the spire to the lip of the opening. For all routine purposes, this is the only measurement required. If the spires of a large proportion of older specimens are eroded, an estimate has to be made of the height.

b) Aquatic snails. Planorbid hosts of *S.mansoni* are disc-shaped. For routine purposes, the only necessary measurement is the greatest diameter of the disc.

Bulinid hosts of *S.haematobium* have a more or less broad spire. Again, the one measurement for routine purposes is the greatest length, i.e. the distance from the tip of the spire to the lip of the opening.

c) Methods for measuring snails. For routine purposes, it is unnecessary to measure the snails with extreme exactness. For the smaller snails, including

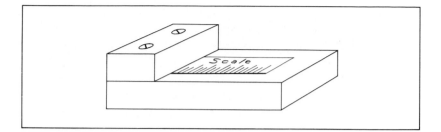

Fig. 10. Snail-measuring device.

the hosts of *S. japonicum* and other hosts up to 6 or 7 mm in greatest dimension, measurement to the nearest 0.5 mm will suffice, while for larger specimens, the dimension to the nearest millimetre will be adequate. A stereoscopic micro-scope can be used in measuring all sizes of the amphibious snails and must be used in measuring the smaller snails of all species, aquatic or amphibious.

One method for measuring snails is to use calipers which show, in milli-metres, the distance between the points. The snail can then be held or laid between the points and measured easily and accurately.

Another device that has been very useful and is quite durable and inex-pensive is a portion of a plastic millimetre rule fastened to a small wooden block having a wooden barrier at one end of the scale. The snail is laid on the scale and moved over until it touches the barrier. In the case of the spiral-shaped shells, the aperture is placed downward with the tip of the spiral toward the barrier. The diameter, or length, is then read on the scale. With this instrument, measurements can be taken more rapidly than with other devices. Estimations to the nearest 0.5 mm can be made, although it is more practical to read to the nearest millimetre (fig. 10).

Laboratory Maintenance
Laboratory Maintenance of Snails for Short Periods

Snails can be held in the laboratory for short periods with the use of relatively simple equipment. Glass containers of almost any sort may be used; amphibious snails can be kept on moist soil, moist filter paper or among moist humus. If proper humidity is maintained, they can be kept for long periods in an icebox (i.e. a few degrees above freezing-point). Aquatic snails may be kept out of water in a humid atmosphere from a few hours to many days or weeks, depending on variation in the capacity of the species to survive out of water.

The aquatic hosts are usually kept in water which should be tested for suitability before use. The snails should not be crowded and, since adequate oxygenation of the water is necessary, the water should be shallow and relatively cool.

The amphibious snails can be fed with decomposing vegetation or filter paper. Fresh lettuce and commercial fish food preparations are favourable food for the aquatic hosts. Since they are more or less omnivorous, local aquatic plants and other materials such as cooked cereal, cooked vegetables, etc., may be tried. Overfeeding may result in fouling the water and death of the snails.

Laboratory Maintenance of a Breeding Colony of Snails

This requires special care, and may require special equipment. Such a colony is usually not needed for snail control operation; it might be required only for the production of uninfected snails for susceptibility experiments.

Transportation of Snails

Transportation of Snails to the Laboratory

When snails are transported from their habitat certain precautions must be observed if they are to be kept alive. Infected snails are more delicate than uninfected ones and certain sizes may be less resistant to unfavourable conditions than others. Therefore, careless handling can result in deaths which may upset the validity of population and infection data gathered after the snails reach the laboratory.

Snails should not be submerged in water while they are being transported. They will survive better if kept out of water in a humid place and in such a way that their temperature is relatively low. It is practical to carry snails in a moistened cloth bag, in a plastic bag through which oxygen can diffuse, packed in moist leafy vegetation, or simply loose in a glass or metal container in which the atmosphere can be kept humid.

In general, aquatic snails require ready access to oxygen and a high humidity. Under such conditions they will survive for hours and even days with very low mortality. For amphibious snails, unless the period of transfer from the field to the laboratory is more than 24 h, the prevention of exposure to extremes of temperature is all that is necessary.

If really good aquarium conditions are not available, snails may be held in the laboratory in a cool, moist atmosphere until they are examined. The longer they are kept, whether in aquaria or in a moist environment, the greater likelihood there is that the usefulness of the snails and the reliability of the data will decrease.

Shipment of Living Snails over Great Distances

Living snails can be sent great distances with relatively little damage if adequately packed. Various types of containers have been used. The hosts of *S.japonicum* are best shipped in an almost dry container which allows access of air to the snails. Perforated sections of bamboo, or perforated or screened wooden or metal boxes have been used successfully.

The aquatic hosts of *S.mansoni* and *S.haematobium* should be shipped in a container without water but in a humid atmosphere. The snails should be layered in moist gauze, paper, moss, or even coarse leaves so that they have access to air, and then placed in a sealed container. For best results the snails should not be crowded and, of course, survival will be more likely if high and very low temperatures are avoided. For this reason shipment in the cabin of an aircraft is greatly to be preferred to shipment in an air cargo compartment.

Preservation of Snails

Snails from a series of habitats should be preserved for identification. The collection from each habitat should include specimens of various sizes, and the date, locality and nature of the habitat should be recorded. All collections should be kept separate.

The snails may be preserved by dropping them into 75% ethyl alcohol or rubbing alcohol. The best method, however, is to preserve the snails in a relaxed state. The snails to be killed are placed in a container of water to which a few crystals of menthol have been added. The container should be covered and left for 10 to 24 h. The snails are anaesthetized by the menthol and become partially extended. They should then be placed in a preservative. Two parts of 75% ethyl alcohol to one part of formalin (40%) is excellent for this purpose. This method provides well-extended animals useful for anatomical study. Some malacologists prefer that for this purpose the shell should be cracked before the snail is placed in preservative.

Identification of Snail Intermediate Hosts

It is not necessary, for purposes of conducting a snail control programme, to know for certain the correct name of the snail species which has been incriminated as the intermediate host in a given area. Such an identification can only be made by a specialist and may require much time. Control efforts need not wait for this. Nevertheless, properly preserved specimens (see above) should be prepared and sent to a specialist for identification.

Incrimination of the Snail Intermediate Host

When a snail species is suspected as the intermediate host, it may be tested in one or more of three ways. First, it may be examined by the method described below to see if it carries cercariae recognizable as the schistosome in question. In a *S. japonicum* area this procedure may be enough to incriminate the snail because *Oncomelania* do not usually carry other schistosome species. In other endemic areas the cercariae of human schistosomes cannot easily be distinguished from those of other mammals, and additional proof is usually necessary.

The second approach is to test schistosome cercariae from a suspected snail to see if they will infect small rodents or other available mammals and develop into adults that can be recognized either by their adult morphology or by the shape of the eggs they produce.

The third approach is to attempt to infect suspect laboratory-reared snails by exposing them to miracidia of the local schistosome. This must be done under controlled laboratory conditions and is usually not attempted by the inexperienced.

a) Examination of snails for schistosome infection. For measurement of prevalence of schistosome infection, freshly collected snails should be used, since infected snails are more likely than uninfected ones to die during laboratory maintenance.

The schistosomes multiply in the snails and, when the cercariae are emerging from the snail (a 'mature' infection) the snail tissues, and particularly the digestive gland, will contain very large numbers of developing and fully developed cercariae.

Isolation method: If the cercariae are needed for infection experiments, such as infection tests in mammals to confirm a tentative indentification based on appearance of the cercariae, the snails can be placed in water either singly or in groups. The water is then checked once or twice a day for the emerged cercariae. If the container is transparent and the cercariae are numerous, they can be seen when the container is held up to the light. The water may also be poured off and examined under low magnification. The cercariae must be distinguished from cercariae of other species and from protozoa and other invertebrates which might be present. If the temperature, water quality and other conditions are not optimal, cercariae may not emerge. There may be considerable variation in the shedding of cercariae by the amphibious snail hosts.

Crushing: If the snails are being examined only to determine whether or not they harbour schistosome infection, they should be examined by crushing the shells and not by placing them in water to see if cercariae will emerge. The latter method is far more laborious than the crushing method, requires more time and equipment, is less reliable since it misses some infections, and gives no more accuracy in specific identification.

Examination of snails by the crushing method is performed as follows:

(1) Place from three to five snails at intervals near the edge of a suitable container – a Syracuse watch-glass for the small species or a Petri dish for the larger ones.

(2) Use a suitable instrument to crush the snails, wiping it before crushing the next specimen to prevent contamination.

(3) Add a drop or two of water to each crushed snail.

(4) Mince each snail with a pair of dissecting needles, which should be wiped after each dissection.

(5) Examine the remains of each snail under the lower power of a stereoscopic microscope.

(6) Questionable objects may be placed on a slide and examined with a compound microscope for identification.

Since cercariae in the snails, or shed by the snails, may be infective to man, persons handling or examining the snails should avoid contact with the water or the snails. Rubber gloves may be used, but they are not essential.

As will be noted in the following section, there are a good many species of trematodes that have cercariae which resemble those of the human schistosomes; earlier stages in the snail resemble one another even more closely. Special care must be taken in attempting to identify immature trematode infections.

The record derived from snail examinations should include the time and place of the collection, the time of examination, the number of snails harbouring each species of cercaria encountered, the number of 'immature' infections that were recognized as 'probable' schistosome infections, and the number of 'immature' infections that could not be identified. It should be remembered that the presence of a large number of immature infections can be used to predict forthcoming periods of transmission.

The prevalence of infections in the snails may vary widely from time to time and often depends on seasonal factors. Therefore, snail examinations should be repeated periodically, preferably for several years, in order to establish the pattern of snail infection prevalence.

b) Identification of cercariae. The hosts of *S. japonicum* are not often infected with other species of trematodes, and schistosome cercariae found in them are unlikely to be misidentified. This is not true of the hosts of *S. mansoni* and *S. haematobium* which may have infections with other schistosome species. Identification of these species may be accomplished by using the cercariae to infect mice for identification of the *S. mansoni* group, or hamsters for the identification of the *S. haematobium* group. When such infections are attempted, it should be remembered that a naturally-infected snail usually produces cercariae, and accordingly adult worms, of one sex. Therefore, the use of cercariae from several infected snails from the same habitat will be necessary for positive results. In some areas this may be complicated by the existence of closely-related schistosome species.

The cercariae of the schistosomes affecting man consist of a body and a long, forked tail. The forks of the tail are shorter than the unforked portion. The body has no dark pigmented spots, called 'eye-spots'. Cercariae meeting these criteria are suspect. However, since recognition of schistosome species requires highly specialized skill, positive identification based on the cercariae alone may not be possible.

When positive identification cannot be made, typical cercariae should be preserved for reference. This is best done by adding an equal volume of hot (60–70 °C) water to the cercaria suspension and then after the cercariae have settled, replacing the water with any good preservative such as 70% alcohol or 5 to 10% formalin. The cercariae need not be stained or mounted on slides. Cercariae placed directly in fixative will be distorted and may stick to the container and be lost.

Snail-Collecting Instruments

a) Forceps. Snails detected visually can be collected with forceps if the water is shallow and clear or if the snails are on the soil surface as is often the case with the snail hosts of *S. japonicum*.

b) Kitchen sieve. Simple, light and effective scoops for casual collecting can be made by fixing a kitchen sieve to a light pole about 1 m long (fig. 11). A strainer about 12 to 14 cm in diameter and made of heavy wire is best. The openings need not be small enough to hold the smallest snails.

c) Brazil sieve. A large sieve used with success in Brazil and other areas consists of a large perforated metal cup having holes about 2 to 3 mm in diameter, attached to a metre-long handle (fig. 12). When made of heavy-gauge

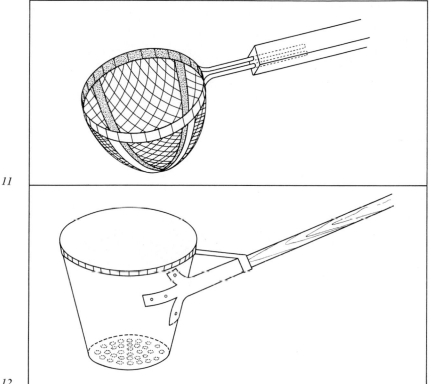

11

12

Fig. 11. Long handled kitchen sieve for snail collecting.
Fig. 12. Snail scoop used in Brazil for snail collecting.

sheet metal and firmly attached to the handle it will survive heavy use and rough handling. Soft metal such as aluminium should be avoided. The diameter of the top is about 20 cm and that of the bottom about 17 cm. This 'scoop' is passed through the water with a rocking motion to keep the debris that falls into the bottom agitated and free the holes for the passage of water and small objects. After passage through the water, it may be held at the surface with the edges exposed, and agitated to wash the debris clean of mud or small sediment.

d) Wire scoop. Another useful device is a rectangular scoop net of millimetre-mesh steel or copper gauze, having a strong iron frame and a long wooden handle made in fitted sections to permit easy transport. The forward edge of the frame may be sharpened so as to facilitate the cutting of water weeds. Such a scoop is not only useful for collecting water plants on which

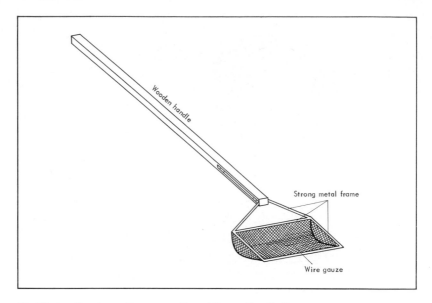

Fig. 13. Another type of scoop or dip-net for snail collecting.

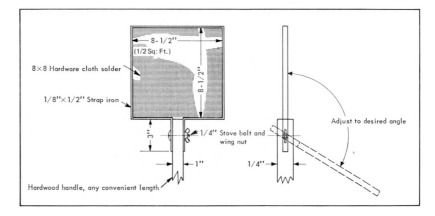

Fig. 14. Adjustable dip scoop.

snails may be feeding, resting or ovipositing, but also for gathering samples of bottom mud in which snails may be buried and from which they may be freed by gentle agitation of the net just below the surface of the water (fig. 13). A modification of this type of scoop in which the angle of the net relative to the handle is adjustable has also been extensively used (fig. 14).

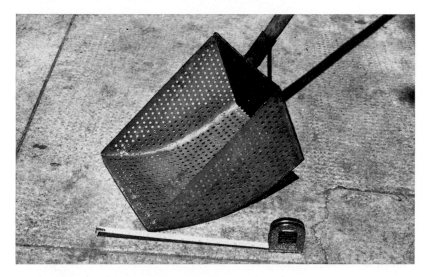

Fig. 15. Snail-collecting scoop used in Brazil.

e) Rectangular sheet metal scoop. A very sturdy and useful scoop designed and used in Brazil is shown in figure 15. Heavy-gauge perforated sheet metal is formed into a rectangular scoop with a forward cutting edge and a deep rear portion.

f) Drag scoop. Another type of collecting instrument which has given satisfactory results is the drag scoop. This consists of a long-handled wire-mesh net with a deep belly, properly braced. The sample is taken by placing the scoop face downwards and dragging it across the bottom and up the side to the water's edge. Here the scoop is inverted and the mud is washed out. The scoop can be used to sample a finite portion of the bottom, but it is comparatively slow and laborious in operation. It finds its principal application where population studies are being undertaken (fig. 16).

g) Bottom grab. It may occasionally be necessary to search for snails in deep water. For this purpose a bottom grab is best. It is essentially a metal box fitted with movable jaws and attached to a long handle. When open, the jaws exactly fit the dimension of the box. The grab is lowered into the water vertically, and while it is firmly pressed against the bottom, the jaws are closed by means of an attached wire. Both box and jaws are fitted with wire-mesh windows to permit water to flow out freely when the sample is raised (fig. 17).

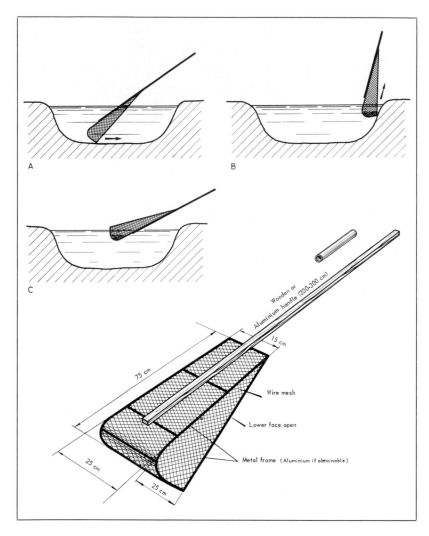

Fig. 16. Details of drag scoop for snail collecting. *A* Start of sampling. *B* End of sampling. *C* Washing the sample.

Snail Population Sampling

Both epidemiological studies and control evaluation require accurate and reproducible techniques for measuring snail population density. Quantitative snail collections are necessary when an intensive study is made of such things as snail population dynamics, life-history, growth, ecology, etc. These studies

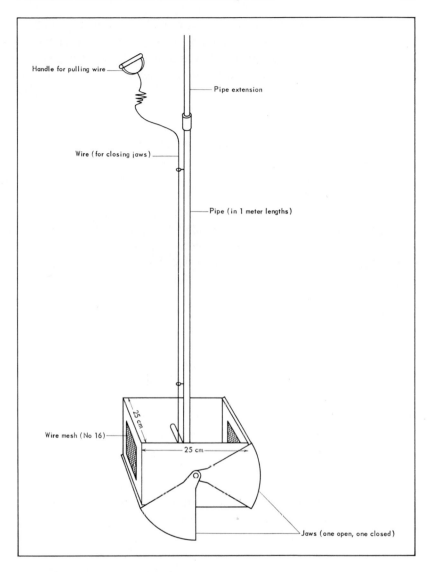

Fig. 17. Bottom grab for aquatic snails.

are in the nature of snail research and are conducted by a specialist. The techniques required are determined by the needs of the researcher but they are
usually highly refined and may require exhaustive collections to determine the
total snail population in selected areas.

Quantitative snail collections are also made to measure the efficacy of snail control measures. One of the aims of snail control is reduction of the snail population and a way must be found to measure this change accurately and usefully. For this purpose an accurate measure of the snail population density in the area in which control is to be attempted must be made and then repeated in exactly the same way after the control measure has been put into effect.

For the purpose of evaluation of control the snail population measurements need not be measures of the total snail population in the focus in which the collections are made. They need only give a reliable indication of a change in population density.

It is not practicable, obviously, to attempt to measure the population throughout the whole area to be controlled. Some method must be devised so that field personnel can measure the relative snail population density of one or more portions of the habitat on the basis of a series of sample snail collections. Such collections must be accurate but must not require complex equipment nor be too time-consuming. Unfortunately, thus far, a highly satisfactory snail sampling method has not yet been found. Those which are employed are discussed below:

a) Techniques for amphibious snails. Populations of amphibious snails are best estimated by the use of numerous small quadrats. In areas where the soil or mud surface is readily accessible to visual inspection, the samples are easy to obtain. In order to keep the area covered by a quadrat constant, a metal ring 10 to 15 cm in diameter may be carried into the field and dropped in the habitat. All snails inside the ring are collected with forceps, counted and measured and returned to the habitat, or placed in a small paper envelope for transportation to the laboratory where counting and measuring may be done.

If the quadrat samples are spaced properly in the habitat, the collecting technique is uniform and enough samples are taken, the average number of snails per quadrat sample is an index of snail density in the sampled area. In habitats with water or densely matted vegetation this procedure cannot be used and it is necessary, if quadrats are to be studied, to remove the contents within the quadrats and screen them for snails. In practice this usually means transporting them to the laboratory, a laborious task anywhere and an impossible one in many situations. A sharpened pipe of the same diameter as the ring is pushed into the mud with the help of handles and the enclosed plug of mud, water and vegetation is removed to a pail. Difficulties in raising the sample can be overcome by tilting the pipe after it has been pushed into the mud and inserting a hoe or similar instrument under the open end. The sample is washed through a series of sieves and the snails recovered from the sieves of finer mesh (6 to 8 meshes per cm). This second method is time-consuming but more accurate than the directly collected quadrat, fewer very small snails being missed.

A regular, repeatable pattern for placement of quadrats should nearly always be used. This has no serious drawbacks provided certain precautions are taken. Line transects of samples at regular intervals are satisfactory for sampling in dry canals, and grid patterns are best employed where broad areas are to be sampled. Two precautions should be observed. The first is that different parts of the area should be properly represented in the samples; this should cause no difficulty as long as the total extent of potential habitat is known. The second precaution is that areas of unusual density or scarcity do not coincide or alternate with transects or rows of samples; proper spacing, based on preliminary observations, should enable the field worker to avoid this difficulty.

b) Techniques for aquatic snails. Populations of aquatic snails are much more difficult to sample than are populations of amphibious snails. No single method of sampling is satisfactory for all habitats. Moreover, each method to be described has defects which should not be overlooked in judging the results. However, all the methods will detect large shifts in population and so, unless the population shift is small, they are useful in spite of their drawbacks.

Drag scoop: In irrigation canals up to 4 m wide and in streams of comparable proportions, it may be possible to measure the number of snails that can be collected per unit of stream-bottom area. A standard drag or scoop (fig. 16) with a known width is pulled or pushed across the bottom, starting at the middle of the stream and continuing to the edge in such a way that all the surface mud, the debris, and the vegetation is picked up. The area in square metres covered by each pass of the drag or scoop can be estimated, and when many passes are made and the snails for each pass of the scoop are counted and recorded, a calculation can be made as to the number of snails collected per square metre of bottom. When successive passes are made along a segment of canal or stream the number of snails collected per linear metre of canal can be calculated. Obviously, vegetation or debris will reduce the reliability of the procedure, and heavy vegetation or an irregular bottom will prevent use of the method. If a large amount of material is caught in the scoop the search for the snails may be very slow and estimations of snail density by this method are costly and laborious. While this method may be useful for population studies, it may be impractical for evaluation of large-scale snail control measures.

Snails per dip: In some situations a standard sieve or scoop may be used to sample a snail population by providing a record of the average number of snails collected with each pass of the instrument. This method has been widely used but has not been evaluated statistically. The method has the advantages of simplicity and usefulness in a variety of habitats, but misses most of the small snails. A sieve or scoop (as shown in figures 11 and 13) may be used. It is essential that the instrument be used in the same way throughout the test area and every time the collection is repeated in that area. The collector must be aware of the importance of consistency in making the samples.

The instrument is passed through the water, through vegetation or along the bottom, and the number of snails captured with each pass is recorded. To facilitate counting, each catch can be emptied into a large, white enamel tray for inspection. Leaves and stems of water plants, pieces of bark, and other vegetable debris in the water are attractive to some species of snails and should be meticulously examined. The average number of snails collected per pass of the instrument can then be calculated. Each sampled area should be limited and clearly recorded so that later collections can be made in the same area. A hundred or more passes can be made in a relatively short time. The number necessary is determined by the number of snails present. Since water depth, amount of vegetation, accessibility and so forth will affect the number of snails collected per pass of the instrument, the collections should be made, when possible, under the same conditions.

Snails per unit of time: It has been shown that there is reasonable statistical reliability if snail population density is measured by counting the number of snails that can be collected in a marked area in a unit of time. An area to be sampled, such as a segment of canal or a portion of the edge of a pool, is selected and its limits are clearly marked. One or more collectors then search for snails for an interval of time, such as 10, 15 or 20 min. Any standardized collecting procedure can be used but the preferred method in aquatic habitats involves the use of a sieve. Hand-picking with forceps can be used for amphibious snails in moist-soil habitats. The method is only applicable to amphibious snails when their presence is not self-evident and search must be made for them in obscure habitats. All snails are placed in a container and counted at the end of the timed period. The length of the timed period depends upon the snail density. The collections of different collectors must be kept and recorded separately. The measure of snail density is the number of snails collected per man per minute. When a collection is repeated in the sample area the same collector and sieve should be used, and the collector should attempt to collect in exactly the same manner as that used in the first collections. The time interval used can be extended if the population density is low. It is better to estimate the snail density by this method in several relatively small areas than to use a single large one. The collector must take particular care to avoid the temptation to increase the number of snails collected by seeking out and collecting longer in areas of greater snail density or greater accessibility of snails. The method has the advantage of being suited to almost every type of habitat and is moreover relatively simple, requires only simple tools, and facilitates reasonably accurate and useful snail population estimates in a short time.

Mapping

A fundamental prerequisite for a study relating either to the molluscan hosts or to the parasite are good field maps. They are just as essential to the team as blueprints are to builders of a structure. It is fortunate if the team has an engineer or a draftsman assigned to its staff to map the area. Often, however, such specialists are not available, and the drawing of the maps must become the responsibility of the field staff. It is not necessary that such a map should be a work of art but it is most essential that it be accurate. It can best be prepared at the time when measurements are made to determine the size of the area to be treated. A scale allowing 1 cm to represent 1 km will be satisfactory for a sketch map, but a larger scale, e.g. 10 cm or more per km, may be essential for marking details. All seepage areas, swamps, rivulets and borrow-pits, both permanent and temporary, should be plotted, besides the major waterways such as river, irrigation systems, reservoirs, drains and ponds. Roads, paths, villages, and isolated dwellings should also appear on the map. Additional details such as contours, and even soil types and vegetation may be useful under certain conditions.

A reasonably accurate sketch map may be prepared by using paper containing a 1-cm grid (graph paper is excellent), attached to a sketch-board with clips. The sketch-board should be 45 to 50 cm², and may be of any light durable material that is smooth. A compass is essential and it should be equipped with a prismatic or other sighting device. For large-scale maps, a tape is used to measure distances, starting from some convenient reference point. For small-scale maps, speedometer or pedometer measures usually suffice. Bearings taken with the compass may be transferred to the map by means of a protractor. Bearings and distances from the primary and all subsidiary reference-points should be taken of all prominent features, especially bodies of water. When these have been entered on the map, details may be added from observations, sometimes with the help of additional measurements.

Of necessity, maps made by field personnel may be relatively crude. Nevertheless, they can be very useful and quite adequate, especially in the early stages of an anti-snail programme. As the programme progresses and the need for more accurate and sophisticated maps increases, more skilled help in map-making may be sought.

Sketch maps are usually adequate for survey work and for snail control by the use of molluscicides. Snail collectors or other field staff can easily be trained to gather the essential data and make the maps.

It may be that maps on a suitable scale will be available in government agencies. However, each agency's maps usually emphasize those features important to its activity. Hence, even where good maps are available, some of the features mentioned above will have to be added by the anti-schisto-somiasis personnel themselves. Check should be made particularly to see if air mapping has been done.

For permanent records, the location at which host snails are collected should be designated by latitude and longitude. This is especially desirable when forwarding specimens to identification centres. Maps showing host distribution should contain latitudinal and longitudinal markings.

Water Flow Measurement

Velocity of Flow
The velocity of flow of a stream can be used to calculate the volume of flow. Water velocity records may also be useful in the study of the relation of snail distribution to velocity.

a) Float method. The average velocity of a stream or canal can be determined approximately from the surface velocity; this is determined by measuring the time taken by a weighted cork or other object to travel a certain distance. The cork must float just below the surface of the water in order to avoid wind effects. In streams, the average velocity varies from 80 to 95%

of the surface velocity. In canals, the average velocity may be as low as 75% of the surface velocity. The average of several estimates should be used. This method is reasonably accurate in unobstructed streams and irrigation canals, but is worthless in vegetation-choked habitats.

b) Flow-meter method. A more accurate measure of average velocity can be obtained with a flow meter having a wheel which rotates as the water passes it. The number of revolutions per unit of time can be used to calculate water velocity and a series of readings at different points in the stream's cross-section can provide a measure of average flow velocity. A variety of flow meters exists. A small meter, the 'Pygmy Meter', is the one most likely to be useful in shallow streams with a relatively small flow. It is attached to the depth-rod by a spring mechanism which allows it to be raised or lowered very quickly to its proper depth. The rod is held in a vertical position upstream from where the operator stands in order to prevent any interference with the current where the flow reading is being made.

In waters deeper than 1 m a larger instrument, e.g. a 'Price Meter', is used. The current is taken by lowering the meter on a metal cable from a bridge.

The following procedure is used to determine the current in flowing waters with a current meter:

(1) Select a straight section of a stream or canal that is free from obstructions, e.g. trees, large boulders, pilings of bridges, etc.

(2) Measure in metres (or feet, depending on whether the metre conversion table is rated in feet or metres per second) the width of the stream.

(3) Make and record depth readings across the width of the stream at sufficient and evenly-spaced intervals so that a reliable average depth may be determined.

(4) At each station where the depth is taken, record the flow of water with a current meter by placing the instrument 0.6 of the depth of the water; more exact readings may be taken by averaging two readings made at each station by placing the meter at 0.2 and 0.8 depths of the water. It is advisable to take the current reading at the same time that the depth is being ascertained.

(5) Total the depth readings and divide the sum obtained by the number of measurements taken. This will give the average depth.

(6) Total the current readings made from each station and divide the sum by the number of measurements taken. This will give the average flow of metres or feet per second (depending on the conversion table used).

(7) Multiply the width of the stream by the average depth.

(8) Multiply this product by the average flow per second. This will give

the number of cubic metres (cubic feet) per second of water flowing past that particular section of stream or canal.

Example:
3.4   m = width of stream
0.93   m = average depth of stream

3.162   m² = area of cross-section of stream
0.18   m/sec = average current of stream

0.56916 m³/sec (569.16 l/sec) = volume of flowing water per second

Volume of Flow

a) Volume from stream velocity measurement. The volume of flow can be calculated if the average stream velocity and the stream's cross-section are known. Volume is derived by multiplying the area of the cross-section in square metres by the average velocity in metres per second to obtain volume in cubic metres per second. Some hydrographers prefer to refer to flow volume in cubic feet per second.

b) Volume by use of weirs and flumes. Since the velocity and cross-sectional area of a stream can only be approximated under most circumstances, it is usually preferable to find flow volume with a weir or flume. Some irrigation systems have permanent structures of this type for flow measurement.

V-notch weir and rectangular weir: The discharge in small water courses may be conveniently measured by means of a rectangular or V-notch weir (fig. 18). For discharges of between 0.1 and 1.0 m³/sec, a rectangular weir with a sharp crest is placed across the channel with the crest level. By measuring the depth of water over the crest and the length of the weir, the discharge can be computed from the following approximate formula:

$$Q = 1,800 \; L H^{\frac{3}{2}},$$

where:

Q is the discharge in litres per second,

L is the length of the weir in metres,

H is the depth of water in metres above the crest of the weir

For example, if

L = 1 m and H = 0.30 m, then

$Q = 1,800 \times 1 \times 0.30 \sqrt{0.30}$

$\quad = 1,800 \times 1 \times 0.30 \times 0.55$

$\quad = 297 \; l/sec.$

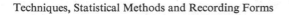

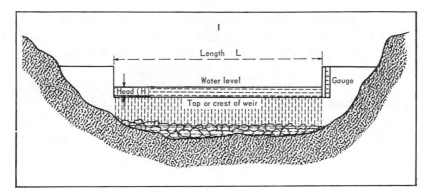

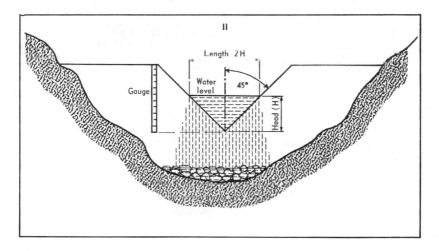

Fig. 18. Rectangular (I) and V-notch (II) weirs.

The following tabulation gives flow volumes for a length of weir of 1 m and various depths of water above the crest:

H, m	Q, l/sec
0.10	57
0.20	161
0.30	296
0.40	455
0.50	635

For other lengths of weir the discharge is in direct proportion. Thus, if the length is only 0.50 m, the discharges are only half the values given above. If the length is 2 m, then the discharges would be double the values given above.

The use of the rectangular weir is limited by practical considerations to about 3 m in length and 0.50 m depth of water above the crest.

For low flows of less than 0.1 m³ sec, a weir with a 90° V-shaped opening or notch in the crest is more accurate. An approximate formula for this type of weir is:

$Q = 1,400 \ H^{2.5}$
where:
Q is the discharge in litres per second,
H is the depth of water above the bottom of the notch.
For example, if
H = 0.20 m, then
$Q = 1,400 \times 0.20 \times 0.20 \ \sqrt{0.20}$
  = 25 l/sec.

Some other discharges for this type of weir are as follows:

H, m	Q, l/sec
0.10	4.5
0.15	12.0
0.20	25.0
0.25	44.0
0.30	69.0

From data obtained in this manner, the average rate of flow may be calculated, and also the volume of flow per unit of time. Either figure may be useful in classifying waters as snail habitats and in calculating amounts of chemical needed for treating flowing water.

Where large discharges are involved, and in calculating the concentration of molluscicides, it is more convenient to have the volume of flow in cubic metres rather than litres. The conversion is readily made by dividing the results obtained from the above formulae by 1,000.

Calculation of Molluscicide Dosage

a) Calculation for flowing water. The calculation of the proper amount and application time of a molluscicide for flowing water involves four steps. Although most of the necessary information for these calculations can be determined before the application, the last step must be performed in the field. These steps are as follows:

Step 1. Calculate the amount of any substance that will give 1 ppm in a 'standard' unit volume of water. This is a constant or arithmetic fact, and is not subject (for these purposes) to experimentation. Its dimensions are determined by the units of measurement used.

Step 2. Obtain from table II on pp. 485 to 487 the rated potency (ppm/h) value of the molluscicide of choice or its formulation.

Step 3. Calculate the total amount of the molluscicide needed to treat the 'standard' unit volume of water (i.e. results from step 1 multiplied by value in step 2).

Step 4. Calculate the total amount of molluscicide needed to treat the habitat in question after measuring its water flow in the same units used in step 1 (i.e. results of step 3 multiplied by number of volume units). Divide this by the desired number of hours of treatment time. The measurements and calculations in this step are done in the field.

Step 1: standard unit volume of water: One gram of chemical in a cubic metre of water produces 1 ppm; the amount of water passing a given point in 1 h in a stream or a canal with a flow of 1 m³/sec would be 3,600 m³ and this would require 3,600 g, or 3.6 kg, of the chemical to give 1 ppm for the total volume. Thus, 3.6 kg can be used as a constant in the calculations given below.

Step 2: ppm/h rated potency: This relationship is first determined experimentally in the laboratory and then under field conditions. For example, if it is found that 10 h of exposure to a concentration of 5 ppm is required to kill the snails, the 'rated potency' is 50 ppm/h. The ppm/h must be accurately established for each compound before it is used in a control programme. As noted in table I, such experiments under different conditions give a range rather than a specific value, i.e. 50 to 80 ppm/h for NaPCP, 2 to 7 ppm/h for niclosamide.

Step 3: determination of the total amount of a formulation required to treat the total volume at a standard rate of flow, 1 m³/sec: The initial determinations of ppm/h are usually made on the basis of the actual amount of active ingredients present. When a compound has reached the stage where it is ready for field use, however, it usually has been mixed with other materials to give it certain qualities which make it easier to apply, more effective, and so on. Therefore, if the formulation used in a control programme is not relatively pure, it is necessary to take this into account. For example, if the amount of an 80-percent formulation of each of the two chemicals just mentioned has to be determined, the following calculations would be made:

NaPCP. As indicated above, it requires 3.6 kg of any chemical to give 1 ppm in an hour's flow, where the rate is 1 m³/sec. Let us say that local experts have determined that it requires 80 ppm/h to kill the snails in the habitats involved. The formulation being used contains 80% of the active ingredient. Therefore, the amount of this formulation required for this standard volume would be determined as follows:

$$3.6 \times 80 \times \frac{100}{80} = 360 \text{ kg.}$$

Niclosamide. If 3.6 kg is again required to treat the standard volume, the determined ppm/h is 7, and 80-percent formulation is used, the total amount of material required would be determined as follows:

$$3.6 \times 7 \times \frac{100}{80} = 31.5 \text{ kg.}$$

Step 4: determination of amount of material to be applied in a given flowing water habitat: Ordinarily only one molluscicide and probably only one formulation will commonly be used in a given area. Therefore, the only figure that the field personnel must keep in mind would be 360, if the above example of NaPCP applies or 31.5 of the above example if niclosamide applies. This figure will vary with the type of snail involved, the chemical used, etc. To determine the amount of formulation required in each flowing water habitat, first calculate the volume of flow (instructions for doing this are given on p. 676). Then the figure calculated in the previous step, given to the field operator by his superiors, and the volume of flow can be used to determine the amount of chemical that will be needed for a particular habitat. The following examples, using the data given above, are for two different volumes of flow:

NaPCP. The field operator has been given the figure 360 for the formulation of this compound. If he is to control the snails in a habitat with a flow of 2.3 m³/sec, he would make the following calculation: 360 × 2.3 = 828 kg of the formulation will be required.

If the chosen treatment time is to be 8 h, the amount to be dispensed per hour would be determined as follows:

$$\frac{828}{8} = 103.5 \text{ kg/h.}$$

If the volume of flow were found to be only 0.15 m³/sec, the calculations would be as follows:

$$\frac{54}{8} = 6.75 \text{ kg/h.}$$

Niclosamide. In this case, the field operator would have been given the figure 31.5. If an 80-percent formulation of this compound is to be used in the habitats mentioned, but the chosen treatment time is to be 9 h, the following calculations would be made:

with a flow of 2.3 m³/sec:
31.5 × 2.3 = 72.45 kg of the formulation required

$$\frac{72.45}{9} = 8.05 \text{ kg/h;}$$

with a flow of 0.15 m³/sec:
31.5 × 0.15 = 4.725 kg of the formulation required

$$\frac{4.725}{9} = 0.525 \text{ kg/h.}$$

In practice, the actual figures for the determined values of ppm/h, the amounts of material required to treat the total 'standard' volume, the measured volume of the flow and the chosen treatment time, would be substituted in place of those given in these examples.

Figure 19 shows the quantity of active molluscicide in kg/h to be dispensed for various durations of application at 5 and 8 ppm/h based on a flow of 1 m³/sec. The figure applies to niclosamide but can be adapted to NaPCP, in which event the quantities of molluscicide will be ten times greater.

b) The calculation of dosage for stationary water. This is a simple procedure compared to the steps necessary for calculating dosage for flowing water. The fact that in still waters the chemical is not as rapidly dissipated as in running water, but will remain active for a much longer time, enables a lower initial dilution to be employed. In most instances, the lower dilutions mentioned for each chemical in table I will suffice for providing effective concentrations for stationary water. For measuring dosage for stationary waters, the same first three steps may be employed. The volume of water can be estimated in cubic metres or other units by taking the product of the average width × the average length × the average depth.

Large ponds and lakes present a special problem. It is often neither necessary nor feasible to treat the entire volume of water. Snail hosts are usually concentrated near the margins and may only occur along certain portions of the shore-line. It is customary in such circumstances to apply molluscicides only to the infested parts of the pond or lake. The calculation of dosage, once the

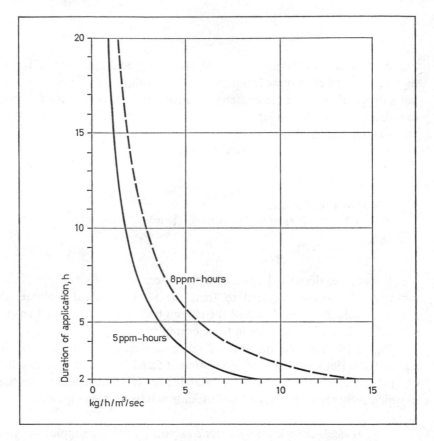

Fig. 19. Quantity of active molluscicide in kg/h to be dispensed for various durations of application at 5 and 8 ppm-hours based on a flow of 1 m³/sec. The ppm-hours shown apply to niclosamide. For NaPCP the ppm-hours would be 50 to 80 and the quantities of molluscicide will be 10 times more.

area of each infested part has been determined, follows the same procedure as that for any body of stationary water.

c) The calculation of dosage for moist-soil habitats. The amphibious snail hosts (*Oncomelania* spp.) of *S. japonicum* frequently must be attacked when they are out of the water habitat. The same applies to certain aquatic species, which may be marooned by the drying-up of rainwater pools or by other means. Some of these snail hosts are markedly resistant to desiccation and may survive the dry season and repopulate the area after the rains begin. Such is the case with *Biomphalaria straminea* in Brazil. It is difficult, if not impossible, to destroy snail hosts under completely dry conditions. However, the application of molluscicides to moist-soil situations is practicable and reasonably effective. The molluscicide may be applied as a spray or, under certain circumstances, dusts might possibly be effective. Table I contains recommendations for dose rates per square metre applicable to moist-soil situations. These rates may be used also in calculating dosage for shallow inundated areas, in which it may not be essential to measure the volume of water.

Field Tests for Estimation of Molluscicide Concentration

a) Test for Sodium Pentachlorophenate and Copper Pentachlorophenate (HASKINS' *method*[3]).

Reagents required

Methylene blue chloride solution: A 0.02-percent solution is prepared from certified dye (CI922). The weight of material taken for the preparation of this solution is corrected for the actual dye content of the dye lot, as stated on the label, so that 100 ml of solution contains 20 mg of actual dye.

Bicarbonate-methylene blue reagent: A mixture of 1 volume of 0.02% methylene blue chloride solution and 1 volume of saturated sodium bicarbonate solution is extracted with successive 1-volume portions of chloroform until the chloroform extract is colourless or nearly so. Usually four or five extractions are sufficient. (The chloroform used for the extractions may be recovered by shaking it with an equal part of dilute hydrochloric acid, then by washing twice with equal volumes of water. The recovered solvent may be used for preparation of the reagent, but not in the test procedure.)

The aqueous phase is stored in a tightly-closed bottle with a minimum of exposure to strong light. It remains usable for about one week or until 1 ml of it, diluted to 5 ml with water and shaken with 5 ml of chloroform, develops an appreciable pink colour in the chloroform layer within a 15-min period.

Dilution factors for preparation of colour standards

5-ml sample, ppm	2	5	10	25	50	100
1 ml of 0.02% methylene blue chloride solution diluted to, ml	60	30	20	10	5	3

3   Reprinted from HASKINS, W.T.: Anal. Chem. *23:* 1672 (1951), by kind permission of the editors.

Colour standards: The colour standards are prepared by suitable dilution of the 0.02-percent methylene blue chloride solution. The values for these dilutions were determined by matching the colours produced by known concentrations of pure sodium pentachlorophenate with the proper dilution of the dye solution. If water is used as the diluent, the life of the standards is short as judged by fading and the deposition of insoluble material. The life of the standards may be increased to 2 or 3 weeks if 0.1 N hydrochloric acid is used as the diluent. The tabulation above gives the dilution factors for the preparation of the standards. The figures on parts per million are based on the use of a 5-ml sample for the test. Approximately 10 ml of each standard are placed in a screw-capped 16 mm × 150 mm culture tube and protected from strong light when not in use. The same standards may be used for the determination of copper pentachlorophenate solutions, as the pentachlorophenol content differs from the sodium salt by only approximately 3%, which is not detectable by this method. (The culture tubes, as supplied by the Kimble Glass Co., have a coated paper liner over a cork backing in the cap. This coating is soluble in chloroform and should be removed and replaced with an aluminium foil disc in the caps on the tubes used for the test. The coated liners should be retained for the caps used for the tubes containing the acidic colour standards.)

Reproducibility of colour standards: In order to test the reproducibility of the colour standards with varying sources of methylene blue chloride, five different lots of the certified dye from various suppliers were obtained. The stock 0.02-percent solution of each was prepared and dilutions were made for the standards as given on page 683. When inspected in the 16-mm tubes, agreement among the different lots was excellent. The bicarbonate-methylene blue reagent was also prepared from each of the stock solutions, and tests were made at 2 and 10 ppm on sodium pentachlorophenate. The colours produced in the tests matched very well with the corresponding colour standards. Thus, it may be concluded that no great variation in results may be expected with different lots of certified dye.

Test procedure: Place 5 ml of water to be tested in a 16 mm × 150 mm screw-capped culture tube and add 1 ml of the bicarbonate-methylene blue reagent and 5 ml of chloroform. Close the tube tightly and shake it vigorously for 15 sec. Place the tube upright and, as soon as separation of the layers is complete, inspect the upper layer. If it is definitely blue the sample contains 10 ppm or less of pentachlorophenate, in which case the colour in the lower layer is compared with the standards to obtain the concentration. (Comparison of the colour of the chloroform layer in the tubes with the colour standards is greatly facilitated by use of a simple wooden comparator block having three holes into which the tubes can be slipped. Transverse slots are cut through the block near the bottom, so that only the chloroform layer is visible when the tubes are in place. A piece of ground glass cemented over one end of the slots will provide more even illumination and freedom from troublesome reflections.)

With concentrations greater than 10 ppm, the upper layer will be colourless or a very pale blue after shaking with 1 ml of the reagent. In this case, add 1 ml more of the reagent and shake the tube as before. Then compare the colour of the lower layer with the standards to estimate the concentration. In general, it will require an additional 1 ml of reagent for samples containing 25 ppm, 2 ml for 50 ppm and 4 ml for 100 ppm, before a definite blue colour is observed in the upper phase. A moderate excess of reagent does no harm. After extraction of the colour into the chloroform, the tests should be read as soon as the chloroform layer is clear (3–5 min) and, in any case, within 30 min. This limit is necessary because a pink colour develops in time in the chloroform, which makes comparison with the standards especially difficult in the range of 1 to 5 ppm. It is advisable to run a blank determination on 5 ml of the water from the stream before treatment with the pentachlorophenate in order to eliminate the possibility of interfering substances. A blank is also useful in estimating concentrations of the order of 1 ppm where the colour will be lighter than the 2-ppm standard but definitely bluer than the blank. The practical accuracy of the method is about 20% error in the region of 5 to 100 ppm and ± 1 ppm below 5 ppm.

Interfering substances: Hard water, water containing appreciable amounts of iron, or copper pentachlorophenate will produce cloudy precipitates with the bicarbonate-methylene blue reagent. The precipitate is usually carried into the chloroform layer as a suspension and makes comparison with the standards difficult. This interference is readily eliminated by dissolving a few milligrams (four or five small crystals) of sodium citrate in the 5-ml sample before adding the reagent. This prevents the metals from precipitating and does not otherwise affect the test.

b) Niclosamide (R. STRUFE Method Revised)
Principle: The principle of the field method is that the active ingredient of niclosamide reacts with Safranin TH to form a red colour complex, which can be extracted with organic solvents from an aqueous alkaline milieu. The

content of niclosamide in the water sample is then determined by measuring the intensity of the red colour of the organic phase.

Instead of the previously employed aqueous solution of a dyestuff-buffer mixture, a solid dyestuff-buffer granulate is being used, which is readily soluble in water. This guarantees easy, quick and sufficiently accurate dosage of the dyestuff-buffer mixture.

Furthermore, diethylcarbonate is now used instead of amyl acetate as the extraction solvent. Diethylcarbonate reacts with the active ingredient-dyestuff mixture to give a deeper colour so that the sensitivity of the colour reaction is increased.

As already described in the original method, the Zeiss Ikon Polytest colorimeter with colour wedge No. 105 is used for the estimation of the colour intensity. The calibration curve is given for use of this instrument. Any other colorimeter or photometer can be used; for this purpose a new calibration curve must be evaluated.

Instruments Required

(1) 1 Zeiss Ikon Polytest colorimeter with colour wedge No. 105 (or any other colorimeter) with 2 glass cuvettes, light pass 10 mm.

(2) 1 Seitz filter bell with a hand pump to produce pressure.

(3) Schleicher and Schull 2017 cardboard filter discs, 60-mm diameter, for use in the filter bell (2)[4].

(4) 1 Stop-watch.

(5) 2 Polyethylene washing bottles, 1 l (each for acetone and tap-water).

(6) 1 Polyethylene washing bottle, 0.5 l (for diethylcarbonate).

(7) 1 Polyethylene graduated cylinder, 100 ml.

(8) 2 Polyethylene graduated cylinders, 50 ml.

(9) 1 Polyethylene graduated cylinder, 10 ml.

(10) 1 Polyethylene bottle, about 60 ml, origin Kautex (see footnote 4).

(11) 1 Stopper for polyethylene bottle (10) (see footnote 4).

(12) 1 Screw stopper for polyethylene bottle (10) with outlet (see footnote 4).

Reagents Required

(13) Safranine granulate, in bags (see footnote 4).

(14) Diethylcarbonate, chemically pure (see footnote 4).

(15) Acetone, for cleaning instruments.

4   Supplied on request by Crop Protection Department of Farbenfabriken Bayer AG, Leverkusen, Federal Republic of Germany.

Test procedure: Clean the inner part of the filter bell (2) by use of acetone, and rinse twice with tap-water. Put one filter disc (3) between the two parts of the filter bell, and screw the nuts to close the lower and upper part of the filter bell.

Measure 100 ml of the water sample using the polyethylene cylinder (7), and pour the 100-ml water sample into the neck of the filter bell. Screw the tube of the handpump on the filter bell, put one 50-ml polyethylene cylinder (8) below the outlet of the filter bell, and begin to pump until the first 40 ml of the water sample have passed the filter bell. Put the other 50-ml polyethylene cylinder (8) below the outlet of the filter bell, and continue with filtering the water sample through the filter by pressure. Avoid passage of any water other than through the outlet of the filter bell. Discharge the first 40 ml of the filtrate and use the next 50 ml of the filtrate for the analysis. Decant the 50 ml of filtrate completely into the 60-ml polyethylene bottle (10), add the contents of a bag of safranine granulate (13), cover the bottle with a polyethylene stopper (11) and shake for about 5 sec until the granulate has been completely dissolved. Open the bottle, add exactly 5 ml of diethylcarbonate (14) using a polyethylene cylinder (9), cover the bottle with the polyethylene stopper (11) and shake vigorously for exactly 20 sec. Let the phases separate for 2 min, close the polyethylene bottle (10) with the screw stopper (12) and isolate the upper (organic) layer by compressing the polyethylene bottle slightly by hand. The upper phase (about 3 ml) is directly carried over into the cuvette, and the colour is read in the polytest colorimeter.

The content of Niclosamide in the water specimen can be evaluated from the calibration curve (fig. 20).

Cleaning the polyethylene bottle (10) after analyses: The bottle (10) is emptied completely, filled with a small quantity (about 10 ml) of acetone (15) and cleaned with a test-tube brush. The acetone is discharged and the polyethylene bottle is rinsed twice with tap-water. The bottle must not be dried for the next estimation.

Standard solution: 100 ppm Stock solution: 30 mg of niclosamide ethanolamine salt or 36 mg of niclosamide 70% wettable powder are dissolved completely in 10 ml of acetone (15) by means of a glass rod in a test tube; 1 ml of 1 N sodium hydroxide is added and the clear yellow mixture is filled up with water to 250 ml in a volumetric flask. This stock solution is stable for one week if kept in the dark.

10 ppm Stock solution: 10 ml of the stock solution containing 100 ppm

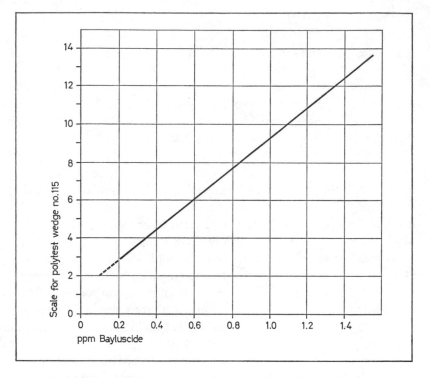

Fig. 20. Calibration curve for estimation of niclosamide.

are diluted and shaken in a volumetric flask with water to give a volume of 100 ml.

1.5 ppm Standard solution: 15 ml of the stock solution containing 10 ppm are diluted in a volumetric flask with the water sample to give a volume of 100 ml.

1.0 ppm Standard solution: 10 ml of the standard solution containing 10 ppm are diluted in a volumetric flask with the water sample to give a volume of 100 ml.

0.5 ppm Standard solution: 5 ml of the standard solution containing 10 ppm are diluted in a volumetric flask with the water sample to give a volume of 100 ml.

c) N-*Tritylmorpholine.* A colorimeter is used to measure the absorbance of the yellow colour of the trityl carbonium ion. Calibration curves are derived by plotting the net absorbance against standard solutions of the compound within the desired range using water from the area to be treated. High organic water content can give high blank values. (Consult Shell Corporation for details of the technique.)

Specifications for a
Weather Data-Collecting Station

Site. Optimally, the site should be a level area of 100 m² without buildings or trees. Where this is not available, the instrument shelter and rain gauge should be placed at least as far from the nearest building or tree as these are high. The site should be a level one away from large areas of concrete and should be covered by short grass.

Instrument shelter. An instrument shelter approximately 77 cm wide × 52 cm deep × 82 cm high (30 × 20 × 32 inches) will be adequate. The shelter should be louvered on all sides so as to provide free circulation of air, and should be kept painted white, including the roof. The door should face north in the northern hemisphere and south in the southern hemisphere, so as to avoid exposure of the instruments to direct sunlight. The instruments should be at a central point in the shelter at least 8 cm (3 inches) from any inside surface. The shelter should be elevated by an amount that will place the instruments 137 cm (4 ft 6 inches) above the ground.

Instruments. The following instruments should be used: a dry-bulb thermometer; a wet-bulb thermometer, a maximum thermometer; a minimum thermometer. A barometer is ordinarily set up in a building near the site, but its usefulness in schistosomiasis work is slight. Instructions for the proper use and maintenance of these instruments will be provided by the manufacturer.

A rain-gauge should be placed 3 or 4 m away from the instrument shelter; instructions for its installation and use will accompany the instrument.

Times of observation. By international agreement, readings at all meteorological stations are made simultaneously at 00.00, 06.00, 12.00 and 18.00 hours, Greenwich Mean Time.

Reference. Satisfactory observations of some features of the weather may be made with improvised instruments. Descriptions of these and general information about weather stations, are to be found in HAYNES [1947].

Techniques for
Measuring Endemicity of Schistosomiasis

The following is a summary of the methods and techniques used by FAROOQ and NIELSEN [1966] to measure the endemicity of schistosomiasis in a portion of the delta near Alexandria, Egypt. With suitable modification to suit local conditions it could be used in any endemic area.

Sampling Procedure

Frame of samples. The specification of the frame, delineating the project area and the categories of the strata to be covered by the survey, was undertaken by a detailed reconnaissance. The boundaries of the area were defined on a 1:25,000,000 scale map and the area was divided into four divisions: rural-agricultural, urban-industrial, reclamation-resettlement, and control based on distinctive features in relation to population characteristics and environmental factors (physical, social and biological). Maps also existed which were sufficiently detailed and accurate for sub-dividing the divisions into 23 clearly defined sections, with their boundaries demarcated by irrigation canals and drains.

The area was chosen following reconnaissance in 1959. This area was believed to be suitable for epidemiological and ecological studies involved in meeting the project objectives. The area covers 422 km². It has a population of nearly a quarter of a million people distributed in its 552 villages. It constitutes a reasonable epidemiological entity with distinctive and characteristic features represented by its four named divisions. Average size of a section is 18.4 km² with 24 villages and an average population of about 9,800.

Based on a list of villages for each section, with population as enumerated in the 1960 national census, a new list was prepared and a Village Register compiled in the first quarter of 1962, with due regard to the minor changes in population which occurred after the census.

Fundamental Domains of Study and Strata

Although the four project divisions constitute the fundamental domains of our study, it was considered necessary to establish prevalence at sectional levels for purposes of evaluating experimental control measures envisaged in certain sections. For this reason is was decided to utilize the sections as strata for purposes of sampling within each division.

Taking into consideration the results of a pre-test carried out in the area during January to March 1962 (referred to later), as well as other operational factors, it was decided that the over-all sampling fraction should be 0.05 for each stratum with the exception of the reclamation-resettlement division. In this division it was decided to draw a 10-percent systematic sample for two reasons: (a) most of the new settlers in the division came during the past few years (1 to 10) from provinces in Egypt with lower rates of schistosomiasis, especially *S. mansoni*, than the expected prevalence for the project area as a whole; and (b) the division has a relatively sparse population.

The population and expected sample size distribution in the four divisions of the project area were as follows:

Division	Population (approximate)	Number of sections	Sample expected (approximate)
Rural-agricultural	92,000	10	4,600
Urban-industrial	73,000	2	3,650
Reclamation-resettlement	18,000	6	1,800
Control	43,000	5	2,150
Total	226,000	23	12,200

The Selection of the Stratified Sample in the Rural-Agricultural, Urban-Industrial and Control Divisions

A two-stage *cluster sample* was drawn from each section (stratum) as follows:

Step 1. An accumulated series of the population was prepared for each stratum, listing village population in the same order as in the Village Register. A random sample[5] of villages (first-stage units), representing 20% of the section's population, was selected, with probability proportional to the size of their population. The last selected village was included in the sample if the accumulated population of the selected villages came closer to the 20% of the total population of the section; otherwise it was excluded. Whenever a random number fell within the same village, it was rejected and another selected.

5   FISHER and YATES: Table XXXIII (i and II) of random numbers (1957).

Step 2. It was not considered necessary to form substrata of villages classified into size groups, but whenever a village with a population of 1,500 or over fell into the sample, it was split into smaller units. A visit was made to the village by the sanitary engineer who, on the spot, estimated the population of each houseblock and, using these figures, split up the village into units of approximately equal size. The borderline of the units was drawn as far as possible in the east-west direction, with each unit containing less than 1,500 persons.

The units were numbered consecutively from north to south. In order to determine the unit selected, the accumulated series of the population was prepared as usual with the population figures for each unit included, in the serial order, in place of the whole village population. The unit in which the random number selecting the village fell, was included in the sample.

It was considered important always to give the borderlines between the units the same direction and also to number the units systematically, as otherwise bias could be introduced when the random number drawn is known beforehand.

The splitting was done in order to reduce the over-representation of larger villages which results from the sampling procedure adopted. This over-representation of larger villages will, however, still remain and this has to be considered in the evaluation of the material collected. It was possible to show that this method of sampling did not bias the frequency rates calculated, since there was no clear relationship between prevalence of schistosomiasis and size of village, in our area of study.

Step 3. A sketch map was prepared of each first-stage unit selected showing the location of every household (dwelling) in it. The definition of a household adopted for the Census of Egypt in 1960 was also used here. The households were numbered consecutively in a spiral pattern and the numbers painted on the doors.

The map of Sidi Ghazi village (fig. 21) is a typical illustration, not only of the splitting mentioned under step 2, but also of the numbering of selected households and other information routinely recorded on each map.

Step 4. A 25-percent sample of households (second-stage units) was randomly selected from each of the selected first-stage units, marked on the map. All persons in the chosen households were eligible for examination.

Thus, each domain of study consisted of a number of sections (strata) and the sample drawn in the two stages described provided a stratified 0.05 (0.25 of 0.20) probability sample of the domain.

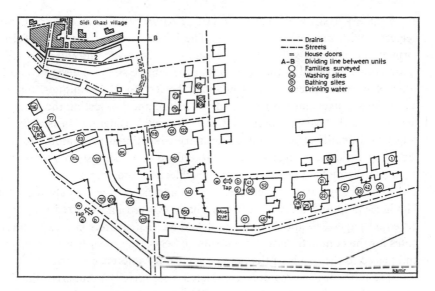

Fig.21. Sidi Ghazi village, unit 1. Division: rural, agricultural. Section: Sidi Ghazi. Inset shows splitting of the village into two units. Unit 1 (shaded) was selected. Number of houses: 128; number of families: 161; population: 828.

Selection of the Systematic Sample in the Reclamation-Resettlement Division

A systematic 10-percent sample was selected separately from each section in this division for reasons mentioned earlier. A complete list of the households in all the villages in the section was prepared and numbered consecutively. One household was then randomly selected out of the first 10 on the list using the table of random numbers. The chosen household was included in the sample and so were all others on the entire list having a serial number ending in the same digit as the household selected. As in the other divisions, all persons in a selected household were eligible for examination.

Pre-Test Study, Record Forms Utilized and Method of Handling Data

Some foreknowledge of approximate epidemiological happenings in the area was sought through an exploratory field survey conducted in one portion of the project, which comprised two sections. The significance of such a study has been often stressed [YATES, 1960; GORDON, 1963] yet too frequently neglected with unwholesome results. The initial survey provided useful information on the variability of the components involved and the rates of infection to be expected in the area so that the sample size and design could be adequately determined. Also it enabled the testing of techniques, making technicians conversant with the field procedure and pre-testing the tentative record forms that were prepared. It further helped considerably in establishing procedural details regarding a preliminary educational programme to gain the co-operation of villagers in order to reduce non-response to a minimum, in standardizing field procedures in the collection and transport of samples, and in finalizing survey schedules. A regular field survey was started later. The household and individual forms finally evolved and utilized are reproduced on pages 740 and 741 (forms 1 and 2). Instructions and explanatory notes for the completion of these forms and checking records were prepared and placed in the hands of the field personnel for reference.

The individual forms duly completed were serially numbered, the data edited and coded and transferred to IBM 8D columns punch cards. Cards were checked and the required data tabulated, utilizing data-processing equipment.

Processing the records was undertaken initially for a few sections to cover the different variables and manifold categories of material collected, before the final formats of tables to be prepared for each division and section were adopted. This facilitated the uniform analysis and interpretation of the data gathered.

The Representativeness of the Sample

The representativeness of the sample drawn in relation to the salient personal attributes of the population, especially of immediate interest in schistosomiasis, is indicated by the close correspondence between the percentage age-group distribution and sex composition of the sample, with that of the project population. Tables I and II show that there was an equal distribution in males and females in the population of the sample area and the examined population. A chi-square test of the difference in age distribution between the project population and the sample shows that this difference is not statistically significant. By coincidence the number of males and females examined happened to be identical. Figure 22, based on tables I and II, illustrates the very close measures of approximation reached.

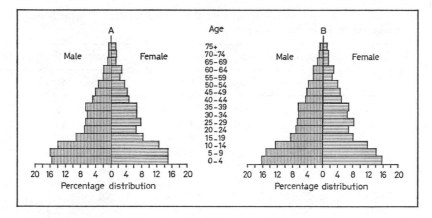

Fig.22. Age and sex distribution of population in Beheira Province (A) and UAR (B), 1960.

Table I. Age and sex distribution of population in the project area, 1962[1]

Age years	Absolute figure			Percentage distribution		
	males	females	total	males	females	total
0–1	3,440	3,295	6,735	3.0	2.9	3.0
1–4	16,034	14,485	30,519	14.2	12.9	13.5
5–9	18,906	18,280	37,186	16.7	16.3	16.5
10–14	15,323	14,667	29,990	13.5	13.0	13.3
15–19	9,607	9,064	18,671	8.5	8.1	8.3
20–24	6,959	7,950	14,909	6.2	7.1	6.6
25–29	7,223	9,388	16,611	6.4	8.3	7.4
30–34	7,690	7,776	15,466	6.8	6.9	6.9
35–39	8,512	7,517	16,029	7.5	6.7	7.1
40–44	5,667	4,822	10,489	5.0	4.3	4.6
45–49	4,165	3,870	8,035	3.7	3.4	3.5
50–54	3,580	3,522	7,102	3.2	3.1	3.1
55–59	1,895	2,111	4,006	1.7	1.9	1.8
60–64	2,031	2,626	4,657	1.8	2.3	2.1
65–69	650	882	1,532	0.6	0.8	0.7
70–74	707	1,184	1,891	0.6	1.1	0.8
75+	702	1,044	1,746	0.6	0.9	0.8
Total	113,091	112,483	225,574	100.0	100.0	100.0

1 UAR Population Census, 1960 (with minor adjustments for changes that have occurred in the area since).

Table II. Age and sex distribution of the sample examined for the prevalence of schistosomiasis in the project area

Age years	Number examined			Percentage distribution		
	males	females	total	males	females	total
0–1	178	175	353	3.0	2.9	3.0
1–4	844	867	1,711	14.1	14.5	14.3
5–9	1,082	1,001	2,083	18.1	16.8	17.4
10–14	828	804	1,632	13.9	13.5	13.7
15–19	513	441	954	8.6	7.4	8.0
20–24	295	398	693	4.9	6.7	5.8
25–29	299	467	766	5.0	7.8	6.4
30–34	406	438	844	6.8	7.3	7.1
35–39	361	345	706	6.0	5.8	5.9
40–44	387	318	705	6.5	5.3	5.9
45–49	249	203	452	4.2	3.4	3.8
50–54	226	186	412	3.8	3.1	3.4
55–59	114	89	203	1.9	1.5	1.7
60–64	118	130	248	2.0	2.2	2.1
65–69	37	59	96	0.6	1.0	0.8
70–74	25	33	58	0.4	0.5	0.5
75+	10	18	28	0.2	0.3	0.2
Total	5,972	5,972	11,944	100.0	100.0	100.0

Similar breakdown of the data of the four project divisions shows insignificant variations in age and sex composition of their populations and that of the samples drawn. The sample, therefore, adequately represented a typical cross-section of the population and eliminated the necessity for the application of any correction procedure for inter-stratum and inter-domain comparisons of rates obtained.

Over-Representation of Larger Villages

As explained earlier, the first-stage units (in the rural, urban and control) divisions) were drawn with probability proportional to their population size. Therefore, it is obvious that the chance of being selected was higher for larger first-stage units than for smaller ones. The second-stage units were selected from each first-stage unit with a constant sampling fraction. Therefore, the

Table III. Number of villages and population in project area, in villages in the sample and for examined population, outside reclamation division, by size of village

Size of village population	Project area (excluding reclamation division)		Villages (first-stage units) selected		Persons examined	
	villages	population	villages	population	villages	examined
– 100	169	9,804	4	274	4	75
100– 199	147	20,873	10	1,379	10	307
200– 499	125	38,243	14	3,853	14	944
500– 999	45	29,722	16	9,658	16	2,226
1,000–1,999	21	28,711	8	7,814	8	1,989
2,000–3,499	9	26,124	5	7,814	5	1,841
3,500–5,499	3	13,347	2	2,718	2	603
7,000–	3	41,004	3	8,493	3	2,128
Total	522	207,828	62	42,003	62	10,113
Percentage distribution						
– 100	32.4	4.7	6.5	0.6	6.5	0.7
100– 199	28.2	10.0	16.1	3.3	16.1	3.0
200– 499	23.9	18.4	22.6	9.2	22.6	9.3
500– 999	8.6	14.3	25.8	23.0	25.8	22.0
1,000–1,999	4.0	13.8	12.9	18.6	12.9	19.7
2,000–3,499	1.7	12.6	8.1	18.6	8.1	18.2
3,500–5,499	0.6	6.4	3.2	6.5	3.2	6.0
7,000–	0.6	19.8	4.8	20.2	4.8	21.1
Total	100.0	100.0	100.0	100.0	100.0	100.0

persons belonging to larger first-stage units had a larger probability of being included in the sample. This is apparent from the distribution in villages in size groups shown in table III.

Table III shows the population of the three divisions, distributed by size of village and a similar distribution of the population of the 62 villages which fell in the sample. The last two columns of the table show the number of persons examined in the sample of villages (first-stage units) selected. It will be noted that more than 60% of the villages had a population of less than 200, but the population of these villages amounted to only about 15% of the total population of the area.

Table IV. Population and distribution of sample (outside reclamation division) in relation to size of village

Size of village	Total population	Population in random sample of villages (first-stage units), % of total population	Persons examined, % of total population	Persons examined, % of population of random sample of villages (first-stage units)
– 100	9,804	2.8	0.8	27.4
100– 199	20,873	6.6	1.5	22.3
200– 499	38,243	10.1	2.5	24.5
500– 999	29,722	32.5	7.5	23.0
1,000–1,999	28,711	27.2	6.9	25.5
2,000–3,499	26,124	29.9	7.0	23.6
3,500–5,499	13,347	20.4	4.5	22.2
7,000–	41,004	20.7	5.2	25.1
Total	207,828	20.2	4.9	24.1

The degree to which the smaller villages were under-represented in the sample is brought out in table IV which has been calculated on the basis of table III.

The population of the sample of villages was 20.2% of the total population of the area, or very nearly the 20% expected. By the sampling procedure adopted, this percentage was smaller for villages with a population of less than 500 and larger for middle-sized villages, but very near 20% for villages with populations over 3,500.

From the villages in the random sample of villages (first-stage units) one household in every four was randomly selected. By this procedure 24.1% of all persons in the random sample of villages were examined, or very nearly the expected 25%. This percentage is, with minor variations, the same in the various size-groups of villages.

The Rate of 'Non-response'

Arrangements for re-visits to households in cases of non-response, especially for young children, were made and out of a total sample size of

12,055 persons, 11,944 were examined, which represents an over-all 'non-response' rate of 0.9%.

Twenty-six infants were not able to produce specimens, and other non-respondents included 15 soldiers drafted on duty. Ten persons were in hospital, 14 had left the village and seven died, during the period of survey. For 39 persons (mostly infants and young children) the reason for non-response is not available, and in the case of six individuals, record forms were not completed due to negligence.

Reliability of Estimates Obtained

In order to obtain data describing the prevalence of schistosomiasis in the project area and its four divisions, and also various relationships between the occurrence of the infection and several environmental factors, it was necessary to resort to sampling procedures due to the fact that it is difficult, time-consuming and costly to collect very large numbers of specimens for examination.

In this study there were, therefore, two kinds of investigations involved. One consisted of the description of the characteristics of the population (enumerative investigations) and here computations were limited to the confidence intervals for the prevalence of schistosomiasis in the four divisions. For the formulae used, reference is made to COCHRAN [1953].

The other kind of investigation may be called analytical, because an attempt was made to find out relationships within the population and the underlying causal factors which may have led to certain observed differences. In this case, we ask whether two or more sets of observations can be regarded as drawn from the same infinite population, and the simple random sampling formulae are applied.

In deciding on the type and size of sample of the population to be examined, consideration of variability of data obtained and costs of providing these data must be made [American Public Health Association, 1954]. Since it was known that the prevalence of infection could be expected to be around 50% it was, as stated earlier, considered that a sample of 5% of the population would yield adequate estimates of the over-all prevalence in the various sections and divisions of the project area. For reasons stated, it was decided to increase the sampling ratio to 10% in the reclamation-resettlement division.

As described above, the sampling procedure applied gives small villages comparatively little chance of being selected in the sample. This fact did not affect the prevalence found, since prevalence in the present area does not vary with village size. However, to avoid disproportionate representation of villages of different sizes in the sample, except for sampling variations, villages may be selected with probability proportional to their population size. This may be done by combining a small village with a neighbouring one so as to obtain villages or groups of villages with about the same population size.

Determination of the Clinical Gradient

For purposes of judging the importance of schistosomiasis in an endemic area and for evaluating the efficacy of a control programme, it is useful to measure the severity of infections by means of the clinical gradient.

A classification of the disease based on parasitological, clinical and pathological aspects is given in table V. Notes on working criteria for the recognition of stages and their sub-divisions according to grades of severity are given in the following pages.

As an illustration, table VI expresses quantitatively the clinical fractions of the disease in the different age groups in Leyte, Philippines. A similar presentation, devised on the basis of an agreed classification, should be undertaken whenever possible. Any shift in the clinical pattern in relation to age or environment, qualitatively or quantitatively, could then be followed from this base-line in subsequent examinations and would provide important indications of the effects of control on the diseases.

For purposes of placing a measure on the severity of human schistosome infection an attempt may be made to grade all infected persons according to severity of symptoms.

The following working criteria for recognition of the various stages of schistosome infection and of their sub-divisions according to grades of severity are merely suggestions to be used as a guide in the development of better criteria. It is recommended that in the early stages of the study an attempt be made to modify the suggestions so as to produce standardized criteria which will be satisfactory in practice.

Stage 1. No practicable criteria of sufficient specificity for exact purposes are available. Recognition depends on clinical appreciation of a skin rash in association with past history of exposure and later history of development of infection. The stage cannot be readily sub-divided. Furthermore, it is not ordinarily recognized in an endemic area except in previously uninfected immigrants.

Table V. A classification of the course of schistosomiasis, based on parasitological, clinical and pathological aspects

Stage	Parasitological	Clinical	Pathological
Stage of invasion	A. Migration and beginning of maturation B. Completion of maturation and early oviposition	Incubation period, including cercarial dermatitis if present Toxaemic stage of the disease (or acute febrile stage) not always recognized or present	Slight inflammatory reactions in skin, lungs and liver Hyperergic reactions, generalized and local, to products of eggs and/or young schistosomes
Stage of established infection	Intensive oviposition accompanied by a corresponding egg discharge	Stage of early chronic disease, characterized for instance by haematuria, or intestinal and other digestive manifestations possibly with cardio-pulmonary or other complications	Local inflammatory reactions due to ova, resulting mainly in granuloma formation. Fibrosis is not a predominant feature
Stage of irreversible effects	Prolonged infection (usually with reduced or discontinued egg extrusion)	Stage of late chronic disease, due to irreversible effects, and/or sequelae or complications	Progressive formation varying with intensity of infection, and possibly other factors, of fibrous tissue, with its consequences according to the organs involved

Stage 2. The characteristic features, a general allergic reaction with eosinophilia, are not specific. The nearest approach to exact recognition lies in the association of this state with the demonstration of a developing infection by evolution of egg output and immunobiological reactions. This stage, like stage 1, cannot be readily sub-divided.

Stage 3. In *S. japonicum* and *S. mansoni* infections egg output may occur associated with splenic enlargment due to other causes, and the probability

Table VI. Clinical gradient of a random sample of 278 schistosome-infected individuals arranged according to age distribution in Leyte, Philippines

Age group years	Number exam-ined	Symptomatic Mild				Moderate		Severe		Very severe
		num-ber	%	num-ber	%	num-ber	%	num-ber	%	
Below 5	1	0	0	0	0	0	0	0	0	
5– 9	23	11	48	4	36	7	64	0	0	
10–14	49	36	73	15	42	18	50	3	8	
15–19	38	11	29	8	73	2	18	1	9	
20–24	23	7	30	6	86	1	14	0	0	
25–29	28	10	36	7	70	3	30	0	0	
30–34	15	5	33	1	20	4	80	0	0	
35–39	22	9	41	6	67	3	33	0	0	nil
40–44	19	4	21	4	100	0	0	0	0	
45–49	20	6	30	5	83	1	17	0	0	
50–54	14	2	14	1	50	1	50	0	0	
55–59	8	1	13	1	100	0	0	0	0	
60 and over	18	3	17	2	67	1	33	0	0	
Total	278	105	38	60	57	41	39	4	4	

of this chance association needs examination. Where it is necessary to overcome uncertainty a specific conclusion can be attempted by rectosigmoidoscopy and identification of inflammatory changes in the mucosa, though no fully specific picture can be described.

Rectal biopsy without a complete rectoscopy can give some supporting information, but may not differentiate between stages 3 and 4. There is preliminary evidence that the specificity of egg-counts for this purpose could be defined by research studies, which are therefore recommended. In S. haematobium infections the criterion of this stage is egg excretion without marked fibrotic changes. An approximate estimation of this criterion can be based on urine exmination and the absence of any history of repeated and marked dysuria or other localizing symptoms, which are typical of stage 4. This approximate estimation is only moderately sensitive as it may include some persons in stage 3 who are in reality in stage 4. Some further approach to accuracy can be made by the exclusion of marked fibrotic changes in the prostate and seminal vesicles by rectal examination. A fully accurate estimation can be made by determining the absence of marked fibrosis of the bladder, or deformation of the uretal orifice, by cystoscopic examination.

Grades of severity in stage 3: *1. Mild:* Occasional abdominal pain, occasional diarrhoea or dysentery and other gastro-intestinal complaints; mild haematuria. *2. Moderate:* Manifestations of grade 1, together with other disturbances causing weakness; with or without hepatomegaly; marked haematuria. *3. Severe:* Manifestations of grade 2, with more frequent diarrhoea and dysentery; presence or absence of hepatosplenomegaly; no other evidence of portal hypertension such as collateral circulation, haemoptysis or ascites. (No comparable example for vesical infection is given because recurrent and marked dysuria is indicative of stage 4 fibrosis.)

Stage 4. This stage is marked in the intestinal infections by splenic enlargement, with or without hepatic enlargement, due to portal hypertension, or by pulmonary, cardio-pulmonary, or pan-visceral involvement, with eggs in the mucosa or stools, or a history of past examination or treatment. A combination of these clinical effects may itself constitute a sufficiently specific syndrome, or diagnosis can be attained by the demonstration in liver biopsy of granulomatous lesions with or without eggs and/or fibrotic interlobular changes, though these latter alone, without granulation changes, are not specific.

References

American Public Health Association: Committee on Sampling Techniques in Public Health Statistics, Statistics Section. Amer. J. publ. Hlth *44:* 719 (1954).

ANDERSON, R.I.: Amer. J. trop. Med. Hyg. *9:* 299 (1960).

ANDERSON, R.I.: Relationship of antibody nitrogen to titer obtained in the cercarial antigen slide flocculation test for schistosomiasis; Ph.D. Thesis, The Catholic University of America, Washington, D.C. (1961).

BAILENGER, J.: Coprologie parasitaire et fonctionnelle (Drouillard, Bordeaux 1965).

BARRETT, P.D. and ELLISON, I.R.: Cent. Afr. J. Med. *11:* 338 (1965).

BELL, D.R.: Bull. Wld Hlth Org. *29:* 525 (1963).

BRADLEY, D.J.: Bull. Wld Hlth Org. *33:* 503 (1965).

BUTLER, J.M., jr.; FERGUSON, F.F., and PALMER, J.R.: Publ. Hlth Rep., Wash. *82:* 250 (1967).

CHEEVER, A.W.: Amer. J. trop. Med. Hyg. *17:* 38 (1968).

COCHRAN, W.: Sampling Techniques (Wiley, New York 1953).

DAZO, B.C.: Bull. Wld Hlth Org. *33:* 861 (1965).

DUVALL, R.H. and DEWITT, W.B.: Amer. J. trop. Med. Hyg. *16:* 483 (1967).

FAROOQ, M. and NIELSEN, J.: Bull. Wld Hlth Org. *35:* 281 (1966).

FISHER, R.A. and YATES, F.: Statistical tables for biological, agricultural and medical research; 5th ed., rev. and enl. (Oliver & Boyd, Edinburgh/London 1957).

GORDON, J.E.: Amer. J. med. Sci. *246:* 354 (1963).

HASKINS, W.T.: Analyt. Chem. *23:* 1672 (1951).

HAYNES, B.C.: Techniques of observing the weather (Wiley, New York/Chapman & Hall, London 1947).

HUNTER III, G.W.; INGALLS, J.W.; and COHEN, M.G.: Amer. J. clin. Path. *16:* 721 (1946a).

HUNTER III, G.W.; DIAMOND, L.S., INGALLS, J.W., and HODGES, E.P.: Anat. Rec. *96:* 19 (1946b).

INGALLS, J.W., jr.; HUNTER III, G.W.; McMULLEN, D.B., and BAUMAN, P.M.: J. Parasit. *35:* 147 (1949).

KAGAN, I.G. and PELLEGRINO, J.: Bull. Wld Hlth Org. *25:* 611 (1961).

KLOETZEL, K.: Amer. J. trop. Med. Hyg. *12:* 334 (1963).

LAYRISSE, M.; MARTINEZ-TORRES, C., and FERRER-FARIAS, H.: Amer. J. trop. Med. Hyg. *18:* 553 (1969).

MARTIN, L. and BEAVER, P.C.: Amer. J. trop. Med. Hyg. *17:* 382 (1968).

MEYLING, A.H.; SCHUTTE, C.H.J., and PITCHFORD, R.J.: Bull. Wld Hlth Org. *27:* 95 (1962).

OLIVIER, L.J.: Amer. J. trop. Med. Hyg. *15:* 875 (1966).

PESIGAN, T.P. and YOGORE, M.G., jr.: Acta med. philipp. *4:* 69 (1947).

RADKE, M.G.; BERRIOS-DURAN, L.A., and MORAN, K.: J. Parasit. *47:* 366 (1961).

RITCHIE, L.S.: Bull. US Army med. Dept. *8:* 128 (1948).

ROWAN, W.B.: Bull. Wld Hlth Org. *33:* 63 (1965).

SADUN, E.H.; WILLIAMS, J.S., and ANDERSON, R.I.: Proc. Soc. exp. Biol. Med. *105:* 289 (1960).

SCOTT, J.A.: Amer. J. Hyg. *25:* 546 (1937).

STRUFE, R.: Pflanzenschutz-Nachrichten 'Bayer' *16:* 221 (1963).

WHO: Measurement of the public health importance of bilharziasis; Report of a WHO Scientific Group, Geneva 1965. Wld Hlth Org. techn. Rep. Ser. 349 (1967).

YATES, F.: Sampling methods for censuses and surveys; 3rd ed., rev. and enl. (Griffin, London 1960).

YOLLES, T.K.; MOORE, D.V.; DE GIUSTI, D.L.; RIPSOM, C.A., and MELENEY, H.E.: J. Parasit. *33:* 419 (1947).

B. Statistical Methods

K. UEMURA

Introduction

The collection and analysis of numerical data should be based upon sound statistical principles in order that scientifically valid conclusions may be drawn. It is essential that statistical considerations should be applied properly from the very beginning of any such project. Even though many refined techniques of statistical analysis have been developed to exploit, to a maximal extent, the information collected, they are rarely conducive to improvements in the quality of the source data. No elaborate statistical analyses can therefore compensate for defective techniques of data collection.

Some of the standard statistical methods as applicable to schistosomiasis data are described in this chapter. They may, however, require adaptation to each specific problem. Statisticians should be consulted whenever the particular circumstance does not fit well in the description given in this chapter.

Statistical techniques deal with measurements which vary, among persons, from one biological specimen to another, between different time periods, and so forth. Methods of describing biological variations are first discussed, followed by an account of how the reliability and usefulness of information affected by such variability should be evaluated. Considerations in the data collection, in particular the statistical sampling methods and the adequacy of sample size, are then discussed. Finally, methods of dose-response analysis on molluscicide are briefly touched upon.

Frequency Distributions

A biological measurement usually varies from individual to individual. In order to examine how the values of measurement are distributed among individual units of study, the frequency distribution is constructed from the data.

Tabular and Graphical Presentations

Table I shows an example of the distribution of the size of skin test reactions in millimetres to a schistosomal antigen on 110 individuals. In this table the frequency of each possible value of the measured size is given.

Often the number of possible categories of measurement is too large to describe the distribution in a form assessable at a glance. In such cases a grouping of categories makes the table concise. Table II gives an example of the distribution of the snail density in a natural habitat. The density is classified into 12 groups. In addition to the number of samples falling into each category, i.e. the absolute frequency, the proportional distribution, i.e. the relative frequency, is also shown in this table.

The frequency distribution may be presented graphically in the form of a histogram. Figures 1 and 2 are histograms drawn from the data shown in tables I and II.

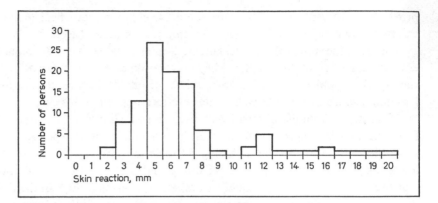

Fig.1. An example of the frequency distribution of the size of skin reaction to a schistosomal antigen.

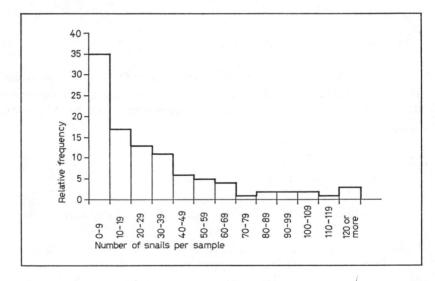

Fig.2. An example of the frequency distribution of the number of snails per sample collected in a natural habitat.

Normal and Lognormal Distributions

The statistical theory has been well developed to deal with a so-called 'normal distribution' which is bell-shaped and symmetrical (fig. 3). This distribution is characterized by the average (indicated by symbol m in fig. 3) and the

Table I. An example of the frequency distribution of the size of skin reaction to a schistosomal antigen

Size of reaction (mm)	Number of persons
1	–
2	2
3	8
4	13
5	27
6	20
7	17
8	6
9	1
10	–
11	2
12	5
13	1
14	1
15	1
16	2
17	1
18	1
19	1
20	1
Total	110

standard deviation (indicated by symbol σ)[1]. About 68% of the distribution is concentrated within the standard deviation from the average and 95% within twice the standard deviation (see fig. 3). For practical purposes, a symmetrical distribution with a single peak may be regarded as approximately normal.

However, frequency distributions observed in biology and medicine are often asymmetrical, with the longer tail to the right of the peak, such as the one shown in figure 2. In many of them the measurements are usually restricted to positive values. A transformation of the measured value by means of a suitable mathematical formula may bring the distribution to an approximately normal one.

1　The mathematical formula for the curve is:

$$\frac{1}{\sqrt{2\pi}\,\sigma} e^{-\frac{1}{2}\left(\frac{x-m}{\sigma}\right)^2},$$

where 0 m stands for the mean, σ for the standard, x for the measurement, $\pi = 3.1416$ and $e = 2.7183$.

Table II. An example of the frequency distribution of the number of snails found in 131 samples in a natural habitat

Number of snails per sample	Frequency	
	absolute	relative, %
0	18	14
1–9	28	21
10–19	22	17
20–29	17	13
30–39	14	11
40–49	8	6
50–59	6	5
60–69	5	4
70–79	1	1
80–89	2	2
90–99	3	2
100–109	2	2
110–119	1	1
120 or more	4	3
Total	131	100

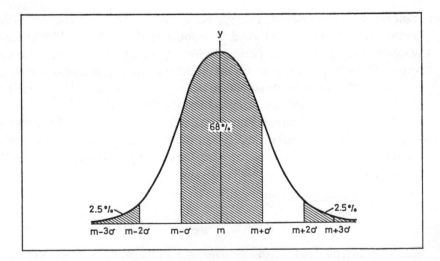

Fig. 3. The normal curve (m stands for the mean, and σ for the standard deviation).

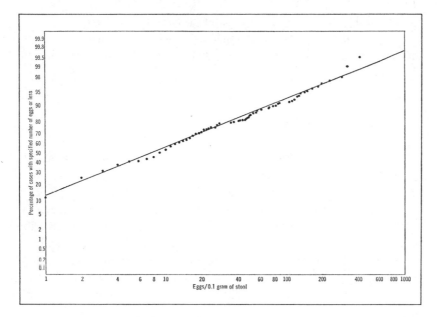

Fig.4. Cumulative frequency distribution of *S. mansoni* eggs found in 0.1 g of stool of lower primary school-children, Mwanza 1963. Dr. BELL's method: 5 g of stool in 50 ml formalin, 1-ml sample examined.

One of the frequently used transformations is to take the logarithm of the measured value. A distribution which can be converted into the normal distribution by means of the logarithmic transformation of individual values is called lognormal. It is convenient to use a special graph paper called the lognormal-probability paper (also called the probability-log paper) for the study of lognormality of the distribution of measurements. On this graph paper, the abscissa is on the logarithmic scale and the ordinate on a scale corresponding to the cumulative frequencies of the normal distribution. By plotting the observed cumulative frequency against each value of measurement, one can see whether or not the plotted points align themselves along a straight line. If they do, the distribution is lognormal. Its use is explained by an example of the *Schistosoma mansoni* egg-count.

In the stool examination of primary school-children (age 5 to 9 years) in Mwanza, Tanzania in 1963, 5 g of stool for each child were suspended in 50 ml of formalin and a 1-ml sample was examined for *S. mansoni* eggs. Eggs were found in specimens from 196 school-children. In order to study whether individual egg-counts follow the lognormal distribution, the data were plotted on the probability-log paper. The data and the computations required are shown in table III and the results of plotting in figure 4. The points fall along a straight line, indicating the lognormality of the distribution of egg-counts from infected children.

Poisson Distribution

A standard distribution which occurs frequently in schistosomiasis studies is the Poisson distribution. It applies to the number of small particles contained in a random sample of a fixed volume of suspension such as the egg-count in the urine specimens of a fixed quantity and the number of cercariae in each of 1-ml aliquots taken from the same water sample. The shape of the distribution varies according to the expected number per sample[2]. As an example, the Poisson distribution is shown in figure 5 for the expected number 2.5.

To study whether the measurements follow the Poisson distribution, the dispersion test is applied. In this test the quantity χ^2 is computed according to formula:

$$\chi^2 = \frac{\Sigma x^2 - \frac{(\Sigma x)^2}{n}}{\bar{x}}, \text{ degrees of freedom} = n - 1,$$

where the x denotes individual measurements, n denotes the total number of measurements, Σ indicates the summation over all values of x, and $\bar{x}$ stands for the mean of the measurements, namely $\bar{x} = \Sigma x/n$. The critical values of χ^2 corresponding to different 'degrees of freedom' and probability levels are found in annex 1. If the computed value of χ^2 is larger than the critical value, it is concluded that the data do not follow the Poisson distribution.

Example 1. S. haematobium egg-counts on the same urine.

The urine specimen collected from a patient was divided into 10-ml portions, and *S. haematobium* eggs were counted on each portion.

Case 1. Twelve 10-ml portions were examined and the egg-counts were 29, 22, 16, 13, 20, 17, 19, 12, 16, 14, 21 and 16. We can then compute:

$n = 12, \Sigma x = 215, \bar{x} = \Sigma x/n = 215/12 = 17.92.$
$\Sigma x^2 = 4093, (\Sigma x)^2/n = 215^2/12 = 3852.08.$

$$\chi^2 = \frac{4093 - 3852.08}{17.92} = 13.44, \text{ degrees of freedom} = 11.$$

2   The mathematical formula for the relative frequency of x is $P(x) = e^{-m} m^x/(x!)$, where m is the expected number per sample, e = 2.7183 and $x! = 1 \times 2 \times 3 \times \cdots (x-1) \times x$. In particular, the relative frequency of x = 0 is $P(0) = e^{-m}$, (0! is mathematically defined as equal to 1).

Table III. S.mansoni egg-counts on 0.1 g stool specimen from 196 infected school-children, Mwanza, Tanzania, 1963

Eggs[1]	Fre-quency	Cumu-lative fre-quency	Relative cumulative frequency, %[2]	Eggs[1]	Fre-quency	Cumu-lative fre-quency	Relative cumulative frequency, %[2]
1	23	23	11.7	46	1	160	81.6
2	26	49	25.0	47	1	161	82.1
3	13	62	31.6	48	1	162	82.7
4	11	73	37.2	49	1	163	83.2
5	6	79	40.3	50	2	165	84.2
6	3	82	41.8	51	1	166	84.7
7	4	86	43.9	54	2	168	85.7
8	4	90	45.9	57	1	169	86.2
9	8	98	50.0	58	2	171	87.2
10	7	105	53.6	63	1	172	87.8
11	6	111	56.6	72	1	173	88.3
12	4	115	58.7	73	1	174	88.8
13	5	120	61.2	79	1	175	89.3
14	2	122	62.2	83	1	176	89.8
15	3	125	63.8	87	1	177	90.3
16	3	128	65.3	89	1	178	90.8
17	4	132	67.3	108	1	179	91.3
18	4	136	69.4	112	1	180	91.8
19	1	137	69.9	117	1	181	92.3
20	3	140	71.4	127	2	183	93.4
21	3	143	73.0	128	1	184	93.9
22	1	144	73.5	131	1	185	94.4
23	1	145	74.0	143	1	186	94.9
24	1	146	74.5	150	1	187	95.4
26	1	147	75.0	169	1	188	95.9
27	3	150	76.5	188	1	189	96.4
28	3	153	78.1	200	1	190	96.9
35	1	154	78.6	235	1	191	97.4
37	2	156	79.6	294	1	192	98.0
41	1	157	80.1	329	2	194	99.0
42	1	158	80.6	417	1	195	99.5
44	1	159	81.1	610	1	196	100.0

1 Represented by the abscissa in figure 4.
2 Represented by the ordinate in figure 4.

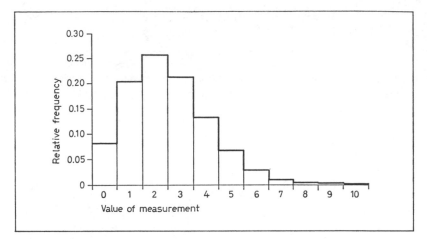

Fig. 5. The Poisson distribution. Mean = 2.5.

According to annex 1, the critical value of χ^2 with 11 degrees of freedom is 19.675 at 5% probability level. The computed value is lower than the critical value, and therefore the observed data are compatible with the Poisson distribution.

Case 2. Nine 10-ml portions were examined and the egg-counts were 156, 189, 162, 125, 146, 205, 139, 173 and 197. In this case: $n = 9, \Sigma x = 1492, \bar{x} = 165.78, \Sigma x^2 = 253\,326$, $(\Sigma x)^2/n = 247\,340.4$. $\chi^2 = 36.11$, with 8 degrees of freedom.

According to annex 1, the critical value of χ^2 with 8 degrees of freedom is 15.507 at 5% probability level and 20.090 at 1% probability level. The computed value of χ^2 exceeds both of these critical values. It is concluded, therefore, that the egg-counts do not follow the Poisson distribution.

Generally the egg-counts repeated on the same specimen follow the Poisson distribution when the count is low, but they often deviate from the Poisson law as the count becomes high. In general, the deviation from the Poisson law indicates the existence of a source of variations in the egg-count besides random fluctuations expected in a homogenous suspension, thus reducing the precision of measurement. Statistical precision is therefore improved by stirring the specimen well to obtain a maximum degree of homogeneity.

The Poisson distribution applies to samples taken from the same urine. Egg-counts on samples collected from different subjects do not follow the Poisson distribution, but follow the lognormal distribution as described on page 706.

Example 2. Cercariae counts in 1-ml aliquots of suspension.

In an animal infection experiment, 5,000 to 10,000 cercariae were suspended in 25 to 33 ml water and 1-ml aliquots were used for infecting animals. To study the uniformity of this procedure, cercarial counts were made on 10 1-ml aliquots. The counts obtained were:

250, 186, 237, 217, 167, 257, 256, 161, 241 and 144.

$n = 10, \Sigma x = 2116, \bar{x} = 211.6, \Sigma x^2 = 464\,566, (\Sigma x)^2/n = 447\,745.6$.

$$\chi^2 = \frac{464\,566 - 447\,745.6}{211.6} = 79.49, \text{ with 9 degrees of freedom.}$$

Since the critical value for χ^2 is 18.307 at 5% probability level and 23.209 at 1% level, the deviation of the cercarial counts from the Poisson law is highly significant.

After further practice the test was repeated, and the counts obtained were:

169, 161, 180, 204, 191, 164, 147, 187, 192 and 170.

$n = 10, \Sigma x = 1765, \bar{x} = 176.5, \Sigma x^2 = 314\,217, (\Sigma x)^2/n = 311\,522.5$.

$$\chi^2 = \frac{314\,217 - 311\,522.5}{176.5} = 15.27, \text{ with 9 degrees of freedom.}$$

The variation between counts was thus reduced to an insignificant level.

Statistical Indices and their Precision

The entity of variable measurements is represented by the frequency distribution. For the sake of convenience, it is desirable to express it in terms of a few characteristic values and, if possible, by a single index. The index most frequently used for this purpose is the average, which indicates the central tendency of the frequency distribution.

Averages

The averages in common use are the arithmetic mean, the geometric mean and the median.

The *arithmetic mean*, or simply called the mean, is the average usually employed. When the frequency distribution is symmetrical, such as the normal distribution, this is the best indicator of average. As is well known, the arithmetic mean is computed by dividing the sum total of the measured values by the number of measurements. For instance, the arithmetic mean of the size of the skin reaction shown in table I is:

$$\frac{2 \times 2 + 3 \times 8 + 4 \times 13 + \cdots + 20 \times 1}{110} = \frac{741}{110} = 6.74 \text{ mm.}$$

When individual measurements are grouped into several classes such as in table II, it is practically precise enough to use the central value of each class interval in the computation of the mean. Thus the arithmetic mean number of snails per sample based on the data of table II is[3]:

$$\frac{0 \times 18 + 5.0 \times 28 + 14.5 \times 22 + \cdots + 124.5 \times 4}{131} = \frac{3712.5}{131} = 28.3.$$

When the frequency distribution is asymmetrical, the arithmetic mean may be largely affected by a few extremely high (or low) values. Nevertheless, it may still be used for certain purposes. For instance, in the evaluation of the risk of transmission of schistosomes in an endemic area, the average number of eggs passed by the inhabitants per unit time and the average number of cercariae shed by snails per unit time, should be estimated. The arithmetic mean is the appropriate average to use in such a case, even though the frequency distributions of eggs passed by different inhabitants and cercariae shed by different snails may be considerably asymmetrical.

On the other hand, the arithmetic mean may not be a suitable indicator of the 'usual' situation. For the assessment of the usual egg output by an infected person, the arithmetic mean tends to give an exaggerated picture, because of very high counts which may be produced by a few persons. The geometric mean or the median are more appropriate indicators in this case.

The *geometric mean* of n values is the n-th root of their products. Mathematically the geometric mean of $x_1, x_2, x_3, \ldots, x_n$ is expressed by:

$$\text{Geometric mean of x} = \sqrt[n]{x_1 \, x_2 \, x_3 \ldots x_n} \, .$$

The computation is usually done by using logarithms:

$$\text{Geometric mean of x} = \text{Antilog of arithmetic mean of log x}$$

$$= \text{Antilog} \left(\frac{1}{n} \, \Sigma \log x \right),$$

where Σ stands for the summation over all the values of x.

The logarithmic tables are found in FISHER and YATES [1963, table XXV]. More detailed tables are published in Chambers' seven figure mathematical tables [PRYDE et al., 1930].

The geometric mean is not computed when the observations include zero or negative values.

Example 3. Number of cercariae shed by infected snails.

The number of cercariae shed during 24 h by 11 infected snails was counted and is shown in the first column of table IV. The geometric mean is 881, while the arithmetic mean is 1,226.

---

3   An arbitrary value of 124.5 was assigned to the last class '120 or more'.

Table IV. Computation of the geometric mean of the number of cercariae shed by 11 infected snails

Number of cercariae shed by each snail x	Log x		
176	2.246		
272	2.435		
324	2.511		
472	2.674		
897	2.953		
1,340	3.127		
1,410	3.149		
1,740	3.241		
1,848	3.267		
2,119	3.326		
2,886	3.460		
Total 13,484	32.389		
Mean 1,226 (arithmetic mean)	2.945 (mean of logarithms)	Antilog ⟶	881 (geometric mean)

The *median* is the value which divides the total frequency distribution into two equal halves. The measurements should first be rearranged in order of magnitude and the middle value should then be found. For example, in the data in table III, the total frequency is 196. The middle values are the 98th and the 99th values. From the cumulative frequency it is found that the 98th value is 9 and the 99th value is 10; 9.5 may be taken as the median.

The median is easy to find and it is useful for a quick appraisal of the average level. It does not take into account the actual magnitude of the other values, and hence it does not make full use of the information provided by the data.

Proportions

Proportions are used frequently in schistosomiasis work. The prevalence rate for example is the proportion of the persons possessing the particular characteristic under study at a fixed time point. Proportions are often expressed in percentages, per mille or per 100,000, etc., in order to arrive at figures of a convenient magnitude.

Variability of Measurements

Variations are commonly observed in biological and medical measurements. First of all there are intrinsic variations in the biological subjects under study. Additional variations are introduced due to inaccuracy and imprecision of the technique of measurement applied and to observer errors. It is important that these variations should be kept within an acceptable magnitude. The development of better techniques and the training of observers will reduce the measurement errors, while proper planning of observations may enable one to obtain measurements under controlled conditions, reducing the biological variations to a minimum. The variations which still remain should be reduced to an acceptable level through replications of observations.

The spread of a frequency distribution may be expressed by several different indices. Those most commonly used are the variance and the standard deviation.

The *variance* is the mean squared deviation from the arithmetic mean and it is computed by the formula:

$$V(x) = \frac{\Sigma(x - \bar{x})^2}{n - 1} = \frac{1}{n - 1}\left\{\Sigma x^2 - \frac{(\Sigma x)^2}{n}\right\},$$

where the x denotes individual measurements and n denotes the number of measurements obtained. The last expression in the above formula is more convenient in practical calculations.

The *standard deviation* is the square-root of the variance:

$$SD(x) = \sqrt{V(x)}.$$

The standard deviation has the same dimension (scale of measurement) as the original measurements. In the normal distribution, 68% of the total frequency is contained within $\pm$ one standard deviation around the mean and 95% within $\pm$ two standard deviations around the mean (see fig. 3). It follows that, in the lognormal distribution, the range within which 95% of the frequency falls can be computed first by finding the logarithmic values which are located at the distances of $\pm$ twice the standard deviation of logarithms around the logarithmic mean and then by taking their antilog.

The ratio of the standard deviation to the arithmetic mean, expressed in percentage, is called the *coefficient of variation*. Thus:

$$CV(x) = \frac{SD(x)}{\bar{x}} \times 100\%.$$

Precision of the Arithmetic Mean

Any statistical index computed from variable measurements is itself subject to some degree of imprecision. The variability of an index can be expressed in terms of its variance or standard deviation. The terms 'error variance' and 'standard error' are used specifically for the variance and the standard deviation of a computed figure instead of the original measurement. For instance, the arithmetic mean is also subject to measurement errors. If one experiment comprises n observations from which the arithmetic mean is computed and if such experiments are repeated independently of each other, the arithmetic mean would vary from one experiment to another. The standard deviation of the arithmetic means which would be obtained from a series of experiments repeated under identical conditions is then the standard error of the arithmetic mean.

According to the theory, the error variance of the arithmetic mean of n observations is n times smaller than the variance of the original measurements, namely,

$$V(\bar{x}) = \frac{V(x)}{n}.$$

Consequently the standard error of the arithmetic mean is reduced by a factor of $1/\sqrt{n}$ from the standard deviation of the original measurements. Thus:

$$SE(\bar{x}) = \frac{SD(x)}{\sqrt{n}}.$$

By using the computed mean and twice the standard error, the range within which the true mean lies with 95% probability (called the 95-percent confidence interval) can be found by:

$$\bar{x} \pm 2SE(\bar{x}).$$

This formula is based on the assumption that the arithmetic mean follows the normal distribution. This assumption holds true when the individual measurements themselves follow the normal distribution. It is known, however, that the distribution of the arithmetic mean tends to approach the normal distribution even when the underlying distribution is different from the normal distribution. In other words, the formula is 'robust' against changes in the shape of the underlying distribution.

For the lognormal distribution better values for the 95-percent confidence interval of the true geometric mean can be obtained by:

$$\text{Antilog of} \left(\text{logarithmic mean} \pm \frac{2 \text{ standard deviation of logarithms}}{\sqrt{n}} \right).$$

Precision of a Proportion

The standard error of the proportion p observed on a random sample of n individuals is:

$$SE(p) = \sqrt{\frac{p(1-p)}{n}}.$$

With an increase of the sample size n, the standard error is reduced in proportion to $1/\sqrt{n}$.

For instance, if in a random sample of 100 snails 20 were infected, then the proportion infected was 0.2 (or 20%) and the standard error would be

$$SE(p) = \sqrt{\frac{0.2 \times 0.8}{100}} = \sqrt{0.0016} = 0.04, \text{ or } 4\%.$$

The exact values of 95-percent confidence interval for a proportion are given in table VIII corresponding to selected values of p and n.

Precision of the Counting of Micro-Organisms in a Suspension

It was mentioned earlier (p. 710) that if micro-organisms are randomly distributed in a suspension, the number of organisms contained in a sample of a fixed volume follows the Poisson distribution. The precision of the average count over replicated specimens can be assessed according to the method described on page 717.

In the detection of persons passing schistosome eggs, the errors due to random sampling of urine or stool specimens occur only in one direction, namely by missing positive cases, since diagnosing a negative case falsely as positive does not arise except through careless operation (contamination or mixing-up of specimens, etc.). Thus, the results are biased due to under-estimation of the prevalence of positive cases. The chances of not detecting a positive case increase as the egg output becomes lower. Some further considerations in this respect are given on page 729.

Comparison of Statistical Indices

Statistical Tests

In comparing two or more values of a statistical index, a hypothesis to test, called a null hypothesis, is established. The usual hypothesis is that there is no essential difference between the groups but that the observed difference between groups has arisen because of random fluctuations in the measurement which did not cancel each other due to a limited number of measurements which were actually taken. Statistical theory has been developed to calculate the range of random errors which could occur with a specified probability. The levels of probability which are commonly used in statistical tests are 95 and 99%, that is, the probability for the random error exceeding the critical range is as low as 5 or 1% (this probability is called the level of significance) if the null hypothesis holds. If the actual observations indicate a difference exceeding the critical limit, it is concluded that the null hypothesis does not hold, namely there is a statistically significant difference between the groups. Reference tables are available for the critical values in statistical tests in common use.

Statistical significance does not necessarily indicate the degree of importance from the health point of view. Since the precision of statistical indices is improved by increasing the sample size, small differences may be judged as statistically significant, if a large number of observations are made. For example, in a therapeutic trial two different treatments may have produced cure rates of 70 and 73% respectively. Usually such a difference is considered of no practical importance from the medical viewpoint, even though the figures were true.

Comparison of Proportions

Proportions may be computed from independent samples or computed on the same subjects at different periods of time. The procedures described below apply to proportions obtained from independent samples.

The difference between two proportions can be examined by the χ^2 test. The general schema of computation is shown below, where a, b, c and d are actual numbers falling into the four categories of 2×2 classification:

	Group 1	Group 2	Total
Number possessing the characteristic	a	c	a + c
Number not possessing the characteristic	b	d	b + d
Total	a + b	c + d	a + b + c + d = n

In order to test whether the proportion $a/(a + b)$ in group 1 is different from the proportion $c/(c + d)$ in group 2, the following value of χ^2 should be computed:

$$\chi^2 = \frac{\left(|ad - bc| - \frac{n}{2}\right)^2 n}{(a + b)(c + d)(a + c)(b + d)} \text{ with 1 degree of freedom,}$$

where the symbol $|\ \ |$ indicates the absolute value.

Example 4. S. haematobium cases by sex.

Thirteen males out of 149 examined (i.e. 8.7%) and 10 females out of 139 (i.e. 7.2%) were found positive for *S. haematobium* eggs in the urine.

Eggs	Male	Female	Total
Positive	13	10	23
Negative	136	129	265
Total	149	139	288

The value of χ^2 is:

$$\chi^2 = \frac{(|13 \times 129 - 136 \times 10| - 144)^2 \times 288}{149 \times 139 \times 23 \times 265} = 0.068.$$

Since the critical value of χ^2 with 1 degree of freedom is 3.841 at 5% level of probability (see annex 1), the computed value of χ^2 is not statistically significant. In other words, the data do not indicate any statistically significant difference in the egg-positive rate between males and females.

The comparison of a proportion between several independent samples can be made also by the χ^2 test. In this case, the general format of data is as follows:

	Group 1	Group 2	Group 3	...	Group k	Total
Number possessing the characteristic	n_{11}	n_{21}	n_{31}	...	n_{k1}	$N_{.1}$
Number not possessing the characteristic	n_{12}	n_{22}	n_{32}	...	n_{k2}	$N_{.2}$
Total	$N_{1.}$	$N_{2.}$	$N_{3.}$	...	$N_{k.}$	N

The purpose of the statistical test is to study whether the differences among the k proportions $n_{11}/N_1., n_{21}/N_2., \ldots, n_{k1}/N_k.$, are statistically significant. The expected frequency is first computed for each cell of the table:

$$E_{11} = \frac{N_1. N_{.1}}{N}, \quad E_{12} = \frac{N_1. N_{.2}}{N}, \ldots, \text{in general}, E_{ij} = \frac{N_i. N_{.j}}{N},$$

where i varies from 1 to k and j varies from 1 to 2.

Then:

$$\chi^2 = \Sigma \frac{(N_{ij} - E_{ij})^2}{E_{ij}}, \text{ with } (k-1) \text{ degrees of freedom.}$$

The summation Σ extends over all the cells.

Example 5. S. mansoni cases by age group.

Age groups	Eggs		Total
	positive	negative	
0– 9	14 (19.99)	87 (81.01)	101
10–19	16 (9.70)	33 (39.30)	49
20–29	14 (15.83)	66 (64.17)	80
30–39	7 (8.11)	34 (32.89)	41
40 and above	6 (3.36)	11 (13.64)	17
Total	57	231	288

The expected frequencies are shown in the brackets. For instance, for positive cases in age group $0 - 9$, $E = (57 \times 101)/288 = 19.99$.

$$\chi^2 = \frac{(14 - 19.99)^2}{19.99} + \frac{(87 - 81.01)^2}{81.01} + \frac{(16 - 9.70)^2}{9.70} + \cdots + \frac{(11 - 13.64)^2}{13.64} = 10.378,$$

with four degrees of freedom. The critical value of χ^2 with four degrees of freedom is 9.488 at 5% probability level (annex 1). The computed value of χ^2 is greater than the critical value; the observed differences between age groups are therefore statistically significant.

The test procedure can be extended to tables with several rows and columns.

The χ^2 test described above applies to the comparison of independent samples. The method is not suitable for the situation in which the same persons are compared between two different time periods. For instance, let us suppose that surveys were carried out in the same village in two successive years and that the results were as follows and the degrees of freedom for χ^2 should be $(k-1)(h-1)$, where k and h stand for the numbers of rows and columns, respectively:

	First year	Second year
Number examined	160	157
Number of cases	15	30
Prevalence rate, %	9.4	19.1

The question asked is whether or not the prevalence rate increased between the two surveys. It often happens in practice that the identification of individuals is difficult with respect to their attendance at the previous examination, and consequently it is not known how many of the 157 persons seen in the second survey were examined in the first survey. Strictly speaking, the χ^2 test is not appropriate for such a situation. However, when the two results are likely to be correlated positively as in the example, that is, when, for a person examined twice, the second results are more likely to be positive (or negative) if the first results were positive (or negative), then the χ^2 test may still be applied, though it is an inefficient method. The above data for instance will give

$$\chi^2 = \frac{(145 \times 30 - 127 \times 15 - 158.5)^2 \times 317}{160 \times 157 \times 272 \times 45} = 5.390.$$

Since the critical value of χ^2 is 3.841, the computed value is statistically significant at 5% probability level.

The best organization for data collection in repeated surveys would be to record the data on each individual and to match the data between the two surveys on the individual basis. Thus, the persons examined should be classified in the following form:

Results at 1st survey	Results at 2nd survey		Total
	positive	negative	
Positive	a	b	a + b
Negative	c	d	c + d
Total	a + b	b + d	a + b + c + d

In this table, the symbols a, b, c and d denote the number of persons falling in each category. A statistical test to be applied is to study whether b and c occurred with the same probability. For example, if in the above-mentioned data all the 157 persons examined at the second survey could have been examined at the first survey and if there were 15 positive cases at the first survey out of which 10 remained to be positive in the second year while 20 new positive cases were seen at the second survey out of 142 negatives at the first survey, the values of a, b, c and d would be:

a = 10, b = 5, c = 20, d = 122.

Annex 2 gives critical values in testing whether the observed values of b and c indicate statistically significant difference between the two groups. In this annex symbol N is used for the total of the two numbers and the larger group is called group A. For the above data we look at N = 5 + 20 = 25 and find that if the number of A's is 18 or more the difference is significant at 5% probability level, while if it is 20 or more the level of significance is 1%. Therefore, the above data would indicate that there was a significant increase (at 1% probability level) in the prevalence rate between the two surveys.

Comparison of Means

When the means computed from two independent samples are to be compared, and if the parent distribution is approximately normal, a test called the t-test is used. The t-test can be applied without much loss of validity to non-normal distributions if the number of observations is large, e.g., more than 30 in each sample.

The t-test is based on the assumption that the two parent distributions have approximately the same variance. If the parent distributions have considerably different variances, a test called WELCH's method should be used. This is, however, outside the scope of this short chapter, and the interested readers are referred to PEARSON and HARTLEY [1966].

When the parent distribution is not normal, attempts should be made to transform the data into the normal distribution. In the lognormal distribution, the geometric means can be compared between the two samples by applying the t-test to the logarithmic values.

If nothing is known about the form of the parent distribution, or if the parent distribution is far from normal and if no transformation can bring it to the normal one, a distribution-free test should be used. The rank order test by WILCOXON is applicable under such circumstances.

A distribution-free method is of general applicability, but when the parent distribution is known to be normal, the t-test or WELCH's test are more efficient methods.

In the t-test the following 't-statistic' is computed:

$$t = \frac{\bar{x} - \bar{y}}{\sqrt{\frac{n_1 + n_2}{n_1 n_2 (n_1 + n_2 - 2)} \left[\Sigma x^2 - \frac{(\Sigma x)^2}{n_1} + \Sigma y^2 - \frac{(\Sigma y)^2}{n_2}\right]}}, \text{ with } (n_1 + n_2 - 2) \text{ degrees of freedom.}$$

where the x and the y are individual values from the two samples and n_1 and n_2 are the number of observations in each group. The critical value of t corresponding to each degree of freedom is found in annex 1.

Example 6. Comparison of two treatments.

Treatments A and B were applied to two groups of 7 patients. The egg-count after the treatment, in percentage of the pretreatment egg-count, was as follows:

Treatment A: 20.0%, 5.7%, 5.1%, 4.0%, 3.8%, 1.7%, 0.0%.
Treatment B: 38.0%, 17.5%, 15.7%, 14.5%, 14.3%, 10.0%, 9.4%.
$n_1 = 7, \Sigma x = 40.3, \bar{x} = 5.76, \Sigma x^2 = 491.83.$
$n_2 = 7, \Sigma y = 119.4, \bar{y} = 17.06, \Sigma y^2 = 2599.84.$

$$t = \frac{5.76 - 17.06}{\sqrt{\frac{7+7}{7 \times 7 \times 12} \left(491.83 - \frac{40.3^2}{7} + 2599.84 - \frac{119.4^2}{7}\right)}} = \frac{-11.30}{\sqrt{19.60}} = -2.55,$$

with 12 degrees of freedom.

According to annex 1, the critical value for t with 12 degrees of freedom is 2.179 at 5% probability level, and therefore the observed difference is statistically significant. (In the computed t-value the sign should be ignored.)

In WILCOXON's rank order test, all the observations in the two groups are taken together and a rank is given to each observation in order of magnitude. If equal observations occur, they should each receive the average of ranks which they should jointly occupy.

The mean rank is then computed for each group and the difference, d, between the mean ranks is divided by its standard error:

$$SE(d) = \sqrt{\frac{T}{6}\left(\frac{1}{n_1} + \frac{1}{n_2}\right)},$$

where n_1 and n_2 are the number of observations in each group, and T is the total rank in the two groups, which is equal to:

$$T = \frac{(n_1 + n_2)(n_1 + n_2 + 1)}{2}.$$

If the ratio d/(SE (d)) is greater than 1.96, the difference is significant at 5% level and if it is greater than 2.58 the difference is significant at 1% level.

Example 7. Comparison of two treatments (same data as in example 6).

The rank assigned to each value and the computation of the test is shown below:

Treatment A		Treatment B	
egg-count after treatment, %	rank	egg-count after treatment, %	rank
20.0	2	38.0	1
5.7	9	17.5	3
5.1	10	15.7	4
4.0	11	14.5	5
3.8	12	14.3	6
1.7	13	10.0	7
0.0	14	9.4	8
Total:	71		34
Average:	10.14		4.86

$T = 71 + 34 = 105, \ d = 10.14 - 4.86 = 5.28.$

$$SE(d) = \sqrt{\frac{105}{6}\left(\frac{1}{7}+\frac{1}{7}\right)} = 2.236.$$

$$\frac{d}{SE(d)} = \frac{5.28}{2.236} = 2.36.$$

Since the ratio is greater than 1.96, the difference between the two groups is significant at 5% probability level.

In the above example, it is suspected that the distribution of the measurements deviates considerably from normal though its form cannot be identified clearly from the 14 observations recorded. It appears, therefore, that the rank order test is the method to be chosen in this particular example.

Paired Comparisons

When the two sets of observations to be compared are not independent, the precision in comparison is increased by making use of the information on the degree of correlation. Thus, if the same individuals were examined twice at different time periods, a comparison should first be made on each individual between the two observations, and a conclusion should be drawn by consolidating all the individual comparisons. An example was quoted on pages 721 to 722 in this regard.

In designing a therapeutic trial on two different treatments, an efficient method is to pair the patients with a similar characteristic, and allocate a different treatment at random to the two patients paired. The results should be compared first within each pair of patients, and the comparison from different pairs should then be accumulated.

The method of analysis of paired data will depend on the type of distribution of the quantity obtained by the individual comparison. If the arithmetic difference between the two observations is used and if it is distributed according to the normal distribution, then a t-test is applicable to test whether the average difference is statistically different from zero. If the distribution is not normal and cannot be transformed suitably into the normal distribution, then a distribution-free method is called for.

Example 8. S.haematobium eggs found in urine samples taken in the morning and in samples taken in the early afternoon.

Two samples of urine were collected from 52 school-children, one during 9.00–9.30 a.m. and another during 1.45–2.15 p.m. The egg-counts per 10 ml urine were compared between the two samples. The data are shown in table V.

The comparison between the morning and the afternoon samples shows that only one case (No. 44) gave a lower egg-count in the afternoon, 34 cases gave higher counts in the afternoon, and 17 cases gave identical results (of which 16 were egg-negative). It is evident, therefore, that the afternoon specimens contained a greater number of eggs than the morning specimens. (To test for the difference, 34 and 1 should be compared as to whether both frequencies could arise by chance when the two events had an equal probability of occurrence. The critical value to be used in this test [called sign test] is tabulated in annex 2.)

In order to evaluate the difference quantitatively, the ratio of eggs discovered in the two samples was computed for each child. Since the comparison is not pertinent to non-infected children, their data were discarded. The ratio computed from each of the 36 children infected was averaged and the variance and the standard error of the arithmetic mean were computed. The successive steps of these computations are:

$$\Sigma \text{ ratio} = 1{,}321, \text{ Mean ratio} = 1{,}321/36 = 36.69, \ \Sigma(\text{ratio})^2 = 71{,}929$$

$$V(\text{ratio}) = \frac{71{,}929 - \frac{(1321)^2}{36}}{35} = 670.16 \qquad SD(\text{ratio}) = 25.9$$

$$V(\text{mean ratio}) = \frac{670.16}{36} = 18.62 \qquad SE(\text{mean ratio}) = 4.31$$

Mean ratio = 36.69%, SE (mean ratio) = 4.31%
95% confidence interval of mean ratio = 36.69% $\pm 2 \times 4.31$
                                        = 28.07%, 45.31%.

Thus the ratio of the egg-counts between morning and afternoon samples is about 37%, with 95% confidence interval from 28 to 45%.

Table V.

Serial No. of child	Eggs/10 ml urine a.m.	p.m.	Ratio % $\left(\frac{am}{pm}\right)$	Serial No. of child	Eggs/10 ml urine a.m.	p.m.	Ratio % $\left(\frac{am}{pm}\right)$
1	15	124	12	27	0	0	NA
2	73	213	34	28	0	0	NA
3	241	653	37	29	0	0	NA
4	17	31	55	30	0	0	NA
5	117	289	41	31	139	523	27
6	292	1,165	25	32	16	26	62
7	63	266	24	33	252	867	29
8	11	103	11	34	0	0	NA
9	96	342	28	35	0	0	NA
10	31	35	89	36	30	633	5
11	3	19	16	37	12	144	8
12	33	93	35	38	10	10	100
13	0	0	NA	39	21	178	12
14	9	35	26	40	0	0	NA
15	74	183	40	41	147	374	37
16	0	0	NA	42	138	458	30
17	236	826	29	43	14	28	50
18	41	329	12	44	11	9	122
19	85	738	12	45	0	0	NA
20	0	0	NA	46	0	0	NA
21	0	0	NA	47	0	0	NA
22	21	57	37	48	0	0	NA
23	5	8	62	49	75	198	38
24	0	0	NA	50	43	106	41
25	66	437	15	51	338	596	57
26	49	326	15	52	146	303	48

NA = Not applicable.

Example 9. Comparison of suppressive treatments on matched pairs.

A trial of two different regimes of treatment, A and B, was carried out by allocating the treatments to pairs of school-children matched for the pretreatment *S. haematobium* egg-counts. The results are shown in table VI.

The ratio of two egg-counts showed a very wide variation. Since obviously it did not follow the normal distribution, a distribution-free method was applied. The treatment which gave a better result is noted under the last column. In 10 pairs treatment A showed a better result and in 16 pairs treatment B was superior, while both treatments were equally effective in three pairs. In order to test whether the difference between the two frequencies 10 and 16 is statistically significant, we look at annex 2 for the sign test. Against 26 obser-

Table VI

Serial No. of pair	Treatment A			Treatment B			Treatment which gave a better result
	before treatment	after treatment	ratio %	before treatment	after treatment	ratio %	
1	3,350	393	12	3,106	40	1	B
2	2,323	2,750	118	2,566	300	12	B
3	1,756	1,010	58	1,313	127	10	B
4	926	300	32	1,043	50	5	B
5	920	253	28	950	77	8	B
6	756	30	4	873	57	7	A
7	703	83	12	890	690	78	A
8	560	193	34	606	123	20	B
9	423	103	24	433	0	0	B
10	413	890	215	373	57	15	B
11	330	70	21	353	3	1	B
12	266	817	317	266	7	3	B
13	206	120	58	223	27	12	B
14	193	83	43	190	63	33	B
15	126	373	296	143	0	0	B
16	136	47	35	143	10	7	B
17	96	3	3	110	17	15	A
18	93	0	0	103	3	3	A
19	70	33	47	86	53	62	A
20	66	23	35	80	3	4	B
21	46	10	22	53	67	127	A
22	46	3	7	50	303	606	A
23	46	87	189	46	83	180	B
24	33	0	0	30	510	1,700	A
25	23	0	0	26	0	0	equal
26	16	0	0	16	0	0	equal
27	13	0	0	13	33	254	A
28	10	0	0	13	0	0	equal
29	10	0	0	6	63	1,050	A

vations (10 + 16) we see that the number of 'A's which is significantly greater than non-'A's, at 5% probability level, is at least 19; thus the difference would be statistically significant between 7 and 19, 6 and 20, 5 and 21, etc. The frequencies in the present example are 10 and 16, and hence the difference is not significant.

Size of Sample Required in Schistosomiasis Study

In dealing with variable measurements the size of the study should be large enough to obtain results with an acceptable degree of precision.

It is, of course, essential that the sample should be representative of subjects which it is intended to study, and that the measurements should be based on valid techniques. Defective sampling techniques and unreliable techniques may introduce bias in the results which cannot be remedied merely by increasing the sample size.

Detection of Schistosome Eggs in Urine and Stool

The detection of schistosome eggs in heavily infected cases does not present statistical problems. The number of eggs passed is large enough to be detected in the examination of a small amount of urine or stool specimens. However, when the egg output is low, no eggs may be contained in small specimens. The chances of missing an egg-positive case is reduced to a minimum if the sample is taken from a specimen in which the distribution of eggs is homogeneous. As discussed on page 710, the distribution of eggs then follows the Poisson law.

Table VII gives the probability of detection of eggs corresponding to the expected number of eggs per count, when eggs are distributed at random. The table also applies to the detection of miracidia, cercariae, etc., in a suspension. It is seen from this table that a low level of infection with less than three eggs per count may sometimes be missed in a single count. An output less than 0.7 egg per count is more likely to be missed than detected in a single count.

Example 10. Direct-smear preparation of faeces for the detection of *S. mansoni* eggs [BELL, 1963].

The standard direct-smear preparation (BEAVER's method) contains about 2 mg of faeces. With a large stool of 200 g weight, 20 direct smears, each of 2 mg, represent altogether 1/5,000th of the total stool; using 20 negative smears as a criterion of cure, the 'cured' patient may still be passing in the region of 5,000 eggs per day. The probability of detecting eggs is found from table VII as follows:

If 200 g stool contains 5,000 eggs, the 20 direct smears of 2 mg each are expected to contain

$$5,000 \times \frac{0.002 \times 20}{200} = 1 \text{ egg.}$$

Table VII indicates that the probability of detection is 63%. If double the number of smears, i.e. 40 smears, are examined, the probability of detection will be 86% (under column

Table VII. Probability of detection of eggs and the expected number of eggs per count

Expected number of eggs per count	Probability of detection of eggs in			
	1 count	2 counts	3 counts	
0.1	0.09	0.18	0.26	
0.2	0.18	0.33	0.45	unsatisfactory detection
0.3	0.26	0.45	0.59	
0.4	0.33	0.55	0.70	
0.5	0.39	0.63	0.78	intermediate degree of
0.6	0.45	0.70	0.83	detection
0.7	0.50	0.75	0.88	
0.8	0.55	0.80	0.91	
0.9	0.59	0.83	0.93	
1.0	0.63	0.86	0.95	
1.2	0.70	0.91	0.97	
1.4	0.75	0.94	0.99	
1.6	0.80	0.96	>0.99	
1.8	0.83	0.97	>0.99	
2.0	0.86	0.98	>0.99	satisfactory detection
2.5	0.92	>0.99	>0.99	
3.0	0.95	>0.99	>0.99	
3.5	0.97	>0.99	>0.99	
4.0	0.98	>0.99	>0.99	
4.5	0.99	>0.99	>0.99	
5.0	>0.99	>0.99	>0.99	

'2 counts' corresponding to one egg, or under column '1 count' corresponding to two eggs). Probabilities for other situations are found in a similar manner.

Estimation of Proportions

The precision of a proportion was discussed on page 718. Table VIII gives the 95-percent confidence interval for various combinations of the observed percentage and the sample size n. This table may be used in the determination of the sample size required on the basis of the required range of the confidence interval and an estimated value of p.

Table VIII gives the sample size theoretically needed for an 'infinite' population. For practical purposes a sample smaller than 1/10th of the population may be regarded as drawn from an infinite population, and the figures shown in this table may be used without modification. If the sample size found is larger than 10% of the population, the following adjustment factor should be applied in order to obtain the sample size for the finite population:

$$f = \frac{1}{1 + \frac{n}{N}},$$

where N is the population size and n is the required sample size for an infinite population.

Example 11. Determination of sample size for a serological survey.

The sero-reactor rate in a child population to be investigated is estimated at about 40%. If the rate should be estimated with a confidence interval of $+5\%$ on both sides of the estimated rate, i.e. 35 to 45%, table VIII gives the required sample size to be 400. This is the sample size required for an infinite population. If, in fact, the child population is about 1,000, the required sample size for this finite population will be:

$$400 \times \frac{1}{1 + \frac{400}{1,000}} = 400 \times \frac{1}{1.4} = 286,$$

that is, about 300 will suffice.

Density of Micro-Organisms

The problem of the presence or absence of schistosome eggs and other micro-organisms was discussed on page 729. Their numerical estimation is now dealt with.

The number of organisms per sample taken from a homogeneous suspension follows the Poisson distribution (p. 710). Table IX shows the 95-percent confidence interval of the true density of organisms on the assumption of the Poisson law.

Example 12. Counting of *S. mansoni* eggs on 0.1 g stool specimen.

If 10 eggs were discovered in a 0.1-g sample taken from a stool specimen of 180 g, the 95% confidence limits would be 4.80 and 18.4, according to table IX. If this finding is to be extrapolated for the 180-g specimen, the estimated number of eggs would be 18,000 (i.e. $10 \times 1,800$) with the confidence interval from 8,640 (i.e. $4.80 \times 1,800$) to 33,130 (i.e. $18.4 \times 1,800$). If three samples of 0.1 g were examined and a total of 30 eggs were found, the confidence interval would be from 20.2 to 42.8 per 0.3 g according to table IX. The estimated number of eggs per 0.1 g stool would then be 10 (i.e. 30/3) with the confidence limits of 6.73

Table VIII. 95-percent confidence intervals corresponding to varying sample sizes and sample percentages

Sample size n	Percentage observed in sample p × 100%						
	1%	2%	3%	4%	5%	10%	15%
100	0.02–5.45	0.24–7.04	0.62–8.53	1.10–9.93	1.6–11.3	4.9–17.6	8.6–23.5
200	0.12–3.57	0.55–5.04	1.11–6.42	1.74–7.73	2.4– 9.0	6.2–15.0	10.4–20.7
300	0.21–2.89	0.86–4.20	1.52–5.50	2.17–6.81	2.8– 8.1	6.8–14.0	11.2–19.6
400	0.27–2.54	0.38–3.81	1.68–5.08	2.38–6.35	3.1– 7.6	7.2–13.4	11.6–18.9
500	0.32–2.32	1.06–3.56	1.79–4.81	2.53–6.05	3.3– 7.3	7.5–13.0	12.0–18.4
600	0.37–2.16	1.13–3.39	1.88–4.61	2.64–5.34	3.4– 7.1	7.7–12.7	12.2–18.1
700	0.40–2.05	1.18–3.26	1.95–4.47	2.73–5.68	3.5– 6.9	7.9–12.5	12.4–17.9
800	0.43–1.96	1.22–3.16	2.01–4.35	2.80–5.55	3.6– 6.7	8.0–12.3	12.6–17.7
900	0.46–1.89	1.26–3.07	2.06–4.26	2.87–5.45	3.7– 6.6	8.1–12.2	12.7–17.5
1,000	0.48–1.83	1.29–3.01	2.11–4.19	2.92–5.36	3.7– 6.5	8.2–12.0	12.8–17.4
2,000	0.61–1.54	1.48–2.67	2.35–3.79	3.22–4.92	4.1– 6.0	8.7–11.4	13.5–16.6
3,000	0.68–1.42	1.57–2.53	2.46–3.63	3.35–4.74	4.2– 5.3	8.9–11.1	13.7–16.3
4,000	0.72–1.36	1.62–2.45	2.53–3.54	3.44–4.63	4.3– 5.7	9.1–11.0	13.9–16.1
5,000	0.74–1.32	1.66–2.40	2.58–3.43	3.49–4.56	4.4– 5.6	9.2–10.9	14.0–16.0
10,000	0.81–1.22	1.76–2.27	2.70–3.33	3.64–4.39	4.6– 5.4	9.4–10.6	14.3–15.7

Sample size n	Percentage observed in sample p × 100%						
	20%	25%	30%	35%	40%	45%	50%
100	12.7–29.2	16.9–34.7	21.2–40.0	25.7–45.2	30.3–50.3	35.0–55.3	39.8–60.2
200	14.7–26.2	19.2–31.6	23.7–36.9	28.4–42.0	33.2–47.1	38.0–52.2	42.9–57.1
300	15.6–25.0	20.2–30.3	24.9–35.5	29.6–40.7	34.4–45.8	39.3–50.8	44.2–55.3
400	16.2–24.3	20.8–29.5	25.6–34.8	30.3–39.9	35.2–45.0	40.0–50.0	45.0–55.0
500	16.6–23.8	21.3–29.0	26.0–34.2	30.8–39.4	35.7–44.4	40.6–49.5	45.5–54.5
600	16.9–23.4	21.6–28.7	26.4–33.8	31.2–39.0	36.0–44.0	41.0–49.1	45.9–54.1
700	17.1–23.2	21.8–28.4	26.6–33.6	31.5–38.7	36.4–43.7	41.3–48.8	46.2–53.8
800	17.3–22.9	22.0–28.2	26.8–33.3	31.7–38.4	36.6–43.5	41.5–48.5	46.5–53.5
900	17.4–22.8	22.2–28.0	27.0–33.1	31.9–38.2	36.8–43.3	41.7–48.3	46.7–53.3
1,000	17.6–22.6	22.3–27.8	27.2–33.0	32.0–38.0	37.0–43.1	41.9–48.1	46.8–53.2
2,000	18.3–21.8	23.1–27.0	28.0–32.1	32.9–37.1	37.8–42.2	42.8–47.2	47.8–52.2
3,000	18.6–21.5	23.5–26.6	28.4–31.7	33.3–36.7	38.2–41.8	43.2–46.8	48.2–51.8
4,000	18.8–21.3	23.7–26.4	28.6–31.4	33.5–36.5	38.5–41.5	43.4–46.6	48.4–51.6
5,000	18.9–21.1	23.8–26.2	28.7–31.3	33.7–36.3	38.6–41.4	43.6–46.4	48.6–51.4
10,000	19.2–20.8	24.2–25.9	29.1–30.9	34.1–35.9	39.0–41.0	44.0–46.0	49.0–51.0

NB: (1) For percentages exceeding 50%, take the complement from 100% and look for the confidence interval for the complement. (2) The figures in this table were extracted from WHO [1961], tables 1.3, 1.4, 1.5, 1.6 and 1.7. More detailed tables are included in the latter document.

Table IX. 95-percent confidence interval of the expectation of the Poisson distribution

Observed number of micro-organisms x	95% confidence interval	Observed number of micro-organisms x	95% confidence interval
0	0– 3.00	14	7.65–23.5
1	0.025– 5.57	15	8.40–24.7
2	0.24– 7.22	16	9.15–26.0
3	0.62– 8.77	17	9.90–27.2
4	1.09–10.2	18	10.7 –28.5
5	1.62–11.7	19	11.4 –29.7
6	2.20–13.1	20	12.2 –30.9
7	2.81–14.4	25	16.2 –36.9
8	3.45–15.8	30	20.2 –42.8
9	4.12–17.1	35	24.4 –48.7
10	4.80–18.4	40	28.6 –54.5
11	5.49–19.7	45	32.8 –60.2
12	6.20–21.0	50	37.1 –65.9
13	6.92–22.2		

NB: For $x > 50$, the confidence intervals are computed approximately by $(\sqrt{x} - 1)^2$ and $(\sqrt{x} + 1)^2$.

(i.e. 20.2/3) and 14.3 (i.e. 42.8/3). The total number of eggs in 180 g specimen would be 18,000 (i.e. 30 × 600) with the confidence limits of 12,120 (i.e. 20.2 × 600) and 25,680 (i.e. 42.8 × 600).

Comparison of Proportions

In determining the sample size needed for the comparison of two proportions, it is necessary to specify the amount of difference it is important to detect. The detection of a smaller difference naturally requires a larger sample size.

Two kinds of error should be considered in this connexion, viz. the error of judging the difference between the two proportions observed as significant when, in fact, there is no true difference (type I error), and the error of not detecting a true difference (type II error).

In as far as the proportions are based on observations on samples, chances of committing either of the two types of error cannot be avoided. An acceptable probability of committing each kind of error should be specified.

Table X. Number of cases required in each of two groups to detect as significant an increase from P_1 to P_2 (or a decrease from P_2 to P_1) when $\alpha = 0.05$ (type I error) and $\beta = 0.10$ (type II error)

P_2	P_1									
	0.05	0.10	0.15	0.20	0.25	0.30	0.35	0.40	0.45	0.50
0.10	551									
0.15	191	826								
0.20	107	256	1,067							
0.25	72	134	272	1,272						
0.30	53	86	157	359	1,444					
0.35	41	61	97	176	397	1,581				
0.40	33	47	68	108	191	427	1,684			
0.45	28	36	50	74	114	203	440	1,753		
0.50	23	30	39	54	78	121	211	462	1,787	
0.55	20	25	32	42	56	81	123	214	465	1,787
0.60		21	26	34	43	58	82	125	214	462
0.65			22	27	34	44	58	82	123	211
0.70				23	27	35	44	58	81	121
0.75					22	27	34	43	56	78
0.80						23	27	34	42	54

NB: If P_1 exceeds 0.50 and/or P_2 exceeds 0.80, we take their complements from 1 and regard the complements as P_2 and P_1 respectively.

The precision of the comparison depends on the magnitude of two proportions. A rough guess is needed on the proportions expected.

Table X gives the sample size needed in comparing two groups, one of which is considered as the control group or the standard group. The chances of committing type I error are specified at 5% and those for Type II error are specified at 10%. Sample sizes for other levels of probability for the two kinds of errors are available in WHO [1961].

Example 13. Comparison of 'apparent' cure rate.
According to a standard treatment regime, about 50% of patients become egg-negative after a specified time period. A new treatment is to be compared with the standard, and a real difference of 20% or greater should be detected by the trial.
Table X indicates that 121 patients will be needed in each group, for $P_1 = 0.50$ and $P_2 = 0.70$.

Dose-Response Analysis on Molluscicides

When testing the toxicity of a molluscicide to a species of snails, the chemical is given to different groups of snails at varying concentrations. It is empirically known that when the mortality of each group is plotted against the concentration of molluscicide on the lognormal probability paper, the points tend to fall along a straight line. This indicates that the lethal concentration of molluscicide for individual snails follows the lognormal distribution (p. 706).

The most frequently used indicator of the toxicity of a chemical to a snail species, or the level of susceptibility of a snail species to the chemical, is the LC_{50}. This is the concentration which is estimated to kill 50% of the snails. Sometimes concentrations corresponding to other levels of kill are also used, such as LC_{90} and LC_{95}.

The simplest method to analyse the dose-response data is to plot the data on the lognormal probability paper, to fit a straight line (regression line) by the eye and to read off the LC_{50}.

Example 14. Mortality of *Biomphalaria* (5 to 7 mm) to Zeram.

Seven groups of 40 snails of size 5 to 7 mm were included in the experiment. Six different levels of concentration of the chemical were allocated to six of the groups and one group was left as the control. The following results were obtained:

Dose in ppm	Number tested	Number dead	% kill
2	40	40	100
1	40	40	100
0.5	40	37	92
0.25	40	27	67
0.125	40	20	50
0.0625	40	9	22
0 (control)	40	0	0

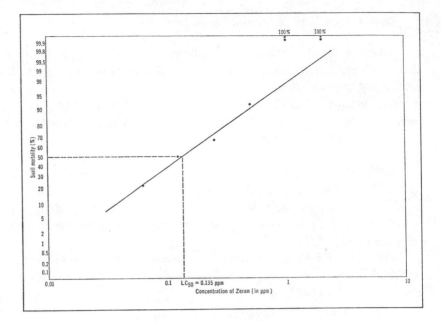

Fig.6. Mortality of *Biomphalaria* to Zeram (data by Dr. R.F. STURROCK).

Footnote to opposite page

The results were plotted on the lognormal probability paper and a straight line was fitted by the eye (fig. 6). The LC_{50} is found by reading, on the horizontal scale, the point on the regression line which gives a 50% mortality, namely 0.135 ppm.

The critical values of χ^2 for large degrees of freedom can be found by the following formula:

For $P = 0.05: \chi^2 = 0.5\,(1.645 + \sqrt{2n - 1})^2.$

For $P = 0.01: \chi^2 = 0.5\,(2.326 + \sqrt{2n - 1})^2.$

This table is based on FISHER and YATES [1963], tables III and IV, except for the values of χ^2 for 120 degrees of freedom which were computed by the above formulae.

Annex 1. Critical values of χ^2 and t for different degrees of freedom at 5 and 1% significance levels

Degrees of freedom n	χ^2		t		Degrees of freedom n
	P = 0.05	P = 0.01	P = 0.05	P = 0.01	
1	3.841	6.635	12.706	63.657	1
2	5.991	9.210	4.303	9.925	2
3	7.815	11.345	3.182	5.841	3
4	9.488	13.277	2.776	4.604	4
5	11.070	15.086	2.571	4.032	5
6	12.592	16.812	2.447	3.707	6
7	14.067	18.475	2.365	3.499	7
8	15.507	20.090	2.306	3.355	8
9	16.919	21.666	2.262	3.250	9
10	18.307	23.209	2.228	3.169	10
11	19.675	24.725	2.201	3.106	11
12	21.026	26.217	2.179	3.055	12
13	22.362	27.688	2.160	3.012	13
14	23.685	29.141	2.145	2.977	14
15	24.996	30.578	2.131	2.947	15
16	26.296	32.000	2.120	2.921	16
17	27.587	33.409	2.110	2.898	17
18	28.869	34.805	2.101	2.878	18
19	30.144	36.191	2.093	2.861	19
20	31.410	37.566	2.086	2.845	20
21	32.671	38.932	2.080	2.831	21
22	33.924	40.289	2.074	2.819	22
23	35.172	41.638	2.069	2.807	23
24	36.415	42.980	2.064	2.797	24
25	37.652	44.314	2.060	2.787	25
26	38.885	45.642	2.056	2.779	26
27	40.113	46.963	2.052	2.771	27
28	41.337	48.278	2.048	2.763	28
29	42.557	49.588	2.045	2.756	29
30	43.773	50.892	2.042	2.750	30
40	55.759	63.691	2.021	2.704	40
60	79.082	88.379	2.000	2.660	60
120	146.291	158.171	1.980	2.617	120
∞	∞	∞	1.960	2.576	∞

Annex 2. Table of critical values in the sign test

Number of observations	Number of A's which is significantly greater than non-A's at probability level of		Number of observations	Number of A's which is significantly greater than non-A's at probability level of	
N	5%	1%	N	5%	1%
1	–	–	37	25	27
2	–	–	38	26	28
3	–	–	39	27	28
4	–	–	40	27	29
5	–	–	41	28	30
6	6	–	42	28	30
7	7	–	43	29	31
8	8	8	44	29	31
9	8	9	45	30	32
10	9	10	46	31	33
11	10	11	47	31	33
12	10	11	48	32	34
13	11	12	49	32	34
14	12	13	50	33	35
15	12	13	51	33	36
16	13	14	52	34	36
17	13	15	53	35	37
18	14	15	54	35	37
19	15	16	55	36	38
20	15	17	56	36	39
21	16	17	57	37	39
22	17	18	58	37	40
23	17	19	59	38	40
24	18	19	60	39	41
25	18	20	61	39	41
26	19	20	62	40	42
27	20	21	63	40	43
28	20	22	64	41	43
29	21	22	65	41	44
30	21	23	66	42	44
31	22	24	67	42	45
32	23	24	68	43	46
33	23	25	69	44	46
34	24	25	70	44	47
35	24	26	71	45	47
36	25	27	72	45	48

Annex 2. (continued)

Number of observations	Number of A's which is significantly greater than non-A's at probability level of		Number of observations	Number of A's which is significantly greater than non-A's at probability level of	
N	5%	1%	N	5%	1%
73	46	48	87	54	56
74	46	49	88	54	57
75	47	50	89	55	58
76	48	50	90	55	58
77	48	51	91	56	59
78	49	51	92	56	59
79	49	52	93	57	60
80	50	52	94	57	60
81	50	53	95	58	61
82	51	54	96	59	62
83	51	54	97	59	62
84	52	55	98	60	63
85	53	55	99	60	63
86	53	56	100	61	64

NB: For N greater than 100, compute the critical number of A's by the following formulae:

at 5% probability level: $0.5 N + 0.98 \sqrt{N}$,

at 1% probability level: $0.5 N + 1.29 \sqrt{N}$.

References

BELL, D. R.: Bull. Wld Hlth Org. *29:* 525 (1963).

FISHER, R. A. and YATES, F.: Statistical tables for biological, agricultural and medical research; 6th ed., rev. and enl. (Oliver & Boyd, Edinburgh/London 1963).

PEARSON, E. S. and HARTLEY, H. O. (ed.): Biometrika tables for statisticians, vol. 1, 3rd ed. (Cambridge University Press, London 1966).

PRYDE, J.; ROBINSON, W. F., and MILNE, A. (ed.): Chambers' seven-figure mathematical tables (Chambers, Edinburgh/London 1930).

World Health Organization: Adequacy of sample size. Unpublished document MHO/PA/220.63 (1961).

C. Recording Forms
L.J. OLIVIER and K. UEMURA

Schistosomiasis Prevalence Survey – Egypt-49

Serial number . . .

Serial number	Name	Sex (M or F)	Age	Relationship to head of household	Occupation School	Individual form filled		Remarks
						Date	Recorder	

Date . . . .

Enumerated by . . . .

Form 1. Household Form.

I

Division . . . .

Section. . . . .

Village . . . .

Household number. . . . .

Individual number . . . .

II

Name . . . .

Age   Sex | 1 M | 2 F |

Religion | 1 M | 2 Chr | 9 Other |

Marital status | 1 S | 2 M | 3 Prev. M | 9 No inf. |

III Occupation

None or other	0
Landowner	1
Farmer	2
Farm labourer	3
Fishing	4
Boatman	5
Water carrier, washerman	6
Domestic servant	7
Skilled labourer	8
Other manual	9
Clerical	X
Professional	Y

IV Education

Pre-school age	0
School (attending school)	1
age (not attending school)	2
Does not read or write	3
Reads only	4
Reads and writes	5
Primary	6
Preparatory	7
Secondary	8
Higher	9
No information	X

V Housing, Sanitation

Type	Stone, redbrick	1
	Mud, mudbrick	2
	Other	3
Latrine	Present and used	1
	Present, not used	2
	Not present	3
Stable	Present, separate	1
	Present, not separate	2
	Not present	3
Water supply	Drain	1
	Canal	2
	Lake	3
	Well	4
	Pump	5
	Piped	6
	Other	7
Swimming	Drain	1
	Canal	2
	Lake	3
	Other	4
	Not swimming	5

Washing clothes and utensils

Drain	1
Canal	2
Lake	3
Well	4
Pump	5
Piped	6
Other	7

Washing cattle

Drain	1
Canal	2
Lake	3
Well	4
Pump	5
Piped	6
No cattle	7

Fishing

Drain	1
Canal	2
Lake	3
Other	4
None	5

VI Examination of stool

Collected
  date . . . .
  hour . . . .
Examined
  date . . . .
  hour . . . .
Stool
consistency

Formed	1
Mushy	2
Liquid	3

S. mansoni

Pos.	1
Neg.	2
Ova No./s	

Smear + 1
  1
Smear + 2
  2
Sedimentation
  + 3

S. haematobium

Pos.	1
Neg.	2
Ova No./s	

Ancylostoma

Pos.	1
Neg.	2

Ascaris

Pos.	1
Neg.	2

Trichuris

Pos.	1
Neg.	2

Oxyuris

Pos.	1
Neg.	2

Taenia

Pos.	1
Neg.	2

Heterophyes

Pos.	1
Neg.	2

Other (specify)
. . . .

Pos.	1
Neg.	2

Other (specify)
. . . .

Pos.	1
Neg.	2

VII Examination of urine

Collected
  date. . . . .
  hour . . . .
Examined
  date. . . . .
  hour . . . .

Haematuria

Mild	1
Moderate	2
Severe	3

S. haematobium

Pos.	1
Neg.	2
Ova/smear	

S. mansoni

Pos.	1
Neg.	2
Ova/smear	

VIII Previous treatment for schistosomiasis

Not received	1
Received	2
Last course received year	
Complete	1
Not complete	2

Recorded by

	Date	Signature
I–IV	. . . . . .	. . . .
V	. . . . . .	. . . .
VI–VII	. . . . . .	. . . .
VIII	. . . . . .	. . . .

Form 2. Individual Form.

Schistosomiasis Clinical Survey – Egypt-49

I. General

Section	Name	Present ☐
Village	Occupation	Absent ☐
P.S. Household No.	Age	Left Village ☐
P.S. Individual No.	Sex ☐ M ☐ F	Dead ☐

II. Helminthic Infections

Previous P.S. Record: ☐ Yes   ☐ No.   Date of examination

Haem · · · · · · · · · · · · Man · · · · · · · · · · · Anky · · · · · · · · · · · · · Asc. · · · · · · · · · · · Other (specify) · · · · · · · · · · · · · · ·

Present examination date   If not examined, state reason
· ·

Haem.: No. ova[1] · · · · · · · · · · · · Hatched · · · · · · · · Man.: No. ova[2] · · · · · · · · · · · · Hatched · · · · · · · · · ·

Anky. · · · · · · · · · · · · · · · · · · Asc. · · · · · · · · · · Other (specify) ·

1. In 50 ml urine sedimented. Early afternoon specimen.   2. Per-gram of faeces. Morning specimen.

III. Signs and symptoms noted on the day of examination

Particulars	None	Mild	Moderate	Severe	V. Severe	Past history only
Cercarial dermatitis						
Febrile reaction						
Glandular enlargement						
Weakness						
Anorexia						
Hypo-gastric pain						
Haematuria						
Frequent micturition						
Dysuria						
Renal colic						
Abdominal pain						
Diarrhoea						
Dysentery						
Cough						
Haemoptysis						
Dyspnoea						
Cardiac enlargement						
Haematemesis						
Sup. abdominal veins						
Ascites						
Anasarca						
Others (specify)						

Mild   : Subjective impairment of working capacity not exceeding 25%
Moderate   : Subjective impairment of working capacity not exceeding 50%
Severe   : Partial absence from work or school. Impairment of working capacity 75%
Very severe : Total absence from work or school. Impairment of working capacity 100%

IV. Nutritional status, general condition and other clinical information

(a) Particulars	None	Mild	Severe	Not examined	(b) General condition				
Oedema					V. good	Good	Fair	Poor	V. poor
Poor turgor									
Bitot's spots					(c) Haemoglobin				
Night blindness					g/100 ml				
Angular stomatitis									
Gums swollen or bleeding					(d) Any other conditions (including pregnancy)				
Dental caries									
Others (specify)									

Form 3. Disease and Disability.

V. Degree of enlargement of liver and spleen and related information

Hepatomegaly	0	1	2	3	4	5	not examined
Splenomegaly	0	1	2	3	4	5	not examined

LIVER   SPLEEN

History of malaria				History of jaundice			
None	During past 3 months	Earlier	No information	None	During past 3 months	Earlier	No information

VI. Stages of infection and estimated degree of severity (clinical gradient) based on band III

	I Stage of invasion	II Stage of maturation	III Stage of established infection	IV Stage of irreversible effects
Absent				
Past history only				
Present			—	—
mild	—	—		
moderate	—	—		
severe	—	—		

VII. Disability relating to conditions under III and VI during the past three months and estimated econimic loss

Number of days

1. Mild_____ : Not well, but carrying out normal duties, not seeking medical care   . . . .
2. Moderate_____ : Not well, but carrying out normal duties, seeking medical care   . . . .
3. Severe_____ : Normal activity partially limited (partial absence from school or work)   . . . .
4. Very severe_____ : Normal activity severely limited, staying at home or at hospital   . . . .

Estimated economic loss incurred from disability during past three months, based on information provided by head of household, including wages and other estimated loss: L.E. . . . .
. . . .

VIII. Treatment status during past three months

	Schistosomiasis			Any other conditions	
Treatment status	check if applicable	period	expenses incurred by patient L.E.	not specified	specified
None					
Hospital					
Health Centre					
Other institution					
Private practitioner					
Other (specify)					

Were any anti-schistosomiasis drugs taken during last three months? Yes☐   No☐   If 'yes' complete ☐   Incomplete ☐

State name of drug if known . . . .

Examined, date and signature   Checked, date and signature

Form 3. Continued.

Standard Operating Protocol for Schistosomiasis

Investigating centre . . . .

Clinical record No. . . . . *Post mortem* No. . . . . . .

Name . . . .

Column	Locus		
1–6		Centre No.	Schistosomiasis autopsy No.

Column 1–6: Centre No. (boxes 1 2)   Schistosomiasis autopsy No. (boxes 3 4 5 6)

Column	Locus		
7	Y	Male	
	0	Female	Sex
	1	Unknown	
	2	0 days	
	3	1 day	
	4	2 days	Time since death
	5	3 or more days	
	6	Unknown	
	7	Known	
	8	Estimated	Age
	9	Unknown	
8 & 9	→	Age in years	(boxes 8 9) (use 99 for 99 and over) (use no + X for estimated to nearest ten)
10	0	Endemic area	
	1	Non-endemic area	Place of recent residence
	2	Unknown	
	3	Endemic area	
	4	Non-endemic area	Place of birth
	5	Unknown	
11	0	Pagan	
	1	Christian	
	2	Muslim	Religion
	3	Buddhist	
	4	Other	
	5	Unknown	
12	0	Farmer with irrigation	
	1	Farmer without irrigation	
	2	Plantation employee with irrigation	
	3	Plantation employee without irrigation	
	4	Fisherman	Occupation
	5	Other specially relevant occupation	
	6	Other rural occupation	
	7	Other urban occupation	
	8	Not known	
13	0	Unknown	
	1	Caucasian	
	2	Mongolian	
	3	Negroid	
	4	Other	Ethnic Group
	5		
	6		
	7		
	8		

Major anatomical diagnoses

(List all major findings using preferably SNOP (Standard Nomenclature of Pathology) or the international list of causes of death. Then code the specific things listed below as well.)

Column	Locus		
14	0	Uraemia	
	1	Hepatic failure	
	2	Haematemesis	
	3	Cor pulmonale	
	4	Acute schistosomiasis.	Some specific possible causes of death
	5	Calcification of the bladder	
	6	Possibly one of these	
	7	None of these	
15	0	Main disease	
	1	Schistosomiasis therapeutic death	
	2	Associated disease	Schistosomal infection
	3	Incidental finding	
	4	Not present	
	5	Not known	

Form 4. Post-Mortem Studies.

Column Locus

16	0	S. haematobium
	1	S. japonicum
	2	S. mansoni
	3	Mixed
	4	Other
	5	Uncertain
	6	Nil

Species of schistosome

17	0	Survey case
	1	Hospital patient
	2	Medicolegal case
	3	Other (specify)

Origin of subject

Origin of infections (uncoded)

Other relevant data (uncoded)
(ante mortem egg count to be recorded later)

18	0	Known
	1	Not known
	2	Nil

Treatment

19 & 20	Body weight kg	
21–23	Body length cm	

(99=99 and over) (X=unknown)

24	0	Good
	1	Fair
	2	Poor
	3	Unknown

Nutritional state

	4	Present
	5	Absent
	6	Unknown

Jaundice

	7	Present
	8	Absent
→	9	Unknown

Oedema

Ante and *post mortem* excreta, compression preparations, digests
compressions — taken by biopsy forceps

	Not done	Not counted	Nil	1–3	4–15	16–	64–	250–	1000–	4000–	16,000–	64,000–
	X	Y	0	1	2	3	4	5	6	7	8	9
25 . . . . Rectum												
26 . . . . Sigmoid												
27 . . . . Trans. colon												
28 . . . . Ileum												
29 . . . . Mid-jejunum												
30 . . . . Bladder												

Egg counts in life

	Not done	2nd half	Nil	1– 2–	4– 8–	16– 32–	64– 125–	250– 500–	1000– 2000–	4000– 8000–	16,000– 32,000–	64,000– 128,000–
	X	Y	0	1	2	3	4	5	6	7	8	9
31 . . . . Urine/g												
32 . . . . Stool/g												

Egg counts after death

	Not done	2nd half	Nil	1– 2–	4– 8–	16– 32–	64– 125–	250– 500–	1000– 2000–	4000– 8000–	16,000– 32,000–	64,000– 128,000–
33 . . . . Urine/g												
34 . . . . Stool/g												

Form 4. Continued.

Column	Locus
	Digests

35 . . . . Whole bladder
36 . . . . Rectum
37 . . . . 20g liver
38 . . . . 20g lung
39 . . . . Spleen
40 . . . . R. kidney
41 . . . . L. kidney
42 . . . . Pancreas
43 . . . . Appendix
44 . . . . Cerebella
45 . . . . Cervix
46 . . . . Colon
47 . . . . Fallopian tube
48 . . . . Prostate
49 . . . . R. testis
50 . . . . L. testis
51 . . . . R. ureter
52 . . . . L. ureter
53 . . . .
54 . . . . . .
55 . . . . . .

Histology

56	X	Not done	⎤
	0	Normal	
	1	R.V. hypertrophy	
	2	L.V. hypertrophy	
	3	Both V. hypertrophy	⎬ Heart
	4	Other	
	5	Ova seen	
	6	Ova not seen	⎦

57 & 58 ➝ Weight in 10s of grams [ ][ ]

59	X	Not done	⎤
	0	Normal	
	1	Hashem's diffuse fibrosis	
	2	Pipestem fibrosis	
	3	Nutmeg	
	4	Cirrhotic	⎬ Liver
	5	Other	
	6	Ova present	
	7	Ova absent	
	8	Pigment present	
	9	Pigment absent	⎦

60 & 61 ➝ Weight in 100s of grams [ ][ ]

62	X	Not done	⎤
	0	Normal	
	1	Obstructive arteritis	
	2	Atheroma	⎬ Lungs
	3	Other infection	
	4	Ova present	
	5	Ova absent	⎦

63	0	No ascites	⎤
	1	1–500 ml ascites	
	2	500–2000 ml ascites	⎬ Abdominal cavity
	3	Over two litres ascites	⎦

64	0	Normal	⎤
	1	Thrombosis	
	2	Other	⎬ Portal vein
	3	Not examined	⎦
	4	Normal	⎤
	5	Thrombosis	⎬ Splenic vein
	6	Other	
	7	Not examined	⎦

Form 4. Continued.

Column	Locus			

Column Locus

65   X   Not done
      0   Normal
      1   CVC
      2   Lesions
      3   Ova present
      4   Ova not present
      5   Weight 0–1 kg
      6   "   1–2 kg   } Spleen
      7   "   2–3 kg
      8   "   3–4 kg
      9   "   4 kg and over

66 & 67 ⟶ Weight in 10s of grams

68   X   Not done
      0   Normal
      1   Pseudotubercles
      2   Ulcers
      3   Sandy patches
      4   Polypi
      5   Calcification
      6   Hypertrophy   } Bladder
      7   Diverticula
      8   Bladder neck fibrosis
      9   Stone

69   1   Fibrosis
      2   Malignancy
      3   Others
      4   Ova present
      5   Ova absent

70   X   Not recorded
      0   No lesions
      1   Trigone
      2   Apex   } Site of main bladder lesion
      3   Anterior wall
      4   Posterior wall
      5   Diffuse

71 & 72   71R   72L
      X   X   Not examined
      0   0   Normal
      1   1   Stricture lower third
      2   2   Stricture middle third
      3   3   Stricture upper third
      4   4   Calcification   } Right and left ureters
      5   5   Stone
      6   6   Ova present
      7   7   Ova absent
      8   8   Dilated up to 10 mm
      9   9   Dilated over 10 mm

Form 4. Continued.

Column	Locus			
73 & 74	73R	74L		

	73R	74L		
	X	X	Not examined	
	0	0	Normal	
	1	1	Nephrosclerosis	
	2	2	Glomerulonephritis	
	3	3	Acute pyelonephritis	Right and left kidneys
	4	4	Chronic pyelonephritis	
	5	5	Hydronephrosis	
	6	6	Other	
	7	7	Ova present	
	8	8	Ova absent	

Column			
75	X	Not examined	
	0	Normal	
	1	Varices with bleeding site	Oesophagus
	2	Varices without bleeding site	
	3	Other	
	4	Not examined	
	5	Normal	Stomach
	6	Tumour present	
	7	Other lesions present	
76	X	Not examined	
	0	Normal	
	1	Lesions present	Small intestine
	2	Ova seen	
	3	Ova not seen	
77	X	Not examined	
	0	Normal	
	1	Fibrosis	
	2	Polypi	
	3	Ulceration	Large intestine
	4	Tumour	
	5	Stricture	
	6	Other	
	7	Ova seen	
	8	Ova not seen	
78	X	Not examined	
	0	None seen	Ectopic schistosomal lesions (specify)
	1	Present	
79	X	Not sought	
	Y	Not counted	
	0	Nil	
	1	1–4	
	2	5–9	
	3	10–	
	4	20–	Adult worms
	5	40–	
	6	80–	
	7	160–	
	8	320–	
	9	640–	

Form 4. Continued.

Chapter 15

Epidemiology and Control of Schistosomiasis, pp. 749–752
(Karger, Basel and University Park Press, Baltimore 1973)

Special Acknowledgements

We wish to acknowledge with thanks the collaboration received from the specialists listed below whose comments on the manuscript have been taken into consideration or who have contributed to other WHO publications used in the preparation of the present manual.

Dr. A. ABDALLAH, Director General, Institute of Research for Tropical Medicine, Department of Endemic Diseases, Ministry of Public Health, Cairo, United Arab Republic

Dr. Z.A. ANDRADE, Head, Department of Pathology, Hospital Professor Edgard Santos, Faculty of Medicine, University of Bahia, Salvador, Bahia, Brazil

Mr. J. DE ARAOZ, Sanitation Services and Housing, Division of Environmental Health, World Health Organization, Geneva, Switzerland

Professor M. M. BADR, Department of Urology, Faculty of Medicine, Cairo University, Cairo, United Arab Republic

Dr. D. R. BELL, Department of Tropical Medicine, Liverpool School of Tropical Medicine, Liverpool, United Kingdom

Dr. A. D. BERRIE, Department of Zoology, The University of Reading, Reading, Berks, United Kingdom

Professor E. G. BERRY, Curator of Medical Malacology, Museum of Zoology, University of Michigan, Ann Arbor, Mich., USA

Dr. D. M. BLAIR, Former Secretary of Health, Ministry of Health, Salisbury, Southern Rhodesia

Mr. R. BLONDEAU, Chief Plant Physiologist, Shell Development Co., Modesto, Calif., USA

Dr. D. J. BRADLEY, Dunn School of Pathology, Oxford University, Oxford, United Kingdom

Dr. D. S. BROWN, British Medical Research Council, c/o Institute for Parasitology, Durban, South Africa

Professor L. BRUMPT, Chair of Tropical Diseases, Faculty of Medicine, University of Paris, Paris, France

Professor E. R. BRYGOO, Director, Institut Pasteur de Madagascar, Tananarive, Madagascar

Dr. J. J. C. BUCKLEY, Emeritus Professor of Helminthology, London School of Hygiene and Tropical Medicine, London, United Kingdom

Dr. A. W. CHEEVER, Senior Surgeon, Laboratory of Parasitic Diseases, National Institutes of Health, Bethesda, Md., USA

Professor E. J. CHRISTIANSEN, Irrigation Engineer, Agricultural Research Service, Utah State University, Logan, Utah, USA

Dr. J. A. CLEGG, National Institute for Medical Research, Department of Parasitology, Mill Hill, London, United Kingdom.

Dr. N. O. CROSSLAND, Product Evaluation Division, Woodstock Agricultural Research Centre, Shell Research Ltd., Sittingbourne, Kent, United Kingdom

Dr. G. M. DAVIS, Malacologist, 406th Medical Laboratory, Department of the Army, San Francisco, Calif., USA

Dr. B. C. DAZO, WHO Scientist (Biologist), Inter-regional Schistosomiasis Research Team, World Health Organization, Geneva, Switzerland

Professor G. M. EDINGTON, Head, Department of Pathology, University of Ibadan, Ibadan, Nigeria

Mr. J. FRANCOTTE, Sanitary Engineer, Bureau Central d'Etudes pour les Equipements d'Outre-Mer (BCEOM), Délégation du Languedoc-Roussillon, La Grande Motte, France

Dr. A. GABALDON, Ministry of Health and Social Welfare, Caracas, Venezuela

Mr. N. GIL, Project Manager, UNDP(SF)/FAO Uplands Development and Watershed Management, Seoul, Korea

Mrs A. GISMANN, 'Malacologia', International Journal of Malacology, Maadi, United Arab Republic

Dr. C. W. GÖCKEL †, Medical Officer, Parasitic Diseases, Division of Communicable Diseases, World Health Organization, Geneva, Switzerland

Dr. A. L. GRAM, G. A. Molina Engineering Consultants, West Covina, Calif., USA

Mr. L. B. HALL, Public Health Engineer, Planetary Quarantine Officer, National Aeronautics and Space Administration, Washington, D. C., USA

Dr. B. HUBENDICK, Director, Naturhistoriska Museet, Göteborg, Sweden

Dr. I. G. KAGAN, Chief, Parasitology Unit, National Center for Disease Control, Atlanta, Ga., USA

Dr. N. H. KENT, Parasitic Diseases, Division of Communicable Diseases, World Health Organization, Geneva, Switzerland

Dr. M. T. KHAYYAL, Department of Pharmacology, Faculty of Pharmacy, Cairo University, Cairo, United Arab Republic

Dr. K. KLOETZEL, Department of Preventive Medicine, Faculdade de Medicina de Mogy das Cruzes, São Paulo, Brazil

Dr. R. E. KUNTZ, Chairman, Department of Parasitology, Southwest Foundation for Research and Education, Southwest Research Center, San Antonio, Texas, USA

Mr. J. N. LANOIX, Chief, Sanitation Services and Housing, World Health Organization, Geneva, Switzerland

Dr. C. W. LAURITZEN †, Project Supervisor, United States Department of Agriculture, Agricultural Research Service, Soil and Water Conservation Research Division, Utah State University, Logan, Utah, USA

Dr. J. LENGY, Department of Parasitology, Faculty of Science, Tel-Aviv University, Tel-Aviv, Israel

Dr. F. C. VON LICHTENBERG, Senior Associate in Pathology, Peter Bent Brigham Hospital, Boston, Mass., USA

†   deceased

Professor ADETOKUNBO O. LUCAS, Head, Department of Preventive and Social Medicine, University of Ibadan, Ibadan, Nigeria

Professor B.G. MAEGRAITH, Dean, Liverpool School of Tropical Medicine, Liverpool, United Kingdom

Dr. E.A. MALEK, Associate Professor, Department of Tropical Medicine and Public Health, School of Medicine, Tulane University, New Orleans, La., USA

Dr. G. MANDAHL-BARTH, Director, WHO Snail Identification Centre, Danish Bilharziasis Laboratory, Charlottenlund, Denmark

Dr. J.H. MIDDLEMISS, Director, Department of Radiology, University of Bristol, Bristol, United Kingdom

Professor H. MOST, Chairman, Department of Preventive Medicine, New York University Medical Center, New York University School of Medicine, New York, N.Y., USA

Dr. F.K. MOSTOFI, Chief, Division of Special and General Pathology, Armed Forces Institute of Pathology and Veterans' Administration Central Laboratory for Anatomic Pathology and Research, Washington, D.C., USA

Professor A.H. MOUSA, Department of Endemic Medicine, Faculty of Medicine, Cairo University, Cairo, United Arab Republic

Dr. R.C. MUIRHEAD-THOMSON, Department of Entomology, London School of Hygiene and Tropical Medicine, London, United Kingdom

Professor K. OKABE, Department of Parasitology, Kurume University School of Medicine, Kurume, Japan

Professor J. OLIVER-GONZALEZ, Head, Department of Medical Zoology, School of Medicine, University of Puerto Rico, San Juan, Puerto Rico

Dr. J. PELLEGRINO, Head, Department of Immunology, Instituto de Biologia, Faculdade de Filosofia, Universidade Federal de Minas Gerais, Belo Horizonte, Brazil

Dr. M.B. RAINEY, Assistant Chief, Encephalitis Section, Public Health Service, Greeley, Colo., USA

Dr. RISK HASSAN F., Under-Secretary of State, Ministry of Public Health, Cairo, United Arab Republic

Professor J. RODRIGUES DA SILVA †, Head, Service of Tropical Medicine and Infectious Diseases, University of Brazil, Rio de Janeiro, Brazil

Dr. W.B. ROWAN, Department of Zoology, University of Montana, Missoula, Mont., USA

Dr. E.H. SADUN, Chief, Department of Medical Zoology, Walter Reed Army Institute of Research, Washington, D.C., USA

Dr. J. ALLEN SCOTT, Chief, Parasitology and Medical Entomology Branch, Extramural Programs, National Institute of Allergy and Infectious Diseases, National Institutes of Health, Bethesda, Md., USA

Dr. C. SHIFF, Blair Research Laboratory, Salisbury, Southern Rhodesia

Dr. O. STANDEN, Director, Laboratory of Tropical Medicine, Wellcome Research Laboratories, Beckenham, Kent, United Kingdom

Dr. B. VELIMIROVIC, Communicable Disease Adviser, WHO Western Pacific Regional Office, Manila, Philippines

Professor H. VOGEL, Bernhard-Nocht-Institut für Schiffs- und Tropenkrankheiten, Hamburg, Federal Republic of Germany

† deceased

Professor J. M. WATSON, Principal Lecturer in Zoology, West Ham College of Technology, London, United Kingdom

Professor T. H. WELLER, Chairman, Department of Tropical Public Health, School of Public Health, Harvard University, Boston, Mass., USA

Dr. C. A. WRIGHT, British Museum (Natural History), London, United Kingdom